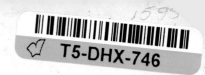

Little, Brown's Paperback Book Series
Little, Brown and Company
34 Beacon Street
Boston, Massachusetts 02106

Basic Medical Sciences

Boyd & Hoerl	Basic Medical Microbiology
Colton	Statistics in Medicine
Hine & Pfeiffer	Behavioral Science
Kent	General Pathology: A Programmed Text
Levine	Pharmacology
Peery & Miller	Pathology
Richardson	Basic Circulatory Physiology
Roland et al.	Atlas of Cell Biology
Selkurt	Physiology
Sidman & Sidman	Neuroanatomy: A Programmed Text
Siegel, Albers, et al.	Basic Neurochemistry
Snell	Clinical Anatomy for Medical Students
Snell	Clinical Embryology for Medical Students
Streilein & Hughes	Immunology: A Programmed Text
Valtin	Renal Function
Watson	Basic Human Neuroanatomy

Clinical Medical Sciences

Clark & MacMahon	Preventive Medicine
Eckert	Emergency-Room Care
Grabb & Smith	Plastic Surgery
Green	Gynecology
Gregory & Smeltzer	Psychiatry
Judge & Zuidema	Methods of Clinical Examination
Keefer & Wilkins	Medicine
MacAusland & Mayo	Orthopedics
Nardi & Zuidema	Surgery
Niswander	Obstetrics
Thompson	Primer of Clinical Radiology
Ziai	Pediatrics

Manuals and Handbooks

Alpert & Francis	Manual of Coronary Care
Arndt	Manual of Dermatologic Therapeutics
Berk et al.	Handbook of Critical Care
Children's Hospital Medical Center, Boston	Manual of Pediatric Therapeutics
Condon & Nyhus	Manual of Surgical Therapeutics
Friedman & Papper	Problem-Oriented Medical Diagnosis
Gardner & Provine	Manual of Acute Bacterial Infections
Iversen & Clawson	Manual of Acute Orthopaedic Therapeutics
Massachusetts General Hospital	Diet Manual
Massachusetts General Hospital	Manual of Nursing Procedures
Neelon & Ellis	A Syllabus of Problem-Oriented Patient Care
Papper	Manual of Medical Care of the Surgical Patient
Shader	Manual of Psychiatric Therapeutics
Snow	Manual of Anesthesia
Spivak & Barnes	Manual of Clinical Problems in Internal Medicine: Annotated with Key References
Wallach	Interpretation of Diagnostic Tests
Washington University Department of Medicine	Manual of Medical Therapeutics
Zimmerman	Techniques of Patient Care

Gynecology
Essentials of Clinical Practice

Gynecology
Essentials of Clinical Practice

Third Edition

Thomas H. Green, Jr., M.D.

Associate Clinical Professor of Gynecology, Harvard Medical School;
Visiting Surgeon, Massachusetts General Hospital, Boston;
Chief of Gynecology, Pondville State Cancer Hospital, Walpole;
Gynecologist, New England Deaconess Hospital, Boston

Illustrations by Edith S. Tagrin

Little, Brown and Company   Boston

Preface to the Third Edition

In the field of gynecology the past five years have seen a continuation of the trend toward a rapidly changing and expanding body of knowledge, a trend shared by all other branches of medicine. Preparation for the third edition of this textbook of clinical gynecology therefore called for a complete updating of each chapter and involved considerable revision of all of them. Furthermore, it was felt important to add a chapter concerning diseases of the breast and the role of the gynecologist in their recognition and management.

These extensive revisions are in keeping with the original purpose of the first edition of this book, which was, and is, to provide a concise yet comprehensive and up-to-date volume covering the fundamentals of clinical gynecology. The lists of selected references for the reader who wishes to delve further into a particular subject were also brought up to date and in some instances lengthened, where it seemed this would prove helpful.

Once again, I would like to thank Mr. Fred Belliveau and his entire staff at Little, Brown and Company for their continued help and encouragement, and once more it should be officially recorded that completion of the project depended heavily on the patience and support of an understanding wife and family.

T. H. G., Jr.

Preface to the First Edition

This volume attempts to present concisely yet comprehensively the basic facts and principles necessary to the sound understanding and proper evaluation and management of gynecologic disorders. Since the trend in medical schools today increasingly is to take the larger part of the teaching of clinical medicine out of the lecture halls and into the hospital wards and outpatient clinics, the student now frequently receives almost his entire exposure to and training in gynecology and other branches of clinical medicine within clinical settings, with the emphasis on actual student participation in the physician-patient relationship. It therefore is hoped that this book, which also approaches the fundamentals of gynecology primarily from a clinical standpoint, will prove helpful to the student obtaining his initial training in gynecology in a hospital setting.

Although there is no intent to place a special emphasis on details of therapy (descriptions of operative techniques are completely omitted), since proper treatment must be based on a complete and broad understanding of the disease process and its relation to the patient as a whole, consideration is given throughout to therapeutic principles and methods. It is hoped that this will prove pertinent not only for students, particularly since they are usually presented the opportunity to learn while working among patients, but also for physicians in internship and residency training and for busy practitioners not necessarily specializing in gynecology, all of whom are constantly called upon to examine and treat women with pelvic disease or dysfunction. The intention is that these discussions of therapy will also serve to recapitulate and reinforce the basic facts and current concepts of gynecologic disorders—both for the benefit of those just beginning in gynecology and those seeking an up-to-date review.

In keeping with this general theme, the fundamental embryology, anatomy, and physiology of the female reproductive tract are not presented in the traditional separate sections. They have been integrated instead into appropriate subject matter, where they can most succinctly contribute to the proper understanding of the underlying pathophysiology as well as the clinical features of various disorders.

Each chapter includes a short list of references for further study. The majority of the references listed were chosen because they represent key articles or monographs of particular significance with respect to a specific subject, either historically or because they are recent and valuable additions to the knowledge of this subject or are excellent and succinct reviews of it. The choice of references was also governed by the ready availability, in even a small medical library, of the various periodicals cited, and the lists have deliberately been kept short to further tempt the reader to use them.

I acknowledge with gratitude the untiring efforts of Miss Sarah Butera, my secretary, in the preparation of the manuscript, the superb illustrative work of Mrs. Edith Tagrin, and the skilled craftsmanship of Mrs. Betty Herr Hallinger, who compiled the index. Thanks also go to Mr. Fred Belliveau of Little, Brown and

Company for his invaluable advice and help throughout the project. Equally important, the obvious fact should be recorded officially that such a project could never
have been completed without the patience, encouragement, and support of an understanding wife and family.

Finally, in a very real sense, this book is dedicated to the memory of the late
Dr. Joe Vincent Meigs, with whom it was my privilege to be closely associated for
twelve years. His teaching, guidance, and stimulating enthusiasm over the years
served as the inspiration and major justification for undertaking this task.

T. H. G., Jr.

Contents

xi

Gynecology
Essentials of Clinical Practice

1
Gynecologic History and Physical Examination

The importance of a thorough preliminary survey of the patient's overall background and current health status cannot be too strongly emphasized. An adequate general medical history, including a careful system review, and a thorough general physical examination are essential because of the frequency with which the gynecologic condition that prompts the patient to consult a physician is the first manifestation of a serious systemic disease. The menstrual irregularities appearing early in the course of thyroid disease and the vulvovaginitis that may be the first clue to a latent diabetes are specific, frequently encountered examples of this relationship. Furthermore, gynecologic disorders may be accompanied by significant, generalized disturbances, either directly related to and resulting from, or entirely incidental to, the primary pelvic disease. These disorders may have a marked influence on the overall plan of diagnosis and therapy. The systemic manifestations of the various primary pelvic disorders will be discussed in more detail in the appropriate sections.

The presence of independent cardiovascular, renal, or pulmonary disease must also be determined, and this information will often affect the choice of treatment where more than one alternative is available. The nature and details of past illnesses or operative procedures are also important, and it may be necessary to write to other physicians or hospitals to obtain accurate information on these points. If the patient is or has been receiving medications, this fact should be known. Certain hormones may cause abnormal bleeding; broad-spectrum antibiotics may result in candidal vaginitis; certain cardiovascular medications and cortisone compounds may have an important bearing on the preoperative preparations and choice of anesthesia, should surgery be indicated. A history of allergy or sensitivity to any medications is important for obvious reasons.

Social and environmental factors that might have a bearing on pelvic symptoms should also be adequately explored. A general idea of the personality of the patient, her mental and emotional attitudes and problems, and the adequacy of her past and present adjustment to various life situations will also prove extremely helpful in evaluating her pelvic complaints, for symptoms arising in relation to the reproductive tract and its function are frequently psychosomatic in origin. The gynecologist must not only make sure to hear what the patient says but also must listen with a "third ear" to what the patient does not say and to nonverbal forms of communication such as body movements, evidences of inner tension or hesitation, and changes in attitude — all of which may be of help in understanding and dealing with the patient's problems.

Finally, inquiry should always be made regarding familial disorders, particularly whether or not there is a family history of malignant disease, diabetes, tuberculosis, or allergies. A strong family history of any of these disorders should alert the physician to be on the lookout for similar conditions in the patient and may make it possible to detect them in an early, asymptomatic phase. For example, most patients with some form of pelvic malignancy show a tendency to a higher-than-normal incidence of malignancy in their family background.

The gynecologist must approach the care of the patient from a broad viewpoint. Although his or her principal function in the overall care of women has been and undoubtedly should remain that of a highly trained specialist-consultant in the field of gynecology, in actual fact the gynecologist has long played another important role. For in many ways the gynecologist serves as a primary physician for women — not in the capacity of one who provides them comprehensive primary care in the way that a physician in general practice does, but in the sense that for a large number of American women the gynecologist is the principle source of medical supervision, advice, and occasionally initial care for nongynecologic problems. Thus the gynecologist represents their initial portal of entry into the total health care system and provides them continuity of care within this system.

THE GYNECOLOGIC HISTORY

The patient should initially be allowed to present her chief complaint and the story of her present illness in her own way and words. However, the physician should eventually, if necessary, begin to guide the conversation so as to avoid the presentation of repetitious or insignificant material. By judicious questioning he should elicit accurately the following points of information, if not spontaneously reported by the patient, in order to complete the gynecologic history:

Menstrual History. Age at menarche; length of cycle; regularity of cycle; premenstrual molimina (e.g., breast pain, tenderness and swelling, skin changes, cramps, headaches, tension, weight gain, edema); duration of flow; associated cramps or pelvic pain and time of occurrence; description of amount (number of sanitary pads required per day provides a rough index, with three to six normal) and character of flow; dysmenorrhea, primary or acquired (characteristics of pain, location of pain, time of onset and subsidence, effective medications); date of last menstrual period and previous menstrual period; description of any prior therapy for menstrual disorders; if postmenopausal, age at menopause and description of menopausal symptoms.

Marital History. Age at first or subsequent marriage; duration of marriage; frequency of coitus; dyspareunia; use of contraceptives; general impression of marital adjustment.

Obstetric History. Number of pregnancies and dates (gravidity); number of deliveries and dates (parity) and whether or not births were normal, full term, or presented complications; type of delivery (normal, vaginal, forceps, section); episiotomy or other procedure; birth weight of babies; postpartum difficulties and complications; number of miscarriages (duration of pregnancy at time, complications, need for curettage).

Special inquiries should be made concerning the following:

Abnormal Bleeding. Character and amount; any associated symptoms (e.g., pain, discharge), relation to periods (premenstrual, postmenstrual, intermenstrual, postmenopausal); frequency, duration, and onset (sudden or slow); whether or not preceded by amenorrhea or other menstrual irregularities.

Abnormal Discharge. Amount, color (yellow, white, mucoid, brown), odor, and consistency (thin, watery, thick, cheesy, mucoid); relation to menstrual cycle (premenstrual or postmenstrual aggravation); associated symptoms (vulvovaginal burning and itching, urinary symptoms).

Abnormal Pelvic or Abdominal Pain. Type (sharp, dragging, aching, pressure or bearing-down, crampy, colicky, burning); sudden or gradual onset; duration; whether steady or intermittent; location and radiation; relation to menses or to phase of menstrual cycle; relation to position (upright versus recumbent); relation to function of other organ systems (gastrointestinal or urinary tracts); associated symptoms (abnormal bleeding or discharge, gastrointestinal or bladder disturbances). Pain referred to the low back or buttocks is commonly associated with disease in the cervix, urethra, bladder neck, or lower rectum and often radiates into one or both legs. Discomfort due to uterine or vaginal disease or associated with inflammatory conditions of the bladder fundus is usually localized in the lower abdomen. Ovarian pain and pain due to disease of the fallopian tubes is most often referred to the lower abdominal quadrants just above the groin and often radiates down the medial aspect of the thighs.

Back Pain. Backache of gynecologic origin is most commonly secondary to endometriosis, chronic pelvic inflammatory disease, large fibroids arising in the posterior uterine wall and wedged in the hollow of the sacrum, or posterolateral extension of carcinoma of the cervix. It is fair to say, however, that most backaches are of musculoskeletal rather than of gynecologic origin.

Infertility. Duration, prior use of contraceptives, frequency and timing of coitus, prior studies, previous marriages of either partner and any resulting pregnancies.

Abnormal Symptoms of Genital Relaxation. Feeling of protrusion, dragging sensation, pressure, bearing-down discomfort, or sense of insecurity.

Associated Bladder Symptoms. Frequency, nocturia, urgency, dysuria, difficult voiding, incontinence (stress, urgency).

Associated Bowel Symptoms. Constipation, diarrhea, pain referred to region of the rectum, vaginal protrusion on straining during defecation.

Past history of any acute abdominal or pelvic illnesses or operations should be elicited.

THE GYNECOLOGIC PHYSICAL EXAMINATION

A complete general physical examination should be carried out first, including determination of the height, weight, and blood pressure, and a survey of the neck, breasts, heart, lungs, abdomen, inguinal and femoral regions, and lower extremities. A nurse or other female attendant should always be present for the physical examination if the gynecologist is male. The presence of another female in the room is comforting to female patients, since for some of them the situation is a source of considerable apprehension and embarrassment. Furthermore, it affords complete protection to the physician against the possibility that a patient with an unsuspected psychotic tendency may subsequently allege improper behavior on his part in the examining room. The patient should be warm, physically comfortable and relaxed, properly draped, and have had an opportunity to void immediately prior to examination. The patient's mental ease and relaxation should also be assured by a conscious effort to gain her confidence and cooperation while obtaining the history and by continued reassurance during the physical examination. If the patient is not comfortable and relaxed, the maximum information will not be gained from the examination.

Examination is conveniently begun with the patient in a sitting position on the edge of the table. The physician first checks the head and neck (including palpation of the thyroid and the cervical and supraclavicular nodes), breasts, axillae, back, and lungs. The patient then lies flat on the table for a further check of the breasts, heart, abdomen, groins, and lower extremities.

In examination of the breasts, it is well to inspect them first with the patient sitting erect, both with her arms at her sides, and again while she raises them. This maneuver frequently discloses breast asymmetry, nipple fixation, or a fixed mass beneath the areolar margin, any of which might go unnoticed in the recumbent position. A careful, methodical examination of all quadrants of the breasts and the adjacent axillary regions should then be carried out with the patient in both the erect and supine positions. Palpation is best performed and breast masses most readily appreciated if the flat, palmar surface of the hand and contiguous palmar surfaces of the apposed fingers are employed rather than the actual tips of the fingers. It is important to learn to distinguish the somewhat finely granular, irregular consistency of normal breast tissue from discrete masses that may represent either neoplasm or benign fibrocystic change. It is also important to be aware of the frequent existence of an axillary extension of normal breast tissue, the "axillary tail," and not to mistake it for a tumor; when present, it is almost invariably bilateral and symmetrical. Finally, the areolar areas should gently be compressed to demonstrate the presence of any abnormal secretion or bloody fluid in the nipple glands and ducts.

Since nearly all breast irregularities or lumps are first discovered by the woman herself, it is well worth the effort to instruct patients in the proper method of self-examination of the breast. Patients can readily be shown the correct technique during the course of the physician's examination and should be urged to examine their breasts every month, just after completion of the menstrual period, at a time when normal premenstrual breast engorgement and tenderness will not be misleading. They should be taught to inspect their breasts in front of a mirror, first with arms at their sides, then with arms overhead, looking for changes in size or contour or for dimpling of the skin. Next, lying flat, they can be shown how to palpate correctly with the right hand all four quadrants of the left breast, preferably with a small pillow under the left shoulder and with the left hand under the head while palpating the inner half of the breast, the left arm down at the side while palpating the outer quadrants. The procedure is then reversed to examine the right breast with the left hand. It is to be hoped that such instruction in proper self-examination of the breast will permit women to recognize any changes more promptly and hence will lead to the earlier detection of breast cancer.

Careful, detailed examination of the abdomen is obviously an integral part of the gynecologic physical examination. It is also particularly important never to neglect examination of both groins, since many gynecologic disorders affecting the vulva and vagina are accompanied by inguinal adenopathy, whether they be inflammatory or neoplastic in type.

The patient is then placed in the lithotomy position with her feet in stirrups and is suitably draped by the nurse. Rarely, the lateral Sims, knee-chest, or standing positions may also be employed, for they are occasionally more suitable than the lithotomy position for determining specific points. The actual pelvic examination begins with inspection; the lower abdomen, the external genitalia (mons veneris, vulvar skin, and labia majora and minora, prepuce and clitoris, introitus, hymeneal or vaginal opening, and the visible portions of the anterior and posterior vaginal walls), the urethral meatus, and the anoperineal area are surveyed first for abnormal distribution or character of hair or pigmentation, clitoral hypertrophy, generalized or local skin lesions, visible subcutaneous or submucosal abnormalities (e.g., inflammation, leukoplakia, ulcers, tumors, or atrophy), and gross displacement and relaxations.

If vaginal smears (cytologic or fresh) are to be obtained, these should be secured prior to the vaginal examination. Although it has long been taught that the left hand should be used to perform bimanual examination, it is not at all necessary to adhere to this ancient tradition. Rather, the hand one is most accustomed to employ or with which one feels most natural and proficient during palpatory examination of any body region should be used, and one should consistently employ this same hand. The examiner stands to the right or left of the patient in employing the right or left hand respectively, rather than directly in front, from which site bimanual examination is difficult and awkward. The labia are gently separated and one or two well-lubricated fingers of the gloved hand are introduced, depressing the perineum and posterior vaginal wall so as to avoid undue and uncomfortable pressure against the more sensitive anteriorly placed structures. With the finger depressing the perineum, the perineal body and pubococcygeal (levator) muscles are palpated. The patient is asked to strain, or cough, or both, which will further reveal any tendency to perineal relaxation, cystocele, rectocele, or prolapse of the uterus or vagina (see Fig. 66). Abnormalities of the structures at the level of the introitus (urethra, Skene's glands, Bartholin's glands) are searched for between the thumb and forefinger. The fingers are then inserted at the proper angle (approximately 30 to 45 degrees above the horizontal) the length of the vagina, palpating the vaginal wall and exocervix and external os as this maneuver is carried out.

Bimanual examination of the uterus and adnexal regions is then carefully done,

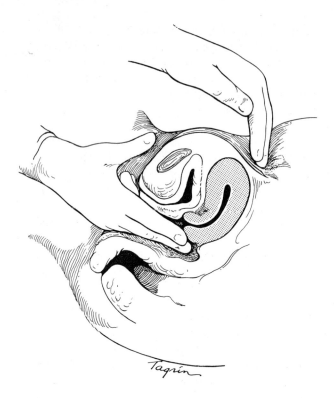

Figure 1
Bimanual abdominovaginal palpation of the uterus.

checking on the size, outline, consistency, mobility, and position of the uterus, ovaries, and any palpable pelvic masses, the vaginal fingers serving to steady and elevate the cervix and uterus anteriorly where the abdominal hand can perform this evaluation (Fig. 1). The vaginal vaults (lateral fornices or adnexal regions) are then palpated, feeling primarily with the vaginal fingers, the abdominal hand being used to sweep the adnexa down to them (Fig. 2). Anterior and posterior (cul-de-sac or pouch of Douglas) fornices are then explored bimanually in the same way, and the fingers then turned and pressed laterally to feel the pelvic walls as well. Normal adnexa are frequently not palpable even under the most ideal conditions (normal fallopian tubes probably never), particularly if the patient is unrelaxed or obese. However, under anesthesia, normal-sized ovaries are nearly always palpable even in an obese patient. Unusually mobile adnexa (with relaxed and elongated infundib-ulopelvic and ovarian ligaments) may result in the ovaries being palpated in the cul-de-sac posteriorly at the time of rectal examination, rather than during vaginal examination. Palpation of "normal-sized" ovaries (e.g., 3.5 × 2 × 1.5 cm) in the premenopausal woman with active ovarian function is to be expected. However,

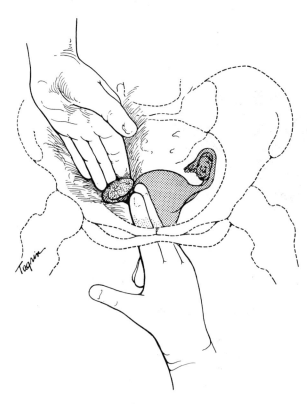

Figure 2
Bimanual abdominovaginal palpation of the adnexa.

as pointed out by Barber and Graber [1], palpation of ovaries of "normal size"
in a woman three to five years after her menopause is not a normal or expected
clinical finding; on the contrary, it suggests that the ovaries are not normal at all,
and may signify early ovarian cancer, which has its peak incidence between the ages
of 45 to 60. (Serious consideration needs to be given to surgical exploration and
removal of the gonads in this situation, since the normal postmenopausal ovary is
usually one-third or less the size of the premenopausal ovary and is ordinarily not
palpable.)

The examiner now sits directly in front of the patient with a suitable flexible
lamp at his disposal and carries out the speculum examination, introducing the previously warmed and well-lubricated blades after separating the labia and depressing
the perineal body in the same manner as for bimanual examination. A Graves bivalve
speculum of appropriate size (small [infant], medium ["regular"], medium with
narrow blades [Pederson], or large, depending on the size of the introitus and the
size and length of the vaginal canal) is inserted at the proper angle and with a slight
rotary motion (Fig. 3). In most instances, even in the presence of an intact hymen,

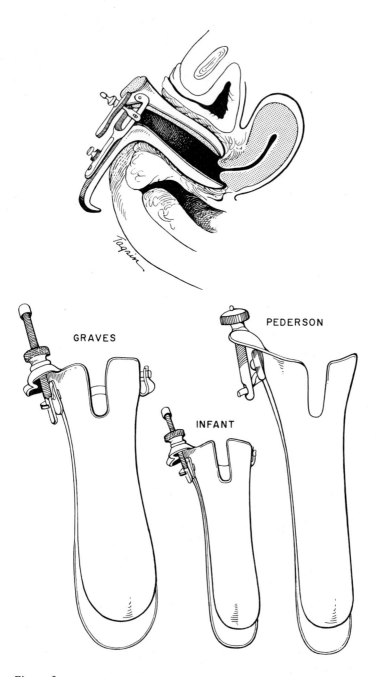

Figure 3
Insertion of vaginal speculum. The various types and sizes of specula are shown.

the hymeneal opening is sufficient to permit both one-finger bimanual vaginal and speculum examinations (usually employing the narrow-bladed instrument) without difficulty, if they are properly and gently done. (If these examinations are not possible, information obtained by a bimanual rectal examination is often sufficient in a young female; otherwise, examination under anesthesia will be necessary.) The speculum is gently but firmly inserted its full length, and the blades then opened, exposing the cervix for inspection, Schiller's test, cervical or endometrial biopsy, or any of the other office diagnostic procedures (see Chap. 2). A little manipulation may be necessary to expose the cervix if the uterus is retroverted or if the vaginal walls are voluminous, lax, and redundant. A cotton pledget grasped at the end of a curved uterine-dressing forceps may be used as a "pusher" to facilitate exposure. As the instrument is withdrawn, the vaginal walls, including the posterior fornix, and any secretions or discharge present are then also examined for evidence of vaginitis, atrophy, or other lesions.

Last, rectal and bimanual abdominal-rectal examinations are done, to look for external and internal hemorrhoids, fissures, fistulas, or anorectal polyps or tumors, and the uterus is palpated bimanually (only now will the fundus be palpable if the uterus is retroverted), together with the ovaries and particularly the cul-de-sac and uterosacral ligament areas and the paracervical and paravaginal regions (so-called anterior parametrium). These areas are best felt rectally, and herein the diagnostic findings of endometriosis or early spread of cervical carcinoma may lie (see Fig. 38). The rectal finger can also explore the surface of each pelvic wall in turn, feeling for enlarged nodes or other abnormalities. At this point, with the index finger already in the rectum, the thumb may be introduced simultaneously into the vagina so that a bidigital, bimanual abdominal-vaginal-rectal examination is done (Fig. 4). The accuracy and precision of the findings are thereby sometimes increased, particularly with respect to the cul-de-sac, rectovaginal septal, uterosacral, and paracervical regions. Furthermore, by having the patient strain or assume the standing position while the examiner maintains the two fingers within the rectum and vagina, the presence of an enterocele (see Fig. 67), perhaps suspected but demonstrable in no other way, may be confirmed by feeling the sac with its contents bulge down between the vaginal and rectal fingers.

At the conclusion of the pelvic examination the patient should be examined briefly in the standing position, checking for the presence of inguinal or femoral hernias and inspecting the lower extremities for varicosities, edema, or skin lesions. If varicosities are present, the various maneuvers useful in the evaluation of their type and extent can be carried out. If there is any question of peripheral arterial insufficiency, the femoral, popliteal, dorsalis pedis, and posterior tibial pulses should also be checked.

Following completion of the physical examination, the patient is allowed to dress in privacy. When she returns to the consultation room, the important features of the history and physical findings should be reviewed for her, their significance explained in easily understood terms, and the suggested plan of further study and treatment outlined, again explaining the need and rationale for the proposed program so that

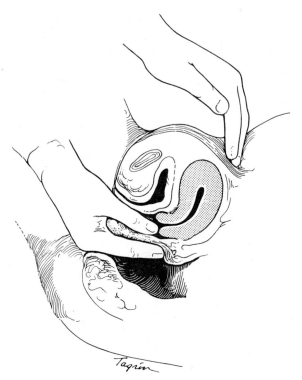

Figure 4
Bidigital rectovaginal examination.

she can readily comprehend its importance and cooperate completely. If the husband, mother, or other close relative has accompanied the patient, it is often wise — but always with the patient's agreement and permission — to invite them to sit in on this final summation. In this way, the member or members of the family most vitally interested in and concerned with the patient's welfare will obtain the information about her current medical situation directly and therefore more accurately, and their assistance, if needed, to support her and ensure her understanding of and cooperation in the subsequent course of study and therapy is thereby usually guaranteed.

PSYCHOSOMATIC MECHANISMS AND DISTURBANCES
IN THE GYNECOLOGIC PATIENT

In a reasonably concise presentation of the field of gynecology, it is impossible even to begin to do justice to the many facets of the various psychosomatic mechanisms and disturbances that may be encountered in the gynecologic patient. Acute or chronic emotional disorders, through interference with the normal, delicately balanced neuroendocrine control of the cyclic activity of the female reproductive tract, may often cause fundamental disturbances in this cyclic function, with the result that distressing symptoms arise on a purely psychosomatic basis. Such psychosomatic mechanisms are almost invariably important in the comprehension and management of many of the functional gynecologic disorders discussed in Chapter 5 and elsewhere in the book: essential dysmenorrhea, so-called hypothalamic amenorrhea, the premenstrual tension syndrome, the "pelvic congestion" syndrome and related types of functional pelvic pain, idiopathic pruritus vulvae, and so on. Undoubtedly, they also play an important etiologic role in many instances among the large group of women with recurring functional menstrual irregularities as well as in some patients suffering from infertility or habitual abortion. Certainly, the significance of psychological factors in the production of many of the disabling menopausal symptoms experienced by a few women is well recognized.

On the other hand, among the various manifestations of organic disease of the reproductive tract are usually to be found secondary symptoms arising on a psychological basis. This is because disturbed function of or complaints localized to the region of the pelvic viscera invariably are the source of considerable anxiety to the woman — they may raise the specter of premature loss of or failure to completely fulfill childbearing potential, cause concern over possible loss of sexual function, or arouse the fear that cancer or a "shameful social disease" may be present. In fact, pelvic symptoms often suggest to the patient a serious threat to her very integrity as a female, either as a result of what the disease itself will do to her or as a consequence of the treatment that may be required, e.g., hysterectomy. Thus emotional factors must also be taken into account and sympathetically dealt with by explanation and reassurance in the patient with obvious organic disease as well as in the woman who proves to have functional complaints.

Some of the more frequently encountered psychosomatic mechanisms and resulting gynecologic disturbances will be considered more fully later on in the appropriate chapters, but it is important at the very outset to emphasize their potential significance in the evaluation and management of any patient with pelvic disease or symptoms. For exploration of this subject in greater depth, the publications of Sturgis [11], Gardiner [4], and McLennan [8] can be specifically recommended to the reader as being particularly instructive and succinct.

PROGRAM FOR THE EARLY DETECTION OF GYNECOLOGIC CANCER

Since at least 25 percent of all malignant disease in women arises in the genital tract, and since female genital cancer is particularly susceptible to simple methods of early detection, the opportunity to carry out such a program of early recognition during the process of securing the gynecologic history and performing a complete gynecologic examination should never be neglected, regardless of the patient's chief complaint. Through the educational programs sponsored by a variety of both medical and lay organizations, women (and their physicians) have become increasingly aware of the value of annual checkups and yearly Papanicolaou smears in the discovery of early asymptomatic pelvic malignancy at a stage when, if treatment is prompt and adequate, cure rates are potentially the highest of any area of the body. In the decade from 1964 to 1974, an American Cancer Society survey showed that the percentage of women who had had a routine Papanicolaou smear rose from 48 percent to 78 percent, and the percentage of women who had a smear during the year immediately preceding this American Cancer Society study had risen from 23 percent in 1963 to 52 percent in 1974. In spite of tremendous advances in surgical techniques, radiation treatment, cancer chemotherapy, and so on, during the past 15 to 20 years, the only malignancy to show a significant decline in mortality in the United States has been carcinoma of the cervix. The absolute, overall improvement in the cure rate for cervical cancer is definitely due to the fact that it is now being detected at a much earlier stage far more often than formerly. (In the past 20 to 25 years, a decrease in the death rate from cancer of the cervix as much as 50 to 60 percent has been observed in several areas of the country where long-term, ongoing Papanicolaou smear screening programs involving 90 to 95 percent of the local population have been in existence.)

The habit now adopted by many women of reporting for a vaginal smear each year has had equally important secondary dividends in the form of opportunities to carry out a complete medical examination. Thus a neoplasm arising elsewhere in the pelvis (e.g., ovary) or in other body regions (e.g., breast, thyroid, rectum), as well as significant benign disorders, both in the pelvis and in other body regions or systems, can also be discovered early and dealt with expeditiously and often successfully. It was noted in a 1970 study [12] that when a cervical cancer screening program was extended to include a complete gynecological examination as well as clinical examination of the breasts, 26 new, unsuspected malignant tumors (including 7 breast cancers) were found in 4000 patients seen, and 23 percent of all patients examined were felt to be in need of treatment or further investigation of other, nonmalignant abnormalities. Because it has been the obvious value of the yearly vaginal smear that has made women "checkup-conscious," much of the responsibility for carrying out routine annual examinations has fallen on the shoulders of the gynecologist. This burden can, should, and must be shared by other physicians if the benefits of annual checkups are to be extended to a larger segment of the female population.

Yearly pelvic cancer detection procedures should probably be offered to all women over the age of 18 or 20 (the teenager should certainly be included if she is sexually active) and are particularly feasible on a broad scale in obstetric patients, nearly all of whom are now under regular medical supervision and thus readily available for a routine screening program. Any physician's office may be simply and inexpensively equipped to carry out a complete gynecologic cancer detection study. The only materials needed are:

1. Bivalve vaginal specula, preferably of assorted sizes.
2. A cervical biopsy punch (Gaylord, Younge, etc.).
3. A small endometrial biopsy curet.

4. A uterine tenaculum.
5. A uterine sound.
6. An endometrial aspiration cannula (optional).
7. Curved glass pipettes and a rubber suction bulb, for obtaining vaginal cytologic smears.
8. Throat sticks (or a special spatula) for securing cervical cytologic smears.
9. Small bottles of 10% formalin solution to be used as tissue biopsy fixative.
10. Small bottles of Papanicolaou's fixative (equal parts of ether and 95% alcohol) (as an alternative, pure 95% alcohol may also be employed), which serves as the fixative for cytologic smears. Smears may be submitted in the original bottle of fixative, or, if more convenient, the glass slides may be left in the fixative for at least 30 minutes, then air-dried and forwarded to the laboratory in simple cardboard mailing containers.
11. A bottle of Schiller's solution (see Chap. 2).
12. Glass slides, paper clips, a diamond marking pencil for labeling glass slides.

Routine screening of the patient with no apparent symptoms referable to the pelvic organs should include:

1. Inquiry regarding abnormal bleeding or discharge (particularly significant if the occurrence is postcoital, intermenstrual, or postmenopausal); menstrual irregularities, pelvic or lower abdominal discomfort; change in or abnormalities of bowel or bladder function; pruritus or lesions of the vulvar skin.
2. Cytologic examinations: vaginal smears and cervical scrapings.
3. Pelvic examination (a careful general examination, including a survey of the neck, breasts and axillae, abdomen, groins, and legs, should of course be done prior to the vaginal and rectal examinations), which involves:
   a. Inspection and palpation of the external genitalia.
   b. Bimanual abdominal-vaginal examination.
   c. Speculum examination of the cervix and vagina.
   d. Rectal examination, including bimanual abdominal-rectal examination.

The following additional office procedures are indicated in patients in whom any of the abnormal symptoms are elicited during the interview, in whom examination reveals any suspicious findings (e.g., cervical "erosion," a questionable adnexal mass, a vulvar lesion of unknown nature), or in whom doubtful or positive vaginal or cervical smears are reported:

1. Cervical and endocervical smears (scrapings), if not previously obtained.
2. Schiller's test of the cervix (see Chap. 2).
3. Cervical biopsy of grossly abnormal areas or of grossly normal areas that do not stain with Schiller's solution.
4. Colposcopy if available and colposcopically guided biopsies of the cervix if indicated.

5. Endometrial biopsy; endometrial-aspiration cytologic smears (optional).
6. Biopsy of any suspicious vulvar or vaginal lesion; toluidine blue test of vulvar skin (see Chap. 2).
7. Careful, repeated follow-up observations in all patients with presumed fibroids, physiologic ovarian enlargements, vulvar leukoplakia, etc.

If the source of suspicious symptoms or the abnormal vaginal smear remains undetected, or if the nature of any abnormal finding is not completely clarified by the office diagnostic survey, further gynecologic evaluation becomes essential and will usually involve hospitalization for examination under anesthesia, fractional curettage of the endocervix and endometrial cavity, more extensive cervical biopsies or cold-knife total cone biopsy of the cervix, or for culdoscopy, laparoscopy, or exploratory laparotomy if an ovarian tumor is suspected. In other words, the office tests, even if absolutely negative, cannot be relied on to exclude completely the presence of pelvic cancer in patients with suggestive symptoms or findings, or with suspicious vaginal cytologic findings.

If, on the other hand, any of the office procedures yield positive results and disclose definite malignancy, immediate hospitalization is indicated for a more complete evaluation of the exact extent of the disease and for the subsequent institution of appropriate therapy.

The value of such routine cancer detection programs, whether carried on by the individual physician or within the framework of large medical institutions or special cancer detection clinics, has been amply demonstrated in numerous published reports. For more detailed data concerning the typical results of such programs, the reader may be interested in consulting the work of Day [2] and of Scott [10], the first of which contains a more extensive bibliography on the subject.

EXAMINATION OF THE RAPE VICTIM

Because it represents a specialized examination situation involving the obtaining and recording of specific historical details and clinical findings, together with certain specific laboratory studies, all of which are very important from a medicolegal standpoint as well as for the proper care of the patient, it seems appropriate to include a special section in this chapter on examination and management of the patient who has been sexually assaulted. In the current climate of violence within our society, physicians, especially gynecologists, are called on more often than formerly to examine and counsel the unfortunate victim of rape, as well as to treat the medical and emotional complications associated with it.

By definition, rape is coitus without the consent of the woman, and legal determination of rape requires (1) proof of force, (2) proof of labial penetration, with or without emission, and (3) proof that the act was performed without consent. Statutory rape is coitus with a female "below the age of consent" (usually this is age 16 or 18, but it has varied in different states over a range of 14 to 21). Sexual molestation is noncoital sexual contact without consent.

For the sake of her emotional health, the victim of rape needs the positive reassurance from the very beginning that those caring for her medically are well aware that she has indeed been criminally assaulted and is not, as has often been presumed in the past, a consciously or subconsciously willing participant in the sordid event. An accurate history of the alleged rape should be recorded, quoting the patient's own words and indicating the time, place, and circumstances of the alleged incident. The patient's emotional state and whether or not she may have been intoxicated (and hence legally incapable of giving consent) should be clearly noted in the record.

A thorough physical examination, including vaginal and rectal examinations, is obviously necessary (for which the patient's consent should be obtained in writing — and a parent's if the victim is a minor) to rule out possible physical injury, as well as for the purpose of obtaining and recording the following: (1) evidence of the use of force (torn or bloody clothing; bruises or abrasions of the thighs; vulvar, perineal, or vaginal trauma); (2) evidence of penetration, with or without ejaculation, on the part of the rapist (see the following paragraph); (3) proof that the act was committed against the woman's will, which, together with (2), will be essential in the legal determination of rape and the subsequent prosecution of the attacker.

Torn and soiled clothing should be saved as evidence and the cloth leached with saline and tested for semen or examined for sperm, as indicated. Vaginal and cervical secretions should be obtained by cotton swab or aspiration and slides made and examined immediately under the microscope for the presence of motile sperm. Additional slides should also be made from saline washings of the vagina and vulva, and smears and slides from the anal area may also be useful. All specimens should be carefully made and labeled, so that they may be retained as permanent evidence. Swabs should also be made and kept in sterile test tubes for police laboratory examinations for (1) acid phosphate (a fairly accurate indicator of the presence of semen); (2) blood group antigens of semen; and (3) precipitin tests against human sperm and blood.

Potential medical complications of rape, in addition to soft-tissue injuries that might require immediate treatment (these should be repaired under general anesthesia), include venereal disease and pregnancy. Smears and cultures should be taken in an attempt to identify gonorrheal organisms, if present, and these should be repeated in 7 to 10 days. A blood test for syphilis is also done and is repeated in six to eight weeks. Majority opinion advocates giving prophylactic penicillin therapy — e.g., 4.8 million units of procaine penicillin intramuscularly — since this is adequate treatment for both gonorrhea and incubating syphilis. If the patient is allergic to penicillin, appropriate dosages of tetracycline or spectinomycin can be given (see also Chap. 8).

The possibility of pregnancy can usually be avoided by a postcoital contraceptive regimen such as 25 mg of diethylstilbestrol twice daily for five days (see also Chap. 20); failures following this program are extremely rare. However, should pregnancy occur as a result of rape, therapeutic abortion can easily be performed. The patient should be reassured that there are cogent compassionate, moral, and ethical grounds and a firm legal and a sound medical basis for abortion in her case, and that it can be done in any accredited institution without the need to specify rape as the reason for the abortion request.

Equally important, if not more so, is attention to the emotional state of the patient. In many instances a sympathetic ear on the part of the physician and social worker and an opportunity to talk freely about this most frightening and traumatic experience allow the patient to ventilate her fears and anxieties and recover satisfactorily from the emotional shock. Sometimes this may require several follow-up visits with a sympathetic physician or social worker who can lend the much-needed emotional support and reassurance. However, approximately 10 percent of rape victims may require more prolonged counseling and psychiatric consultation because of persistence of adverse psychological or emotional reactions.

REFERENCES

1. Barber, H. R. K., and Graber, E. A. Postmenopausal palpable ovary syndrome. *Obstet. Gynecol.* 38:921, 1971.
2. Day, E. Evaluation of exfoliative cytology as a screening method for pelvic cancer. *Clin. Obstet. Gynecol.* 4:1183, 1961.
3. Evrard, J. R. Rape: The medical, social, and legal implications. *Am. J. Obstet. Gynecol.* 111:197, 1971.
4. Gardiner, S. H. The role of the gynecologist in psychosomatic illness. *Clin. Obstet. Gynecol.* 5:298, 1962.
5. Good, R. S. The third ear: Interviewing techniques in obstetrics and gynecology. *Obstet. Gynecol.* 40:760, 1972.
6. Hayman, C. R., and Lanza, C. Sexual assault on women and girls. *Am. J. Obstet. Gynecol.* 109:480, 1971.
7. Koss, L. G., and Hicklin, M. D. Standards of adequacy of cytologic examination of the female genital tract. *Obstet. Gynecol.* 43:792, 1974.
8. McLennan, H. Tension and stress in gynecology. *Am. J. Obstet. Gynecol.* 94:477, 1966.
9. Pearson, J. W. The obstetrician and gynecologist: Primary physician for women. *J.A.M.A.* 231:815, 1975.
10. Scott, J. W., Gilpin, C. A., and Blake, T. F. Cancer detection in private practice. *Obstet. Gynecol.* 20:814, 1962.
11. Sturgis, S. H. *The Gynecologic Patient: A Psycho-Endocrine Study.* New York: Grune & Stratton, 1962.
12. Thomas, B. A. Screening for breast and gynecological lesions. *Lancet* 2:409, 1970.

2

Laboratory Tests and Special Procedures in Gynecologic Diagnosis

A complete, thoughtfully elicited history and a thorough, carefully performed physical examination, with obvious emphasis on the recognition and proper interpretation of significant findings demonstrated by abdominal, pelvic, and rectal examinations, are the two basic and perhaps most important avenues of approach to the diagnosis of pelvic disorders. Information so obtained may be all that is necessary to arrive at an exact diagnosis in some situations; at the very least, the broad outlines of the clinical problem posed by the chief complaint will have been narrowed considerably, so that further investigation of a limited number of the more likely possibilities can now be effectively undertaken. Only in this way can the wide variety of laboratory tests and special procedures that have proved useful in the differential diagnosis of the various general types of gynecologic complaints (e.g., abnormal bleeding, pelvic pain, menstrual irregularities, pelvic tumors, infertility) be efficiently and profitably applied, avoiding delay in diagnosis and treatment and reducing to a minimum the number of unnecessary studies performed.

Once the likely possibilities have been clearly defined, the necessary additional information that will lead to a precise diagnosis can usually be obtained by intelligent use of the various office, laboratory, roentgenographic, and surgical diagnostic procedures that are presented and described in this chapter. In the case of each test, the indications for its use, the manner in which it is performed and interpreted, and its chief clinical applications are presented in some detail, so as to avoid the need for repetition in later chapters. A few special procedures, commonly employed only in connection with a specific problem (e.g., infertility), are described elsewhere in the appropriate chapter.

BASIC OFFICE DIAGNOSTIC TECHNIQUES

Cytologic Technique (Papanicolaou Smear)

Use of the cytologic technique is one of the most valuable recent additions to the diagnostic methods available to the gynecologist.

VAGINAL SMEARS

To be certain of obtaining a satisfactory vaginal smear, the patient should not have douched or undergone pelvic examination during the preceding 24 hours, and vaginal bleeding should be absent or minimal. With the patient in lithotomy position and prior to digital or speculum examination, the labia are spread, and a clean, dry glass pipette with attached rubber suction bulb (the latter is compressed before introducing the pipette into the vagina) is inserted gently into the posterior vaginal fornix (Fig. 5A).

17

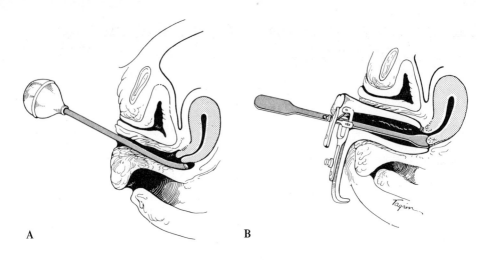

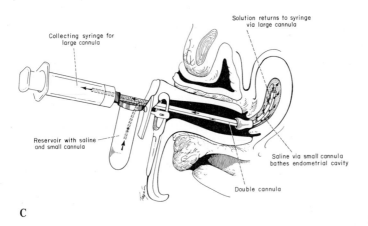

Figure 5
Technique for obtaining cytologic smears. A. Vaginal pool smear from the posterior
fornix. B. Cervical scraping smear. C. Artist's drawing of the Gravlee Jet Washer,
a disposable kit for the negative-pressure lavage technique of obtaining endometrial
aspiration specimens for cytologic and histologic study.

The manual compression of the bulb is slowly released and the pipette simultaneously gradually withdrawn, aspirating vaginal secretions from the pool in the posterior fornix. These are promptly ejected and carefully smeared out with the tip of the pipette on a clean glass slide previously marked with the patient's name and identifying number. The slide should be quickly placed in a bottle of fixative before drying of the secretions occurs, because drying prior to fixation frequently results in cellular distortion and unsatisfactory smears. Multiple slides can safely be placed in the same bottle of fixative by simply attaching a paper clip to each slide, thus preventing contact and transfer of cells from one slide to another. Papanicolaou's original fixative was a mixture of equal parts of 95% alcohol and ether, but many laboratories have found pure 95% alcohol equally satisfactory. Slides may be transported in the bottle of fixative to the cytologist; or after 30 minutes they may be removed from the fixative, air-dried, and mailed in ordinary cardboard slide containers.

It is generally agreed that any woman over age 20 (or sexually active women of any age) should have a routine vaginal smear and careful pelvic examination annually if the ideal goal of achieving diagnosis of all cervical cancer in the carcinoma in situ or very early invasive phase, when it is still potentially 100 percent curable, is to be realized. Commencing yearly cytologic screening as early as age 20 is not unreasonable; 10 to 15 percent of new cases of cervical cancer (carcinoma in situ or invasive carcinoma) have been appearing in the 20- to 29-year age group in recent years. There have also been reports of a small but definite incidence of cervical cancer in sexually active teenagers in recent years. The screening of large populations of women for gynecologic malignancy, particularly early cervical cancer, by means of annual examinations and vaginal smear tests has been conclusively demonstrated to be effective in detecting the early, asymptomatic, unsuspected cases in a number of well-controlled studies throughout the country in which such a program has been instituted on a citywide, countywide, and in some instances, statewide basis. In populations screened for the first time, reports of the number of abnormal smears encountered have ranged from 3 to 12 women per 1000.

In view of the success of such trial programs, efforts to make at least the annual cytologic test available to all women through the development of "do-it-yourself" techniques involving special diagnostic tampons, irrigation and aspiration kits, and the like are currently under study and trial. The principal drawback – and a serious one – to such an approach is that it will tend to reduce the number of women who actually receive a thorough examination by their physicians, with the result that the "smear test at home" may defeat its own purpose. There has also been some question regarding the diagnostic accuracy of do-it-yourself methods. However, the irrigation smear, done at home by the patient herself, has definitely proved its worth in several pilot studies of mass screening, each accomplished entirely by mail. A gratifying response rate of 85 percent of the populations surveyed was observed, and the programs achieved an increasing accuracy (80 to 95 percent) in detecting the preinvasive and invasive cervical cancers, ultimately shown to be present, in the thousands of women responding. This "mail-order" approach is infinitely less expensive than similar surveys utilizing cancer detection clinics and, unlike the latter, is potentially capable of reaching the entire female population at risk. If automated cytologic analyzers become a reality, they will greatly enlarge the possible scope of such mass population screening techniques — in fact, they will be essential for expanding such programs. (Optical scanners capable of registering both cell size and total cell counts are now being developed which, by automatically plotting cell-size frequencies, will permit recognition of the characteristic cell-size distribution patterns of both pre-malignant and malignant lesions.)

Routine cytologic study may also disclose unsuspected carcinoma of the endometrium, fallopian tube, ovary, and vagina, and positive vaginal smears may even be obtained in the presence of vulvar carcinoma. Rarely, a positive vaginal smear may occur in the presence of an extrapelvic malignant tumor arising elsewhere in the peritoneal cavity (e.g., stomach or pancreas); desquamating malignant cells travel through the fallopian tubes and uterus to appear in the vaginal secretions, or, in the case of bladder or renal tumors, arrive as the result of the admixture of small amounts of urine to the vaginal contents. In addition to its use as a screening procedure and as an adjunct to diagnosis in patients with symptoms, the vaginal smear may be extremely helpful in detecting early asymptomatic recurrences at a stage still amenable to further therapy in patients previously treated for pelvic cancer by surgery or radiation.

The two commonly employed methods of classifying and reporting cytologic smears with regard to the presence or absence of malignant cells are:

Negative	Class I: Negative.
	Class II: Atypical, not suspicious for tumor cells.
Doubtful (atypical and suspicious)	Class III: Atypical, suspicious for tumor cells.
	Class IV: Probable tumor cells.
Positive	Class V: Definite tumor cells.

If the smear was obtained or fixed improperly, so that sufficient numbers of well-preserved and adequately fixed and stained cells are not available for study and interpretation, the test will be reported "Unsatisfactory." Occasionally, doubtful (and, rarely, even positive) smear reports will be rendered in the presence of severe chronic cervicitis, trichomonal or other types of vaginitis, or in postmenopausal women who have recently received a sizable amount of estrogenic hormones. The incidence of false-positives is very low, however, running less than 0.5 percent in most laboratories. The cytologist is ordinarily readily able to distinguish between smears positive for squamous carcinoma and those positive for adenocarcinoma. Furthermore, as experience in the field of cytologic interpretation has increased, many cytologists now find it possible, on the basis of the cellular picture in the vaginal or cervical smear, to predict accurately which one of the three probable stages in the evolution of epidermoid carcinoma is present in the patient's cervix: severe anaplasia or dysplasia of the squamous epithelium, carcinoma in situ, or invasive carcinoma. In addition, when adenocarcinoma cells are seen in the smear, certain cytologic criteria are present in some instances that enable the cytologist to suggest the most likely source: adenocarcinoma of the endometrium, adenocarcinoma of the endocervix, or ovarian or tubal carcinoma. More rarely, sarcoma cells may be seen and correctly identified by the cytologist.

With regard to the accuracy with which a single cytologic smear will detect malignancy if present, it averages 90 to 95 percent or better in the case of both invasive and in situ squamous carcinoma of the cervix (especially if both vaginal fornix and cervical-endocervical scrape and aspiration smears are made), 70 to 80 percent in cervical dysplasia, and only 70 to 80 percent at best, often considerably less (25 to 50 percent), in adenocarcinoma of the endometrium. The reduced accuracy of vaginal smears in detecting endometrial carcinoma is important to note; it presumably is due to failure of some of these lesions to shed cells, or to cytoplasmic and nuclear deterioration before the cells reach the vaginal pool. Obviously, cytologic accuracy increases if multiple smears are taken on different days. However, for the purposes of annual screening to detect incipient malignant change in the cervical epithelium, even a potential 10 percent false-negative rate on the initial smear is essentially reduced to zero so rapidly within the first few years of the annual checkup program that the chances of failure to detect the preinvasive stage of cervical cancer are remote. The important point, however, is that the performance of the smear test should always be simply a part of the complete pelvic and speculum examination, and any suspicious cervix should receive the benefit of a Schiller's test, biopsy, and, if available, colposcopy. It should also be stressed that a final diagnosis is determined only by biopsy and rests on histologic evidence of malignancy and its type, not on cytologic criteria alone, a point strongly and repeatedly emphasized by cytologists themselves.

Another important, often neglected use of the vaginal smear is in the evaluation of the endocrine status of the patient. The vaginal mucosa is another of the target organs that responds cyclically to the fluctuating levels of female steroid hormones, and the desquamated vaginal epithelial cells are readily available for study and accurately reflect this changing hormonal pattern. If smears are to be used for this purpose, they are best obtained from a scraping of the lateral wall of the midportion of the vagina rather than from the posterior vaginal pool. In this way, fresh cells that reflect more precisely the endocrine picture of the moment and are relatively uncontaminated by cells from other portions of the reproductive tract are secured from the segment of the vagina most sensitive to hormone level changes. Although there are a number of readily discernible cytologic changes, some or all of which may be taken into account in arriving at an estimate of the hormone activity present in a given patient at a particular time, the fundamental criterion employed in most laboratories is the determination of the percentages of the various types of normal vaginal epithelial cells that ordinarily appear in the smear. By noting the relative proportions of parabasal (sometimes abbreviated to basal), "precornified," and "cornified" epithelial cells desquamated by the normal vaginal mucosa, a qualitative estimate of estrogen levels may be obtained.

Some laboratories have felt that the presence of deeply pigmented nuclei in the so-called cornified cells has been the most reliable manifestation of estrogen effect and hence have referred to the **karyopyknotic index**. The International Committee on Terminology in Exfoliative Cytology has pointed out that true cornification of the vaginal mucosa does not normally occur and that the term *cornified cell* is a misnomer when applied to vaginal cytology. The committee has therefore recommended that the designations **superficial cell** and **intermediate cell** be used instead of **cornified cell** and **precornified cell**, and that the term **maturation index** be employed in place of **cornification index**. Thus the maturation index describes the relative percentage of parabasal, intermediate, and superficial cells seen in the smear, is estimated after identifying and counting several hundred vaginal cells, and is denoted by three numbers, with the parabasal percentage on the left, the intermediate percentage in the center, and the superficial percentage on the right. For example, in a patient with adequate to marked estrogen effect it might be 0/10/90; poor estrogen effect might be 20/75/5; complete absence of estrogen effect might be 100/0/0; maximum progesterone effect in the presence of adequate estrogen might approach 0/100/0. As a rough guide, the significance of the percentage of superficial ("cornified") cells is as follows:

Percentage of Superficial ("Cornified" or Karyopyknotic) Cells	Estrogen Effect
1–10%	Slight estrogen effect.
10–30%	Moderate estrogen effect.
Over 30%	Marked estrogen effect.

If 50 percent or more of the cells are basal cells, low estrogen effect is also indicated. The relative percentage of intermediate ("precornified") cells is highly variable and not significant except when over 90 percent of the cells are of this type; either pregnancy (suppression of estrogen effect by progesterone) or relative estrogen lack is then indicated. The presence of inflammation (e.g., chronic cervicitis, vaginitis) will disturb the cornification pattern and render it unreliable as an index of estrogen effect.

Serial smears in women of menstrual age may be used in this fashion to determine the occurrence and timing of ovulation and the accompanying progesterone effect, although the method is often too cumbersome for routine clinical use, since it requires daily vaginal smears. Because of the characteristic cytologic changes of progesterone effect that persist in the amenorrhea of early pregnancy, as contrasted with the lack of such changes in the amenorrhea of ovulatory failure, the vaginal smear can be utilized in the diagnosis of early pregnancy, as well as for an index of failing corpus luteum function and the probability of an incipient abortion in early pregnancy. However, again, its use here is often impractical because of the need for serial smears to achieve any degree of reliability.

In a postmenopausal woman not receiving estrogenic medication, the vaginal smear should show a low maturation index. Therefore, evidence of marked estrogen effect in such a patient might suggest the possibility of an estrogen-secreting granulosa cell or theca cell tumor of the ovary. However, it should be noted that an abnormal estrogenlike effect on vaginal cytology has also been observed in postmenopausal women taking digitalis and related cardiac glycosides, and a markedly elevated maturation index is regularly seen in the majority of women who have been on digitalis for two or more years.

Typical maturation indexes for various stages in the female life cycle are set forth in the following table, although it must be remembered that these are average values and that individual variation is great:

	Parabasal	Intermediate	Superficial
At birth (due to hormonal stimulation from mother)	0	95	5
Childhood (1 month to 8 years)	90	10	0
Prepuberty (variable)	30	50	20
Childbearing age:			
Ovulation	0	40	60
Menstruation	0	70	30
Pregnancy	0	95	5
Lactation	90	10	0
Menopause (variable)	30	60	10
Postmenopause (atrophic)	100	0	0

Finally, a number of the common organisms responsible for the occurrence of vaginitis and cervicitis can be recognized in cytologic smears, including *Trichomonas vaginalis, Candida,* and the viral inclusion bodies of herpes simplex type 2.

CERVICAL SMEARS

In the hands of some cytologists, cervical smears have been slightly more accurate in demonstrating abnormal cervical epithelial cells than have simple vaginal smears. Material for a cervical smear is obtained by exposing the external os with an unlubricated speculum and aspirating directly from the cervix, or preferably scraping in a rotary manner completely around the squamocolumnar junction within the cervical os (Fig. 5B). A special (Ayre) spatula may be used as a scraper, but an excellent substitute, always available and with the added virtue of disposability, can be quickly fashioned by splitting a throat stick longitudinally. A simple cotton-tip applicator may also be used but is less satisfactory because the cells tend to adhere to it. The cervical scrapings are smeared out on a slide, which is then handled in the same manner as for a vaginal smear.

ENDOMETRIAL (ASPIRATION) SMEARS

Tumor cells have been reported to be absent from the vaginal smear in from 25 percent to as high as 75 percent of patients with endometrial carcinoma in various published series. The accuracy of the cytologic diagnosis of this lesion may be improved by preparing smears in the usual way from material aspirated directly from the endometrial cavity by means of a special aspiration cannula attached to an ordinary syringe. The cannula is of the same size and shape as a uterine sound or endometrial biopsy curet, and the technique of insertion is identical (see Fig. 10). Isaacs [29] has designed a simple, inexpensive, disposable instrument kit (Curity Endometrial Sampling Set, Kendall) for this purpose that has proved highly accurate. A further refinement of the aspiration technique has been developed by Gravlee [23] and employs a negative-pressure lavage type of aspirator that is also suitable for use in the physician's office. The Gravlee Jet Washer, a disposable kit marketed by Upjohn, utilizes a double cannula and a stopper that is firmly seated in the cervical os to create negative pressure in the uterine cavity. This closes the fallopian tubes and allows approximately 30 ml of sterile normal saline solution to be drawn through the uterus to lavage the entire endometrial surface, without fear of forcing uterine contents into the abdominal cavity (Fig. 5C). Both cells and tissue fragments are obtained in the lavage fluid sample, so that the specimen can be used for both cytologic and histologic studies. Many thousands of asymptomatic as well as symptomatic patients have been studied using the Gravlee Jet Washer, with a diagnostic accuracy of 95 to 100 percent, essentially no false-positive results, and few false-negative reports. (**Note:** It cannot be emphasized too often that, even in the face of negative cytologic smears and endometrial biopsies, a dilatation and curettage are essentially mandatory in any woman with postmenopausal bleeding or other symptoms suggestive of endometrial carcinoma.)

Simple Fresh or "Wet" Vaginal Smears

Simple fresh or "wet" vaginal smears are much more useful for diagnostic purposes than is generally appreciated. They are obtained as follows: Prior to vaginal examination a drop of vaginal secretion is aspirated by pipette in the usual manner, placed on a glass slide, mixed in a drop of saline, and a coverslip applied. Examination of a fresh or "wet" vaginal smear under low- and high-power microscope will determine, confirm, or suggest the presence of any of the following:

1. **Trichomonal vaginitis.** The typical moving, flagellate organisms are usually obvious (Fig. 6A).
2. **Candidal vaginitis.** The long thin, septate hyphae and the small, oval budding yeast forms are characteristic but may be difficult to identify in a simple saline preparation. Their recognition is greatly facilitated by the use, instead of saline, of one or two drops of the following readily prepared solution: 10 ml of Parker 51 Superchrome blue-black ink are mixed with 20 ml of a 10 to 20% potassium hydroxide (KOH) solution. The stained smear is allowed to stand for 5 minutes before examination under the microscope. With dissolution of most of the rest of the cellular debris in the smear by the 10 to 20% KOH solution, the darkly stained hyphae and yeast forms become clearly visible (Fig. 6B).
3. **Nonspecific vaginitis or cervicitis.** In the absence of *Trichomonas* or *Candida* on microscopic examination, the presence of bacteria and leukocytes in abundance suggests a nonspecific vaginitis or cervicitis.

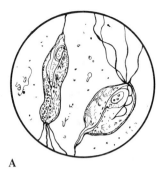 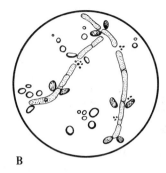

A   B

Figure 6
Fresh vaginal smear preparations. A. Microscopic appearance of *Trichomonas vaginalis* organisms. B. Microscopic picture in candidal vaginitis.

4. **Atrophic vaginitis.** The absence or rarity of "potato-chip" superficial vaginal cells and the finding of essentially only small, round basal cells usually indicate the presence of an atrophic vaginal mucosa and, in the absence of any visible pathogens, suggests that the patient's vulvovaginal symptoms, if any, may be on this basis alone. Conversely, if significant estrogen effect is present, many of the vaginal cells seen in the smear will be of the superficial ("cornified") type.

5. **Pyometrium.** If a purulent-appearing vaginal discharge is found on examination of a fresh smear to consist almost entirely of crenated, deteriorating red blood cells, possibilities to be considered are pyohematometrium or, less often, bleeding and secondary infection superimposed on atrophic vaginitis.

Culture Studies

VAGINAL CULTURES

1. **Trichomoniasis.** Culture media are available but are rarely necessary because of the ease with which a diagnosis can be made on examination of a fresh smear.

2. **Candidiasis.** Since identification by smear is often difficult, if the clinical diagnosis is in doubt, the cultural method using Nickerson's medium is simple, accurate, and very helpful in establishing a definite diagnosis. The culture medium is inexpensive and commercially available for office or clinic use in small slant tubes from the Ortho Company. Incubation is at room temperature with a color end point in one to five days.

3. **Routine bacteriologic cultures.** When the presence of trichomonal or candidal vaginitis has been excluded, and a nonspecific bacterial vaginitis is suspected, routine cultures and antibiotic-sensitivity studies are indicated to identify the organism and determine the appropriate antibiotic therapy.

4. **Genital herpesvirus type 2 cultures.** Herpetic infections can be recognized easily and rapidly by appropriate cultures for this organism from vaginal (or cervical or vulvar) lesions.

CERVICAL CULTURES

Culture swabs taken directly from the cervical os are useful in definitely establishing a diagnosis of gonorrhea. Formerly, these were planted on ascitic and blood agar plates and incubated anaerobically. However, a newer technique now used by most bacteriology laboratories employs the Thayer-Martin culture medium and permits rapid and extremely reliable identification of the gonococcus. (A gram-stained smear should also be made and examined in the hope of demonstrating immediately the presence of gram-negative intracellular diplococci.) Cervical cultures are frequently also invaluable in determining the organisms involved and their antibiotic sensitivities in patients with postpartum or postabortal sepsis.

UTERINE CULTURES

Uterine cultures are employed chiefly in attempts to establish a diagnosis of pelvic tuberculosis. Menstrual discharge should be used and is aspirated from the endo-cervix or lower fundus and submitted for tuberculosis cultures, guinea pig inocula-tions, and stained smears for tubercle bacilli.

Cervical Mucus Arborization Test (Fern Test)

The phenomenon of arborization (the formation of fern patterns) in dried cervical mucus is dependent on the presence in cervical secretions of sodium chloride and other electrolytes, together with various protein substances in certain definite pro-portions. Because control over these proportions appears to be exerted exclusively by ovarian steroid hormones through their effects on the secretory activities of the endocervical glands, the presence or absence of fern patterns at any given moment is directly dependent on the ovarian hormonal status of the patient at that particular time. The fern phenomenon is seen in its typical form only when adequate amounts of estrogen are available. Furthermore, progesterone inhibits or completely abolishes it, even in the presence of sufficient estrogen. Minor variations (atypical fern pat-terns) are also recognizable in the presence of fluctuations in the relative amounts of estrogen and progesterone that may occur during a normal menstrual cycle, in patients with ovarian dysfunction, during pregnancy, and so on. In view of its rather direct correlation with ovarian hormone levels, the fern test has proved very useful for their qualitative evaluation.

   The test, which is easily performed in the office or clinic, is carried out as follows: After the cervix is exposed and gently swabbed clean, a sample of endocervical mucus is obtained with a completely dry glass pipette that has been sterilized in distilled water, or by a cotton-tipped applicator or cupped metal forceps, and is spread on a clean glass slide. If the secretion is spread too thinly, or if blood is present, arbor-ization will not occur, even when adequate estrogen levels exist. The slide is air-dried for at least 10 to 20 minutes (drying must be absolutely complete) and then is read under both low- and high-power magnification on the microscope. If true arborization

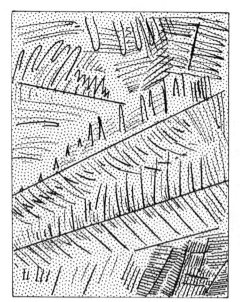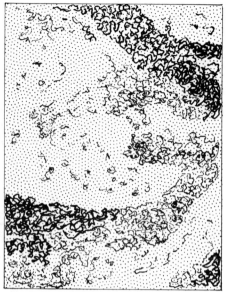

Figure 7
Cervical mucus arborization test (fern test). The fern phenomenon indicative of
good estrogen effect is illustrated on the left; a progesterone effect (or lack of or
failure of the cervix to respond to estrogen) is shown at right. (From T. H. Green,
Jr. Gynecology. In G. L. Nardi and G. D. Zuidema [Eds.], *Surgery: A Concise
Guide to Clinical Practice* [3rd ed.]. Boston: Little, Brown, 1972, Chap. 39.)

with crystallization is present, it is indicative of a predominant estrogen effect, and
the test is positive (Fig. 7, left). If a cellular pattern without crystallization and
arborization is seen (Fig. 7, right), the test is negative and indicates either little or
no estrogen effect or, more commonly, suppression of estrogen activity by progesterone. Actually, Figure 7 represents a drastic oversimplification, since a great
variety of typical and atypical patterns may actually be encountered and at times
present difficulties in interpretation. Fortunately, in the vast majority of instances,
if the slide has been properly prepared, the results are clear-cut and unequivocal.

DIAGNOSTIC USES

Ovulation

Since, within a few days, ovulation and the production of progesterone by the
corpus luteum normally result in a shift from the positive fern test characteristic of
the preovulatory phase to a negative test typical of the latter half of the menstrual
cycle, this simple office procedure can be employed as an index of ovulation and
normal corpus luteum function. (Since both low estrogen levels as well as chronic
endocervicitis may lead to a continually negative test throughout the cycle, at least

two tests must be done, one in each half of the cycle, for a valid conclusion to be reached.)

Pregnancy

In the case of a woman who has recently missed a period, the presence of a positive fern test would be strongly in favor of an anovulatory cycle (predominant estrogen effect) with a delay in onset of flow and would argue against the existence of pregnancy. A negative test would be consistent with pregnancy but not absolutely diagnostic unless a previous test showing arborization had been done in the first half of the same menstrual cycle.

Disorders of Early Pregnancy

There is increasing evidence that patients with persistence or reappearance of the cervical mucus arborization phenomenon in early pregnancy will show a high incidence of abortion. Such a change in the fern test reflects the development of a progesterone inadequacy.

Schiller's Test

Schiller's test is performed as follows: The cervix is exposed by speculum. Avoiding any trauma whatsoever to the cervical epithelium, any mucus or vaginal secretions are gently removed by allowing them to adhere to a soft cotton pledget. (The cotton may be moistened in a solution that rapidly dissolves mucus and is marketed commercially as Alkalol by the Alkalol Company, Taunton, Massachusetts.) Schiller's iodine solution (formula: iodine, 1 part; potassium iodide, 2 parts; water, 300 parts; because of photosensitivity and rapid deterioration, it must be stored in a brown bottle and a fresh solution made up every four to six weeks) is then either poured into the vagina to inundate the cervix and vaginal fornices or is gently painted on the cervix with a soft cotton pledget saturated in the solution. The abundant glycogen in the normal squamous cervical and vaginal epithelium takes up the stain, with the production of a homogeneous mahogany-brown color. If the entire squamous epithelium of the cervix and vagina takes up the stain, the test is normal. If the even grossly normal-appearing squamous epithelial covering is microscopically abnormal in any area (e.g.: carcinoma in situ or very early invasive cancer; basal cell hyperplasia or similar epithelial atypicalities; squamous metaplasia; leukoplakia), the stain is not taken up, and a light-colored, unstained island results and signifies an abnormal or positive Schiller's test. It should be noted that the normal columnar epithelium of the endocervix does not stain, so that one must first carefully visualize the unstained cervix and identify the squamocolumnar junction to interpret Schiller's test properly and avoid miscalling abnormal the exposed normal columnar epithelium so often visible in a lacerated, everted cervix or routinely seen in the presence of a congenital cervical erosion (Fig. 8).

Schiller's test has three valuable applications:

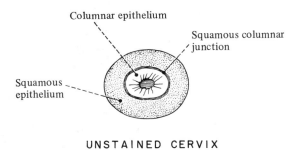

UNSTAINED CERVIX

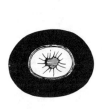

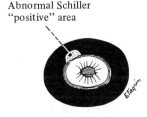

NORMAL TEST   ABNORMAL TEST

Figure 8
Schiller's test. (From T. H. Green, Jr. Gynecology. In G. L. Nardi and G. D. Zuidema [Eds.], *Surgery: A Concise Guide to Clinical Practice* [3rd ed.]. Boston: Little, Brown, 1972, Chap. 39.)

1. It may be used independently as a simple office screening test. Biopsies should be done of all abnormal nonstaining areas, and although cancer will not be found in the majority, carcinoma in situ or early microinvasive cervical cancer is detectable in this fashion.
2. If a positive smear is obtained in a patient with a cervix that clinically appears benign, Schiller's test may be used to pinpoint likely areas for biopsy to obtain a histologic diagnosis.
3. During preparation for hysterectomy for carcinoma in situ or for radical surgery for invasive carcinoma of cervix, the vaginal vault may be stained with Schiller's solution to define the limit of possible microscopic vaginal extension, thus ensuring that an adequate area of vagina is excised with the specimen.

Vulvar Staining and Biopsy

A number of diffuse disorders of the vulva (e.g., leukoplakia, lichen sclerosus et atrophicus, various chronic inflammatory processes) may either raise the suspicion of an underlying malignancy or actually be associated with a premalignant epithelial dysplasia, carcinoma in situ, or early invasive cancer. When one encounters such suspicious vulvar skin changes, biopsy is clearly indicated. Collins and associates [11] have developed a clinical stain for use in selecting biopsy sites in patients with this type of vulvar disease. This simple test, employing toluidine blue, does for the vulva what Schiller's test accomplishes for the cervix. A 1% aqueous solution of toluidine blue is thoroughly applied with cotton-tipped applicators, staining the entire vulva a deep blue. After it has been allowed to dry briefly, the skin is sponged with a 1% acetic acid solution. This results in decolorization of all normal areas of skin. Any areas that retain the deep-blue stain represent abnormal epithelium and are considered "positive." All such areas should be examined by biopsy, and in women over the age of 50, roughly 50 percent will prove to be carcinoma (intra-epithelial or early invasive); the remainder usually show either dysplasia or chronic inflammatory changes, and from a cancer detection standpoint are thus false-positives. False-negative tests are extremely rare, however, so the technique has real value in evaluating the diseased vulva.

Cervical Biopsy

Biopsy should always be done in the presence of any suspicious area on the cervix or in the event of an abnormal Schiller's test, employing any of the several punch-biopsy instruments available (Gaylord, Younge, Kervorkian). To make certain that the pathologist receives tissue most suitable for histologic study and diagnosis, a sample should be obtained large enough to include a segment of squamocolumnar junction (for this is the region where most cervical neoplasms arise) and deep enough to permit differentiation between intraepithelial and invasive carcinoma, if carcinoma is present. However, biopsy excision need not be so deep that subsequent bleeding becomes excessive. The normal slight resulting ooze is readily controlled by light cauterization with a silver nitrate stick and placement of a vaginal tampon that the patient removes in a few hours. If brisk arterial bleeding is encountered, as happens occasionally, a mattress type of suture is usually necessary for hemostasis.

If one is dealing with a clinically benign-appearing cervix in a patient with abnormal cytologic findings, a biopsy specimen may be taken as indicated by the Schiller's test, but, thereafter, additional random cervical biopsy specimens (e.g., the so-called four-quadrant biopsy technique illustrated in Fig. 9) are no longer considered adequate for proper evaluation of a cytologically suspicious cervix. Rather, colposcopy should be done, together with selective cervical biopsies taken under colposcopic guidance and/or cold-knife cone biopsy (conization) of the cervix where this is indicated by the colposcopic findings or when facilities for colposcopy are not available. (See Colposcopy and Colpomicroscopy and Diagnostic Operative Procedures.) In addition, the endocervical canal should be scraped with a small, sharp curet and any tissue obtained submitted separately. (**Note:** Pieces of tissue obtained by biopsy [either cervical or endometrial] are best placed on small squares of filter paper and then promptly immersed in a small bottle of 10% formalin solution for transport to the laboratory.)

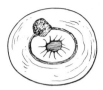

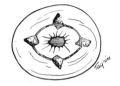

Simple Biopsy   4-Quadrant Biopsy

Figure 9
Cervical biopsy. (From T. H. Green, Jr. Gynecology. In G. L. Nardi and G. D.
Zuidema [Eds.], *Surgery: A Concise Guide to Clinical Practice* [3rd ed.]. Boston:
Little, Brown, 1972, Chap. 39.)

Colposcopy and Colpomicroscopy

By means of brightly illuminated, elaborately designed optical instruments, the
colposcope and colpomicroscope, a moderately magnified (10 to 20 times with the
colposcope) to highly magnified (up to 400 times with the colpomicroscope) three-
dimensional view of the stained or unstained cervical epithelium in situ may be
obtained. A number of enthusiastic workers have found these instruments valuable
in research on the cervix and its abnormalities and increasingly useful in office or
clinic as the primary diagnostic procedure for the detection and recognition of
cervical disease. The instruments are moderately expensive ($3000 to $5000), and
special training and experience are required for their proper use, but the precision
and accuracy of diagnosis achieved with colposcopy more than offset these features,
and the technique is simple, painless, and without complications for the patient.
The time involved in carrying out each examination precludes the use of colposcopy
for routine screening programs, but routine cervicovaginal cytologic screening has
and will continue to fulfill this role admirably.

Colposcopy, however, is ideally suited for the evaluation of all patients with
cytologic abnormalities suggesting dysplasia, carcinoma in situ, or early invasive
carcinoma, particularly when there is no obvious cervical lesion to examine by
simple biopsy for a definitive diagnosis of frankly invasive carcinoma. Colposcopy
is also useful in the evaluation of vaginal and vulvar epithelial abnormalities detected
on clinical examination or by cytologic studies, e.g., vaginal adenosis or vulvar epithelial dystrophies. Colposcopic observations are important in themselves in arriving
at a diagnosis, but colposcopically guided biopsies of the most suspicious and most
extremely abnormal areas of epithelium provide the final, definitive histological
diagnosis. Such guided biopsies of the ectocervix and squamocolumnar junction,
supplemented by sharp curettage of the endocervical canal, should permit a final,
definitive diagnosis of either dysplasia, carcinoma in situ, or invasive carcinoma in
all but a small percentage of patients. The chances that a lesion exists that is more
severe than the one recognized by colposcopy with selected biopsies are probably
less than 0.5 percent at most.

In roughly 10 percent of patients, it will not be possible to visualize or obtain colposcopically guided biopsies from all the cervical epithelium that appears to be at risk, and these patients will require diagnostic cone biopsy (see Diagnostic Operative Procedures and Chap. 13).

The technique of colposcopy is simple, but its detailed description here is not feasible. (The interested reader can consult any of the several excellent atlases of colposcopy currently available.) The examination involves observation of both the unstained cervix and, most important, of the cervix treated with 3% acetic acid to accentuate some of the important morphologic features. A colposcopic diagnosis is based on an evaluation of the vascular pattern, intercapillary distance, surface contour, color tone, and clarity of demarcation of the lesion. Final confirmation is obtained by direct biopsy under colposcopic guidance of the most extreme abnormality to be visualized.

Endometrial Biopsy

The ease with which a sample of endometrium can usually be obtained for histologic study is of tremendous help in the office evaluation and management of a variety of pelvic disorders; in functional menstrual disturbances and infertility, two outstanding examples, endometrial biopsy nearly always proves absolutely essential. The cervix is exposed by speculum, the external os swabbed free of mucus and painted with Schiller's solution, and the anterior cervical lip grasped with a tenaculum a slight distance from the external cervical os. A uterine sound is passed to determine the length and direction of the cervical canal and endometrial cavity. The patient is warned to expect slight discomfort similar to a menstrual cramp, and a curved endometrial biopsy curet is introduced to the top of the fundus (Fig. 10). The curet is pressed firmly against the wall of the fundus anteriorly, posteriorly, or laterally and is then withdrawn, the cupped, spoonlike end removing a strip of endometrium. (Some prefer a suction or aspiration biopsy instrument such as the Vacurette [Berkeley Bio-Engineering], a biopsy cannula with a blunt-tipped plastic aspirator and an attached collecting container including disposable vacuum tubing and vacuum bottle or syringe adapter. With this technique the tissue samples are removed by suction rather than by actual curettage.) Details of the recent menstrual history should accompany the pathology laboratory requisition, since the pathologist is able not only to render a diagnosis of proliferative or secretory endometrium but, on the basis of certain histologic criteria, is also actually able to "date" the progestational phase of the endometrial sample submitted for comparison with the known actual day of the patient's current cycle.

Endometrial biopsy is most often utilized as an index of ovulation and progesterone effect in the course of a sterility study or as an aid in the diagnosis and further management of dysfunctional (anovulatory) bleeding. Obviously, biopsy must be performed in the immediate premenstrual phase or on the first day of menstruation to be of any help in either situation. Endometrial biopsy is also useful as a diagnostic maneuver in patients suspected of harboring endometrial cancer; a positive report facilitates the diagnosis, but a negative report is of little value and does not

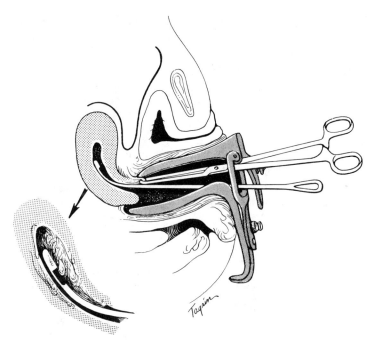

Figure 10
Endometrial biopsy.

alter the need for a diagnostic curettage in women with symptoms suggestive of this lesion.

Fertility Evaluation

Tubal insufflation (Rubin's test), the postcoital cervical mucus test (Sims-Huhner test; "PK test"), and the basal body temperature (BBT) chart are discussed in Chapter 11.

Office Tests for Early Pregnancy

There are several office tests useful **in the presumptive diagnosis of early pregnancy** during the month immediately following the first missed period, at a time when the diagnosis is usually impossible on the basis of physical examination alone. Not all the tests are absolutely diagnostic.

BASAL BODY TEMPERATURE CHART

If the basal body temperature chart shows a typical biphasic ovulatory temperature curve and if the temperature remains elevated following the first missed period, an anovulatory cycle has been completely ruled out as a cause of the delayed period, and pregnancy is essentially certain (see Fig. 40). This probably represents the earliest means by which a diagnosis of pregnancy can be made with certainty. (Conception while the patient is maintaining a record of her basal body temperature curve occurs fairly often during the course of an infertility investigation.)

CERVICAL MUCUS TEST

Although the cervical mucus test yields indirect or circumstantial evidence only, as previously noted in this chapter, it is actually fairly reliable; and it is highly so if a preovulatory test in the same cycle had been done and showed a typical fern pattern that has subsequently disappeared completely and remained suppressed.

PROGESTERONE TEST

The progesterone test involves the administration of progesterone, either orally (10 to 20 mg daily for five days) or intramuscularly (25 to 50 mg in a single dose) in women with a prior history of normal, regular cycles whose regular period is overdue. If the missed period is due to failure of or delay in ovulation, the administration of progesterone will result in the onset of flow, usually within the next two to four days, the progesterone acting to produce endometrial maturation followed by withdrawal bleeding as the progesterone effect subsides. If the missed period is due to early pregnancy, no flow will occur.

NEOSTIGMINE TEST (SOSKIN TEST)

The neostigmine test is based on the theory that a significant number of delayed periods in the absence of pregnancy are not due to failure of ovulation but to an inhibition of the normal premenstrual neurovascular reaction in an otherwise suitably ripened premenstrual secretory endometrium. The use of neostigmine (Prostigmin) with its acetylcholinelike action allegedly overcomes this inhibition and restores the normal neurovascular changes necessary for the ischemic vasoconstriction of the spiral arteriolar network.

Neostigmine methylsulfate, 1 ml of a 1:1000 solution, is injected daily for one to three days. If the patient is not pregnant and is not suffering from an endocrine dysfunction, bleeding will occur following a time interval varying from a few hours after the first injection to as long as 72 hours after a third injection. If the patient is pregnant, bleeding will not occur. It is essential that the patient have a history of perfectly normal menses prior to missing the period in question since the test is not valid in the presence of endocrine disturbances, ovarian disorders, or at the menopause. In spite of these limitations, because of the frequency of "missed periods" of neurogenic origin, and because the chance of a false response in the presence of pregnancy is practically nil, the test is of some practical value.

SPECIAL LABORATORY PROCEDURES

Pregnancy Tests

Laboratory tests for pregnancy are all based on the detection of chorionic gonado-tropin in urine or serum. Formerly, a variety of bioassay techniques employing laboratory animals (mice, rats, rabbits, frogs, and toads) were widely used. However, these various biologic tests for chorionic gonadotropin have been almost completely abandoned and replaced by an immunologic test for pregnancy. This method involves use of a latex particle preparation sensitized to human chorionic gonado-tropin (HCG), together with a standardized human chorionic gonadotropin antiserum. Based on an agglutination inhibition reaction, the test is carried out on a freshly voided morning urine specimen, and the results of the standard laboratory test-tube procedure are usually available in two to three hours. (Simple and fairly accurate latex agglutination inhibition immunologic slide tests that can be performed in 2 minutes in the physician's office are commercially available: e.g., Gravindex Slide Test for Pregnancy [Ortho Diagnostics] ; Pregnosticon Dri-Dot Test [Organon] , Gest-Stage [Lederle Diagnostics] , UCG-Slide Test [Wampole Laboratories] . These slide tests are not as accurate as the 2-hour test-tube laboratory procedures, however.) The immunologic test for pregnancy has proved to have a precision and reliability equal to, if not greater than, that of any of the biologic tests and is much more easily and rapidly performed. The sensitivity of the immunologic test is such that it is often positive as early as four or five days after the first missed menstrual period.

A radioimmunoassay method, based on the competition for anti-HCG serum between a known amount of radioactive iodine—labeled gonadotropin and the un-labeled HCG in the sample to be tested, represents a further development in this field. An even more sensitive and rapidly performed radioimmunoassay specific for HCG is now available that uses an antiserum prepared with an antigen that is a highly purified beta subunit of HCG. Finally, the latest development in the field of preg-nancy testing and still under investigation is a radioreceptoassay of HCG in blood, employing plasma membranes as the receptor. This new test is highly sensitive and has shown 100 percent accuracy on the first day after the missed period. This further refinement in laboratory technique allows greater precision and sensitivity in quantitative measurements, even in handling small amounts of gonadotropin, such as are present in samples of serum.

In interpreting the results of these tests and applying them to specific clinical problems, it is important to be aware of the following points:

1. The standard immunologic latex agglutination inhibition tests can be relied on for definitely positive or negative evidence of pregnancy 10 to 14 days after the first missed period, although the radioimmunoassay approaches 100 percent accuracy even a few days after the first missed period. Tests performed earlier than this carry a high rate of false-negative and indefinite results. The overall accuracy of the latex agglutination inhibition tests approaches 95 to 98 percent, with less than 5 percent false-negative and less than 5 percent false-positive results.

2. The chorionic gonadotropin level rises rapidly thereafter until the tenth or twelfth week of pregnancy, when it may again fall rapidly, reaching levels low enough after the twentieth week to give negative tests (perhaps 50 percent or more of the time) after the fifth or sixth month, even in a normal pregnancy.
3. Quantitative determination using either immunologic or bioassay methods can be done. In the first and second trimesters of pregnancy:
   a. Abnormally low levels may indicate the likelihood of impending abortion; early in pregnancy, they may indicate the possibility of an ectopic gestation.
   b. Abnormally high levels suggest the presence of hydatidiform mole, choriocarcinoma, or, occasionally, multiple pregnancy.
4. Since chorionic gonadotropin usually disappears completely within a few days (one to six) after delivery, persistence of positive tests indicates the likelihood of either retained placental tissue, mole, or a chorionic tumor of some type.
5. False-positive biologic and rarely even false-positive immunologic pregnancy tests may occasionally be observed in patients receiving phenothiazine compounds such as chlorpromazine, promazine hydrochloride, and similar tranquilizers and antidepressants. It is believed that the neuroendocrine effect of these drugs is the result of an increased production of pituitary gonadotropins.

Other laboratory tests for pregnancy include the Guterman test for urinary pregnanediol excretion, and the determination of serum estrogen level. The levels of both rise to a peak in the latter half of pregnancy, and because under ordinary circumstances only pregnancy is associated with such elevated levels, either determination is highly diagnostic for pregnancy, though they are a little too complicated to be practical for routine use. (It should also be mentioned that a plain abdominal x-ray film will usually show fetal skeletal structure beginning at about 4½ months and hence is a possible diagnostic maneuver whenever a pregnancy of five to six months' duration is suspected in spite of a negative pregnancy test, which many merely reflect the frequent fall in gonadotropin levels in the later part of pregnancy.)

HORMONE ASSAYS OF SPECIAL SIGNIFICANCE IN GYNECOLOGY

Pituitary Gonadotropins

Quantitative determination of the levels of activity of the various tropic or stimulating hormones produced by the pituitary are frequently of great help in the differential diagnosis of abnormalities of reproductive tract function; in fact, such information is essential in distinguishing between primary ovarian disorders and disturbances of pituitary function. Aside from their use in individual clinical situations, the ability to carry out these pituitary hormone assays with increasing ease and accuracy in recent years has resulted in the accumulation of a large amount of clinical and laboratory research data of great significance to a better understanding of the biochemical nature and pathophysiology of many of the endocrine disorders that involve the reproductive tract or affect its function.

FOLLICLE-STIMULATING HORMONE

To obtain a measure of the total daily pituitary output of follicle-stimulating hormone (FSH), a 24-hour urine sample is required. A radioimmunoassay technique that is specific for FSH as well as highly accurate is now available in many laboratories. Nevertheless, some laboratories continue to use a bioassay method.

In the biologic method, the assay animals commonly employed are the mouse and rat, the end points being an increase in mouse uterine weight or rat ovarian weight, with the increases in weight varying in response to variations in the FSH content of the urine samples tested.

Normal values of urinary FSH excretion in mouse and rat units (m.u. and r.u.) are:

Mouse Bioassay

Puberty:	2–3 m.u./24 hours
Maturity:	5–80 m.u./24 hours
Menopause (early):	80–250 m.u./24 hours

Rat Bioassay

Normal males and females:	5–10 r.u./24 hours
Postmenopausal females:	Over 25 r.u./24 hours

Since these bioassay methods are relatively insensitive at low levels, 24-hour urinary pituitary gonadotropin determinations alone cannot reliably distinguish between a patient with hypopituitarism and a significant number of women, many of whom are menstruating normally, whose gonadotropin levels happen to be in the low-normal range, despite normal pituitary function. Therefore the chief value of 24-hour urinary pituitary gonadotropin assays lies in clinical situations in which it is important to determine whether gonadotropin output is either high or low. Thus, in a 19-year-old girl with primary amenorrhea, it is essential to know whether the pituitary is hypoactive (low or absent urinary gonadotropins), or whether the problem is one of primary gonadal deficiency (in which case a high level of urinary gonadotropin excretion will be observed).

An even more precise 24-hour urine FSH determination, as well as measurements of the level of FSH in the blood at any given time, can now be performed by a radioimmunoassay technique entirely similar to the one now employed for serum HCG and serum LH determinations. Random serum FSH determinations are not so meaningful or helpful in the clinical study and management of an individual patient as is a total 24-hour urinary FSH output assay because of the great variation in FSH secretion at different times during a 24-hour interval in the same person. (However, serial serum FSH determinations have proved very useful to the research investigator studying the physiology of the normal menstrual cycle and the abnormal hormonal patterns of the various endocrine disorders of the reproductive system.)

RADIOIMMUNOASSAY

24-hour urine FSH excretion in females:

Follicular phase:	5–20 IU/24 hours
Midcycle:	15–60 IU/24 hours
Luteal phase:	5–15 IU/24 hours
Menopause:	50–100IU/24 hours
Serum FSH levels:	0.10–0.46 μU/ml

LUTEINIZING HORMONE OR INTERSTITIAL CELL–STIMULATING HORMONE

In combination with FSH, the production of luteinizing hormone (LH) by the pituitary is presumed to initiate the secretion of estrogen by the follicular cells of the ovary. Development of a radioimmunoassay technique for LH determinations has provided and undoubtedly will continue to provide data of increasing significance in the elucidation of the underlying mechanisms involved in a number of gynecologic endocrine disturbances. The immunologic method for the quantitative measurement of LH is entirely similar to the one developed for the detection of HCG and in fact is based on a cross-reaction to this same HCG immunologic system. This immunologic test is specific and accurate, and its increasing use has served to confirm its simplicity, reliability, and accuracy for routine clinical use. The radioimmunoassay modification of this test for LH is also entirely similar to that previously described for HCG. Its sensitivity and precision appears to be considerably greater than that reported for all other methods for detecting and quantitating LH.

Radioimmunoassay ranges of serum or plasma LH in the female are as follows:

Preovulatory or postovulatory:	5–22 μU/ml
Midcycle peak:	30–250 μU/ml
Menopause:	20–100 μU/ml

PROLACTIN (HPRL)

Pituitary secretion of prolactin (formerly known as the luteotropic hormone, or LTH) is presumed to aid in stimulating progesterone production by the corpus luteum. Serum prolactin levels can be measured by a radioimmunoassay test that utilizes immunochemical human prolactin and rabbit antihuman prolactin. Serum prolactin determinations are especially helpful in the investigation of patients with galactorrhea or the combination of amenorrhea and galactorrhea (see Chaps. 5 and 6).

LUTEINIZING HORMONE–RELEASING HORMONE (LH-RH) TEST

A neurohormone, luteinizing hormone–releasing hormone (LH-RH), produced by the hypothalamus, is responsible for triggering the production of LH (and probably FSH as well) by the pituitary. If 50 to 100 μg of either the synthetic or the purified natural decapeptide LH-RH is administered intravenously, a rapid and significant rise in both LH and FSH should occur in patients with amenorrhea and hypogonadal syndromes, provided no fundamental pituitary abnormality exists. This test is thus very helpful in distinguishing between hypothalamic, pituitary, and central nervous system causes for secondary hypogonadism.

Steroid Hormones

From the standpoint of gynecologic diagnosis, determination of the steroid hormones normally produced by the ovary, namely, estrogen and progesterone (or their urinary metabolites), is obviously of greatest concern. However, because disorders of adrenal function frequently have a profound effect on ovarian physiology as well, and because the ovary under certain circumstances can also be the site of formation of both adrenal steroids and androgens, it is usually important to be able to obtain as complete a measurement of the steroid hormone pattern as is currently possible. This is particularly true in any clinical situation in which an endocrinologic disorder involving abnormalities of steroid metabolism in either ovary, or adrenal, or both, is suspected. The assays currently available for routine use, which will be outlined, have become increasingly useful and valuable in recent years, both in the diagnosis and clinical management of patients as well as in the research investigation of the various diseases and biochemical mechanisms involved. It must constantly be borne in mind, however, that the four principal types of steroid compounds — estrogens, progesterone, androgens, and the corticoids — though chemically separable and quantitatively measurable in terms of the urinary output of certain specific compounds, are actually interrelated in a very complicated fashion. The interpretation of the results of urinary steroid hormone assays is therefore sometimes fraught with difficulties and often provides only limited information as to the exact nature of the physiologic disturbance in the patient. These difficulties result from the facts that (1) any one of the four main steroid-secreting glands (ovary, testis, adrenal cortex, and placenta) may produce any or all of the four principal types of steroid hormones, and (2) interconversion among the four principal and chemically separable types of steroid compounds frequently takes place during their catabolism and excretion. Thus, simple measurement of the urinary excretion products is not invariably an index of the original nature and biologic activity of the steroid hormones being secreted nor of the organ or type of glandular tissue in which they were initially produced. Fortunately, in many disorders in which grossly abnormal function of a specific organ (e.g., ovary or adrenal) is involved, the steroid hormone excretion pattern is characteristic, and urinary assays are of great value as diagnostic procedures.

ESTROGEN

Indirect estimate of estrogen levels may be obtained by vaginal smear, endometrial biopsy, and by the response to progesterone injection in the patient with amenorrhea.

Several bioassay methods employ the rat as the test animal; the end points are the degree of vaginal cornification in oophorectomized adult rats or the amount of increase in uterine weight in immature rats. Determinations are made on 24-hour urine specimens except during pregnancy, when serum may be used. Chemical assay is also possible. However, currently, a quantitative radioimmunoassay technique has replaced the bioassay or chemical assay techniques in many laboratories. The radioimmunoassay also makes it feasible to obtain plasma estrogen levels at any given time (Table 1).

Table 1
Common Steroid Hormone Assays as Performed on 24-Hour Urine Sample, with
Corresponding Test on Plasma Sample: Average Normal Values in Females

24-Hour Urine Specimen	Normal Range (per 24 hours)	Plasma Sample	Normal Range (ng/ml)
17-Ketosteroids	4–16 mg	Dehydroepiandrosterone sulfate:	
		Premenopausal	1250–1950
17-Hydroxycortico-steroids (Porter-Silber chromagen)	2–7 mg	Postmenopausal	230–370
		Cortisol	70–90
Pregnanediol:		Progesterone:	
Preovulatory	0–1 mg	Premenopausal	0.45–0.50
Postovulatory	3–8 mg	Postmenopausal	0.15–0.20
Pregnanetriol	0.1–1.8 mg	17-Hydroxyprogesterone:	
		Premenopausal	0.35–0.45
		Postmenopausal	0.2–0.25
17-Ketogenic steroids	5–18 mg	Cortisol + 17-hydroxypro-gesterone (closest approximation)	
Total estrogens	4–100 μg		
Estradiol	0–10 μg	Estradiol-17 beta:	
		Premenopausal	0.045–0.055
		Postmenopausal	0.012–0.014
Estrone	2–25 μg	Estrone	0.05–0.09
Testosterone	0–20 μg	Testosterone	0.3–0.95

PROGESTERONE; PREGNANEDIOL URINARY EXCRETION

Bioassays for progesterone are available, but the chemical assay for pregnanediol, its principal excretion product, is simple and highly accurate, and determination of the 24-hour urinary output of pregnanediol is the test usually employed as an index of progesterone production. Refinements in technique have been introduced involving paper and gas chromatography. Measurements of pregnanediol excretion have been shown to correlate extremely well with the appearance and rising level of progesterone during the luteal phase of the normal menstrual cycle, and with the high levels of progesterone occurring during pregnancy (Table 1). Hence pregnanediol determinations may be utilized as an index of ovulation and may also serve as a diagnostic test of pregnancy. In this regard, a falling level of pregnanediol in early pregnancy has been employed by some in the evaluation of the possibility of impending abortion and as an indication for supplementary progesterone medication in its treatment and prevention.

It should be noted that the liver has been shown to be the site of conversion of progesterone to pregnanediol, and that the latter appears to be at least partially excreted in the bile. Hence, in certain primary liver diseases, this conversion may be blocked, with a decrease in pregnanediol excretion, whereas there may be an apparent increase in urinary excretion in the presence of biliary tract obstruction.

A quantitative radioimmunoassay technique is also available now to determine plasma progesterone levels at any given time (Table 1). Progesterone levels determined in this way are highly accurate, and this method has proved to be of great value in research and clinical investigative work.

ANDROGENS AND ADRENAL STEROIDS

Indirect measurement of the level of production of 17-ketosteroids, 17-hydroxy-corticosteroids, testosterone, and other related androgens and corticoids is possible by differential chemical assays of the 24-hour urinary excretion of their various metabolites; direct measurement of the plasma levels of these compounds is now possible using radioimmunoassay and competitive protein-binding techniques.

It is important to remember that the 17-ketosteroid determination is a measure not only of androgen metabolites but also of certain metabolites of the adrenal steroid cortisol as well. Hence the 17-ketosteroids will be elevated in situations in which an abnormally increased production of either androgens or cortisol occurs. On the other hand, and although it does not detect all steroids of adrenal origin, the 17-hydroxycorticosteroid determination reflects more specifically adrenocorticoid production. Thus if one suspects adrenal hypofunction, either primary, or secondary in association with pituitary deficiency, determination of the 24-hour urinary excretion of 17-hydroxycorticoids would be the only screening test necessary. This would also be true for the patient suspected of having Cushing's syndrome, because a marked elevation would be diagnostic, and a normal value would essentially exclude the possibility. Conversely, in patients who present with symptoms and findings suggesting virilization, one is primarily interested in androgen levels, and a 24-hour 17-ketosteroid determination would be the proper screening test. However, both 17-ketosteroid and 17-hydroxycorticoid determinations may well be indicated when the clinical picture suggests a mixture of excessive androgen and glucocorticoid production. The range of normal values for the 24-hour urinary excretion of these two steroid assays is as follows:

17-Ketosteroids (mg/24 hours)

Age	Males	Females
10	1−4	1−4
20	6−21	4−16
30	8−26	4−14
50	5−18	3−9
70	2−10	1−7

17-Hydroxycorticosteroids (mg/24 hours)

Females: 2−7
Males: 3−8

Just as in the case of estrogen and progesterone, radioimmunoassay techniques are now available for the measurement of plasma androgens and adrenal steroids

(Table 1). Of these, the two of greatest significance in the evaluation of gynecologic endocrinopathies are plasma testosterone and plasma cortisol determinations.

Plasma testosterone levels in the normal female fall within the range of 0 to 0.08 μg per 100 ml or 30 to 95 ng per milliliter (1 ng = 0.001 μg). Elevated levels, often in the range of 100 to 300 ng per 100 ml and sometimes greater than 1000 ng (1 μg) per 100 ml, are usually indicative of excessive testosterone production of ovarian origin (arrhenoblastoma, hilar cell tumor, polycystic ovary [Stein-Leventhal syndrome]); less often, the excessive production is of adrenal origin. If the 17-ketosteroids and 17-hydroxycorticosteroids are normal, and if adrenal suppression tests with corticosteroids (e.g., dexamethasone) fail to cause a fall in plasma testosterone, an ovarian source is definitely indicated.

It is now also possible to do rapid plasma cortisol (17-hydroxycorticosteroid) assays using a method based on competitive protein binding. Bearing in mind that estrogens, pregnancy, and liver disease elevate plasma cortisol (but not the 24-hour excretion), and that tranquilizers and diphenylhydantoin also interfere with the test, normal ranges of plasma cortisol for standard times and conditions are as follows:

Time and Conditions	Range (ng/100 ml)
8 A.M.	5–25
8 P.M.	0–10
8 A.M. after 1 mg dexamethasone at midnight	0–5
4 hours after start of ACTH infusion, 20 U/4 hours	30–45
8 hours after start of ACTH infusion, 40 U/8 hours	Over 45

Thyroid Function Tests

Because of the frequency of disorders of thyroid function and the fact that the majority occur in women during the years from menarche to menopause, and because of the known interference of either hyperthyroidism or hypothyroidism with normal pituitary-ovarian reciprocal relationships, an evaluation of thyroid function is essential to, and should be one of the first steps in, the program of investigation of patients with disorders of menstrual function or infertility. Often, disturbances of ovarian function are the first or only manifestation of a mild thyroid disorder, the presence of which will not be detectable on the basis of the clinical signs and symptoms ordinarily associated with the full-blown picture of hypothyroidism or hyperthyroidism. Thus, unsuspected mild thyroid dysfunction must be searched for by employing the several reliable tests of thyroid function now available in any patient who complains of amenorrhea, oligomenorrhea, and related menstrual irregularities, or who suffers from infertility or repeated abortions. No single thyroid function test will invariably yield a complete and valid picture of the functional thyroid status of a given patient. Thus it is often advisable to use two or more such tests to be absolutely certain that a thyroid disturbance is or is not present.

BASAL METABOLIC RATE

The basal metabolic rate (BMR), when properly carried out by a reliable laboratory, is perhaps the simplest of all tests of thyroid function, albeit an indirect one, since it measures peripheral utilization of thyroid hormone. The normal range is customarily considered to be from −15 to +10.

SERUM PROTEIN-BOUND IODINE

The measurement of serum protein-bound iodine (PBI) more or less directly assesses the quantity of circulating thyroid hormone, the normal range being 3.5 to 7.5 μg per 100 ml. The test is of no value in anyone taking thyroid medication and will be artificially elevated and completely invalid in patients who have taken any of a variety of drugs containing iodides or have undergone x-ray studies employing iodinated radiocontrast substances (e.g., a cholecystogram, intravenous pyelogram, hysterosalpingogram) within the preceding weeks, or, in the case of radiocontrast substances, months. Among the iodide-containing drugs, which include many cough syrups and several of the tranquilizers, the gynecologist should particularly remember diiodohydroxyquin (Floraquin), a vaginal suppository commonly used in the treatment of trichomonal vaginitis, as well as Schiller's solution and povidone-iodine solution (Betadine), which are antiseptic solutions often employed in preoperative vaginal preparation; the use of any of these preparations may cause an elevation of the PBI for several days.

RADIOACTIVE IODIDE UPTAKE TEST

The radioactive iodide (RAI) uptake test measures the capacity of the thyroid to remove iodide from the blood and is an excellent index of thyroid function, the normal range of accumulation of ^{131}I within the thyroid in a 48-hour period being 20 to 55 percent. Values above or below suggest hyperthyroidism or hypothyroidism, respectively. Prior administration of iodide-containing compounds in any form will of course yield falsely low values.

BUTANOL EXTRACTABLE IODINE

The butanol extractable iodine (BEI) measures essentially only circulating protein-bound thyroxine, whereas the PBI measures not only the level of circulating thyroid hormone but also the level of all other iodinated protein substances present in serum. Hence the BEI (normal range is 3.0 to 6.5 μg per 100 ml) has replaced the PBI as a test of thyroid function in many laboratories and is probably one of the best screening tests for routine use. Both PBI and BEI may be falsely elevated during pregnancy or in patients taking estrogens or oral contraceptives, because in either case the level of thyroxine-binding globulin is elevated. Conversely, the PBI and BEI may be depressed in patients receiving drugs such as testosterone or cortisone, which lower the thyroxine-binding protein level in the plasma.

RESIN UPTAKE OF TRIIODOTHYROXINE

The resin triiodothyroxine (T_3) uptake test is particularly useful in establishing a diagnosis of hyperthyroidism during pregnancy, since no radioactive substance is involved. The normal level of the T_3 uptake by a resin column in most laboratories falls within the range of 25 to 35 percent. In the euthyroid pregnant patient with a typically falsely elevated BEI (due to high serum estrogen level and the resulting increase in thyroid-binding globulin [TBG] level), the T_3 uptake is depressed; however, if the patient is actually hyperthyroid, it will be in the normal or slightly elevated range.

DIRECT ASSAY FOR THYROXINE

In many laboratories the thyroxine (T_4) assay (more properly the total thyroxine [TT_4] assay) has completely supplanted the PBI and BEI assays, because it is not affected by previous intake of inorganic iodides, mercurial diuretics, or by iodine-containing contrast media employed in diagnostic radiology. It is influenced by changes in the concentrations of the thyroxine-binding proteins (TBG), however, just as in the case of both the PBI and BEI, and therefore may be elevated (1) during pregnancy, (2) in patients taking estrogens, oral contraceptives, or phenothiazines, (3) in patients who have liver disease, and (4) in rare cases of congenital excess of TBG. Conversely, the T_4 level may be abnormally low in (1) patients with severe liver failure, nephrotic syndrome, or congenital TBG deficiency, (2) in patients receiving androgen or corticosteroid therapy, or (3) in patients who are on large doses of diphenylhydantoin. In the absence of any of these situations in which the level of TBG is abnormal, the T_4 assay is elevated only in hyperthyroidism and depressed only in hypothyroidism. It is also possible to measure only the free thyroxine in the blood (free T_4 level, or FT_4); here, abnormal levels are encountered only in the presence of either hyperthyroidism or hypothyroidism. The normal range for the FT_4 assay is 0.8 to 2.4 mμg per 100 ml. The normal range for the T_4 (TT_4) assay is 4 to 11 μg per 100 ml.

DIRECT ASSAY FOR TOTAL TRIIODOTHYRONINE

The direct assay for total triiodothyronine (TT_3) offers a measurement of the other major product of thyroid hormone biosynthesis. Normal serum concentrations range from 150 to 250 ng per 100 ml. A radioimmunoassay for TT_3 is also under development. T_3 secretion usually correlates with T_4 secretion except in the following: "T_3 hyperthyroidism," a type of thyrotoxicosis in which only TT_3 (not TT_4, FT_4, or TBG) is elevated; dietary iodine deficiency (when T_3 is preferentially synthesized and may be normal or elevated, despite a low T_4); or following either Hashimoto's thyroiditis or medical or surgical treatment of thyrotoxicosis, when TT_3 levels maintain a euthyroid state despite lowered T_4 levels.

RADIOIMMUNOASSAY FOR PITUITARY THYROTROPIN

The normal range of serum TSH is 0.5 to 4.0 μU per milliliter, with 10 percent of normal individuals having undetectable levels and essentially all hyperthyroid patients having undetectable levels. In patients with primary hypothyroidism or in those with diminished thyroid reserve due to Hashimoto's thyroiditis, previous radioiodine therapy, or surgery for hyperthyroidism, the serum TSH is invariably elevated. Conversely, in secondary hypothyroidism due to pituitary or hypothalamic disease, the serum TSH is low. Serum TSH determinations are thus most useful in diagnosing hypothyroidism, in differentiating primary from secondary hypothyroidism, in the early detection of diminished thyroid reserve, and in monitoring thyroid replacement therapy for hypothyroidism.

ANTITHYROID ANTIBODIES ASSAY

The antithyroid antibodies assay is a tanned red cell agglutination test that is particularly helpful in confirming the diagnosis of Hashimoto's thyroiditis, in which considerably elevated antibody titers are the rule.

TESTS FOR EVALUATION OF HEMORRHAGIC TENDENCIES

It is estimated that in approximately 10 to 20 percent of all serious hemorrhagic disorders in women, the earliest, most significant, or sole manifestation is the occurrence of excessive menstrual flow or prolonged uterine bleeding. It is therefore important to keep this possibility in mind in the study and management of women suffering from menorrhagia, particularly when no response to the usual measures for control of so-called dysfunctional bleeding on a hormonal basis is obtained, and when the presence of local uterine abnormalities that might cause excessive bleeding has been excluded. In this situation, investigation of the possible existence of an abnormal bleeding tendency is clearly indicated.

A useful, simplified approach to the study of these possible hemorrhagic disorders has been suggested by Jacobson [30] and assumes that serious organic disease with secondary hemorrhagic tendencies has been ruled out. The approach is outlined in the paragraphs that follow.

Evaluation of Platelets (Platelet Count and Blood Smear)

If the platelet count is low (thrombocytopenia), bone-marrow aspiration and further hematologic studies are done to determine the etiology of the thrombocytopenia. If the platelet count is normal, the bleeding time is determined.

It should also be mentioned that several even more sophisticated platelet function tests are now available that can aid in the detection of thrombotic disorders and abnormalities of the hemostatic mechanism. These tests include techniques to demonstrate reduced platelet coagulation capacity as well as to identify abnormally increased platelet adherence and platelet aggregations characteristic of the presence of intravascular thrombotic processes and tendencies.

Bleeding Time

If the bleeding time is also normal, the chances that any fundamental hemorrhagic disorder is present are remote in the female. If the bleeding time is prolonged, a diagnosis of von Willebrand's disease in the female is strongly suggested. Approximately 75 percent of all women with this disorder have menometrorrhagia as a prominent symptom (see Chap. 5).

JACOBSON METHOD FOR DETERMINATION OF BLEEDING TIME

1. With the patient reclining and one forearm supported at the level of the heart, an area of the volar aspect of the forearm (avoiding superficial veins) is sterilized by placement of a sponge soaked in acetone (no rubbing).

2. A blood pressure cuff placed on the upper arm is inflated and maintained at 40 mm Hg during the test.

3. Employing a new No. 11 Bard-Parker blade that has been sterilized by soaking in acetone for several minutes, a longitudinal incision 3 mm deep and 3 mm long is made in the previously prepared area on the forearm (a 3-mm longitudinal ink mark is made on the forearm, and a transverse ink mark is also made 3 mm from the tip of the scalpel blade to ensure complete accuracy and uniformity in the dimensions of this incision).

4. The arm is tilted to allow blood to flow away from the incision, and the blood is picked up by filter paper every 30 seconds until the bleeding ceases, taking care not to allow the filter paper actually to touch the incision. (Bleeding ordinarily does not begin for 30 to 60 seconds, and if an immediate flow of dark, venous blood occurs, a superficial vein has been entered, the test is invalid, and the incision should be repeated elsewhere on the forearm.)

5. At the conclusion of the test, the edges of the incision are approximated by an adhesive bandage that is left in place for 48 hours.

The average bleeding time by this method is 3½ to 5½ minutes, with the upper limit of normal at 6½ minutes. (**Note:** Certain medications, especially aspirin, but also including chlorpromazine and related phenothiazines, phenylbutazone, and glyceryl-guaicolate [an ingredient of most cough syrups and cold remedies], may prolong the bleeding time, and the test is not valid or reliable if any of these drugs has been taken by the patient within the preceding 10 days.)

Partial Thromboplastin Time

Finally, if a coagulation disorder rather than an abnormality of platelets or vascular fragility is suspected, a partial thromboplastin time (PTT) determination can be made. This is a very sensitive and reliable indicator of the integrity of the entire so-called intrinsic pathway of normal blood coagulation and is vastly superior to the clotting time as a screening test for the presence or absence of a coagulopathy. (The PTT has a normal range of 22 to 37 seconds.) It will be abnormally prolonged in patients with clotting disorders due to liver disease or vitamin K deficiency, in patients receiving heparin or coumadin anticoagulants, and in patients in whom a "consumption coagulopathy" develops in association with defibrination-fibrinolysis syndromes secondary to disseminated intravascular coagulation. Of special interest to the gynecologist among the disorders that can produce the latter situation are gram-negative endotoxemic shock such as is encountered in septic abortion, retained dead-fetus syndrome, and incompatible blood transfusion reaction. Rarely, the PTT may be slightly elevated in patients with von Willebrand's disease.

If these three screening tests are normal, the likelihood of a general hemorrhagic disorder is completely ruled out. The other commonly employed battery of tests (e.g., capillary fragility test, clotting time, clot retraction, prothrombin time) rarely, if ever, add any useful information, may even be misleading, and are unnecessary.

(**Note:** The prothrombin time remains useful in monitoring anticoagulant therapy with either heparin or coumadin. Rarely, clotting time determinations may be helpful in monitoring heparin therapy in patients with disseminated intravascular coagulopathy, for in this disorder the PTT and prothrombin times are abnormal and are useless as monitoring indexes.)

DETERMINATION OF NUCLEAR SEX CHROMATIN PATTERN

Of the various cytologic techniques, the oral or buccal smear is the one now most commonly employed for determining the nuclear sex chromatin pattern; it may be studied more easily and rapidly than blood smears or skin biopsies. Vaginal smears may also be employed for this purpose but are somewhat less satisfactory. The test is based on the recognition of a chromatin mass (sex chromatin body) in the cell nucleus adjacent to the nuclear membrane in females and its absence or virtual absence in the cell nuclei of tissue or desquamated cells in males (Fig. 11). The sex chromatin body will be present in about 65 to 75 percent of all nuclei in suitably prepared histologic sections (e.g., skin) of female tissues and in 20 to 80 percent of satisfactorily preserved nuclei in buccal smears from genetic females. In buccal smears from normal males, less than 4 percent of nuclei will have sex chromatin bodies. However, in the case of genetic disorders involving sex chromosome mosaicism such as XO, XX (see Chap. 3), the nuclear sex chromatin count may be in an intermediate range, e.g., 10 to 15 percent, and this should raise the suspicion of some form of gonadal dysgenesis with mosaicism. (In some of the sex chromosomal disorders described in Chapter 3, more than one chromatin body may be present.) Discovery of an abnormality of nuclear sex chromatin should, of course, be followed up with a chromosome analysis.

A more recent application of nuclear sex chromatin determination has been the essentially 100 percent successful prediction of fetal sex in utero by carrying out

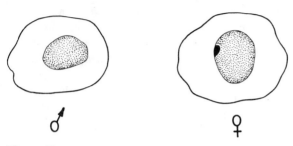

Figure 11
Nuclear sex chromatin determination. Note chromatin mass (Barr body) adjacent to the nuclear membrane in the normal female cell nucleus and absence of this sex chromatin mass in the normal male nucleus. (From T. H. Green, Jr. Gynecology. In G. L. Nardi and G. D. Zuidema [Eds.], *Surgery: A Concise Guide to Clinical Practice* [3rd ed.]. Boston: Little, Brown, 1972, Chap. 39.)

sex chromatin counts on fetal cells present in amniotic fluid, now readily and safely obtained by amniocentesis. A male fetus can be predicted if the nuclear sex chromatin count is less than 3 percent, a female if it is 12 percent or higher (usually 20 to 40 percent). However, it is not recommended that this be done simply to satisfy the curiosity of the parents-to-be. On the other hand, amniocentesis for the purpose of complete chromosomal and enzymatic studies, including chromosomal karyotyping as well as simple nuclear chromatin determination, has proved far more important and significant in the prenatal recognition of chromosomal or genetic-linked abnormalities that either might be treatable and/or preventable in utero or, on recognition, might be an indication for therapeutic interruption of the pregnancy. Equally or perhaps even more important, a recent analysis of the results of second-trimester diagnostic amniocenteses in over 2000 pregnant women in whom the risk of a birth defect in the fetus was felt to be high revealed that over 97 percent of these women could be assured that the suspected disorder was not present. On the basis of a national collaborative study involving many thousands of amniocenteses, performance of the procedure early in the second trimester, though not completely free of potential complications, appears to be eminently safe in skilled hands, with the risk of fetal loss probably considerably less than 0.5 percent.

As will become apparent in the next few chapters, there are certain more or less obvious clinical situations in which nuclear sex chromatin studies as well as chromosome analyses are clearly indicated. These are as follows:

1. Primary amenorrhea in apparent females.
2. Presence of ambiguous external genitalia at any age.
3. Prepubertal girls with pronounced shortness of stature.
4. Male infertility.
5. Mental retardation and/or psychotic or antisocial behavior in either females or males.
6. Aggressive, antisocial behavior in males of excessive height.

Because of the multiple factors involved in assigning a person a gender role, it is strongly suggested that the use of the terms *chromatin-positive* (for female-type nuclei) or *chromatin-negative* (for male-type nuclei) be employed in reporting the results rather than genetic male or female, or chromosomal male or female. Furthermore – and of more fundamental significance – the nuclear sex chromatin pattern is not necessarily synonymous with genetic sex; nor, in the case of sex chromosome abnormalities, does it necessarily coincide with a specific sex chromosomal pattern, as will become obvious from the more detailed discussion in Chapter 3.

Technique of Buccal Smear

1. A large area of buccal mucosa is firmly scraped with a wooden or metal spatula, and the material is transferred to a small area of a slide coated with a thin film of egg albumen. A relatively thick smear being the most satisfactory, several are made to obtain one of optimal thickness.

2. The slides are immediately fixed in Papanicolaou's fixative (equal parts of 95% alcohol and ether) for a half-hour or more and then immersed for 5 minutes each in 70% alcohol, 50% alcohol, and distilled water (two changes).

3. Staining: 1% cresylecht violet for 5 minutes; 95% alcohol (two changes) for 5 minutes; absolute alcohol until cleared (check with microscope).

4. Cleared further in two changes of xylene and mounted in balsam.

(Some cytology laboratories prefer to employ the technique of Feulgen's reaction, using Schiff's reagent [basic fuchsin], which stains nuclear detail more specifically than either cresyl violet or hematoxylin.)

X-RAY AIDS IN GYNECOLOGIC DIAGNOSIS

It is axiomatic that every effort should be made to avoid the unwitting use of elective diagnostic pelvic and abdominal x-ray studies in the presence of an early and unsuspected, normal intrauterine pregnancy. Bearing this point in mind, the following roentgenologic studies are frequently of great value in completely evaluating many gynecologic disorders.

Kidney, Ureter, and Bladder

A plain x-ray film of the abdomen (kidney, ureter, and bladder [KUB]) may show the following: a pelvic mass; calcified fibroids (see Fig. 45); a dermoid cyst with recognizable teeth (see Fig. 57) or with the characteristic layering pattern of the cyst's contents of liquid sebaceous material; calcified ovarian tumors (occasionally psammoma bodies are seen); fetal skeletal structure after 4½ months of pregnancy; lithopedions; or bony changes characteristic of osteoporosis or metastatic cancer. It may reveal or confirm the presence of ascites or intestinal obstruction secondary to disease of the pelvic organs.

Intravenous Pyelogram

In addition to any of the preceding findings, an intravenous pyelogram (IVP) may disclose ureteral displacement or obstruction secondary to gynecologic disease (Fig. 12), a pelvic kidney, or other urinary tract anomalies that are frequently associated with congenital anomalies of the reproductive tract. Retrograde pyelograms only rarely add any additional information pertinent to the gynecologic problem.

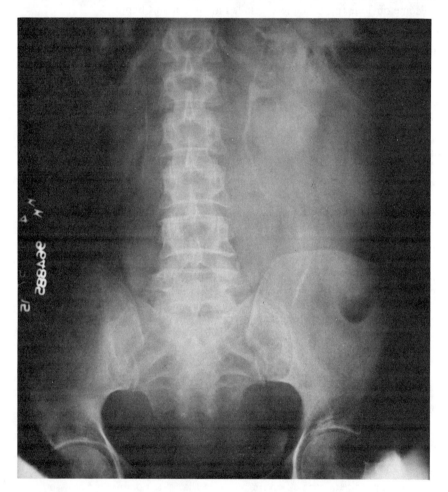

Figure 12
Intravenous pyelogram showing displacement of the left ureter by a pelvic mass. At laparotomy, the tumor proved to be an ovarian cystadenocarcinoma that had expanded retroperitoneally between the leaves of the broad ligament.

Barium Enema

X-ray examination of the large bowel may reveal rectosigmoid involvement by disease primary in the reproductive tract, such as cancer of the cervix, endometrium, or ovary or pelvic endometriosis (see Fig. 39). Or it may disclose a primary disturbance in the colon that is either masquerading as a disorder of the uterus, or adnexa, or both, or is involving them secondarily (e.g., diverticulitis, carcinoma of the rectum or sigmoid).

Chest Film (and Metastatic Series or Skeletal Survey)

Aside from its help in the general medical evaluation of a patient, a chest film is necessary in the presence of pelvic malignancy in an effort to secure evidence of metastatic spread, if such exists, to reveal signs of old pulmonary tuberculous foci in patients suspected of harboring pelvic tuberculosis, or to detect the pleural effusion characteristic of Meigs' syndrome in a patient with ascites and palpable ovarian tumor (see Fig. 58).

Special X-Ray Procedures

HYSTEROSALPINGOGRAM (UTEROTUBOGRAM)

It should be noted that hysterosalpingography is useful not only in assessing the anatomy and patency of the fallopian tubes (see Chap. 11) but also in studying the anatomy and configuration of the uterus and endometrial cavity (e.g., in the discovery of congenital anomalies or intracavitary lesions such as polyps and fibroids), and the cervix and endocervical canal (e.g., in the demonstration of an incompetent internal cervical os). (Note: Use of a special balloon catheter placed in the endocervical canal and lower fundus and then inflated with an aqueous dye such as sodium acetrizoate [Urokon] yields particularly excellent x-ray films of the cervical canal and internal os and would seem to be superior to the standard uterotubogram in demonstrating an incompetent internal cervical os.)

URETHROCYSTOGRAM

See Chapter 18.

GYNECOGRAPHY

The technique of gynecography is as follows: Approximately 1000 cc of carbon dioxide is introduced intraperitoneally by transtubal insufflation if the tubes are patent; or, more simply, cul-de-sac cannulation is done in the knee-chest position, allowing air to enter directly into the peritoneal cavity via the cannula. Films made with the patient either in the knee-chest or the prone Trendelenburg position permit identification of the soft-tissue shadows of the pelvic viscera or any abnormal pelvic masses adjacent to them, which are outlined by the surrounding pelvic pneumo-peritoneum. Further contrast can be obtained by performing a simultaneous hystero-salpingogram. This technique has been used in the past primarily for the demon-stration of the enlarged, bilateral polycystic ovaries of the Stein-Leventhal syndrome and in an attempt to differentiate between fibroids and ovarian tumors. As a diag-nostic method for these purposes, it has largely been replaced by culdoscopy or laparoscopy.

PRESACRAL PNEUMORETROPERITONEUM (ADRENAL PNEUMOGRAM)

Through the introduction of carbon dioxide as a contrast medium into the retroperi-toneal periadrenal areas, the outlines of the adrenal glands may be more precisely visualized by x-ray and the presence of an adrenal tumor frequently demonstrated. Although the procedure may be utilized in either male or female patients, it is often of particular value to the gynecologist, especially when combined with culdoscopic or laparoscopic study of the ovaries, since he is the physician usually called on to investigate the frequently encountered obese, hirsute, or slightly virilized female with amenorrhea or oligomenorrhea in whom it is necessary to differentiate between ovarian or adrenal disorders.

Technique. The patient is placed in the knee-chest position as for culdoscopy. A No. 20 lumbar puncture needle is passed into the presacral, retrorectal area of the retroperitoneal space, piercing the skin 1 cm lateral to the midcoccyx and directing the needle at an angle such that, when introduced, it will lie just beneath the sacrum in the midline. (The position of the needle should be checked by rectal examination.) After aspiration to assure that the needle is not in a blood vessel or the epidural canal, and with the patient remaining in the knee-chest position, 1000 to 1500 cc of carbon dioxide (a Rubin tubal insufflator serves as a handy source) is introduced slowly over a 10- to 15-minute period. The patient is placed in the upright position for 5 to 10 minutes, and then anteroposterior, lateral, and oblique x-ray films (and tomograms if indicated) are obtained. This has proved to be a simple, safe technique that yields excellent bilateral simultaneous roentgenograms of the adrenal areas.

LYMPHOGRAPHY (LYMPHANGIOGRAPHY OR LYMPHANGIOADENOGRAPHY)

The technique for the radiographic demonstration of lymph vessels and lymph nodes was devised and perfected in the 1960s in the belief that it might be helpful in evalu-ating the presence or absence of lymphatic spread in patients with pelvic cancer. However, as experience has accumulated, the method has proved to be less accurate and reliable than had been hoped. In several sizable reported series of patients with cervical cancer so studied, for example, a 25 to 30 percent rate of error in the attempt to make an early diagnosis of lymph node metastases was observed. Of significance was the fact that false-positive results were just as frequent as false-negative results.

Technique for Pelvic Lymphography. A preliminary intradermal injection in the four intermetatarsal dorsal web spaces of both feet of 2 ml of an aqueous solution of Patent Blue V-F dye permits ready identification of lymph vessels when small transverse incisions are made on the dorsum of each ankle 1 hour later. One lymph vessel on each side is cannulated with a small needle connected by a polyethylene catheter to a syringe containing the radiopaque medium. Ethiodized oil (Ethiodol) has proved a most satisfactory medium, and approximately 12 ml is injected slowly over a period of an hour into each lower extremity. Anteroposterior roentgenograms are then obtained of the legs, thighs, pelvis, abdomen, and chest and demonstrate not only the lymph channels but the lymph nodes as well (inguinal, femoral, external and common iliacs, and paraaortic chains). Additional x-rays taken 24 to 48 hours later frequently show the architecture of the lymph nodes to even better advantage (Fig. 13).

When lymph nodes contain metastatic tumor, a characteristic marginal filling defect is seen, and their differentiation from normal nodes or from lymphadenitis or lymphoma is usually readily accomplished. The technique has been valuable in the diagnosis of lymph node metastasis in patients with cervical carcinoma. It can also be utilized in determining the completeness of pelvic lymphadenectomies by

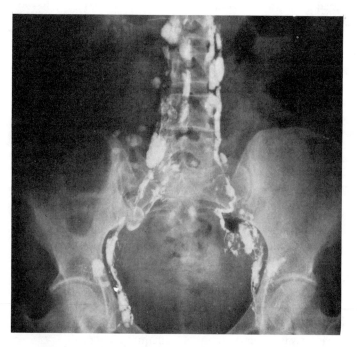

Figure 13
Pelvic lymphography. This 24-hour x-ray film of a patient with cervical cancer shows the excellent visualization of the pelvic wall and paraaortic nodes usually obtained. A filling defect in the right pelvic wall node at the level of the pelvic brim is clearly demonstrated. This node was subsequently proved at laparotomy to contain metastatic disease.

comparison of preoperative and postoperative films. Furthermore, it is now possible to add an effective color dye to the radiopaque medium used for injection, a feature that may prove helpful in visualizing and identifying the lymphatic channels and nodes during the actual performance of radical pelvic operations.

PELVIC VENOGRAPHY (INFERIOR VENA CAVAGRAMS)

Venographic study of the iliac and inferior vena cava system may sometimes provide valuable information concerning the status of the retroperitoneal lymph nodes of the pelvis and lower abdomen.

Technique. Both femoral veins are catheterized percutaneously, and with the catheter tips placed in the common iliac veins just below their junction, 20 to 30 ml of contrast medium (e.g., Hypaque Sodium) is injected simultaneously through each catheter. Using a rapid-exposure technique, serial roentgenograms are made during the injection.

Enlarged lymph nodes will be seen to displace or indent the inferior vena cava or the iliac veins in a characteristic way. At times, thrombosis of normal venous trunks with development of dilated collaterals not ordinarily visualized provides an additional clue to the presence of retroperitoneal disease. Since lymph nodes completely replaced by cancer may not be visualized by lymphography, venography may sometimes prove more reliable in demonstrating metastatic spread. The use of both lymphography and venography may therefore prove extremely helpful in the study of patients with lower-extremity edema of uncertain cause, in whom silent retroperitoneal malignant disease, either new or recurrent, must always be suspected. However, pelvic venography is probably not indicated as a routine maneuver in evaluating patients with pelvic malignancy because of limitations in the diagnostic accuracy as well as potential thrombotic complications.

PELVIC ARTERIOGRAPHY

By means of percutaneous, transfemoral, retrograde aortography, the pelvic arterial blood supply can be accurately delineated.

Technique. Under light sedation, a percutaneous femoral artery puncture is made with a short 16-gauge needle with stylet. A guide wire is introduced into the artery and the needle removed. An intraarterial perfusion catheter is then threaded into the arterial lumen over the guide wire, the latter removed, and the catheter advanced under image-intensifier control to a point just above the aortic bifurcation. Thereafter, 30 to 50 ml of contrast medium is injected over a 2-second interval during which 10 to 12 serial x-ray films are made, using a rapid-exposure technique.

The vascular pattern and the course, distribution, luminal diameter, and any deviation or displacement of major branches of the uterine, ovarian, or hypogastric arteries may sometimes be helpful in the demonstration and differential diagnosis of pelvic masses and in the recognition and localization of metastases or extension from known pelvic tumors. However, the correlation between arteriographic patterns and a specific pathologic condition is not reliable enough to make this a worthwhile procedure except in special situations. There is a small but definite incidence (roughly 0.5 percent) of complicating arterial thrombosis following arteriography by any route.

Radioisotope Scanning Techniques

A variety of nuclear scintillation scanning procedures is available to study a number of organs, tissues, or tumors. In appropriate cases, such procedures may add valuable information to the total workup of a patient with a gynecologic malignancy or suspected pelvic tumor.

BONE SCAN

Radioisotope bone scanning is a very helpful supplement to and is usually more sensitive than a routine metastatic skeletal x-ray survey in patients known to have or suspected of having skeletal metastases. Various radioisotopes have beem employed for this purpose, including sodium fluoride F-18, strontium, and, more recently, 99m-labeled technetium (Tc) phosphate compounds, currently the most widely used agents. There is ordinarily a clearly visible increased radioisotope uptake in areas of bone involved by metastatic tumor, not because of tumor cell uptake but because of increased vascularity, or increased calcium metabolism, or both, so the results of the study have to be interpreted carefully and correlated with the clinical picture. In gynecologic cancer patients without symptoms or signs of skeletal metastases, a bone scan is not indicated as a routine screening procedure because the yield of positive scans will be extremely low. It should also be borne in mind that routine skeletal x-ray films sometimes reveal lesions not demonstrated by radioisotope skeletal imaging, that the reverse may also be the case, and that some lesions in their initial stages escape detection by either method.

BRAIN SCAN

A similar procedure employing ^{99m}Tc pertechnetate is available for brain imaging with the high-performance gamma scintillation camera. Again, this scan should be employed only in gynecologic cancer patients who have signs or symptoms suggestive of cerebral metastases, since the incidence of cerebral metastases from primary cancers of the pelvic organs is very low.

LIVER SCAN

Liver scanning has been used clinically since 1955. The current procedure provides imaging of both liver and spleen and employs ^{99m}Tc sulfur colloid as the radioisotope. Liver-spleen scanning is potentially more useful in the overall evaluation and screening of patients with gynecologic cancer, since liver metastases are more likely to occur as cancers of the reproductive tract become more extensive and begin to spread. However, it must be remembered that, despite technical advances in the procedure, the number of patients with small hepatic metastases not visualized by liver scanning remains high (20 to 25 percent false-negative results); furthermore, there is a significant, 10 to 15 percent incidence of false-positive results.

GALLIUM CITRATE (^{67}Ga) SCAN

^{67}Gallium is a radiopharmaceutical that accumulates in inflammatory tissues and in some tumors as well. Hence scintiscanning of the abdomen 48 hours following the administration of ^{67}gallium can be helpful in establishing the presence and location of an intraabdominal abscess, either secondary to an underlying pelvic inflammatory disease or occurring in a postoperative patient. Occasionally, a gallium scan may be used to supplement the standard bone, liver-spleen, and brain scans and may contribute additional information in patients with known or suspected metastatic disease, because it is often picked up by metastases, not only in liver and bone but also in lymph nodes as well as in more obscure, nonosseous sites.

ULTRASOUND AS A PELVIC DIAGNOSTIC AID

Ultrasonic scanning equipment has been perfected to the point where it is now available for routine clinical use in many centers. Diagnostic ultrasonic techniques utilize pulsed ultrasound waves of a frequency exceeding 20,000 cycles per second, scanning the abdomen and pelvis in linear fashion and recording the reflected sound wave, or echo, on an oscilloscope screen. Reflection occurs whenever the sound meets a material of different acoustical density, and a cross-sectional impression, or "somagram," of the area being scanned is obtained. Hence it is possible to outline and define soft-tissue masses and often to distinguish between solid and cystic tumors and between free fluid (ascites) and encapsulated (within a cyst or abscess cavity) fluid. This information, together with the KUB and IVP findings, often supplements the clinical findings sufficiently to permit the preoperative distinction between benign and malignant pelvic tumors and cysts, the monitoring of the response of pelvic tumors undergoing radiotherapy, and the localization of pelvic abscesses and wandering intrauterine contraceptive devices. Diagnostic ultrasound studies are especially helpful in obese patients, in whom both an adequate pelvic examination and conventional x-ray studies are often difficult and unsatisfactory.

Diagnostic sonar has become even more widely used in clinical obstetrics and has the obvious advantage that no ionizing radiation need be employed. It has proved to be a very safe and reliable technique in the early diagnosis of pregnancy (a gestational sac can be visualized at six weeks), in the diagnosis of hydatidiform mole and multiple pregnancy, and in the detection of hydramnios. It is equally useful and precise in localizing the placenta as well as in determining the fetal presentation and the degree and normality or abnormality of fetal development, including accurate measurement of the biparietal diameter of the fetal head (cephalometry), which correlates well with gestational age. It is thus also helpful in the determination of fetal death and occasionally in the differential diagnosis between ectopic and intra-uterine pregnancy.

RADIOLOGIC EXAMINATION OF THE BREASTS

Mammography

Conventional mammography using ordinary soft-tissue x-ray techniques was first attempted in the 1930s, but not until the 1960s, with improved methodology and greater experience, did this approach to the diagnosis of breast disease become reli-able and widely used. Accuracy in diagnosis by mammography hinges on good-quality films, experience in interpretation on the part of the radiologist, and the age of the patient. In premenopausal patients, especially women under the age of 35, there is a low fat content in the breasts, and the accuracy of discovery and diagnosis in such radiographically dense breasts may be no more than 50 percent; on the other hand, the accuracy may be 90 percent or better in postmenopausal women, whose breasts ordinarily have a high fat content. Mammography is especially helpful as a screening test in women at higher-than-normal risk (e.g., who had previous cancer in the opposite breast; have a strong family history of breast cancer) and is an inval-uable aid in the evaluation and management of women with diffuse, bilateral irregu-larities due to fibrocystic disease of the breast in whom random biopsy obviously will not totally exclude the possibility that one of the palpable "irregularities" is an early cancer. In a patient with a single, dominant lump, biopsy is clearly indicated, even though the lesion may appear benign on mammography; mammography is not really necessary to make that decision. Nevertheless, mammography may well be useful, even in this situation, in screening the opposite breast and other areas of the breast containing the palpable lump for occult cancer.

Xeromammography

Since the early 1970s, xeroradiography has gradually begun to replace conventional mammography in many institutions, since it is probably even more accurate, the films easier to interpret, and the radiation exposure to the breast lower. A correct diagnosis will be achieved in 95 percent of women with breast cancer, and the so-called false-positive rate of "suspicious lesions" in women whose breast lesions are actually benign will be about 10 percent. Xeromammography involves a photocon-ductive imaging process that uses routine x-ray equipment but a special cassette that is dry-developed (no film is involved) to produce a paper radiograph. All the image densities occur on the paper in sharp contrast and are easy to interpret (see Fig. 77).

DIAGNOSTIC OPERATIVE PROCEDURES

Dilatation and Curettage

To be adequate, a thorough diagnostic or therapeutic dilatation and curettage usually requires **general** anesthesia (thiopental is usually very satisfactory) and should always be a **fractional curettage**.

STEPS

1. Vaginal antiseptic preparation, catheterization of the bladder, anesthesia examination, draping, final preparation with Schiller's solution, and Schiller's test of the cervix.

2. The anterior lip of the cervix is grasped with a tenaculum, and the endocervical canal is scraped with a curet first, preferably with minimal or no preliminary dilatation, to ensure that any endocervical scrapings obtained are not contaminated by fragments of endometrial tissue dislodged from above by too forceful dilatation of the internal cervical os. The scraping is done from the external to the internal os, using a small, sharp curet, and the endocervical specimen is placed in a separate jar of formalin.

3. A uterine sound is then passed to determine the length and direction of the intrauterine canal.

4. The cervix and internal os are completely dilated, and a thorough curettage of the endometrial cavity is then accomplished (separate curettage of the lower uterine segment adjacent to the internal os is also advisable if endometrial carcinoma is suspected). At the time of curettage it is possible to check for the presence of submucous fibroids by the "feel" of the curet as it is passed over the walls of the uterus.

5. Exploration of the fundus with "polyp forceps" (a common bile-duct-stone forceps is the ideal instrument for this maneuver) is now done; opening, closing, and withdrawing the instrument in various parts of the endometrial cavity usually permits extraction of any polyps present. Endometrial polyps are often missed completely by curettage alone.

In the case of high-risk patients, a standard D&C can often be accomplished under local anesthesia by means of a paracervical block and adequate premedication. Suction curettage for early incomplete spontaneous abortion or for therapeutic abortion in the early weeks of pregnancy by means of a suction aspirator tube of appropriate size rather than a curet can also be done under light general or regional block anesthesia as an emergency room or transient operating room procedure.

Finally, a disposable kit (Vabra Aspirator, Cooper Laboratories) is now available for the performance of outpatient or office diagnostic aspiration curettage that requires no cervical dilatation and hence no premedication or anesthesia. It is particularly useful in screening women at high risk for, or actually suspected of harboring, early invasive endometrial carcinoma or one of its precursors, atypical endometrial hyperplasia or endometrial carcinoma in situ. The prepackaged, sterile, disposable vacuum aspirator-cannula ("curet") with attached collection chamber is simply connected to a vacuum pump and introduced into the uterine cavity after preliminary sounding of the fundus. Gentle passage of the tip over the mucosal surfaces of the uterus yields adequate and representative samples of endometrial tissue from the entire cavity, and various investigators report 90 to 100 percent agreement between aspiration "curettage" and a conventional surgical D&C as far as histologic findings are concerned.

The Karman catheter is another commercially available instrument for effective evacuation of endometrium or intrauterine contents without the need for anesthesia and often without the need for cervical dilatation (the latter can be done under paracervical block if necessary). Vacuum aspiration of the intrauterine contents is accomplished using either an ordinary 50-ml syringe or an electrical vacuum pump.

Total Cone Biopsy of Cervix

Cone biopsy of the cervix is indicated in patients with an abnormal cytologic smear and/or cervical biopsy findings suggesting the existence of a premalignant or malignant lesion of the cervix but in whom additional cervical biopsies (including also sharp curettage of the endocervical canal), either of clinically suspicious areas, at random, or colposcopically directed, yield insufficient information on which to plan therapy for any of the following reasons:

1. If colposcopy has been employed, the visible epithelial abnormality is large, or is seen to extend out of view and potentially outside the range of simply biopsy, or both.
2. If the clinically prompted, random, or colposcopically directed biopsies reveal a lesion histologically less serious than is suggested by the cytologic abnormality.
3. If the additional biopsies reveal early stromal invasion in what otherwise would be considered a focus of carcinoma in situ.

In (1) and (2), cone biopsy is essential to diagnose or rule out the presence of invasive cancer. In (3), cone biopsy is mandatory to determine the degree of microinvasion, for only in the case of minimal stromal invasion should the lesion be treated by conization or simple hysterectomy as if it were merely carcinoma in situ; a true microinvasive cancer should be treated either by radiation therapy or by radical hysterectomy. Obviously, if any of the additional biopsies reveal frankly invasive carcinoma, cone biopsy is both unnecessary and contraindicated.

When colposcopy is available and is supplemented by colposcopically guided cervical biopsies plus endocervical curettage, cone biopsy can be avoided in approximately 90 percent of patients with abnormal cytologic smears suggesting some form of cervical neoplasia or dysplasia.

Cone biopsy is not without its complications in 10 to 15 percent of patients. The most frequent complications are uterine perforation during the procedure, early or delayed hemorrhage, postoperative pelvic infection, and posthealing cervical stenosis. The resulting injury to the cervix may give rise to subsequent infertility, an incompetent cervical os, prematurity, or dystocia. However, it is fair to say that the complications in nonpregnant patients can be kept low in the hands of experienced and skillful operators. The morbidity is higher (20 to 30 percent) in pregnant patients in many reported series. Furthermore, the procedure requires hospitalization and anesthesia, adding to the patient's expense and inconvenience. Thus, although conization may be mandatory and extremely important in the management of some patients, the need for it can and should be avoided by proper use of colposcopy and

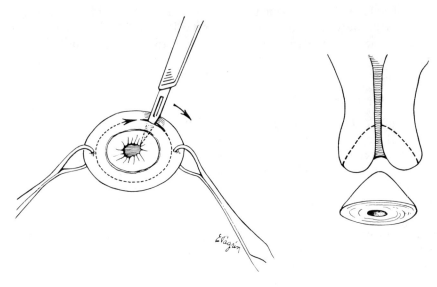

Figure 14
Cone biopsy of cervix. (From T. H. Green, Jr. Gynecology. In G. L. Nardi and G. D. Zuidema [Eds.], *Surgery: A Concise Guide to Clinical Practice* [3rd ed.]. Boston: Little, Brown, 1972, Chap. 39.)

colposcopically guided biopsies in the majority of patients with clinical or cytologic abnormalities suggesting cervical neoplasia or premalignant epithelial abnormalities.

Technique. Cone biopsy is usually accompanied by, but should always precede, a fractional curettage; minimal or no vaginal preparation should be done to avoid any preliminary trauma to the cervical epithelium. The procedure (Fig. 14) is done in the following steps:

1. The cervix is grasped with two tenacula placed at the 9 and 3 o'clock positions on its extreme lateral aspect, and these are drawn down by an assistant to expose and steady the cervix.

2. The cervix is dilated only if necessary because of a tight external os and canal, and then only minimally.

3. A narrow, pointed scalpel blade (e.g., No. 11 Bard-Parker blade) is inserted into the exocervix approximately 1.0 to 1.5 cm from the center of the external os at 6 o'clock and is directed inward at a suitable angle so that the point reappears in the endocervical canal 0.5 to 1.0 cm above the squamocolumnar junction.

4. The scalpel is then advanced with a sawing motion (similar to the action used in coring an apple) in a clockwise, circular direction around the cervix, removing the desired cone. (Starting the incision at 6 o'clock prevents blood from running down ahead of the knife and obscuring the projected course of the blade as it is advanced.)

5. It is important to secure and handle the specimen as atraumatically as possible. A silk suture placed at 12 o'clock on the anterior lip of the cone, with its location indicated on the pathology laboratory requisition, serves to orient the pathologist, who ordinarily prepares multiple blocks and makes sections from several parts of each block.

6. Bleeding from the raw surfaces of the cervical defect is usually only moderate and is readily controlled by light cauterization or occasionally by a few sutures. In general, however, extensive cauterization should be avoided, in case further biopsies are necessary later on.

Cul-de-Sac Aspiration (Colpostomy or Culdocentesis)

Cul-de-sac aspiration is comparable to the peritoneal tap often used as a diagnostic aid in the evaluation of acute upper abdominal disorders; it is done to determine the presence of free blood or pus in the pelvis. If the cul-de-sac is bulging, aspiration may be performed with the patient in the lithotomy position (Fig. 15). In general, however, it is easier and safer, and the tap is uniformly more successful, if the aspirating needle is inserted with the patient in the knee-chest position, returning the patient to the dorsal recumbent position for aspiration. Ordinarily, no anesthesia is required, although local procaine hydrochloride may be injected first at the puncture site. A small thoracentesis cannula with trocar makes an excellent aspirating needle, though a special culdocentesis cannula is commercially available. It should

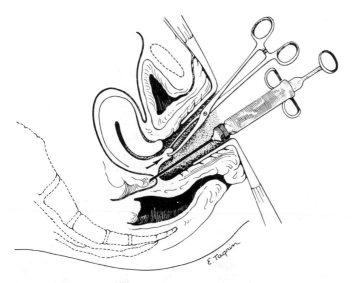

Figure 15
Technique of cul-de-sac aspiration (culdocentesis or colpocentesis). (Reproduced by permission from F. M. Ingersoll. Operations for tubal pregnancy. *Clin. Obstet. Gynecol.* 5:853, 1962. New York: Hoeber Med. Div., Harper & Row.)

be pointed out that the information provided by culdocentesis is limited, and a definite diagnosis can never be established in this manner. However, the absence of cul-de-sac fluid or the character of any fluid obtained, whether bloody or purulent, is helpful information that may suggest the most likely diagnosis when integrated with the overall clinical picture. Nevertheless, failure to obtain bloody fluid by no means rules out ectopic pregnancy, nor does aspiration of blood definitely establish its presence. If blood is obtained, it should be observed for coagulation for 10 minutes; failure to clot indicates that free-lying intraperitoneal bloody fluid has been aspirated, whereas normal subsequent coagulation of the sample would indicate that accidental pelvic venipuncture had occurred. Actually, the accuracy of the method when used to screen patients suspected of having ectopic pregnancy is only in the neighborhood of 75 to 80 percent.

Posterior Colpotomy

In posterior colpotomy, an actual surgical incision is made in the posterior vaginal fornix to permit diagnosis by direct intraperitoneal palpation and, at times, actual inspection of the pelvic organs. The procedure requires general anesthesia and is a formal operative technique. It has the advantage that once a definite diagnosis is established, surgical treatment can sometimes be done through the same incision (e.g., a small early ectopic pregnancy in a mobile, readily accessible tube). However, it has the disadvantage that in many patients, for anatomic reasons, exposure is so difficult and limited that visualization is impossible and even palpation unsatisfactory for accurate diagnosis.

Pelvic Endoscopy

Both culdoscopy and laparoscopy (pelvic peritoneoscopy) enable the gynecologist actually to inspect the pelvis and pelvic viscera and thus avoid exploratory laparotomy when confronted by puzzling diagnostic problems that may or may not require surgical intervention. Since the early 1970s, laparoscopy has tended to replace culdoscopy in most clinics, because it provides a superior visualization of the entire pelvis, especially the cul-de-sac, and permits a more complete visualization of the abdominal cavity. Further, it has proved easier for the physician to develop technical proficiency and diagnostic accuracy with the laparoscope than with the culdoscope. Finally — and perhaps most important — laparoscopy affords the ability to do a number of frequently indicated minor intraperitoneal operative procedures (e.g., tubal ligations) that are not as easily done by the culdoscopic route.

Laparoscopy has the disadvantage of nearly always requiring general anesthesia (it is the decided preference of physician and patient alike from the standpoint of the patient's comfort and the ease and completeness of the examination); culdoscopy can nearly always be done under local anesthesia without significant discomfort to the patient or any limitation to the completeness and thoroughness of the procedure itself. It is also fair to state that culdoscopy is basically the simpler, quicker, and safer of the two methods and requires a minimum of considerably less expensive equipment. Furthermore, the view of the pelvis afforded by culdoscopy is usually just as complete as that with laparoscopy, provided the operator is skilled and experienced, pays attention to the important features of proper patient positioning, and has mastered the technique of cul-de-sac puncture in the knee-chest position.

It should be kept in mind, however, that in the presence of a pathologic condition in the pelvis that is associated with obliteration or fixation of adjacent organs to the cul-de-sac (e.g., some patients with extensive endometriosis, pelvic inflammatory disease, or large pelvic tumors), it will not be possible to perform culdoscopy, whereas laparoscopy may often be readily done. On the other hand, a history of previous abdominal surgery with the possibility of adherence of loops of intestine to the anterior abdominal wall may make laparoscopy both unsafe and technically impossible. Or the patient's general cardiopulmonary condition may prohibit the combination of general anesthesia, a sizable pneumoperitoneum, and the Trendelenburg position and thus also contraindicate laparoscopy. In these situations, culdoscopy can conveniently be substituted.

Ideally, both endoscopic approaches to intraperitoneal gynecologic diagnosis should be available when possible. Therefore, the techniques employed in carrying out both these diagnostic operative procedures will be described, even though in most clinics laparoscopy has become — and undoubtedly will remain — the most widely used of the two endoscopic methods.

CULDOSCOPY

Culdoscopy is the simplest technique for the visualization of the pelvis and pelvic viscera and adjacent organs and structures required in the solution of diagnostic problems. It is also a highly accurate, almost universally applicable, and routinely successful technique. Although, since the early 1970s, there has been a revival of interest in the use of peritoneoscopy (laparoscopy) for the diagnosis of pelvic disorders, many gynecologists continue to find culdoscopy the simpler and safer of the two techniques and also find it capable of providing equally good visualization in most instances. The most frequent indications include the following: suspected ectopic pregnancy; endocrine problems (recognition of primary ovarian disorders); unexplained acute or chronic pelvic pain; infertility when routine studies do not reveal its cause; and the presence of pelvic masses of unknown nature.

Contraindications to or complications following the procedure are extremely rare, and as a result it is widely used for differential diagnosis in a variety of clinical situations, its use frequently obviating laparotomy for diagnosis only.

Anesthesia

The vast majority of culdoscopies can be done using only 1 to 2 ml of procaine infiltrated locally in the apex of the posterior cul-de-sac. Slow intravenous administration of 50 to 100 mg of meperidine immediately before puncture is often helpful in an apprehensive patient; occasionally, low spinal or caudal anesthesia may be indicated.

The procedure may also be done in patients already under general anesthesia, employing steep Trendelenburg in the lithotomy position rather than the preferred knee-chest position.

Preoperative Preparation

Preoperative preparation consists of the following: a perineal shave; an enema unless the procedure is to be done as an emergency; emptying of the bladder by voiding; explanation of the nature and purpose of the procedure, giving the reasons for and instruction in how to assume the knee-chest position; and routine preanesthetic medication if, pending the nature of the lesion discovered, laparotomy is contemplated immediately following culdoscopy.

Position

The knee-chest position is an essential part of the procedure and permits a superior view of the pelvis. A standard operating table is readily adjusted for this purpose.

Technique

After the usual vaginal preparation and draping, a single-blade speculum is inserted and retracted posteriorly (upward) by an assistant. The posterior lip of the cervix is grasped with a tenaculum and retracted anteriorly (not caudally) to stretch and tense the posterior fornix. Air enters the vagina, and the negative pressure in the peritoneal cul-de-sac created by the knee-chest position should result in an inward ballooning of the pouch of Douglas, indicating a free cul-de-sac and an easy, safe cul-de-sac puncture.

After formation of a procaine wheal (1 to 2 ml) in the exact center of the apex of the ballooned-out cul-de-sac, the culdoscopy trocar-cannula is introduced by a firm thrust, angling the instrument anteriorly to avoid the sacrum. The trocar is then removed, permitting air to enter the peritoneal cavity (1000 to 1500 cc), and the observation culdoscope is inserted. Inspection, combined with abdominal palpation to move various surfaces of the pelvic viscera into direct view, permits excellent detailed visualization of the following: uterus, tubes, and ovaries; round, ovarian, uterosacral, infundibulopelvic, and broad ligaments; cul-de-sac; bladder flap; parietal pelvic peritoneum; rectum and sigmoid; ureters; pelvic vessels and nodes; terminal ileum and frequently the cecum and appendix (Fig. 16A). Tubal patency may also be unequivocally determined during the procedure by instillation of sterile indigo carmine solution with the tubes under direct culdoscopic vision.

Aftercare

Before the cannula is removed, the patient is placed flat on the table, and most of the air introduced within the peritoneal cavity is expressed by abdominal pressure and manipulation of the cannula. Suture of the puncture site is unnecessary (rarely, bleeding is sufficient to require placement of a mattress suture for hemostasis), and no antibiotics are indicated. An occasional patient may have distress from residual air for a few days. Patients should not douche or have intercourse for approximately two weeks following the procedure.

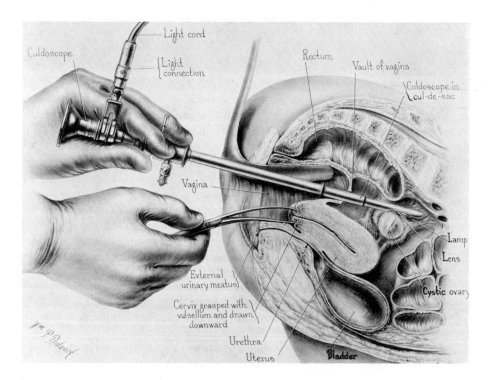

A

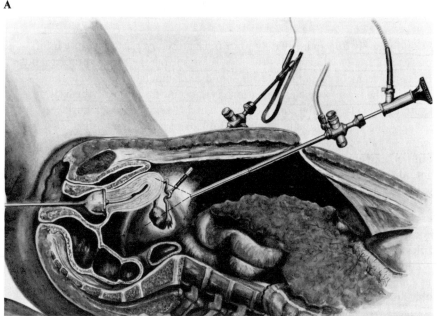

B

Figure 16
A. Culdoscope in place, illustrating the excellent view of the pelvis and pelvic viscera
obtained by culdoscope. (Courtesy of American Cystoscope Makers, Inc.) B. Artist's
drawing of patient undergoing laparoscopy combined with tubal sterilization by
electrocoagulation with high-frequency current. Note cannulated intrauterine sound
in place. (Courtesy of Richard Wolf Medical Instruments Corporation.)

LAPAROSCOPY

The indications for diagnostic laparoscopy are identical to those already discussed for culdoscopy. In addition, a number of straightforward, minor operative procedures can be done via the laparoscopic route, including tubal sterilization, ovarian biopsy, aspiration of physiologic ovarian cysts, lysis of peritubal adhesions, and extraction of intrauterine devices that have perforated the uterine wall, to name a few.

The principal contraindications to laparoscopy are a previous lower abdominal operation (a relative contraindication depending on the nature and extent of the previous surgery and the disease for which it was done), and serious cardiac or pulmonary disease with impaired cardiopulmonary reserve.

The preoperative preparation is also entirely similar to that for culdoscopy.

Anesthesia *almost Always*

Laparoscopy almost always requires general anesthesia, both to alleviate the discomfort of the 3- to 4-liter carbon dioxide pneumoperitoneum, as well as to assure adequate ventilation in the face of the pneumoperitoneum combined with the necessary steep Trendelenburg position. In very skilled hands and with adequate preoperative and intraoperative sedation, laparoscopy can occasionally be done under local anesthesia, but for most patients the latter is inadequate and hence unsatisfactory.

Position

A D&C is ordinarily done immediately prior to laparoscopy, partly because information gleaned from a curettage is often helpful in solving the clinical problem, but also because placement of an intrauterine sound to manipulate and elevate the uterus during the laparoscopic examination is important for optimal visualization of the uterus, adnexa, and the adjacent parietal and visceral peritoneal surfaces. Accordingly, the position usually employed for laparoscopy is a modified low lithotomy with the table tilted in a moderately steep Trendelenburg position, so that the small bowel, omentum, and mobile portions of the colon will fall back out of the way into the upper abdomen, thus providing a clear field of view of the pelvic organs.

Technique

Under general anesthesia with endotracheal intubation, the patient is placed in low lithotomy position with minimal knee and hip flexion. The bladder is catheterized, and pelvic examination is performed under anesthesia. Thereafter, separate sterile preparation of the abdominal skin and of the vaginal-perineal area is done and the drapes applied so as to expose both areas. After the diagnostic curettage is done, a double-lumen suction–uterine sound apparatus (Kahn cannula) is inserted into the uterine cavity, and the attached metal cup that snugly fits and surrounds the cervix is firmly applied to the latter by suction using a hand vacuum pump and clamping off the connecting tube when the desired amount of negative pressure is attained. This apparatus is left covered with a sterile towel to permit manipulation of the uterus by means of the intrauterine sound during the laparoscopy itself.

shld not be done for ... Expo - J of Rep. Med July 1980

After a change of gloves, a midline, slightly curved skin incision about 2 cm wide is made just below the umbilicus. While the operator is elevating the anterior abdominal wall by upward traction on two towel clips that are placed on each side an inch or two lateral to and below the umbilicus, a Verres cannula attached to the carbon dioxide reservoir is introduced into the peritoneal cavity through the center of this small subumbilical skin incision, and a 3½- to 4-liter pneumoperitoneum is achieved, removing the needle when this amount of carbon dioxide has been introduced. The operator watches the pressure gauge carefully; the initial pressure should be only 10 to 20 cm (if higher, the Verres needle has either failed to enter the free peritoneal cavity or is partly occluded by omentum or an adjacent abdominal viscus), and the pressure should not rise more than a few centimeters during the insufflation. Percussion of the lower abdominal wall during the insufflation should evoke easily recognizable tympany if the pneumoperitoneum is developing properly.

The laparoscopy trochar-cannula is then introduced through the skin incision, tunneling down under the skin for 2 to 3 cm before penetrating the rectus fascia and underlying peritoneum (this prevents gas leaks around the cannula later on). When penetration has been made, the cannula is connected to the carbon dioxide reservoir tubing, setting the dial on "Automatic" to maintain a steady flow of carbon dioxide as needed to replace any leak, and the trochar is removed. The laparoscope, prewarmed in hot saline to prevent fogging of the lens by exposure to intraperitoneal temperature and moisture, is then inserted through the cannula (the latter has a built in air lock to minimize leakage of gas) into the peritoneal cavity. Visualization of the pelvis and lower abdomen and the visceral contents thereof is then carried out in detail (Fig. 16B).

If the procedure is being done as part of an infertility investigation, methylene blue dye can be instilled through the intrauterine Kahn cannula while the surgeon watches through the laparoscope for spillage of dye from the fallopian tubes. A second incision, 0.5 cm wide, can be made in either the right or left lower quadrant of the abdomen (avoiding the epigastric vessels by first transilluminating the abdominal wall with the laparoscope), and a small, secondary trochar can be inserted. Through this, one may introduce the tubal ligation instrument, as shown in Figure 16B, or a special probe to manipulate the tube and ovary or other intraperitoneal structures for better inspection (a biopsy forceps or an aspiration cannula).

Aftercare

When the diagnostic laparoscopy and any ancillary procedure have been completed, the trochars are removed, first expelling the carbon dioxide through the primary trochar, and the primary skin incision is closed with a running subcuticular stitch and covered with a Band-Aid. Ordinarily, the patient is ready for discharge as soon as her recovery from anesthesia is complete. However, she should be kept under observation for a sufficient length of time to be certain that she has not encountered one of the following potential complications of the procedure: bleeding from the abdominal wound or from biopsy, coagulation, or inadvertent injury of an intraperitoneal structure; perforation of the intestinal tract by the pneumoperitoneum needle or by the laparoscope trochar-cannula; electrical burns of the skin, abdominal incision, or internal structures (including the intestine) if the electrocoagulation instrument has been used. Postoperative infections are rare.

HYSTEROSCOPY

Although the hysteroscope has been available for a number of years, it has never been widely used. The original instrument was similar to a cystoscope in design and use, permitting an endoscopic view of the interior of the uterus and using continuously running water as the observation medium. However, the apparatus was cumbersome to use and the view frequently unsatisfactory and difficult to interpret. A further modification was developed employing a saline-filled, transparent rubber balloon mounted on the endoscope and inflated after its insertion in the uterine cavity and was felt to provide a superior view without the trauma and bleeding caused by the old model. However, this modification made direct biopsy of visualized lesions impossible and has largely been abandoned.

Modern hysteroscopes are equipped with a fiberoptic lighting system and employ either 5% glucose in water, highly viscous dextran solutions (e.g., 30% dextran-70), or carbon dioxide as the uterine-distending medium. Since adequate dilatation of the uterine cavity is absolutely essential to obtain a clear view of the endometrial surface, pressures of 50 to 100 mm Hg or higher are usually necessary. Rinsing of the uterine cavity is also frequently required to clear away blood and secretory debris that tend to obscure the field. Considering the high cost of the equipment, the need for extensive special training and experience, the frequently less-than-satisfactory view, the danger of tumor cell dissemination if a uterine malignancy is present, and the relatively small increment of additional knowledge likely to be obtained that is not already obtainable by the far simpler, inexpensive, standard diagnostic investigations, it seems unlikely that hysteroscopy will ever be widely utilized solely for diagnostic purposes. Rather, use of one or more of the following will probably remain simpler for most physicians: hysterosalpingography, endo-metrial smears and biopsies, anesthesia examination, and formal curettage. Further-more, the latter will always yield a histologic diagnosis as well as a presumptive gross anatomic diagnosis and, in the case of benign lesions such as polyps or endometrial hyperplasia, permits their simultaneous complete removal.

However, use of the hysteroscope to permit intrauterine closure of the fallopian tubal ostia by chemical injury, electrocauterization, or cryosurgical techniques may well represent the least complicated, least expensive method of the future for tubal sterilization. When and if such a technique is perfected and is consistently reliable, it would certainly be even safer as well as simpler and easier as an outpatient, ambu-latory procedure than laparoscopic tubal sterilization would be, and it might readily supplant this and all other techniques for tubal sterilization.

Related Diagnostic Operative Procedures

Some related operative procedures of great value in the overall evaluation of many gynecologic problems include cystoscopy, proctoscopy, and occasionally ureteral catheterization and retrograde pyelography. They are most commonly employed in determining whether or not the adjacent urinary tract structures or large bowel has been involved by a pelvic cancer, or whether or not, on the other hand, disease primary in the colon, bladder, or ureters is giving rise to symptoms suggestive of gynecologic disease.

REFERENCES

1. Abraham, G. E. The Application of Steroid Radioimmunoassay to Gynecologic Endocrinology. In M. L. Taymor and T. H. Green, Jr. (Eds.), *Progress in Gynecology,* Vol. VI. New York: Grune & Stratton, 1975. Pp. 111–144.
2. Amarose, A. P., Wallingford, A. J., Jr., and Plotz, E. J. Prediction of fetal sex from cytologic examination of amnionic fluid. *N. Engl. J. Med.* 275:715, 1966.
3. Andrews, G. A., and Edwards, C. L. Tumor scanning with Gallium-67. *J.A.M.A.* 233:110, 1975.
4. Aono, T., Goldstein, D. P., Taymor, M. L., and Dolch, K. A radioimmunoassay method for human pituitary luteinizing hormone (LH) and human chorionic gonadotropin (HCG) using ^{125}I-labeled LH. *Am. J. Obstet. Gynecol.* 98:996, 1967.
5. Averette, H. E., Smith, J. K., Elwood, R. B., Gotz, C. T., and Ferguson, J. H. Lymphangioadenography (lymphography) in study of female genital cancer. *Cancer* 15:769, 1962.
6. Barnett, J. M. Diagnostic suction curettage on unanesthetized patients. *Obstet. Gynecol.* 42:672, 1973.
7. Board, J. A., and Bhatnagar, A. S. Serum prolactin levels in galactorrhea. *Am. J. Obstet. Gynecol.* 123:41, 1975.
8. Brueschke, E. E., and Wilbanks, G. D. A steerable fiberoptic hysteroscope. *Obstet. Gynecol.* 44:273, 1974.
9. Cohen, M. R., and Dmowski, W. P. Modern hysteroscopy: Diagnostic and therapeutic potential. *Fertil. Steril.* 24:905, 1973.
10. Cohn, H. E. Mammography in its proper perspective. *Surg. Gynecol. Obstet.* 134:97, 1972.
11. Collins, C. G., Hansen, L. H., and Theriot, E. A clinical stain for use in selecting biopsy sites in patients with vulvar disease. *Obstet. Gynecol.* 28:158, 1966.
12. Cukier, D. S. The assets and liabilities of mammography. *Surg. Gynecol. Obstet.* 141:896, 1975.
13. Davidson, J. W., and Van Lierop, M. J. Lymphography and prognosis in carcinoma of the cervix. *Am. J. Obstet. Gynecol.* 112:669, 1972.
14. Davis, H. J., and Jones, H. W., Jr. Population screening for cancer of the cervix with irrigation smears. *Am. J. Obstet. Gynecol.* 96:605, 1966.
15. Decker, A. *Culdoscopy.* Philadelphia: Davis, 1967.
16. Donald, I. New problems in sonar diagnosis in obstetrics and gynecology. *Am. J. Obstet. Gynecol.* 118:299, 1974.
17. Edelman, D. A., Brenner, W. E., Davis, G. L. R., and Child, P. *Am. J. Obstet. Gynecol.* 119:521, 1974.
18. Fee, H. J., Prokop, E. K., Cameron, J. L., and Wagner, H. N., Jr. Liver scanning in patients with suspected abdominal tumor. *J.A.M.A.* 230:1675, 1974.
19. Felix, E. L., Sindilar, W. F., Bagley, D. H., Johnston, G. S., and Ketcham, A. S. The use of bone and brain scans as screening procedures in patients with malignant lesions. *Surg. Gynecol. Obstet.* 141:867, 1975.
20. Friedman, S. Clinical uses of serum FSH and LH measurements. *Obstet. Gynecol.* 39:811, 1972.

21. Golbus, M. S., Conte, F. A., Schneider, E. L., and Epstein, C. J. Intrauterine diagnosis of genetic defects. *Am. J. Obstet. Gynecol.* 118:897, 1974.
22. Goldstein, D. P., Pastorfide, G. B., Osathanondh, R., and Kosasa, T. S. A rapid solid-phase radioimmunoassay specific for human chorionic gonadotropin in gestational trophoblastic disease. *Obstet. Gynecol.* 45:527, 1975.
23. Gravlee, L. C. Jet-irrigation method for the diagnosis of endometrial adenocarcinoma, its principle and accuracy. *Obstet. Gynecol.* 34:168, 1969.
24. Green, T. H., Jr. Value of culdoscopy in gynecologic diagnosis. *N. Engl. J. Med.* 254:214, 1956.
25. Habibian, M. R., Staab, E. V., and Matthews, H. A. Gallium citrate GA-67 scans in febrile patients. *J.A.M.A.* 233:1073, 1975.
26. Hartnett, L. J. Venography of the female pelvis. *Obstet. Gynecol.* 41:507, 1973.
27. Hodari, A. A., and Hodgkinson, C. P. Lymphography as a diagnostic aid in female genital malignancy. *Obstet. Gynecol.* 29:34, 1967.
28. Horwitz, C. A. Evaluation of a latex agglutination-inhibition slide pregnancy test (Pregnosis). *Obstet. Gynecol.* 43:693, 1974.
29. Isaacs, J. H. A Simplified Method for Aspiration Cytology of the Endometrium. In M. L. Taymor and T. H. Green, Jr. (Eds.), *Progress in Gynecology,* Vol. VI. New York: Grune & Stratton, 1975. Pp. 203–216.
30. Jacobson, B. M. Effects of cortisone and corticotropin on prolonged bleeding time. *Arch. Intern. Med.* 92:471, 1953.
31. Jones, W. B., Lewis, J. L., and Lehr, M. Monitor of chemotherapy in gestational trophoblastic neoplasm by radioimmunoassay of the beta-subunit of human chorionic gonadotropin. *Am. J. Obstet. Gynecol.* 121:669, 1975.
32. Lamb, E. J. Immunologic pregnancy tests. *Obstet. Gynecol.* 39:665, 1972.
33. Loeffler, R. K., Di Simone, R. N., and Howland, W. J. Limitations of bone scanning in clinical oncology. *J.A.M.A.* 234:1228, 1975.
34. Melby, J. C. Current concepts: Assessment of adrenocortical function. *N. Engl. J. Med.* 285:735, 1971.
35. Milunsky, A. Risk of amniocentesis for prenatal diagnosis. *N. Engl. J. Med.* 293:932, 1975.
36. Nyirjesy, I. Atypical or suspicious cervical smears: An aggressive diagnostic approach. *J.A.M.A.* 222:691, 1972.
37. Papanicolaou, G. N. Cytologic diagnosis of uterine cancer by examination of vaginal and uterine secretions. *Am. J. Clin. Pathol.* 19:301, 1949.
38. Parekh, M. C., Murthy, Y. S., Kosasa, T., and Arronet, G. H. The validity of hysterosalpingography and pneumohysterosalpingography as evaluated by subsequent laparotomy. *Surg. Gynecol. Obstet.* 135:921, 1975.
39. Pent, D. Laparoscopy: Its role in private practice. *Am. J. Obstet. Gynecol.* 113:459, 1972.
40. Queenan, J. T., Kubarych, S. F., and Douglas, D. L. Evaluation of diagnostic ultrasound in gynecology. *Am. J. Obstet. Gynecol.* 123:453, 1975.
41. Quick, A. J. Menstruation in hereditary bleeding disorders. *Obstet. Gynecol.* 28:37, 1966.
42. Sandmire, H. F., and Austin, S. D. Curettage as an office procedure. *Am. J. Obstet. Gynecol.* 119:82, 1974.
43. Smith, R. S. Pelvic arteriography in the differential diagnosis of pelvic mass. *Am. J. Obstet. Gynecol.* 111:952, 1971.
44. Stafl, A., and Mattingly, R. F. Colposcopic diagnosis of cervical neoplasia. *Obstet. Gynecol.* 41:168, 1973.
45. Sugimoto, O. Hysteroscopic diagnosis of endometrial carcinoma. *Am. J. Obstet. Gynecol.* 121:105, 1975.

46. Townsend, D. E., Ostergard, D. R., Mishell, D. R., Jr., and Hirose, F. M. Abnormal Papanicolaou smears: Evaluation by colposcopy, biopsies, and endocervical curettage. *Am. J. Obstet. Gynecol.* 108:429, 1970.
47. White, A. J., Buchsbaum, H. J., and Rodman, N. F. Accuracy of the Gravlee Jet Washer in detecting endometrial adenocarcinoma. *Am. J. Obstet. Gynecol.* 116:1169, 1973.

3
Congenital Anomalies of the Reproductive Tract

Developmental anomalies of the female genital tract are considered separately here, rather than in the discussion of gynecologic problems of infancy and childhood in Chapter 4, because, although present at birth, they are more often not discovered until later in the early adult period. Although this failure to recognize such anomalies at birth is perhaps lamentable and sometimes could be avoided by more careful routine examinations of the newborn or young child, it is often completely understandable. Many of the common congenital anatomic abnormalities do not involve either the external genitalia or the ovaries and hence do not manifest themselves in any way until the menarche, or even until marriage and unsuccessful attempts at conception or childbearing prompt an infertility investigation that reveals their presence. Furthermore, only rarely does a delay in the detection of the more common simple anatomic anomalies have any unfortunate effects on the outcome of their treatment, which in fact is often best postponed until adolescence or even maturity.

The situation is different, however, in the more profound disturbances of fetal genital tract development that originate in fundamental hormonal or chromosomal abnormalities and include the various forms of intersex or pseudohermaphroditism. Here, the anomalies of the external genitalia invariably accompanying these disorders draw immediate attention to their presence at or shortly after birth. This is fortunate, since in the majority of such cases, treatment is most successful if planned and carried out in infancy or early childhood.

ETIOLOGY AND CLASSIFICATION

A complete and accurate classification of the various anomalies that may be encountered according to anatomic type and etiology is certainly not possible at present, because the basic causes of developmental errors are as yet not clearly understood. Furthermore, difficulties in classification may never be totally resolved, since it is apparent even on the basis of present knowledge that similar genital anomalies may occur under widely differing circumstances and have entirely different fundamental etiologies. Finally, a theoretical classification devised on purely embryologic grounds does not suffice, since it cannot take into account etiologic differences that may result in various combinations of reproductive tract abnormalities; nor would it allow for the genital tract anomalies that undoubtedly occur in conjunction with lethal anomalies elsewhere in the embryo and hence are never actually seen in the living female. Thus, for the time being, at least, and perhaps quite suitably for the purposes of this book, it is necessary to resort to a clinical classification and present the common anomalies of various segments of the reproductive tract as they are encountered clinically, discussing the probable etiology of each separately on the basis of presently available information.

A few general concepts concerning etiology may be stated, however, and will serve to orient and integrate the later discussion of individual anomalies. Broadly speaking, there appear to be three fundamental types of developmental errors that give rise to congenital anomalies of the female reproductive tract:

1. **Simple retardation, arrest, or partial or complete failure of occurrence of normal embryologic events involving reproductive tract formation in an otherwise normal female embryo** (that is, a genetically normal female with normally developing female gonads). The commonest anomalies of the female genital organs are of this type and involve varying degrees of failure of the normal union of the originally separate müllerian ducts, as will be discussed later. Persistence of a doubled müllerian system in adult life is normal for some of the lower vertebrates (e.g., rabbits and other rodents), and its occurrence in the human female may in this sense be looked on as a reversion to a more primitive type of embryologic development. However, in actuality, it remains a serious anomaly, often with unfortunate effects on reproductive capacity in the human. This phylogenetic relationship emphasizes, however, that this group of anomalies does represent the result of retardation or arrest of an otherwise normally proceeding embryologic process.

As to the basic causes of these failures of completion of otherwise apparently initially normal embryologic sequences, the possibilities are many and varied. Fetal environmental factors, primarily maternal or placental in locus or origin, are undoubtedly the most likely causes and include such diverse maternal conditions as poor nutrition, metabolic disorders (e.g., diabetes), and certain viral or inclusion-body diseases (e.g., German measles and, less frequently, measles, mumps, chickenpox, toxoplasmosis, cytomegalic inclusion disease, herpes simplex, varicella, and poliomyelitis), and placental abnormalities leading to anoxia or disturbed nutrition (in the broad sense) in the fetus. Since most of the significant events in the embryologic formation of the reproductive tract commence around the fifth or sixth week and are essentially complete by the end of 10 to 12 weeks of fetal life, it is clear that the disturbances in fetal environment, whatever they may be, must have occurred at some time during this crucial interval. Although hereditary factors and germ plasm defects may conceivably also be implicated, most women with this type of anomaly are otherwise normal, and since the anomalies themselves do not seem to appear in families, attributing these defects to hereditary factors does not seem justifiable. (A notable exception to the statement that most of these women are otherwise normal must be made in the case of associated urinary tract anomalies, which are found in 35 to 50 percent of women suffering from müllerian duct anomalies. The explanation for this association probably lies in the anatomic juxtaposition of the urinary and reproductive tracts in the fetus and the occurrence of crucial events in the embryologic development of both systems almost simultaneously.) Other less common, though more obvious, causes might include exposure to toxic drugs or ionizing radiation.

2. **Genetic abnormalities involving the sex chromosomes.** The theory of sex determination that has been accepted for over half a century holds that sex is determined at the moment of conception and depends on whether or not the fertilizing

spermatazoon contains either the X or the Y sex chromosome of the original primary spermatocyte (which contained both) at the time of union with the ovum, which can only contain an X chromosome, derived as it is from the primary oocyte, which in turn always carries two identical X sex chromosomes. Recent rapid advances in the field of genetics (including discovery as late as 1956 that the normal diploid chromosome number in man is 46, not 48 as had been believed for so long), particularly the development of techniques for actual study of human chromosomes, have revealed that the situation with regard to the sex chromosome pattern is not always this simple. With application of the newly acquired ability to count and identify human chromosomes, it has been discovered that some individuals have more than two or less than two sex chromosomes within the nuclei of most if not all of their cells, or have two but with one or both abnormal. Furthermore, many of these individuals characteristically present a typical pattern of anomalous development of the reproductive tract, the particular anomaly tending to be correlated with a specific abnormality of the sex chromosome pattern. One of the two most frequently encountered examples of this type of sex chromosome—related anomaly is gonadal dysgenesis ("ovarian agenesis," or Turner's syndrome), in which, although the individuals appear to be female, 80 percent are genetically neither female nor male, chromosomal study showing only one X sex chromosome and a total chromosome number of only 45 (XO sex chromosome pattern). The second is Klinefelter's syndrome, in which there are typically 47 chromosomes with an XXY sex chromosome pattern. Both these disorders will be discussed in more detail later. Because of the increased interest in this obviously important aspect of sexual differentiation, the basic information concerning the study of sex chromosomes and their abnormalities will also be briefly summarized later in a separate section.

The mechanisms by which these chromosomal abnormalities can arise are varied but usually involve either failure of the members of a chromosome pair to separate properly during the cell divisions necessary to form the ovum or spermatazoon (maternal or paternal origin) or a similar failure or nondisjunction after fertilization during the cell divisions of the early embryonic stages (perhaps as a result of an adverse condition in the fetal environment). The underlying factors that might predispose to disruption of the normal pattern of chromosomal separation during cell division are again even less clear. Parental age has been incriminated, since chromosomal abnormalities in general tend to occur more frequently in children born to older parents. (The higher incidence of Down's syndrome in pregnancies in women in their late reproductive years is a case in point, although an autosomal rather than a sex chromosomal abnormality is involved.) Maternal viral infections (measles, rubella) also seem to be followed by a higher incidence of chromosomal aberrations, and anoxia and radiation have been shown experimentally to produce them.

3. **Fetal endocrine disorders interfering with the normal embryologic development of the reproductive tract** in an otherwise normal female or male embryo (normal female or male sex chromosome pattern and normal female or male gonads). The most common reproductive tract anomaly arising through such a mechanism is female pseudohermaphroditism (or the congenital adrenogenital syndrome), which

occurs as a result of fetal adrenal hyperplasia. This syndrome accounts for well over 50 percent of all so-called intersex problems. This also will be discussed later in more detail. The testicular feminization syndrome is now known to be an anomaly of **male** embryos developing in response to a fetal endocrine-metabolic disturbance. Embryonic pituitary and thyroid disturbances have been long recognized as precursors of more generalized congenital disorders of growth and development, and it is possible that as-yet unknown, more subtle, perhaps even transient fetal endocrine abnormalities may play a role in the production of other anomalies involving the reproductive tract as well as other organ systems. As for the basic causes of these fetal endocrinologic errors, reference can only be made again to potential hereditary constitutional deficiencies and the many possible maternal-fetal environmental factors already mentioned.

SUMMARY OF IMPORTANT EMBRYOLOGIC EVENTS IN THE DEVELOPMENT OF THE FEMALE REPRODUCTIVE TRACT

Although no attempt will be made to present the embryology of the female genital tract completely or in detail, a brief recounting in outline form of the normal sequence of principal events should prove helpful in understanding the manner in which the more common anatomic anomalies come about.

The genital system first makes its appearance during the fifth and sixth weeks of embryonic life and at this point is indifferent, or neuter, in appearance, although the prospective sex of the individual is ordinarily theoretically predictable on the basis of the sex chromosomal pattern irrevocably established at the moment of conception. Four key developmental processes proceeding in the primitive genital tract and a fifth and related, though less important, transition occurring in the adjacent embryonic urinary tract need to be kept in mind.

Gonadal Differentiation

The initially indifferent paired gonads, which make their appearance about the sixth week as medial thickenings in the urogenital ridges, have differentiated sufficiently within one or two weeks to assume the characteristics of ovaries and have begun to receive the migrating primordial germ or egg cells. (These primordial germ cells appear to arise in the caudal end of the primitive streak in all mammalian embryos, and their migration may well be initiated by a chemical attractant secreted by the genital ridge epithelial cells.) In the absence of the Y chromosome, this differentiation, when it occurs, must proceed in the direction of the formation of an ovary; conversely, the presence of a normal Y chromosome is absolutely essential to the development of a normal testis from the indifferent gonad. To be more specific (although it is an obvious oversimplification), the primitive gonad contains both a cortical (potentially ovarian) and a medullary (potentially testicular) component. It is becoming more apparent that the presence of two normal X chromosomes is essential for the proper development of the gonadal cortex to form a normal ovary, and that a normal Y chromosome, together with an X chromosome, is needed for normal growth and maturation of the gonadal medulla, with formation of a normal testis.

Thus Turner's syndrome is primarily an instance of cortical gonadal dysgenesis and Klinefelter's syndrome principally an example of medullary gonadal dysgenesis. The few true hermaphrodites (individuals in whom both ovarian and testicular tissues are present) in whom complete chromosome studies have been done have been shown to have mosaic chromosome patterns (e.g., XX/XY; XO/XY) or, in the case of some with pure XX patterns, are believed to have had elements of the Y chromosome transferred to an X (one X is frequently abnormally large) through "translocation" during nuclear division and are thus the result of a combined corticomedullary gonadal dysgenesis. Hence sex chromosomal abnormalities may give rise to the persistence of completely indifferent gonads (gonadal dysgenesis), rarely, to the formation of gonadal tissues of both male and female type in the same individual (true hermaphroditism), or to various intermediate gonadal aberrations.

Occasionally, arrested or failed embryologic development at this stage may result in complete absence of gonadal tissue on one or both sides, although this is rare.

Finally, it should be noted that the primitive gonads arise fairly cephalad in the urogenital ridges and, in the course of growth of the embryo, undergo a relative descent. In the case of the female, they normally come to assume a more caudal position within the pelvis, and an abnormal ovarian descent is unusual. However, failure to complete the descent to the normal scrotal site is not uncommon in the male. Hence, although they are not strictly speaking genital tract anomalies, it should be remembered that having arisen from the same urogenital ridge area from which the kidney and adrenal form, the ovary may carry with it, during its descent, embryonic rests of kidneys or adrenals that may become manifest later in life as either functioning or nonfunctioning, benign or malignant tissue of renal or adrenal origin.

Müllerian Duct Transformations

During the so-called indifferent stage, and regardless of the genetically predetermined sex, the paired müllerian ducts appear in the lateral portion of each urogenital ridge. Once gonadal differentiation is well under way, they continue their normal development in the human female, and ultimately through a complete caudal union form a single uterine cavity and cervix and a provisional single upper vagina, only the cephalic portions remaining unfused as separate fallopian tubes. In the male embryo, the development of the testis and beginning excretion of both androgen as well as a specific "müllerian inhibiting factor" (now identified as a polypeptide moiety secreted by the normal fetal testis) cause regression of the müllerian duct system, only vestiges of which remain in the adult male genitourinary tract. (This same polypeptide is probably also necessary for wolffian duct stimulation as well as for müllerian suppression.) It should be noted, however, that if normal male gonadal development and embryonic androgen and müllerian inhibiting factor secretion do not take place, even in a genetically indifferent embryo, the müllerian ducts will continue to evolve as if the individual were in fact a chromosomal female. This is an important point in understanding the anomalous anatomy present in cases of gonadal dysgenesis or agenesis (Turner's syndrome), wherein although only one X chromosome is present, there is no Y chromosome (XO chromosome pattern).

As previously mentioned, the most common anomalies of the human female reproductive tract involve failures of varying degrees in the process of normal müllerian duct fusion. Rarely, one or both of the müllerian ducts will simply not appear at all. Because the factors producing these apparently simple embryologic arrests of normal müllerian duct development might be expected to have an effect on simultaneously occurring events in the adjacent fetal urinary tract, the frequent coexistence of anomalies of the kidneys and ureters in patients with genital anomalies of müllerian duct origin is not surprising.

Formation of the External Genitalia

After the appearance of the genital tubercle in the sixth week of embryonic life, early modifications during the next two weeks again result in the development of an "indifferent" external genital area that includes the phallus, a urogenital sinus from which ultimately arise both the urethra and the lower end of the vagina, and the paired labioscrotal swellings. Once gonadal differentiation occurs at about the eighth week, further modifications in this primitive external genital region will result in the formation during the next six to eight weeks of either male or female external genitalia in accordance with the gonadal and hormonal (and normally the chromosomal) status of the embryo.

Obviously, incomplete or imperfect occurrence of this sequence of events due to unknown and nonspecific causes can produce a variety of simple anatomic abnormalities in both the genital and lower urinary tracts in either females or males who are otherwise sexually normal, but these abnormalities are uncommon.

Most important, however, are the more specific anomalies resulting from embryologic errors in the further evolution of the primitive, indifferent set of external genitals caused by imperfect gonadal differentiation. In this regard, the crux of the matter lies in the organizing potential of the embryonic male gonad or primitive testis and its early secretion of androgen. For only in the presence of actively functioning testicular tissue or androgen from some other source will the embryonic modifications necessary to form a male set of external genitalia occur. Thus, even in a genetically indifferent embryo, as long as normal male gonadal differentiation and androgen production fail to take place, a female type of external genitalia will appear (Turner's syndrome, gonadal dysgenesis or agenesis, is again an example). In the presence of intermediate androgenic effects that are insufficient to produce the completely masculine type of external genitalia, varying degrees of partial virilization, often with hypospadias, will result.

Equally significant for the genetically female embryo is the abnormal presence of androgens during this crucial phase of the development of the external genitalia. If androgens are present in large enough amounts in the developing female embryo at this time, a tendency toward male external genitalia and a masculine type of lower urinary tract anatomy will be evident to a greater or lesser degree at birth, even though normal female gonads with a potentially normal functional capacity and a normal müllerian duct system (normal fallopian tubes, uterus, cervix, and upper vagina) are present. The two common examples of this phenomenon are (1) the congenital adrenogenital syndrome (congenital adrenal hyperplasia or female pseudo-hermaphroditism), in which the fetal adrenal of a genetically and gonadally normal female secretes large amounts of androgenic steroids, and (2) the more recently encountered, iatrogenic syndrome of virilization of the otherwise normal female fetus by the administration of androgens or, more commonly, progestational compounds with androgenic activity to the mother during the early months of pregnancy.

Union of the Fused Lower Segment of the Müllerian Duct System with the External Genital Tract

At the caudal end (Müller's tubercle) of the fused müllerian duct systems, a lumen normally develops below the cervix and between the rectum and urethra. When contact is made with the deepening external urogenital sinus, union ordinarily occurs, and the thin membrane so formed becomes the hymen. Usually, the hymen assumes its normal perforate form in the latter months of embryonic life or shortly after birth. Thus the upper two-thirds of the vagina are of müllerian duct origin, while the lower one-third is of external genital or, more precisely, urogenital sinus origin.

A knowledge of these embryologic facts serves to explain the various congenital anomalies of the vagina and vestibule, most of which result either from failure of fusion or partial or complete failure of normal development of one or the other of the two initially independent forerunners of the completely formed, final vaginal tract. The simple abnormalities of imperforate hymen or imperforate vagina are easily understood, and complete absence of the upper vagina in the presence of normal external genitalia and a short, apparently normal lower vaginal canal are equally comprehensible. The mechanisms by which less common anomalies such as congenital rectovaginal and urethrovaginal fistulas might arise are also obvious.

Disposition of the Mesonephric (Wolffian) Duct System in the Female

Although the male embryo appropriates the mesonephric ducts and tubules and converts them into the male genital canals, the mesonephric duct system undergoes atrophy in the normally developing female fetus and largely disappears. However, portions do remain as normal vestigial remnants even in adults (the so-called **rete ovarii,** or complex of epoophoron and paroophoron and their ducts, which lie in the broad ligaments and mesosalpinx and mesovarium). Other mesonephric duct remnants may often be found retroperitoneally, in the ovaries or tubes, or in the walls of the uterus, cervix, vagina, and even the vulva. Although not strictly anomalies, numerous cysts (e.g., the common Gartner's duct cysts of the vagina, the hydatid cysts of Morgagni near the fimbriated ends of the tubes, and the frequently large parovarian cysts) and, more rarely, neoplasms arising from these leftover meso-nephric duct structures are often of considerable clinical interest and significance and are in a sense congenital in origin.

SUMMARY OF CURRENT KNOWLEDGE AND METHODS OF STUDY AND RECOGNITION OF SEX CHROMOSOMAL DISORDERS

This review of basic facts essential to an intelligent understanding of congenital anomalies of the female genital system would be incomplete without a brief résumé of the recent rapid advances in medical genetics, particularly those in the field of the chromosomal disorders that produce some of the more common reproductive tract anomalies.

First of all, the methods currently in use for the study and identification of human chromosomes and sex chromosome patterns should be briefly mentioned. Employing special tissue-culture techniques, leukocytes from an ordinary blood sample (other tissue cells, including bone marrow, have also been used) may be grown in a medium to which colchicine later is added. This drug arrests mitosis at a stage when the individual chromosomes will be scattered widely if the cultured cells are "squashed" on a slide and exposed to hypotonic saline solution to cause cellular swelling and disruption (the "squash preparation"). By photomicrography, the various types of chromosomes can then be separately and accurately identified, paired off, and counted (Fig. 17). In this way the total number of chromosomes and their composition, normal or abnormal, can be precisely determined. It is through the use of this and similar complicated techniques that the exact chromosomal patterns of the various known anomalous clinical entities have been established.

A much simpler approach to the problem of chromosomal evaluation and one readily available for routine clinical use is the determination of the nuclear sex chromatin pattern of an individual's cells. As has already been described in Chapter 2, the buccal smear is ordinarily used, because the surface epithelial cells of the oral mucosa are ideal for the purpose and readily available. The determination depends on the fact that in most cells of normal females a sex chromatin body — the so-called Barr body, the presence and significance of which was first noted by Barr and Bertram of England [3, 4] — can be regularly seen and identified in the cell nucleus at or very close to the nuclear membrane (see Fig. 11). This chromatin body is believed to result from the apposition of certain portions of the X chromosomes and is presumed to be visible in the female cell nucleus by virtue of the considerably larger volume of the XX chromosome pair as contrasted with the much smaller XY chromosome complex. An alternative hypothesis (the Lyon hypothesis) is that the Barr body represents a coiled, temporarily inactivated X chromosome in the nucleus of female cells. This explanation would account for the fact that the Barr body count of female cells is never 100 percent and that it actually fluctuates, particularly in adult women during the monthly menstrual cycle, possibly in response

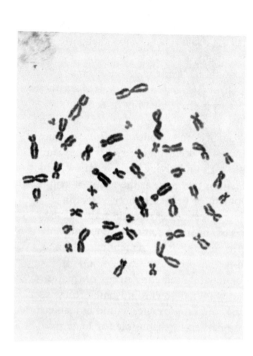
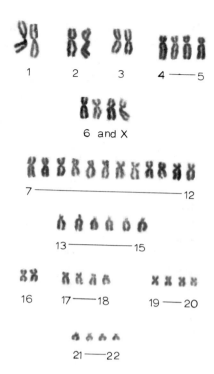

1 2 3 4 —— 5

6 and X

7 ——————————— 12

13 ————— 15

16 17 —— 18 19 —— 20

21 —— 22

Figure 17
Chromosomal analysis by means of the "squash preparation." On the left is shown the "squash smear" of a normal human female cell grown in tissue culture, with cell division arrested at the metaphase. On the right is the normal human female idiogram or karyotype constructed from these individual chromosomes.

to varying estrogen levels. When the majority of cell nuclei show the sex chromatin body, the individual is termed **chromatin-positive**, and an XX sex chromosome pattern can generally be assumed. If three X chromosomes are present, as is the case in certain genetic abnormalities, then two sex chromatin bodies will usually be visible. In other words, the number of Barr bodies is equal to one less than the number of X chromosomes (individuals with as many as four X chromosomes have been reported). However, the presence of a sex chromatin body does not necessarily connote absence of the Y chromosome but rather indicates only that two X chromosomes exist. (In Klinefelter's syndrome, for example, the individuals are chromatin-positive, and the sex chromosomal pattern is XXY.)

On the other hand, absence or virtual absence of sex chromatin bodies in an individual's cells implies that no more than one X chromosome is present, and the individual is termed **chromatin-negative**. This is the situation in a genetically normal male with the normal XY chromosome pattern. But, by the same token, a chromatin-negative status by no means establishes the presence of a Y chromosome, as was originally assumed. Again, for example, in Turner's syndrome or gonadal dysgenesis, the individuals are chromatin-negative, a fact which at one time was believed to indicate that they were genetic males, whereas the usual sex chromosomal pattern is now known to be XO, revealing them to be equally accurately "incomplete females"; perhaps a better descriptive phrase would be "genetically indifferent."

Within these limitations, however, the sex chromatin determination is an extremely helpful clinical test. Since, as will presently be seen, there are only three major sex chromosomal abnormalities of clinical significance, correlation of the clinical picture with the sex chromatin pattern nearly always suffices to establish a definite diagnosis. Through the use of the nuclear sex chromatin test in doubtful cases, it is also readily possible to distinguish between anomalies due to an underlying basic genetic disorder and the far more common congenital abnormalities that arise as the result of simple incomplete or imperfect embryologic development of the reproductive tract in genetically normal females. Knowledge of the nuclear sex chromatin status of the patient frequently permits a definite diagnosis of the more common genetic disorders to be made much earlier in life than heretofore, and this is of tremendous advantage to proper therapy. The use of sex chromatin testing procedures on amniotic fluid cells is also being explored with a view to the prenatal prediction of sex of the fetus.

Although prior to 1956 it was believed that man had 48 chromosomes, it has now been firmly established that the normal number of chromosomes within human cell nuclei is 46. These consist of 22 paired autosomes, each responsible for some specific aspect of the growth and maturation of bodily structure or organ systems and cellular function, and one pair of sex chromosomes, the presence and nature of which determine the genetic sex of the individual and, as a result, whether gonadal differentiation and the subsequent reproductive tract development will be that of a normal male or a normal female. One-half of each pair of chromosomes (a total of 23) is of male parental origin, the other half being of female parental origin, because both male and female germ cells contain only 23 chromosomes as a result of the miotic division that is necessary for the formation of either the ovum or the spermatozoon. At the time of fertilization the two sets of 23 chromosomes unite and pair off again, so that the normal number of 46 chromosomes is once more restored in the nuclear substance of the cells of the zygote. The autosomes are essentially identical regardless of the sex of the individual, but the sex chromosomes differ, normal female cells containing 2 identical X chromosomes, normal male cells containing a similar X chromosome and a smaller Y chromosome, and herein lies the basis for the genetic determination of sex. For from the preceding, it is obvious that all normal female germ cells (ova) will contain one X chromosome, whereas half the normal male germ cells (spermatozoa) will contain an X chromosome and half a Y chromosome. There is thus ordinarily a 50 percent chance at the time of fertilization that the resulting zygote will be genetically female (XX) and an equal chance that the genetic sex and sex chromosome pattern will be male (XY).

The normal nuclear divisions and unions that occur in gametogenesis and conception respectively (Fig. 18) and involve these chromosomal transfers fortunately take place in orderly fashion with the greatest regularity. However, it is now known that abnormal chromosomal transfers may occasionally occur through a number of

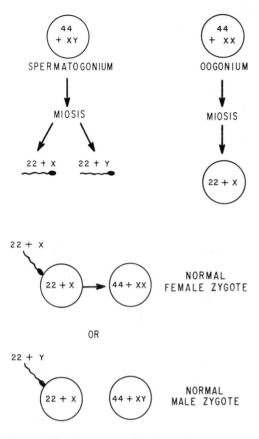

Figure 18
Diagram of the normal germ cell divisions involved in gametogenesis and conception.

mechanisms, and that these may result in a sex chromosome pattern (in either the male or female parental germ cell and/or the fertilized ovum and developing zygote) that is neither male nor female. The various mechanisms by which these chromosomal abnormalities may arise may be listed as follows:

1. Nondisjunction, or failure of the two members of a chromosome pair to separate during the miotic divisions that occur in the formation of ova or spermatozoa.
2. Reciprocal translocation, or exchange of portions of their chromatin material by members of two different chromosome pairs during either miosis or the embryonic mitotic divisions.
3. Deletion or loss of part or all of a chromosome.
4. Reduplication or nondisjunction of only a part of a chromosome.
5. Finally, the phenomenon known as mosaicism, in which nondisjunction occurs during the mitotic divisions of the early embryonic stages, with persistence of

more than one type of nuclear chromosomal pattern, the various cell types having different total chromosome numbers.

On the basis of a worldwide collaborative study, it is now appreciated that about 0.56 percent of the total population of newborn babies have major chromosomal abnormalities; that is, such abnormalities occur in slightly more than 1 in every 200 live births. Further analysis of these data reveals that sex chromosome abnormalities occur in 0.2 percent (in 1 in every 400 newborn males and 1 in every 680 newborn females). Abnormalities of autosomal chromosome number (e.g., trisomies) occur in 0.12 percent, and structural abnormalities of autosomal chromosomes (e.g., translocations) occur in 0.24 percent. To date the one major and clinically significant abnormality involving the autosomal chromosomes to be identified is the consistent finding of 47 chromosomes in mongoloid infants, where an extra autosomal chromosome (derived from number 21) is present, hence the descriptive phrase, the trisomy-21 syndrome (Down's syndrome). Several other trisomies involving autosomes have also been discovered (trisomy 13, or Patau's syndrome; trisomy 16–18, or Edwards' syndrome), but these have involved only a small number of patients with relatively rare clinical syndromes. This paucity of known autosomal abnormalities may well exist because loss or any other major abnormality of an autosome is more often lethal.

The contrary is true in the case of the sex chromosomes, in which abnormalities are not only frequently compatible with life but also are now recognized to be the basic cause of some of the more common reproductive tract anomalies. Currently, the three most common abnormal sex chromosomal patterns that have been encountered are the following:

1. The XO sex chromosomal constitution in phenotypic females with 45 chromosomes, which is the usual situation in the anomaly of gonadal dysgenesis with Turner's syndrome. (A buccal smear is chromatin-negative.)
2. The XXY sex chromosomal constitution in phenotypic males with 47 chromosomes, or Klinefelter's syndrome. (A buccal smear is chromatin-positive.)
3. The XXX sex chromosomal constitution in phenotypic but mentally retarded females, the so-called superfemale, or poly-X syndrome. (A buccal smear reveals that the majority of cells contain two sex chromatin bodies.)

Numerous variants of these three basic abnormal sex chromosome patterns have been identified in individuals presenting any one of the three typical clinical pictures. These variants involve the presence of abnormal or additional X and/or Y chromosomes as well as sex chromosomal mosaics (several different sex chromosome patterns in various cells of the same individual). (For example, in Klinefelter's syndrome, although the 47-XXY chromosomal pattern is the most frequent, various other patterns have also been encountered and reported, including 48-XXXY, 48-XXYY, 49-XXXXY, and a variety of mosaic patterns. Similarly a 48-XXXX "superfemale" type has been observed, and mosaics of various types, as well as some individuals

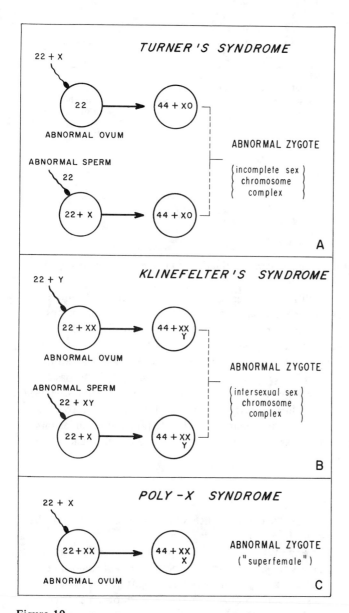

Figure 19
Diagrams of the types of abnormal germ cell divisions that may lead to (A) Turner's syndrome, (B) Klinefelter's syndrome, or (C) the poly-X syndrome.

Table 2
Nuclear Sex Chromatin and Sex Chromosome Patterns in the Principal Genetic
Disorders Associated with Reproductive Tract Anomalies

Clinical Picture	Nuclear Sex Chromatin Pattern as Determined by Buccal Smear	Sex Chromosome Pattern as Determined by "Squash Preparation"	Total Number of Chromosomes
Normal female	Positive	XX	46
Normal male	Negative	XY	46
Turner's syndrome[a]	Negative	XO	45
Klinefelter's syndrome[a]	Positive	XXY	47
"Superfemale"[a]	Positive[b]	XXX	47

[a]Only the most common chromosomal patterns are indicated.
[b]Two chromatin bodies.

who are chromatin-positive, have been encountered in 20 percent of patients with Turner's syndrome.)

Although considerably simplified, the diagrams in Figure 19 indicate the gross mechanisms by which these three principal types of sex chromosomal aberrations might arise. A summary in outline form of the essential features of these sex chromosomal disorders is presented in Table 2.

Finally, with the intense interest in precise study of sex chromosomal abnormalities in recent years and the application of the findings to clinical problems, basic information as to specific chromosomal functions and variations and their correlation with particular features of the resulting gross anatomic and functional disturbances has been accumulating. Some of the information is valuable for a better understanding of the various clinical entities, as well as useful in their differential diagnosis, and may be summarized as follows:

X Chromosomes

1. Two normal X chromosomes are definitely necessary for differentiation of the primitive, indifferent gonads into normal functioning ovaries.

2. The genes abnormalities responsible for the well-known sex-linked conditions of hemophilia and color blindness are known to be carried by the X chromosomes.

3. The gene or genes that determine a person's ultimate height appear to be located on the X chromosomes and most probably on one or both of the shorter arms of the X. Evidence for this rests in the observation that stature in the majority of patients with Turner's syndrome is markedly shorter than normal, and their chromosome pattern is either XO or the second X is abnormal and small, with one or both of the short arms of the second X partially or completely absent. In a smaller number of patients with otherwise typical gonadal dysgenesis, the sex chromosome pattern is an apparently normal XX, and these individuals are normal in height.

4. Where too many X chromosomes are present, as in the "superfemales" or

poly-X syndrome (XXX, XXXX), or as in Klinefelter's syndrome (XXY), the individuals are always mentally deficient. (This is also true where an excess of autosomes is present, as in the case of Down's syndrome.)

5. Early in embryonic life, one of the two X chromosomes may well be rendered physiologically inactive in the somatic cells of normal females, although it is not yet clear whether or not this is also true for cells of the germ line (the so-called Lyon single active X chromosome hypothesis proposed by Mary F. Lyon of Great Britain). Similarly, it appears that even when too many X chromosomes are present, only one tends to remain active.

6. Based on several reported series, the incidence of X chromosome abnormalities varies from 1 in every 200 to 400 live-born infants to an estimated 1 in 1800 in a general population of adults. Klinefelter's syndrome, the triple-X syndrome, and Turner's syndrome are by far the most common anomalies, in that order.

Y Chromosomes

1. The Y chromosome unquestionably contains genetic material strongly determinant for the male phenotype, or masculine appearance and developmental tendencies. Thus, even in Klinefelter's syndrome, the presence of two X chromosomes along with the Y chromosome still results in a masculine-appearing individual.

2. The Y chromosome (especially the short arm) is in general absolutely essential for differentiation of the primitive gonad into a functioning testis. There may be infrequent exceptions to this rule, for the rare, true hermaphrodites so far studied have always shown an XX or, more rarely, an XO sex chromosome pattern. Furthermore, a few cases of an even rarer "male XX syndrome" have been recorded. However, it is also possible that a small, very abnormal Y chromosome is actually present but cannot as yet be identified (it may even be located on an X chromosome or on an autosome), or that a Y chromosome had been present at an early period of fetal life but was subsequently lost. Even more rarely, a female phenotype has been observed in the presence of a 46-XY karyotype and bilateral streak gonads; this syndrome appears to be a familial genetic disorder.

3. The chromosomal opposite of Turner's syndrome, a YO sex chromosome pattern, is probably not viable, since no living individuals with this pattern have ever been encountered. Nevertheless, tissue from early abortions is currently being studied with a view to establishing whether or not such a chromosomal disorder might in fact occur occasionally. However, it is now known that the Y chromosome carries loci, either in its short pairing segment or on its long arm, that are homologous with the loci on the short arm of the X chromosome, the absence of which is responsible for the short stature and congenital anomalies seen in Turner's syndrome. (It seems obvious that these homologous loci on the Y chromosome guarantee normal height and absence of congenital anomalies in normal 46-XY males.) Therefore, as might be predicted, a few individuals have been encountered with probable Y chromosome aberrations (X—abnormal Y) who have short stature and other stigmata of Turner's syndrome as well as defective testicular development.

4. The occurrence of an XYY sex chromosome complement in some individuals has recently been discovered and is discussed in more detail later in the chapter.

SIMPLE EMBRYOLOGIC DEVELOPMENTAL ANOMALIES: CLINICAL ASPECTS

The basic underlying genetic and embryologic mechanisms responsible for their development having been considered, the common genital anomalies will now be presented from the clinical standpoint. In the case of the simpler specific developmental abnormalities, it seems most convenient to consider them according to their anatomic location. Some of the more complex, generalized congenital reproductive disorders of genetic or fetal endocrine origin, particularly those associated with either true or pseudointersexuality, will be discussed separately.

Vulvar Anomalies

Invariably, true congenital vulvar anomalies are encountered only in connection with pseudohermaphroditism.

Vaginal Anomalies

Vaginal anomalies may be of urogenital sinus origin (imperforate hymen, female hypospadias or persistent urogenital sinus membrane) or müllerian duct origin (congenital absence or atresia of the vagina, double or septate vagina).

IMPERFORATE HYMEN

Imperforate hymen is the simplest and perhaps most frequent genital anomaly. It may not be recognized until the menarche, when cyclic monthly distress is experienced, but no overt menses occur. At this point, the vagina behind the intact and bulging hymeneal membrane may be distended with old menstrual secretions (hematocolpos). In the late stages, with further backing up of secretions, secondary distention of the uterus (hematometrium) or even of the tubes (hematosalpinx) may occur, with palpable abdominal and adnexal cystic "masses." The diagnosis is usually now readily apparent, and the treatment is simple hymenotomy or hymenectomy.

Rarely, distention of the vagina by simple mucoid vaginal secretions produced by maternal hormone stimulation may occur in a newborn infant or young child (hydrocolpos), and because of pressure or secondary infection the vagina may require drainage at this time. In this situation, both the differentiation from congenital absence of the vagina as well as the safety of hymenotomy are afforded by the vaginal distention. It is important to note that the hydrocolpos occurring in a newborn infant may be of considerable size and may not only interfere with bladder emptying, but, more significantly, may present as an abdominal mass. The possibility of hydrocolpos must therefore always be kept in mind in this situation, lest an ill-advised, unnecessary laparotomy be undertaken for an "abdominal tumor." Once catheterization has eliminated bladder retention as the sole source of the mass, abdominal roentgenograms following injection of a small amount of iodized oil (Lipiodol) into the distended vaginal portion of the mass will nearly always reveal the true nature of the abdominal component, and simple incision of the hymenal membrane will effectively deal with the problem.

If discovered early in infancy or childhood, and if it is asymptomatic, an imperforate hymen is best treated expectantly until the anatomic structures are sufficiently developed and large enough to distinguish it definitely from congenital vaginal absence and to permit a safe hymenectomy. If it becomes necessary to perform hymenotomy in the absence of distention in a child, the presence of an intact vaginal canal above the imperforate hymen should be assured by rectal examination and by roentgenograms after injection of radiopaque dye through the hymen; at operation, a finger in the rectum and a sound in the urethra and bladder should be used to guide and control the incision.

A variant of imperforate hymen is the so-called microperforate hymen. In infants and young children, this may be a cause for both recurring vulvovaginitis and recurring urinary tract infections due to retention of a pool of infected urine behind the hymenal membrane. The condition is promptly relieved by a hymenoplasty.

Occasionally, variation in aperture size or in the thickness and rigidity of the hymen may require dilatation or formal hymenectomy under anesthesia before maturity, but these are not considered true anomalies.

CONGENITAL ABSENCE OF THE VAGINA

Congenital absence of the vagina most frequently involves only its upper two-thirds, the lower one-third usually being normal. It is one of the commoner anomalies and is usually associated with an absent or rudimentary uterus and tubes; the ovaries, however, are invariably present and normal. Less often (in roughly 10 percent of these patients), a normal uterus and tubes are present, and with the onset of menstrual function a situation analogous to that of the hematocolpos behind an imperforate hymen may develop, except that only hematometrium and hematosalpinx result. At this point, if the diagnosis is made and treatment carried out early, fertility may be preserved by avoiding irreparable damage to the tubes and uterus. When the uterus and tubes are normal, this anomaly is usually not accompanied by anomalies of the urinary tract. If it is discovered in infancy or early childhood, further diagnostic maneuvers and treatment should be delayed because of possible damage to adjacent structures by ill-advised probing or exploration in the tiny patient.

If cyclic menstrual phenomena suggesting the presence of a normally functioning uterus appear at the menarche, prompt laparotomy or peritoneoscopy to prove this, followed by plastic reconstruction of the vagina, is indicated in order to prevent the development of a significant hematometrium and/or hematosalpinges that might interfere with attempts to preserve normal reproductive function. If the anomaly is discovered either before or after the menarche but in the absence of any signs of a normally functioning uterus, creation of an artificial vagina should be delayed until maturity has been reached, and preferably until sexual activity is imminent or likely. The surgeon can then count on the normal functional use of the artificially created vagina postoperatively to maintain its integrity and functional capacity.

Types of Repair

1. Surgical dissection of the perineum and rectovaginal septal area (the space between the bladder and rectum), with placement of a full-thickness skin graft temporarily held in position by a suitable plastic mold, is now the favored method.

2. An ingenious and entirely different approach to vaginal reconstruction has been devised by Williams [34]. It consists of a vulvovaginal plastic procedure creating a new vaginal pouch lined by vulvar skin. The operation is easily performed, is notably free of complications, and the results in terms of coital function have been most satisfactory. Although equally useful in patients with congenital absence of the vagina, this procedure would appear to be especially applicable to the problem of vaginal reconstruction after any radical pelvic cancer operation that of necessity includes a total vaginectomy.

3. Use of an isolated loop of small or large bowel in place of a skin graft. After the preliminary perineal and rectovaginal septal dissection, the mobilized segment of gastrointestinal tract is brought down to the introitus with its mesenteric blood supply intact, the upper end is closed, and the lower end sutured to the perineal skin edges.

4. Various sliding and pedicled skin flaps are transported from the perineum and thighs, and these are sutured in place in the previously dissected space between bladder and rectum.

5. The method of Frank, in which simple pressure at the proper perineal site is used to form a skin pit slowly. By means of a bluntly rounded, solid tube of plastic or metal, the patient gradually produces progressively deeper indentation of the skin by daily pressure for several months until a reasonably satisfactory, functioning vaginal canal is created. Although successful in a few, this method has not proved feasible for the majority of patients.

CONGENITAL VAGINAL ATRESIA

Although seen rather infrequently, membranous or partial fibrous obliteration may occur at various levels of the vaginal canal. The manifestations and physical findings may be indistinguishable from those of either imperforate hymen or congenital absence of the vagina, and the final differential diagnosis may depend entirely on the findings at the time of surgical exposure.

DOUBLE OR SEPTATE VAGINA

Double or septate vagina rarely, if ever, occurs in the absence of one of the uterine duplications (usually uterus didelphia) and is discussed later.

HYPOSPADIAS

Isolated instances of female hypospadias due simply to faulty urogenital sinus development are extremely rare, as are congenital urethrovaginal and rectovaginal fistulas, which presumably arise through similar mechanisms. However, a characteristic type of hypospadias is encountered in association with congenital adrenal hyperplasia and is discussed with that entity.

Uterotubal Anomalies (Müllerian Duct Origin)

For reasons already discussed, uterotubal anomalies of müllerian duct origin are frequently accompanied by congenital anomalies of the urinary tract (e.g., double ureters, absent kidney), but the gonads are usually normal.

FAILURE OF FORMATION

Unilateral Absence

In unilateral absence (uterus unicornis), the vagina and cervix are invariably normal, but the uterus possesses only one cornu and one tube, and usually only one ovary is present.

Bilateral Absence

Bilateral absence may be complete or partial (congenital absence of the uterus and vagina [except the lower third] , with or without rudimentary tubes, and usually with normal ovaries). Although the presence of normal ovaries assures normal female secondary sex characteristics, obviously these patients suffer from primary amenorrhea. Before the menarche, it may be impossible to distinguish them from patients with simple congenital vaginal absence, and laparotomy may therefore be necessary to establish the diagnosis. As previously noted, in the absence of a uterus, it is usually wiser to delay construction of an artificial vagina until sexual activity is contemplated.

Congenital absence of the cervix, with an otherwise normal uterus and a normal vagina, is an extremely rare anomaly. In actuality, it represents cervical atresia due to failure of the normal process of canalization. The clinical picture is one of a pseudoprimary amenorrhea, with the appearance of cyclic, monthly bouts of abdominal pain and the eventual development of a hematometrium behind the obstruction produced by the absence of a normal cervix. As the retained menstrual secretions accumulate, a palpable suprapubic mass becomes evident; hematosalpinges may also develop, and associated pelvic endometriosis has been reported, presumable secondary to tubal reflux and intraperitoneal spillage of viable endometrial cells. This developmental disorder was formerly treated by hysterectomy. However, successful operative correction has been reported in a few cases by the simple technique of creating a fistula between the endometrial cavity and the vagina below it and then allowing this fistulous tract to epithelialize and heal in over a rubber or polyethylene plastic tube.

FAILURE OF FUSION, OR IMPERFECT FUSION

Failure of fusion, or imperfect fusion, constitutes the largest group of müllerian duct anomalies, the so-called duplications, or double uterus. Although a number of nomenclatures and systems of classification have been devised, the following seems the simplest, most accurate and descriptive, and most helpful, particularly with reference to selection of proper surgical treatment.

Double Uterus (Symmetrical Duplications)

1. Externally unified, with two internal chambers formed by an intracavity septum.
   a. Uterus subseptus (Fig. 20).
   b. Uterus septus (with or without a double or septate vagina) (Fig. 20).
2. Externally divided, with two cavities formed by two hemiuteri.
   a. Uterus arcuatus (heart-shaped uterus, often of no significance) (Fig. 20).
   b. Uterus bicornis unicollis (or, more simply, the bicornuate uterus) (Fig. 20).
   c. Uterus bicornis bicollis (didelphia). A double or septate vagina is frequently associated with this anomaly (Fig. 20).

Asymmetrical Duplications

In an asymmetrical duplication, the embryologic development of one müllerian duct proceeds along normal lines, but on the opposite side there is arrested or imperfect development at some phase in the evolution of the upper portion, as well as a variable degree of failure of fusion at the level of the uterus. This results in the development of a rudimentary hemiuterus or horn; the vagina and cervix are usually normal. These rudimentary horns may vary considerably in size as well as in the nature of their communication with the normal horn, or definitive uterus and cervix. In some instances the connecting lumen is extremely tiny; in others it is totally absent. If the rudimentary horn is small and communicates by a wide opening with the uterus, it may remain totally asymptomatic and unsuspected throughout the life of the individual. If it is large enough to permit the implantation and growth of an early pregnancy, a surgical emergency may arise during the childbearing age due to progressive distention and the inevitable rupture and hemorrhage that often follows — in a sense, a form of ectopic pregnancy. A similar acute abdominal emergency may arise in connection with a rudimentary horn that lacks an adequate communication with the main uterus, cervix, and vagina; here, distention and ultimate rupture secondary to the accumulation of menstrual secretions in the postmenarchal female may occur. The mechanism by which such patients might also have acquired and progressively increasing dysmenorrhea and the gradual development of a "lateral pelvic mass" or a "uterine tumor" is also apparent, and this condition must be borne in mind in the differential diagnosis of either of these clinical pictures in the younger woman.

SYMPTOMS OF DUPLICATIONS

Approximately 25 percent of women with the various uterine duplications will have no symptoms whatsoever, exhibiting a normal menstrual pattern, normal fertility,

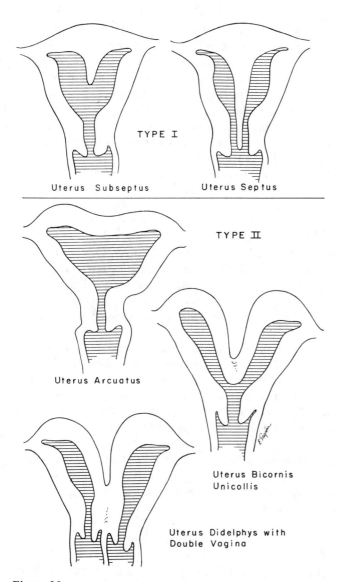

TYPE I

Uterus Subseptus

Uterus Septus

TYPE II

Uterus Arcuatus

Uterus Bicornis
Unicollis

Uterus Didelphys with
Double Vagina

Figure 20
Types of double uteri. (From T. H. Green, Jr. Gynecology. In G. L. Nardi and
G. D. Zuidema [Eds.], *Surgery: A Concise Guide to Clinical Practice* [3rd ed.].
Boston: Little, Brown, 1972, Chap. 39.)

and having uncomplicated pregnancies and deliveries. Far more often, however, symptoms will appear after the menarche and tend to increase in severity. The more commonly encountered manifestations include dysmenorrhea, menorrhagia, irregular bleeding, dyspareunia, infertility, the occasional surgical emergencies mentioned earlier, and repeated bouts of pelvic inflammation secondary to hematometrium and hematosalpinx in a rudimentary horn. Perhaps the most common complications — ones that should immediately suggest the possible existence of a uterine duplication — are repeated abortions, miscarriages or premature deliveries, and difficult labors with malpositions, dystocia, and postpartum hemorrhages. Such a history strongly indicates the need for appropriate studies to confirm or rule out the presence of a uterotubal anomaly.

DIAGNOSIS OF DUPLICATIONS

A history of repeated abortions and menstrual disorders and discomfort may be the initial clue; physical examination, if carefully done, should certainly reveal the presence of uterus didelphia, and a bicornuate uterus or the presence of a rudimentary horn may sometimes be detected on a bimanual pelvic examination, particularly if the index of suspicion is high. The externally unified, septate uterus obviously cannot be recognized in this way.

In the majority of cases, however, definite and anatomically precise diagnosis depends entirely on the findings by hysterosalpingography. Actual x-ray visualization of the anatomic configuration of the uterus and tubes will invariably establish the presence and nature of the anomaly, except in the case of a rudimentary horn that does not communicate with the main uterine cavity. Here, in the face of symptoms, exploratory laparotomy may actually be necessary before a definite diagnosis can be made.

It is essential to include intravenous pyelography in the total diagnostic evaluation, in order to discover any of the frequently associated urinary tract anomalies. Often, no treatment for the urologic abnormality is indicated or necessary, but it is nevertheless important to be aware of its presence.

TREATMENT OF DUPLICATIONS

Symmetrical duplications of all types can nearly always be corrected by the so-called unification operation of Strassman [30], of which there are now several technical variations. As depicted in Figure 21, the separate horns are united by a plastic surgical procedure, and any septum present in the fundus, cervix, or vagina is divided or resected. It should be emphasized that no corrective surgery should ever be undertaken until endocrine or metabolic causes for menstrual disorders, infertility, and repeated abortions have been completely ruled out. The results with regard to relief of symptoms and, more important, improvement in fertility and reduction in fetal mortality, have been highly satisfactory. In the group of 128 operated patients collated by Strassman, only 4 percent had carried a pregnancy to term prior to

Septum

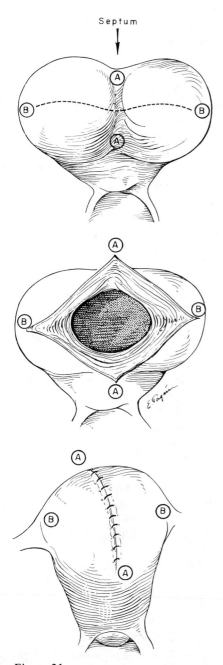

Figure 21
Uterine unification operation of Strassman. (From T. H. Green, Jr. Gynecology.
In G. L. Nardi and G. D. Zuidema [Eds.], *Surgery: A Concise Guide to Clinical Practice* [3rd ed.]. Boston: Little, Brown, 1972, Chap. 39.)

corrective surgery, the abortion or miscarriage rate having been 70 percent and the incidence of premature deliveries, 15 percent. Following the plastic unification operation, however, 85 percent carried pregnancies to term, and the incidence of abortion was only 12 percent. Of considerable further interest and significance from an obstetric standpoint is that the majority of these patients can safely and easily be delivered vaginally, in spite of the previous rather extensive uterine surgery, provided there are no other contraindications to vaginal delivery. In Strassman's own patients, 85 percent were subsequently delivered vaginally, and there were no cases of uterine rupture and no maternal deaths.

In the case of asymmetrical duplications, the symptomatic rudimentary horn should be totally excised; unification procedures are usually both impossible and unnecessary, since the larger hemiuterus is nearly always functioning normally and capable of carrying a normal pregnancy to term.

Obviously, simple resection is all that is required in the case of vaginal or cervical septa unaccompanied by any uterine abnormality.

Hypoplasia of the Uterus (Infantile or Juvenile Uterus)

Hypoplasia of the uterus is often more apparent than real and is probably not a true anomaly. It is sometimes, but by no means always, associated with relative infertility and various menstrual disorders. Such a diagnosis has customarily been made in the past when a tiny uterus with a cervical-fundal length ratio of 2:1 or 1:1 was encountered, instead of the normal 1:2 ratio of the mature adult female. Its significance, if any, is debatable. Most often, it is simply a reflection of ovarian inadequacy.

Congenital Absence or Hypoplasia of the Ovary

Bilateral absence of the ovaries is extremely rare. Occasionally, women are encountered in whom there is unilateral absence of the ovary, and this is nearly always associated with absence of the fallopian tube on the same side, with a normal uterus and normal adnexa on the opposite side. Presumably, an embryonic vascular accident of some type during gonadal descent best explains this abnormality, which is usually of no clinical significance.

Exstrophy of the Bladder

Although the genital tract in females is usually entirely normal, exstrophy of the bladder, which is primarily a musculoskeletal and urologic anomaly, results in a shift of the vaginal canal anteriorly into the suprapubic area. There is also poor support due to absence of the musculature of the lower abdominal wall and pelvic floor. Consequently, the development of uterine and vaginal prolapse may require surgical correction.

ANOMALIES DUE TO GENETIC OR FETAL ENDOCRINE DISORDERS; INTERSEX PROBLEMS

Our understanding of the true nature of genetic or fetal endocrine disorders, as well as the interrelationships between them, has grown rapidly in the past decade. In many, the individuals have features formerly regarded as hermaphroditic, and yet modern chromosomal studies indicate that such is not genetically the case, although clinically the problem of morphologic and functional intersexuality must frequently be dealt with in this group. The problem of meaningful classification by use of the old nomenclature becomes even more insoluble when one considers that congenital adrenal hyperplasia, which is responsible for 50 percent of all the cases of apparently abnormal sex differentiation, is in actuality a simple fetal endocrine disorder in a genetically and gonadally normal female (or male) with a basically normal reproductive tract. Further, with the aid of modern hormone therapy, it is potentially always reversible to the point of restoring normal genital tract function and fertility. The old terms **true hermaphroditism** and **female** and **male pseudohermaphroditism** have lost much of their significance and nearly all their meaning except as a traditional way of describing the more common clinical entities. It seems time to suggest that the qualifying adjectives **male** and **female** be eliminated, because it is becoming apparent that many, if not all, of these individuals are genetically and gonadally neither basically male nor basically female but are in fact something in between, having too many or too few sex chromosomes to be called more one than the other with accuracy. Finally, because of our present ability to determine the sex chromosomal status of these individuals, it is no longer necessary to utilize a purely descriptive classification that was rooted primarily in Greek mythology and completely sidestepped the question of fundamental nature and etiology.

Accordingly, in the subsequent discussion of these disorders, the common intersex problems of genetic origin will be presented as a group of separate syndromes, in most instances now eponyms, followed by the known fetal endocrine-metabolic disorders, the testicular feminization syndrome, and congenital adrenal hyperplasia. Where applicable, the old hermaphroditically oriented nomenclature formerly used will be indicated in parentheses after the name of each syndrome or disorder, primarily to serve as a point of reference for correlation with the older literature as well as with current and future communications in which the old terminology may continue to be employed.

Genetic Disorders Due to Sex Chromosome Abnormalities

GONADAL DYSGENESIS (THE BROAD SPECTRUM)

In normal gonadal genesis, the XX sex chromosome constitution is accompanied by the development of normal ovaries and a normal female genital tract and phenotype; the XY sex chromosome constitution is accompanied by the development of normal testes and a normal male genital tract and phenotype. A variety of abnormal sex chromosomal patterns leads to different degrees of abnormal gonadal development, or gonadal dysgenesis, the spectrum of which ranges from mere vestigial streaks of primitive stroma (usually accompanied by an XO sex chromosomal complement) to structures that may be thought of as hypoplastic ovaries (in association with abnormal "female" types of sex chromosome constitution, e.g., X—abnormal X and various mosaics such as XO/XX or XO/XX/XXX) or that may more properly be looked on as dysgenetic testes (in association with abnormal "male" types of sex chromosome patterns, e.g., X—abnormal Y and various mosaics such as XO/XY or XO/XYY). Thus, individuals with gonadal dysgenesis may have been potentially either female or male from a sex chromosomal—genetic standpoint. But a normally functioning testis is essential for repression of müllerian activity and development of the male genital tract and phenotype, and in its absence — and regardless of whether or not normal ovarian tissue is present — the development of the genital tract and the body configuration or phenotype will proceed along feminine lines. Thus, with rare exceptions (some patients with mixed gonadal dysgenesis and some patients with dysgenetic male pseudohermaphroditism), patients with the various forms of gonadal dysgenesis are generally phenotypic females, and the subject is of obvious importance to the gynecologist. Only the more frequently encountered major forms of gonadal dysgenesis will be discussed; the more obscure variants are extremely rare.

TURNER'S SYNDROME (GONADAL DYSGENESIS)

Turner's syndrome, formerly termed *ovarian agenesis* because its genetic origin in an underlying sex chromosomal abnormality had yet to be elucidated, is the most common clinical form of gonadal dysgenesis, occurring about once in every 10,000 normal female births. In this disorder there is complete aplasia, with all germ cells absent and no development of either the cortical or the medullary components of the gonads; the latter are represented only by thin streaks of fibrous connective tissue in the broad ligaments, the **streak gonads**. The presence of streak gonads is the characteristic feature of all forms of gonadal dysgenesis. In the case of Turner's syndrome, the accompanying short stature and frequently associated spectrum of congenital anomalies outside the pelvis set it apart as a distinct, readily recognizable clinical entity. The genetic abnormality in Turner's syndrome involves either complete absence or partial deletion of one X chromosome. It is now known that loss of the short arm of one X chromosome is the specific cause of the short stature and possibly a contributing factor in the other congenital malformations.

Turner's syndrome (and, much less often, some of the other variants of the abnormality of gonadal dysgenesis) and testicular feminization (see p. 106) are responsible for approximately 50 percent of all cases of primary amenorrhea in apparent females. The importance of performing a buccal smear for the determination of somatic nuclear sex chromatin type in any patient whose chief complaint is primary amenorrhea is therefore obvious. For, as previously noted, the most common chromosomal pattern (in 60 to 80 percent) associated with Turner's syndrome is 45-XO, yielding a negative sex chromatin pattern. In the other 20 to 40 percent, the pattern is either 46-X—abnormal X or a variety of mosaic types (e.g., XO/XX; XO/X—abnormal X), and the nuclear sex chromatin pattern is positive. However, the nuclear sex chromatin smear may yield clues to the presence of an abnormal X in the discovery of Barr bodies that are either smaller or larger than normal, or in the finding of a chromatin count that is intermediate between normal male (less than 2 percent) and normal female (greater than 20 percent). The chromosomal pattern for the testicular feminization syndrome is always a normal 46-XY, and therefore it, too, will be accompanied by a negative sex chromatin pattern. The two syndromes are usually readily distinguished from one another on more or less obvious clinical points but can be precisely differentiated in doubtful cases by the "squash smear" with chromosome count and analysis. In genetically normal females with primary amenorrhea on some other basis, the positive sex chromatin pattern of the normal female would be present on buccal smear; these patients are also invariably of normal height.

In addition to showing primary amenorrhea and other evidences of hypoestrinism (e.g., lack of breast development), patients with Turner's syndrome are of decidedly short stature (the majority being less than 4 feet 8 inches in height). As might be predicted, the müllerian duct system is usually normally developed, with uterus, tubes, and vagina present, though small due to lack of the growth-stimulating effects of estrogen; there are, however, only rudimentary fibrous tissue nubbins present in the anatomic location normally occupied by the gonads (ovaries). In general, these individuals continue to maintain a feminine appearance, although the lack of estrogen prevents the development of adult secondary sex characteristics. Rarely, although no true gonadal tissues or germinal cells are ever present, there may be functioning hilus cells in the rudimentary fibrous nubbins. In this case, hilus cell activity will occasionally be sufficient to produce hirsutism and even true virilization, with clitoral enlargement and a masculine habitus. Although this may result in a confusing clinical picture, the basic features of the syndrome remain the same, and diagnosis is still not difficult if these basic features are integrated with the results of a buccal smear ("squash smear" also, if available), and if culdoscopy, laparoscopy, or laparotomy reveals the typical internal genital appearance.

In addition to the anomalous genital tract due to the sex chromosomal disorder, these patients show a high incidence of other congenital anomalies elsewhere in the body: webbing of the neck; high, arched palate; deformed ears; low posterior hairline; cubitus valgus; shield chest, coarctation of the aorta and other cardiovascular defects; and kidney malformations. (With the exception of the typical short stature, these other anomalies probably arise on some basis other than the sex chromosomal aberration per se, for they are also seen in both males and females of normal sex chromosome pattern.) These patients are usually of normal intelligence.

A few cases of "unilateral gonadal dysgenesis" (female patients with many of the features of Turner's syndrome but with a streak gonad on one side and a normal or hypoplastic ovary on the other) have been reported. In all these patients there was essentially normal secondary sexual development at puberty, including the appearance of regular, ovulatory menstrual cycles. Ultimately, however, oligomenorrhea that progresses into complete, secondary amenorrhea or precocious menopause develops in the majority of these patients. It is also of interest that although in Turner's syndrome with the XO chromosome pattern, the patients have primary amenorrhea and are sterile, a few patients with the clinical features of Turner's syndrome but with the mosaic chromosome pattern XO/XX have exhibited menstrual activity and occasionally have been fertile. In an even less common variant of this disorder associated with either an XX or an XY chromosome pattern (Noonan's syndrome), the patient is relatively fertile, is often taller (e.g., 5 feet tall), and may have minor or no somatic abnormalities.

Diagnosis

The association of short stature with primary amenorrhea and poorly developed breasts, when accompanied by webbed neck, cubitus valgus, low-set ears, and the other somatic congenital abnormalities, frequently renders the diagnosis of gonadal dysgenesis obvious on clinical grounds alone. In infancy and early childhood, the condition may also be suspected by virtue of the multiple, characteristic anomalies present and the retarded growth rate, and in new-born infants, by a characteristic, diffuse lymphedema involving both upper and lower extremities. The nuclear sex chromatin pattern (usually negative) confirms it absolutely (however, the sex chromatin pattern in rare instances may be positive in the presence of mosaicism such as XO/XX); there is also frequently an elevation of the urinary pituitary gonadotropins after puberty. Culdoscopy, laparoscopy, or laparotomy to establish the nature of the pelvic organs and confirm the presence of gonadal agenesis is probably no longer necessary in any but the exceptional, doubtful case, as, for example, in a patient in whom hilus cell activity may have produced some virilization.

Treatment

Because these individuals are invariably of feminine psychological orientation and have a feminine appearance and functioning vagina, and because they have invariably been or will be easily raised as females, no problem arises as to assignment of sex. Treatment by cyclic hormone therapy with estrogen and progesterone not only produces the further development of normal female secondary sexual characteristics but also results in fairly normal, although artificially induced, cyclic menstrual function. Even in the face of absolute infertility, monthly menstrual flow may be of tremendous psychological import to the young woman. However, it is essential to postpone cyclic therapy until after epiphyseal closure and maximum growth have been obtained. (The use of estrogens except in small doses prior to this event will lead to premature epiphyseal closure and further depression of growth in a person already tending toward short stature.) An additional therapeutic measure consisting of the administration of one of the anabolic steroids, norethandrolone (Nilevar), has undergone trial and appears to increase considerably the skeletal growth rate and ultimate height attained.

Because the risk of malignancy developing in the dysgenetic gonads associated with Turner's syndrome (streak gonads in patients with a sex chromatin complement of 45-XO, 46-X—abnormal X, or any form of mosaicism not involving the presence of a Y chromosome) is apparently remote, surgical removal is not necessary or indicated. As discussed in the next section, the contrary is true for all forms of gonadal dysgenesis in which the sex chromosome constitution is XY or any form of mosaicism involving the presence of a Y chromosome.

PURE GONADAL DYSGENESIS

Far less common is the syndrome of pure gonadal dysgenesis in which streak gonads are present in phenotypic females who are of normal height and who lack the associated congenital anomalies and other stigmata of Turner's syndrome. These patients are also of normal intelligence and have good general health. Almost all of them prove to have a 46-XY (normal male) karotype and are correspondingly chromatin-negative. Rarely, a 46-XX complement or XO/XX and other more complex types of mosaicism have been seen, so that occasional individuals with the syndrome are chromatin-positive. The multiple occurrence of the XY form of pure gonadal dysgenesis in one or more sibships in the same family has frequently been recorded. This strong familial tendency (entirely similar in nature to that noted for the testicular feminization syndrome) suggests that it is a genetic disorder transmitted by ostensibly normal female carriers, with the abnormality either in an X-linked gene or in an autosomal dominant gene (abnormal autosomes have been noted in some of these patients) capable of expression only in chromosomal males. It is not known whether the abnormal genes directly suppress testis-determining loci on the Y chromosome or block some early stage of testicular development. In view of these features, the most common example of this syndrome has sometimes been termed **familial XY pure gonadal dysgenesis.**

Diagnosis

As in Turner's syndrome, these patients possess uteri and fallopian tubes (underdeveloped though they may be). They neither menstruate nor spontaneously undergo any pubertal changes. They completely lack any normal secondary sexual development, and the pituitary gonadotropin levels are usually elevated. However, their normal height and the absence of any of the other features of Turner's syndrome, together with the results of chromosomal analysis, make the distinction between the two syndromes an easy one.

At first glance, pure gonadal dysgenesis is more apt to be confused with the testicular feminization syndrome, to be described in more detail later. In both instances the disorders show a strong familial tendency, the general appearance is feminine, the patients are normal in height, there is failure of spontaneous menstrual function (the usual reason for seeking medical attention), and the karyotype is XY, with a negative nuclear sex chromatin pattern (always in testicular feminization, almost always in pure gonadal dysgenesis). However, here again, the differential diagnosis is usually readily made on the basis of several fundamental and obvious differences, as follows:

1. In patients with the testicular feminization syndrome, there has been a complete suppression of müllerian development in the embryo, and examination discloses

absence of the uterus and the fallopian tubes. Furthermore, although imperfectly developed and cryptorchid in location, functioning male gonads are present, **not** dysgenetic streak gonads. These imperfect testes are nevertheless capable of the normal secretion of both androgen and estrogen. However, because of the androgen insensitivity of the normal target tissues, the fetal external genital tract development is forced to take place along feminine lines, and only the effects of estrogen are manifested clinically later on when, with the onset of puberty, gonadal stimulation and secretion of both androgen and estrogen ensue. Thus these patients undergo pubertal changes with normal female secondary sexual transformation, including excellent breast development, and the pituitary gonadotropin levels are normal, as would be predicted. Furthermore, examination reveals normal vulvar and clitoral development and a normal lower vaginal tract, the result of estrogen acting on the normal female type of external genitalia formed during fetal life.

2. In contrast, in patients with pure gonadal dysgenesis, the uterus and fallopian tubes, though hypoplastic and infantile in type, are always found present on examination, and artificial menstrual flow can be induced by cyclic hormone administration. The fundamental and most distinguishing feature, however, is obviously the presence of the dysgenetic or streak gonads; these consist of undifferentiated embryonic stroma totally lacking in normal germ cells, ovarian or testicular elements, and hence incapable of the estrogen (or androgen) secretion required to initiate any normal pubertal events. (Laparotomy is usually necessary for confirmation of the presence of streak gonads as well as for proper treatment of the patient, as is discussed shortly.) Hence, these patients never undergo spontaneous puberty and exhibit minimal or complete lack of breast development. The basically female type of external genitalia remain infantile, but many of these patients tend toward a eunuchoid body build and frequently show mild degrees of virilization, with clitoral hypertrophy and a masculine type of hirsutism. The latter features are believed due to activity of the hilar Leydig cells usually present in dysgenetic gonads, for these virilizing manifestations tend to regress following the removal of the streak gonads and institution of cyclic estrogen-progesterone therapy.

Treatment

Once the diagnosis has been tentatively established, the first step in treatment involves laparotomy, both to confirm the diagnosis definitely and, of equal importance, to remove the abnormal streak gonads completely, usually with the accompanying fallopian tubes. Removal is strongly indicated because of the very frequent presence, or subsequent development, of malignancy in dysgenetic gonads, especially in patients with an XY chromosomal complement or any form of mosaicism involving the presence of a Y chromosome. Estimates of the incidence of malignant change have varied between 30 to 50 percent or higher. Gonadoblastomas and dysgerminomas are the tumors most often encountered, and they are frequently bilateral. Bilateral gonadectomy and salpingectomy, preserving the uterus, are also helpful in that they remove the source of hilar Leydig cell activity and will therefore usually cause at least partial regression of any tendency to hirsutism or virilization present.

Thereafter, cyclic estrogen-progesterone therapy is instituted to promote normal female secondary sexual development. With the uterus still present and intact, the resulting artificial menstrual cycles offer important psychological benefits to these young patients. Since they have invariably been reared as females, there is no problem in gender identity. Except for the absolute infertility, they are perfectly able psychologically, physiologically, and anatomically to function as normal adult females. Any abnormal uterine bleeding in these patients should be promptly investigated, since endometrial carcinoma is reported to have developed in several young women with gonadal dysgenesis after prolonged estrogen therapy. (For this reason, some advocate hysterectomy at the same time the dysgenetic gonads are removed in order to facilitate the safe use of long-term estrogen therapy in these women.)

MIXED GONADAL DYSGENESIS AND DYSGENETIC MALE PSEUDOHERMAPHRODITISM

Mixed gonadal dysgenesis and dysgenetic male pseudohermaphroditism are the two remaining, somewhat similar and obviously closely related forms within the broad spectrum of gonadal dysgenesis so far identified; both are rare. In mixed gonadal dysgenesis a streak gonad is found on one side and a poorly developed dysgenetic testis on the other. In dysgenetic male pseudohermaphroditism, bilateral dysgenetic testes are present. Thus, from the gonadal standpoint, these abnormalities are intermediate between gonadal dysgenesis with bilateral streak gonads on the one hand and true hermaphroditism with normal testicular and ovarian tissue on the other. As has been found true for all dysgenetic testicular tissue, gonadal tumors frequently develop in these patients.

In both disorders, testicular development is abnormal, and although the dysgenetic testes are capable of secreting androgen, the testicular inducer or the müllerian inhibitor factor is deficient, either in amount or embryonic timing. Hence müllerian duct suppression is minimal or absent, and wolffian duct stimulation as well as masculinization of the external genital tract is incomplete. Almost all these patients have a uterus and at least one fallopian tube, although occasionally a vas deferens will be present on one side. At birth, the partially masculinized external genitalia vary from an essentially female type, with clitoral hypertrophy, to an essentially male type, with or without hypospadias and cryptorchidism. At puberty, almost all these patients will undergo further virilization, with a masculine type of hirsutism, deep voice, and phallic enlargement. Clinically, these patients are thus either first recognized as newborns with ambiguous sexual development or are seen later in adolescence because of primary amenorrhea, or virilism, or both.

Both disorders are usually associated with XY/XO mosaicism, and hence patients with either abnormality are invariably chromatin-negative. This is a valuable diagnostic point in evaluating any patient, especially a newborn infant, who presents with ambiguous external genitalia and sexual development. For, as will presently be seen, in considering the two other most likely causes for sexual ambiguity, particularly in the newborn, it is helpful to remember that all patients with female pseudohermaphroditism (congenital adrenal hyperplasia in the female) and 80 percent of all true hermaphrodites are chromatin-positive.

The general approach to management of these and other disorders accompanied by ambiguous sexual differentiation is discussed in the final section of this chapter. However, in any case, treatment will include removal of the dysgenetic gonads because of the high rate of occurrence of gonadal tumors.

TRUE HERMAPHRODITISM

The occurrence of true hermaphroditism, or the presence of both ovarian and testicular tissue in the same individual, is rare. Such patients may be either chromatin-positive or chromatin-negative and present a chromosome pattern of either XX or XY, although recently the occurrence of mosaicism (e.g., XY/XO, XY/XX) has been reported in some true hermaphrodites. In actual fact, however, roughly 80 percent are chromatin-positive with an apparent 46-XX karyotype. There is now good evidence that the second X chromosome in these individuals probably contains the portion of a Y chromosome carrying loci normally determining testicular differentiation and that this transfer could have taken place during the meiotic divisions of gametogenesis, when the pairing of X and Y chromosome occurs. Thus, during spermatogenesis, an X spermatozoon containing a testis-determining factor could result, and the resulting 46-XX zygote would have genetic material capable of inducing both ovarian and testicular development. In the case of the less common mosaic forms, it is postulated that double fertilization occurred (two spermatozoa fertilizing two ova, or one ovum and its polar body), the resulting double zygote fusing to evolve into a true hermaphrodite instead of separating to form fraternal twins of opposite sex. As a result, in these individuals, either a testis or an ovotestis develops on one side and an ovary or an ovotestis on the other. Usually, the gonads remain in an intraabdominal position, but occasionally a testis may migrate to an inguinal or labioscrotal location.

Depending on the degree of function or malfunction of the gonads during both embryonic and postnatal life, the development of the internal and external genitalia and the subsequent endocrine status, body type, and probable parental choice of sex of rearing will vary considerably. Usually, a uterus is found, and at least one fallopian tube is present on the ovarian side; on the side of the testis there may be just a vas deferens, occasionally with an epididymis; or there may also be a second tube. Because the presence of functioning testicular tissue usually produces some degree of external genital tract masculinization, most of the true hermaphrodites have been reared as males. However, the external masculinization is rarely complete, and hypospadias and cryptorchidism are frequently present and serve as potential clues to the actual situation. Gynecomastia as well as ovulatory menstrual function usually appears at puberty in the majority of these patients. However, there is often nothing particularly characteristic about the obvious clinical manifestation in cases of true hermaphrodites that will absolutely distinguish them from the other, more common types of ambiguous sexual differentiation due to specific sex chromosomal abnormalities or congenital fetal endocrine disorders. Hence, a definite diagnosis can only be made by laparotomy (and/or inguinal and labioscrotal exploration in some cases), with biopsy and histologic study of gonadal tissue from any and all apparent gonads present, including careful bisection to assure that an ovotestis is not overlooked as a result of inadequate sampling.

It is important that the disorder be recognized as soon after birth as possible, so that the optimal choice of gender can be made and appropriate therapy begun early. Further discussion of the definitive treatment of true hermaphrodites will be covered in the concluding section in this chapter, in which the general principles of management of all the conditions associated with sexual ambiguity are discussed.

KLINEFELTER'S SYNDROME

Patients with Klinefelter's syndrome are phenotypic males, and the abnormality is therefore of no clinical significance to gynecologists. However, a brief summary of the salient features of the syndrome is of considerable academic interest, particularly since it is the commonest major chromosomal anomaly in masculine-appearing individuals (about 1 in every 1000 normal male births).

The syndrome was first described by Klinefelter, Reifenstein, and Albright in 1942 [18] and was felt to be due to acquired testicular atrophy, with resulting palpable small testes, sparse pubic hair, sterility, azospermia, gynecomastia, and even eunuchoidism. The associated increased urinary excretion of pituitary gonadotropins and decreased excretion of 17-ketosteroids was felt to complete the diagnostic picture. When, 15 years later, nuclear sex chromatin tests and actual chromosome analysis began to be done on patients with the syndrome, it was discovered, as previously discussed, that all these apparent males were chromatin-positive, and the majority had 47 chromosomes, with an XXY sex chromosome pattern. In some of the others, 48-XXXY, 48-XXYY, 49-XXXXY, and various mosaic chromosome patterns have been reported. The gonads are definitely male in type on microscopic examination but show atrophy and hyalinization of the seminiferous tubules, with complete absence of spermatogenesis but with normal interstitial or Leydig cells, sometimes increased in number. Mental deficiency is frequently an associated feature, and this has been shown to be consistently true of any of the sex chromosomal disorders that involve the presence of "too many" X chromosomes. Both external and internal genitalia are of the male type, and it is only following puberty that a tendency to eunuchoidism or even slight feminization (absent beard, high-pitched voice, gynecomastia, feminine fat distribution) occurs. Androgen therapy frequently corrects this and allows the individual to function normally as a male with the exception of the usually associated infertility. However, an occasional patient with an otherwise typical Klinefelter's syndrome has been fertile, possibly due to unrecognized mosaicism, with an XY as well as an XXY cell line.

"SUPERFEMALE" SYNDROME (TRIPLE-X AND POLY-X SYNDROMES)

Since the situation of triple-X chromosome pattern was known to occur in the fruit fly *Drosophilia,* it was postulated that a similar human sex chromosomal disorder might also exist. This hypothesis has subsequently been proved true, but the apparent females in which it has been discovered, far from being superior examples of femininity, have tended to be sexually infantile, with amenorrhea or infertility and underdeveloped external genitalia and breasts, as well as severely retarded mentally. In fact, the majority of such patients have been discovered in mental institutions. It is estimated that the condition occurs once in every 1000 normal female births, so that it is actually a common genetic abnormality, not accompanied by a recognizable clinical syndrome. Aside from a tendency to infantilism, the presence of the extra X chromosome does not appear to result in any major anatomic anomalies of the genital tract, presumably because of the capacity for functional suppression of X chromosomes when they are present in excess (Lyon hypothesis). This, of course, is in marked contrast to the severe adverse effects on embryonic development produced by autosomal trisomy.

Many of these women menstruate, although often abnormally, and some have been fertile; but as pointed out previously, the extra X chromosome is apparently responsible for the subnormal intelligence. The chromosome pattern is 47-XXX (a few examples of 48-XXXX have also been reported in patients with similar clinical characteristics), and the nuclear sex chromatin pattern is positive but with two (or three) Barr bodies visible in the cells of a buccal smear.

XYY AND RELATED YY SYNDROMES

Sex chromosomal surveys carried out on male populations in prisons and mental institutions have uncovered another male sex chromosomal disorder, the YY syndrome. The majority have been XYY, though a few XXYY or XXXYY have been found. This chromosomal abnormality was originally linked with violent criminal and antisocial behavior, high-grade mental retardation, and excessive height, two-thirds or more of those affected being over 6 feet tall. Aside from tallness, no other distinguishing physical characteristics are usually present, though a tendency to persistent acne and to a slightly increased frequency of genitourinary anomalies has been mentioned in some reports.

As more routine population studies are made, it becomes apparent that the YY syndrome may represent one of the more common sex chromosome disorders. The observed incidence in recent surveys of over 46,000 unselected newborns places its probable frequency at 1 per 1000 live-born male infants. More recent ongoing studies of these individuals suggest that although they are impulsive and overreact to both internal and external environmental stimuli (poor impulse control or decreased ability to restrain themselves), the majority, in fact, do not actually exhibit criminal or out-and-out antisocial behavior. Many are apparently of normal intelligence, and only a small percentage are confined in penal or mental institutions.

Genetic Disorders Due to Fetal Endocrine-Metabolic Abnormalities

TESTICULAR FEMINIZATION OR ANDROGEN INSENSITIVITY SYNDROME (MALE PSEUDOHERMAPHRODITISM)

Testicular feminization (androgen insensitivity) syndrome is another form of male pseudohermaphroditism, also familial in type. Originally it was believed to be a form of gonadal dysgenesis. However, it is now known to be a fetal endocrine-metabolic disorder in which there is usually a complete, occasionally a partial, androgen insensitivity on the part of target tissues and organs that should be responding to the normal secretions of the fetal testes in such a manner as to result in the development of a normal male. Because this response is not forthcoming, and despite the fact that there is no sex chromosomal disorder (these individuals have a genetically normal male XY karyotype), patients with this disorder are characterized by a female phenotype, complete absence of female internal genitalia, and cryptorchid testes as gonads. The differentiation of this syndrome from XY pure gonadal dysgenesis and dysgenetic male pseudohermaphroditism has already been presented.

Appearance

Most of these individuals are completely feminine in external appearance, are of normal height, have normal fat deposits and breast tissue (sometimes underdeveloped), have sparse or absent pubic and axillary hair, exhibit normal female external genitalia but have a vagina that is shorter than normal and ends in a blind pouch. The gonads are not dysgenetic in the true sense at all and often grossly resemble testes, although invariably they contain only rudimentary testicular tissue in which spermatogenesis is absent but in which tubular adenomas and other testicular neoplasms sometimes develop. These gonads may be located either intraabdominally or within the inguinal canals. Neither müllerian nor wolffian maturation occurs, and the internal genital tract is either completely absent or represented only by rudimentary structures. As previously mentioned, the sex chromosome pattern is XY, with a total chromosome count of 46. There is a strong familial tendency, and the disorder is probably genetic in origin, though a definite sex chromosomal disorder has not been identified. It seems more likely that a sex-linked recessive or sex-linked autosomal dominant factor is involved. The nuclear sex chromatin pattern is negative; this fact, together with the clinical picture, suggests the diagnosis, but confirmation by laparotomy is usually necessary.

It was initially assumed that the "dysgenetic" male gonads in this syndrome secreted estrogen and little or no androgen, thus accounting for both the female and phenotype (with absence of male internal genitalia and feminization of the external genital tract present at birth) as well as for the subsequent appearance of female secondary sexual characteristics at puberty (for example, the breast development is often strikingly normal). However, recent steroid analyses of gonadal venous blood as well as incubation studies of gonadal tissue from a number of patients with testicular feminization have clearly shown that **both** androgens and estrogens are secreted, and androgen levels are as high as those of normal male controls. Furthermore, the fact that embryonic müllerian duct development in these patients is completely suppressed strongly suggests that the fetal gonads were capable from the start of secreting not only androgens but also the "müllerian inhibiting factor" (müllerian regressor). The latter has been identified as a polypeptide secreted by normal fetal testes that acts entirely independently of fetal androgens and appears essential for both müllerian suppression and wolffian duct stimulation. (Androgen excretion alone is incapable of müllerian duct suppression and has only a partial effect on wolffian duct development; however, androgen secretion alone is capable of causing masculine development of the embryonic external genital tubercle.)

Thus it appears more likely that the syndrome of testicular feminization is the result of an end-organ insensitivity to androgen rather than of an absence of circulating androgens. The precise mechanism of this tissue nonresponsiveness is not yet clear. However, recent work suggests that this failure to respond to circulating androgen (primarily testosterone) on the part of the various target organs (wolffian duct structures [vas deferens, seminal vesicles, epididymis], as well as prostate, penis, breast, hair follicles, larynx, and so on) may be the result of inability at the cellular level in the local tissue sites to convert testosterone into the biologically active androgen dihydrotestosterone, and that this inability is due to the inherited lack of a specific 17-ketosteroid reductase enzyme. In the face of androgen insensitivity in the tissues of the internal and external genitalia, as well as in the secondary sex organs and other accessory sex-linked structures, the effect of estrogen secretion dominates the picture, and feminization results.

These individuals, too, are both morphologically and psychologically oriented as females and, except for absolute infertility, can function satisfactorily as such and are usually anxious to do so. Because of the significant incidence (4 to 10 percent or more) of malignant change in these "imperfect testes," the abnormal gonads should be removed surgically after puberty, following which these patients will also require cyclic estrogen therapy. The vaginal pouch is usually of adequate length for satisfactory function and will elongate further with regular intercourse, so vaginal reconstruction is rarely necessary.

It is possible that excessive amounts of estrogen present during the crucial embryologic period of genital tract development may occasionally be the mechanism involved in the pathogenesis of this syndrome. A similar type of sexual anomaly has been produced in the offspring of pregnant laboratory animals by the administration of estrogen during early pregnancy. Furthermore, a few instances of its presence at birth in human infants born of mothers who had received large doses of estrogen during the critical phase of fetal gonadal differentiation have also been reported. In this respect, the situation is exactly analogous to the iatrogenic masculinization of the female fetus, which may follow the maternal administration of androgens or progestins with androgenic activity and which simulates congenital adrenal hyperplasia (female pseudohermaphroditism).

Finally, it should be noted that not all patients with this syndrome are feminized, although the majority seem to be, and obviously those seeking advice from a gynecologist invariably are. Some have either partially or completely male-appearing external genitalia, with either a male or female type of internal genitalia, have gynecomastia at puberty, and have been raised as males. Possibly these patients suffer from partial degrees of androgen insensitivity, or perhaps there was an initial partial response to androgens coupled with deficiency of the müllerian inhibiting factor during early fetal life. In these cases, efforts at treatment should be directed along lines that will permit the patient to continue in the male gender role already assumed and to function as satisfactorily as possible as a male. (This treatment may involve repair of hypospadias, orchiopexy, gonadectomy, androgen therapy, and occasionally mastectomy.) In many instances, sexual function is possible, although affected persons are, of course, sterile. This special category is sometimes referred to as the Reifenstein syndrome, or as the "incomplete form" of the testicular feminization syndrome.

CONGENITAL ADRENAL HYPERPLASIA, OR CONGENITAL ADRENOGENITAL SYNDROME (FEMALE PSEUDOHERMAPHRODITISM)

Although congenital adrenal hyperplasia may affect males (in whom it produces a precocious and overvirilizing type of masculine puberty), it is most commonly seen and recognized in newborn females. When it is mild in degree, the gross anatomic genital abnormalities may be so minimal that the condition is not recognized until later in childhood or at puberty. (An acquired form also developing later in life exists but is more often due to tumor than to hyperplasia.) It is an important entity, because it is responsible for about 50 percent of all cases of apparently ambiguous sexual differentiation and because it is nearly always correctable.

There is a strong familial tendency (the disorder has even been reported to occur in identical twins), and the condition is undoubtedly genetic in origin, but the sex chromosome and nuclear sex chromatin patterns are always normal female in type i.e., 46-XX and chromatin-positive. (When it is encountered in males, the 46-XY and chromatin negative patterns are just as uniformly present.)

At birth, the characteristic anatomic abnormality consists of clitoral enlargement, sometimes to the point of simulating the penis of a newborn male, with a varying amount of apparent hypospadias, so that the urethra opens directly into the vaginal canal at a level somewhat higher than the usual site of the normal female urethral meatus, creating the effect of a partial urogenital sinus (Fig. 22). This is often accompanied by varying degrees of vulvar ("labioscrotal") fusion. Rarely, the urethra may actually be phallic in type, and the infant or child may be mistakenly assumed to be a bilaterally cryptorchid male unless a nuclear sex chromatin study is done. The uterus, tubes, ovaries, and upper vagina are invariably normal, so that it is obvious that an abnormal androgenic hormone stimulus during the critical phase of the development of the external urogenital tract has been at work in an otherwise normally developing female embryo. If untreated, the newborn child will subsequently exhibit manifestations of continuing excessive androgenic stimulation: increased growth rate; increasing signs of virilization, including progressively enlarging phallus formation or clitoral hypertrophy; and markedly elevated urinary 17-ketosteroid excretion.

Since the gonads are normal ovaries, both histologically and functionally, the source of the androgens in the spontaneous form of the disease is known to be the fetal adrenals. The mechanism for the excessive secretion of androgens by the fetal adrenals is an indirect one and involves a basic biochemical defect, with lack of the proper enzyme system (probably a deficiency in the hydroxylating enzymes, especially 21-hydroxylase) to complete the synthesis of hydrocortisone and related adrenal steroid compounds. As a result of the low levels of hydrocorticoids, the fetal pituitary attempts to promote their production further by the liberation of

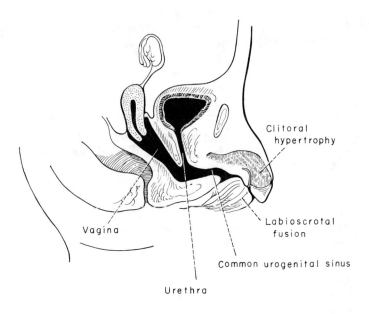

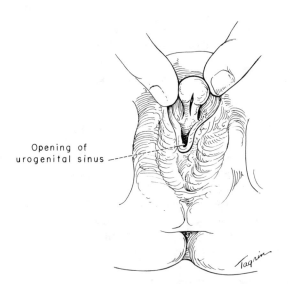

Figure 22
Diagram of the typical urogenital tract anomaly encountered in congenital adrenal hyperplasia of the female (female pseudohermaphroditism).

increasingly larger amounts of adrenocorticotropic hormone (ACTH). Although the adrenal is still unable to respond with the formation of hydrocorticoids, hyperplasia does result, with increased production of other adrenal steroids and, in particular, precursors of compounds with androgenic activity (Fig. 23A). Apparently the embryologic timing is such that this usually occurs or has its maximum effect during the maturation of the external urogenital tract but after the normal gonadal and müllerian duct development has taken place. Following birth, the abnormal androgen production continues to increase, with progressively more pronounced virilization of the infant.

Dangerous electrolyte disturbances of a salt-losing type may also develop in these infants because of the frequently associated deficiency of the enzymatic mechanism (again involving 21-hydroxylase and possibly other hydroxylating enzymes) required for the production of adrenal hormones such as desoxycorticosterone and aldosterone, which are concerned with electrolyte metabolism. An addisonian type of crisis may occasionally be encountered, with vomiting, diarrhea, dehydration, and circulatory collapse in acute adrenal insufficiency with the typical low-sodium, high-potassium serum electrolyte disturbance. Since such a course of events is often fatal, it becomes extremely important to bear this possibility in mind in newborns with this genital anomaly, to anticipate and prevent it if possible, and to treat it early, correctly, and vigorously should it appear.

Diagnosis

The diagnosis is based on the presence of the typical anatomic configuration in a female infant showing a normal positive nuclear sex chromatin pattern on buccal smear and with an elevated urinary excretion of 17-ketosteroids, which, however, will not consistently be increased until after two or three weeks of life. Cystoscopic examination of both the urethra and vagina, and the vaginal introduction of radiopaque dye for the purpose of x-ray visualization for definite confirmation of the presence of a vagina, are frequently very helpful maneuvers in the recognition of the characteristic external urogenital anomaly in newborn infants and young children. In the older child, pelvic or rectal examination will confirm the presence of an essentially normal vagina, cervix, and uterus. In the face of this clinical picture, laparotomy to determine the status of the gonads or internal genital tract should rarely be necessary.

Treatment

Treatment with cortisone or any of the related corticosteroid preparations now available is usually dramatically successful. The administered corticoids substitute for the endogenous failure of the adrenals to produce them in natural form; the excessive ACTH formation and adrenal stimulation are suppressed, and the production of androgens promptly falls to normal levels (Fig. 23B). If the 17-ketosteroid excretion levels do not fall rapidly, the possibility that an adrenal cortical tumor is present should be considered, although this is rare. If an associated electrolyte disturbance is also present, this must be corrected by the administration of desoxycorticosterone,

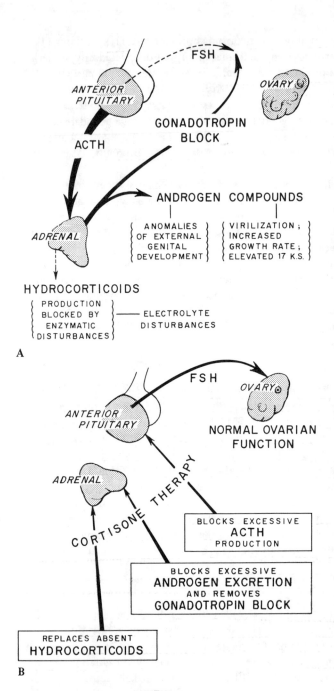

Figure 23
Congenital adrenal hyperplasia. A. Biochemical mechanisms involved in pathogenesis. B. Biochemical mechanisms involved in successful therapy.

and careful attention must be paid to sodium, potassium, and fluid balance in these young, particularly vulnerable patients. Continued lifelong maintenance on cortisone will result in subsequent normal growth and development, normal puberty and adolescence, and continued normal ovarian function in adult life. Ovulation, normal estrogen and progesterone production, fertility, normal pregnancy, and delivery can be anticipated in most instances, though the menarche appears to be somewhat delayed in some patients.

The external genital anomaly itself can of course be corrected only by an appropriate operative procedure. This ordinarily consists of relatively minor local surgery and will usually include a total resection of the phallus and a simple vulvovaginal plastic operation to restore the normal female relationship between the urethra and the vaginal canal. The best psychological results for both the patient and her family are achieved when the operation is performed early, usually at around 18 months of age, before the child develops an awareness of the genitalia and gender role and after she has grown sufficiently to permit easy identification of the vaginal canal, so that it can be properly exteriorized at the time of surgery.

MASCULINIZATION OF THE FEMALE FETUS BY ADMINISTRATION OF ANDROGENIC HORMONES TO THE MOTHER

An iatrogenic type of "female pseudohermaphroditism" has recently been encountered and is being recognized with increasing frequency. The condition is characterized by the presence of the identical external genital anomalies seen in the true congenital form of adrenal hyperplasia, but with a different etiologic mechanism. Adrenal function is entirely normal, the source of the abnormal androgens temporarily present during early fetal life being the administration of certain steroid hormones with androgenic activity to the mother during the early months of the pregnancy. Obviously, testosterone itself might be expected to have this effect, but certain progestational agents frequently employed in the management of women with symptoms of a past history of threatened or habitual abortion and usually administered during the first two or three months after conception have been definitely incriminated. These close chemical relatives of testosterone known to have produced this picture include progesterone itself, if given at the right time and in large doses, members of the 17-ethinyl testosterone group, such as Enovid, and nortestosterone compounds, such as Norluton or Norlutate, all of which are used primarily for their progestational effects. Rarely, large doses of estrogens given prenatally may result in masculinization of the female fetus; the mechanism is not clear, but estrogen may well act indirectly, stimulating the fetal adrenal in some manner to cause excessive androgen production. (It has already been noted that large doses of estrogen given to the mother may cause feminization of the masculine fetus, but in this case the mechanism seems more obvious.) Even more rarely, a maternal arrhenoblastoma or other androgen-producing ovarian tumor, luteoma or theca lutein cyst, or a virilizing adrenal tumor might result in masculinization of the female fetus through the same mechanisms, and such cases are occasionally reported.

These iatrogenically masculinized infants do not show any further tendencies to virilization or abnormalities of growth and development, nor is there any disturbance of electrolyte balance. The diagnosis rests primarily on the finding of a normal 17-ketosteroid urinary excretion, a normal female sex chromatin pattern, and, of course, a history of prenatal administration of any of the compounds mentioned. Because adrenal function is actually normal, no hormone therapy of any kind is necessary, and normal subsequent growth and development are assured. Again, minor vaginal plastic surgery will be indicated to correct the external urogenital anomalies.

It should be noted that only a minority of women receiving prenatal steroid therapy will give birth to infants with masculinized external genitalia. Whether or not this simply reflects the critical role of dosage and timing, or whether some abnormality of maternal metabolism or placental permeability to these steroid compounds must also be presumed, is not clear. At any rate, the possibility should by no means be construed as a contraindication to the proper use of supportive steroid hormone therapy during pregnancy in diabetic women or other women with progestational deficiencies who might otherwise not carry successfully to term. Caution is indicated, however, particularly when some of the newer, more potent, more androgenic compounds are employed, and careful consideration should be given to details of dosage as well as timing, perhaps avoiding their use until after the tenth or twelfth week of pregnancy.

The Management of Intersex Problems

It is apparent that several different disorders may result in ambiguous sexual development. To recapitulate, these include true hermaphrodites, the majority of patients with mixed gonadal dysgenesis, most patients with dysgenetic male pseudohermaphroditism, most patients with congenital adrenal hyperplasia (female pseudohermaphroditism), and some patients with the testicular feminization syndrome (familial male pseudohermaphroditism). Once a definite diagnosis has been established, a decision regarding the optimal management must be made for each patient. Except in the case of congenital adrenal hyperplasia, fertility can never be restored, and thus the chief goal of treatment will be to create the endocrine and anatomic foundation for as satisfactory function as possible later on as either a male or a female. The success of treatment in turn depends primarily on an intelligent decision as to which gender should be assigned.

In making this decision in the infant, the sex chromatin pattern (or genetic or chromosomal sex) is of little significance. Far more important is the anatomic configuration and potential functional capacity of the external genitalia. If they are essentially male in type, with an adequate phallus, then regardless of the chromosomal sex, the child should be reared as a male. Having reached this decision, further treatment will involve removal of all ovarian tissue and any other undesirable female internal structures (this may require complete removal of all gonads in the case of ovotestis formation, though at times the testicular and ovarian components can be separately dissected and one or the other preserved) and surgical repair of any external genital defects such as hypospadias or bifid scrotum that might interfere with the normal male outward appearance and function. It is important to remove all nonconforming gonadal tissue, lest it function at puberty and produce undesirable feminization or masculinization. On the other hand, if the external genitalia are essentially female in type, with a vagina present, then similar surgery to make the internal gonadal picture conform, if possible (otherwise, gonadal removal), and excision of a phallus, if present, should be done, and the infant raised as a female. In either case, appropriate substitution hormone therapy (androgenic or estrogenic) will be indicated at puberty to assure the development of as nearly normal secondary sex characteristics and sexual function as possible. Ideally, the decision and necessary surgical transformations should be completed before the age of 1½ to 2 years; after that time, an attempt at reversal of the already parentally assigned sex of rearing, if it differs from the optimal gender role dictated by the external genital tract configuration, will usually create extremely serious psychological problems.

In the older child or young adult, the sex of rearing or psychologically assumed gender role will play the dominant role in the decision as to therapy, and attempts to reverse either should rarely if ever be made. Both surgical and hormone therapy should consist of procedures and medication that might help the patient function more effectively sexually, physically, and psychologically in the gender role already assumed.

In summary, then, there are basically six aspects to sex determination in the broad, total sense: the chromosomal pattern (genetic); the three morphologic factors (the status of the gonads and the anatomic configuration of the internal and external genital tracts); the endocrine pattern (hormonal status); and, finally, the psychological orientation (the sex of rearing or spontaneously assumed gender role). In the normal female or male, all conform with each other. In the person with an intersex problem or ambiguous sexual differentiation, one or more of these six aspects fail to conform with the others to a greater or lesser extent. In the case of congenital adrenal hyperplasia of the female (female pseudohermaphroditism), the disharmony is often minimal: the genetic sex, the internal genitalia, and the gonads are normally female. Because the endocrine disorder is reversible, the hormonal status and reproductive capacity can also be brought into line with proper therapy. The external genitalia are also basically female, except for the phallic enlargement, and this can be corrected by simple plastic surgery. Finally, if the phallic enlargement is pronounced, medical advice and treatment are sought early; if it is not, most of these children are raised as females, and hence there is rarely, if ever, any psychological conflict in the matter of gender role, regardless of the age at which therapy is undertaken. At the other extreme are the true hermaphrodites and the various other intersex disorders in which there may be profound disharmony among the six basic aspects of sex determination, with no possibility of bringing more than two or three of them into conformity and usually no hope of restoring fertility. In these situations, as already emphasized, the functional potential of the external genitalia and, if the patient is beyond 2 years of age, the psychological orientation are the two key factors to be considered in deciding which will be the most satisfactory permanent gender role for the patient to assume. Once this decision has been made, additional treatment to bring as many of the other modifiable factors into conformity as possible can be done, whether it be surgery on the gonads or internal genital tract, plastic reconstructions of the external genitalia, or hormone substitution therapy. In any case, in the older patient who has already assumed a gender role, the psychological orientation will almost without exception be the sole determining factor in gender assignments, regardless of the status of the external genitalia. These basic principles apply with equal force to the problems of management of either "true" hermaphrodites or "pseudohermaphrodites."

It is perhaps obvious, but should nevertheless be emphasized, that these fundamental genetic disorders of ambiguous sexual development are entirely unrelated to the purely psychological disorders of sexual ambiguity such as transsexualism, transvestism, homosexuality, and neurotic or psychotic problems accompanied by confusion or anxiety regarding sexual identity. All of these occur in persons whose chromosomal, anatomic, and endocrinologic status are completely in accord and entirely consistent with one or the other sex. A detailed consideration of these purely psychological ambiguities in sexual development and role fulfillment are beyond the scope of this textbook, but an excellent summary of the problem, especially of the role the gynecologist may play in the treatment of male transsexualism, has been prepared by Jones, Money, and Meyer [14].

REFERENCES

1. Baker, D., Telfer, M. A., Richardson, C. E., and Clark, G. R. Chromosome errors in men with antisocial behavior. *J.A.M.A.* 214:869, 1970.
2. Barakat, B. Y., and Jones, H. W., Jr. Gynecologic and cytogenetic aspects of gonadal agenesis and dysgenesis. *Obstet. Gynecol.* 36:368, 1970.
3. Barr, M. L. Some notes on the discovery of the sex chromatin and its clinical application. *Am. J. Obstet. Gynecol.* 112:293, 1972.
4. Barr, M. L., and Bertram, E. G. A morphological distinction between neurones of the male and female. *Nature* (London) 163:676, 1949.
5. Barr, M. L., Segovich, F. R., Carr, D. H., and Shaver, E. L. The triple-X female: An appraisal based on a study of 12 cases and a review of the literature. *Can. Med. Assoc. J.* 101:247, 1969.
6. Boczkowski, K., Teter, J., and Sternadel, Z. Sibship occurrence of XY gonadal dysgenesis with dysgerminoma. *Am. J. Obstet. Gynecol.* 113:952, 1972.
7. Buttram, V. C., Jr., Zanotti, L., Acosta, A. A., Vanderheyden, J. S., Besch, P. K., and Franklin, R. R. Surgical correction of the septate uterus. *Fertil. Steril.* 25:373, 1974.
8. Carr, D. H. Chromosomal errors and development. *Am. J. Obstet. Gynecol.* 104:327, 1969.
9. Dewhurst, C. J. The XY female. *Am. J. Obstet. Gynecol.* 109:675, 1971.
10. Farber, M., and Marchant, D. J. Congenital absence of the uterine cervix. *Am. J. Obstet. Gynecol.* 121:414, 1975.
11. Federman, D. D. *Abnormal Sexual Development: A Genetic and Endocrine Approach to Differential Diagnosis.* Philadelphia and London: Saunders, 1967.

12. Greenblatt, R. B., Byrd, J. R., McDonough, P. G., and Mahesh, V. B. The spectrum of gonadal dysgenesis. *Am. J. Obstet. Gynecol.* 98:151, 1967.
13. Heine, M. W., Fontana, J., Jr., and Green, J. R., Jr. Mosaicism in patients with secondary amenorrhea or oligomenorrhea. *Am. J. Obstet. Gynecol.* 113:119, 1972.
14. Jones, H. W., Jr., Money, J. W., Jr., and Meyer, J. K. An Appraisal of the Role of the Gynecologist in the Treatment of Male Transsexualism. In J. P. Greenhill (Ed.), *Year Book of Obstetrics and Gynecology.* Chicago: Year Book, 1972.
15. Jones, H. W., Jr., and Verkauf, B. S. Surgical treatment in congenital adrenal hyperplasia. *Obstet. Gynecol.* 36:1, 1970.
16. Jones, H. W., Jr., and Verkauf, B. S. Congenital adrenal hyperplasia. *Am. J. Obstet. Gynecol.* 109:292, 1971.
17. Jones, H. W., Jr., and Wheeless, C. R. Salvage of the reproductive potential of women with anomalous development of the müllerian ducts. *Am. J. Obstet. Gynecol.* 104:348, 1969.
18. Klinefelter, H. F., Jr., Reifenstein, E. C., Jr., and Albright, F. Syndrome characterized by gynecomastia, aspermatogenesis, without A-leydigism, and increased excretion of follicle stimulating hormone. *J. Clin. Endocrinol.* 2:615, 1942.
19. Lewis, B. V., and Brant, H. A. Obstetric and gynecologic complications associated with müllerian duct abnormalities. *Obstet. Gynecol.* 28:315, 1966.
20. McDonough, P. G., Byrd, J. R., and Freedman, M. A. Gonadal dysgenesis with ovarian function. *Obstet. Gynecol.* 37:868, 1971.
21. Moore, K. L., and Barr, M. L. Smears from the oral mucosa in the detection of chromosomal sex. *Lancet* 2:57, 1955.
22. Morris, J. M., and Mahesh, V. B. Further observations on syndrome, "testicular feminization." *Am. J. Obstet. Gynecol.* 87:731, 1963.
23. Park, I. J., Jones, H. W., Jr., and Bias, W. B. True hermaphroditism with 46,XX/46,XY chromosome complement. *Obstet. Gynecol.* 36:377, 1970.
24. Price, W. H., Strong, J. A., Whatmore, P. B., and McClemont, W. F. Criminal patients with XYY sex chromosome complement. *Lancet* 1:565, 1966.
25. Riddick, D. H., and Hammond, C. B. Long term steroid therapy in patients with adrenogenital syndrome. *Obstet. Gynecol.* 45:15, 1975.
26. Schellhas, H. F. Malignant potential of the dysgenetic gonad. *Obstet. Gynecol.* 44:298, 1974, Part I; 44:455, 1974, Part II.
27. Scully, R. E. Gonadoblastoma: Review of 74 cases. *Cancer* 25:1340, 1970.
28. Slotnick, E. A., and Goldfarb, A. F. Unilateral streaked ovary syndrome. *Obstet. Gynecol.* 39:269, 1972.
29. Sternberg, W. H., Barclay, D. L., and Kloepfer, H. W. Familial XY gonadal dysgenesis. *N. Engl. J. Med.* 278:695, 1968.
30. Strassman, E. O. Fertility and unification of double uterus. *Fertil. Steril.* 17:165, 1966.
31. Teter, J. Prognosis, malignancy, and curability of the germ-cell tumor occurring in dysgenetic gonads. *Am. J. Obstet. Gynecol.* 108:894, 1970.
32. Weisberg, M. G., Malkasian, G. D., and Pratt, J. H. Testicular feminization syndrome. *Obstet. Gynecol.* 39:269, 1972.
33. Wilkins, L., Jones, H. W., Jr., Holman, G. H., and Stempfel, R. S., Jr. Masculinization of the female fetus associated with administration of oral and intramuscular progestins during gestation: Non-adrenal female pseudo-hermaphroditism. *J. Clin. Endocrinol.* 18:559, 1958.
34. Williams, E. A. A Simple Method of Vaginal Construction. In M. L. Taymor and T. H. Green, Jr. (Eds.), *Progress in Gynecology,* Vol. VI. New York: Grune & Stratton, 1975. Pp. 671–687.

35. Wilson, J. D., Harrod, M. J., and Goldstein, J. L. Familial incomplete male pseudo-hermaphroditism, type 1. *N. Engl. J. Med.* 290:1097, 1974.
36. Zourlas, P. A. Surgical treatment of malformations of the uterus. *Surg. Gynecol. Obstet.* 141:57, 1975.

4
Gynecologic Problems in Infancy, Childhood, and Adolescence

Largely because the female reproductive tract normally remains anatomically immature and functionally inactive during infancy and the childhood years before puberty, pelvic disorders are relatively uncommon in this age group. Aside from the various congenital anomalies already discussed, some of which have important manifestations at this time in life, many of the problems are relatively trivial and include primarily minor vulvovaginal inflammations, either infectious in origin or due to trauma or the presence of vaginal foreign bodies. Less frequently, serious disease may be present, either in the form of one of the rare but often highly malignant childhood tumors or secondary to one of the fundamental endocrine disturbances occasionally encountered in infants and children. In any case, symptoms referred to the genital tract in the young child, regardless of their origin, are extremely disquieting to the parents, and the gynecologist must sympathetically accept the responsibility for parental care and reassurance as well as for the diagnosis and treatment of the disorder present in the young female patient herself.

During the adolescent years the situation changes coincident with the menarche and the beginnings of a more adult anatomic and physiologic maturation. Functional activity of the ovaries, so recently awakened from their long state of relative dormancy, is sometimes inadequate and imperfect during the transition, and menstrual irregularities are not uncommon during this period in life. (They appear again with increased frequency at the time of the menopause, during the years of reverse transition from normal, full-blown adult activity to the final state of dormancy.) Menstrual disorders of a functional type thus account for most of the gynecologic problems encountered in adolescent females. Although any of the pelvic diseases that afflict the mature woman may also appear, they are, in general, uncommon during adolescence.

SPECIAL POINTS REGARDING PELVIC EXAMINATION AND GENERAL MANAGEMENT IN INFANTS AND CHILDREN

As should be the rule in carrying out pelvic examination on females of any age, a nurse or female attendant should be present, but preferably not the mother, who usually volunteers. The history will probably be obtained primarily from the mother, but the child should be present, and when old enough should be frequently included in the conversation during the interview, so that a definite physician-patient relationship can be established before she enters the examining room. The child will usually be more relaxed and at ease during the examination without the mother present, and the mother will be spared the sometimes disturbing psychological effects of witnessing the examination of her young daughter, the impact of which she frequently unwittingly transmits to the little patient, with disastrous results.

Following a careful general examination, which can usually be kept brief and straightforward, evaluation of the pelvis can then be accomplished as casually as possible by abdominal and suprapubic palpation (to detect the occasional large ovarian cyst or tumor or the rare uterine neoplasm), followed by inspection of the external genitalia (in search of signs of inflammation, anomalies, or endocrine disturbances), and finally by rectal examination in either the lithotomy or Sims position (preferably the former) to detect the presence of palpable adnexal or uterine abnormalities.

When vaginal infections or foreign bodies are suspected on the basis of symptoms and the physical findings thus far, the infant or child may be placed in either the lithotomy or knee-chest position, in which actual visual examination of the vaginal canal is frequently possible using either a small vaginal or ear speculum, a small proctoscope, or even a cystoscope or female urethroscope. Material for smears and cultures may be obtained directly at this time and the vagina gently probed with a blunt metal sound (simultaneous rectal palpation may be of help in this maneuver) to determine the presence of a foreign body, which can then usually be extracted with a small clamp or forceps. It should not be forgotten that urinary tract infections may give rise to pelvic symptoms, and a clean-catch urine specimen for analysis and culture is frequently helpful in this regard and usually readily obtained. Only rarely, when these office examination techniques cannot be satisfactorily carried out or have failed to explain completely the presence of bleeding or other symptoms and signs of a potentially serious condition, will examination under anesthesia be necessary or indicated.

When the examination has been completed and while the child is dressing, the findings and the nature of the diagnosis, which is usually now apparent, should be explained to the parent or parents. Reassurance must be given liberally and all their unfounded fears and suspicions allayed. The mother should be especially cautioned against persistent questioning of the child and examination of her genital area at home during the treatment phase, if any. The parents should be strongly urged to adopt a casual attitude about what is usually a trivial problem, to avoid any possibility of undesirable psychological side effects in the child or child-parent relationship. For the same reason, repeated follow-up visits to the physician's office or clinic should also be discouraged and avoided. For, in spite of the physician's reassurance, these serve only to fix in the minds of both child and parents the belief that a serious and unpleasant disorder exists, when in fact the condition is usually transient and inconsequential and invariably responds rapidly to simple therapy or requires none at all. It goes without saying that when she rejoins her parents in the consulting room, the child herself, if old enough to comprehend, should also be fully reassured in a matter-of-fact way, with a simple, brief explanation of the symptoms and the plan of treatment, if any is required. Both child and parents should leave with the idea firmly implanted that all is essentially well, that what is a minor problem will respond quickly to simple management, and that no future problems are to be anticipated. On the extremely rare occasions when a serious disorder is found, usually one requiring hospitalization for study and treatment, the approach will obviously have to be entirely different.

GYNECOLOGIC PROBLEMS IN INFANCY AND CHILDHOOD

In addition to the congenital anomalies described in Chapter 3, certain other diseases, abnormalities, or general types of symptomatology are seen often enough and either are of sufficient importance to require therapy or are significant from the standpoint of the differential diagnosis of the rarely encountered more serious conditions to warrant consideration in some detail. Particular attention will be paid to those occurring almost exclusively in infancy or childhood.

Vulvovaginal Conditions

LABIAL AGGLUTINATION (LABIAL ADHESIONS)

Although often termed **vulvar fusion,** the common adherence of the labia minora of infants and young children is not accompanied by any anatomic union of the deeper tissues. It is not a true anatomic congenital anomaly at all but rather is an acquired postnatal condition produced by the simple sticking together of the epithelial surfaces that normally lie in close apposition to each other in the young female. It is therefore very important to recognize the situation for what it actually is and to distinguish it from imperforate hymen, congenital absence of the vagina, or the anomaly of congenital adrenal hyperplasia without the need for any elaborate diagnostic procedures. This should not be difficult, since only the labia minora are involved, and a careful examination reveals the genital tract to be perfectly normal.

Adherent labia frequently cause no symptoms whatsoever, and normal separation will usually occur spontaneously as the infant or young child grows older. They frequently are noted by the parents, however, and their harmless nature should then be thoroughly explained. Why these adhesions form in some children and not in others is not known; their appearance bears no relation to the local hygiene of the child nor to the presence of antecedent vulvovaginitis.

The labial adhesions should never be forcibly separated. Occasionally, if the extent of agglutination is considerable, difficulty in voiding, painful urination, and local vulvovaginal irritation due to the constant presence and accumulation of small amounts of urine and vaginal secretions in the area may result. If these symptoms should arise, the labia should be carefully separated by the physician (only in rare instances will anesthesia be required for this). Should symptoms recur, the mother should be instructed to keep them separated by occasional gentle manipulations at home until the tendency to readherence is no longer present. Permanent separation in patients with recurring symptoms can sometimes be promoted by oiling the labial surfaces with bland petrolatum ointments or estrogenic creams. In any event, the condition ultimately disappears completely in later childhood. If it is asymptomatic, no treatment at all is necessary or recommended.

VULVOVAGINITIS AND VAGINAL DISCHARGE

A variety of relatively minor conditions may produce vaginal discharge in infants and young children with or without an accompanying vulvovaginal irritation. Frequently, the symptoms are of greater concern to the mother than to the child. The more common entities follow.

Neonatal Leukorrhea

Neonatal leukorrhea is a transient and physiologic type of vaginal discharge seen in the newborn infant and is composed of abundant mucoid secretions and desquamated cornified vaginal epithelial cells. It occurs in response to the high levels of circulating maternal estrogens and ordinarily subsides within a few weeks following delivery.

Vaginal Foreign Body with Secondary Inflammation and Infection

The innate curiosity of infants and young children has from time immemorial led them to explore and insert objects into various body orifices, and the vaginal canal in the female has not escaped attention. Perhaps the commonest cause of vaginal discharge is the presence of a foreign body, not noticed by the mother and even forgotten by an older child. As described previously, it can usually be discovered and removed during a simple office examination if this possibility is kept in mind and the offending object carefully sought. The associated secondary irritation or infection usually subsides, with rapid disappearance of the discharge.

True Vulvovaginitis

Actual vulvovaginal infections may be due to a variety of organisms, either bacterial, protozoan, parasitic, or fungal.

Nonspecific Vaginitis. Perhaps the most frequent low-grade vaginal infection with irritating discharge occurs as the result of poor toilet hygiene following bowel evacuation, the child wiping the anal and perineal areas in a posteroanterior direction and introducing a mixed bacterial flora of colon origin (e.g., *Escherichia coli*) into the vaginal canal. Ill-fitting underclothes, simple lack of soap-and-water cleanliness, and masturbation may also be precipitating factors, as well as the previously mentioned insertion of foreign bodies. Once the mixed bacterial, nonspecific nature of the infection has been established by careful examination and bacteriologic studies, therapy is directed primarily toward improvement in local vulvovaginal and perineal hygiene. As in the case of the specific infections to be discussed, antibiotic therapy may also be necessary, the selection being based on the organisms and their antibiotic sensitivities. Sulfonamides, penicillin, or other antibiotics may be given by mouth; however, they are frequently more effective when used locally as vulvovaginal ointments or suppositories. In stubborn infections resistant to these measures, it may be necessary to employ estrogen creams or suppositories for a brief period, to stimulate the vaginal mucosa to cornify and thicken temporarily, thus increasing its resistance to the bacterial invasion.

Gonorrheal Vulvovaginitis. Formerly a very common problem, gonorrheal vulvovaginitis is rarely seen today. It is seldom actually venereal in origin in childhood but is highly contagious from child to child. The initial infection in a child usually follows an indirect contact with the discharge from an infected adult. The thin, atrophic vaginal mucosa of older infants and children is highly susceptible to surface invasion by the gonococcus, and inflammation of the vulva, vagina, and urethra is often intense, with a profuse, creamy, highly irritating discharge. The systemic reaction is minimal, and involvement of the reproductive tract above the level of the vagina rarely, if ever, occurs.

Diagnosis depends entirely on culture of the gonococcus from the discharge; gram-stained smears in search of the characteristic intracellular gram-negative organisms are unreliable, since other varieties of gram-negative intracellular diplococci are commonly present in the vaginal secretions of children. Treatment with penicillin usually suffices, and, as in adults, a prompt response is ordinarily obtained. In refractory cases, estrogens should also be employed to increase the local resistance of the vaginal mucosa to the organism.

Other Specific Forms of Bacterial Vaginitis. Other bacterial organisms causing vulvovaginitis may be of the coliform, streptococcal, staphylococcal, or pneumococcal type; more rarely, they are of typhoid, paratyphoid, or diphtherial origin. The inflammatory process and symptomatology are usually acute in onset and of short duration. Diagnosis rests on accurate identification by culture of the specific organism and treatment with the appropriate antibiotic as indicated by sensitivity studies, together with attention to any deficiencies in local hygiene and to the possible presence of more generalized factors, including poor nutrition or systemic illness.

Trichomonal Vaginitis. For reasons not entirely clear, trichomonal vaginitis is relatively rare in childhood, although it is seen a little more frequently in the immediate prepubertal years. A diagnosis is established in the same manner as in the adult female. The symptoms and gross appearance of the discharge are identical, and the motile organism is easily identified on examination of a fresh saline smear. Therapy is often more complicated in childhood, however, since douching is likely to be out of the question; even the insertion of vaginal suppositories frequently proves difficult. However, it is usually possible for the young patient, with or without the mother's help, to instill acidifying gels and ointments that are available in tubes with attachable, blunt, syringe-type applicators. Nightly applications for a few weeks often clear up the condition.

Candidal Vaginitis. Vulvovaginal *Candida albicans* infection is uncommon in infancy and childhood. It is most often encountered following intensive therapy with one of the broad-spectrum antibiotics or in juvenile diabetic patients; in connection with the latter, it should be remembered that the appearance of a candidal vulvovaginitis may be the earliest manifestation of an unsuspected diabetes, and all such patients should be carefully screened for this possibility. The characteristic thick, pasty discharge and the associated intense pruritus and inflammation usually suggest the diagnosis, but confirmation is readily obtained by special examination of a fresh smear (see Chap. 2) and, even more reliably, by culture on Nickerson's medium. Therapy is the same as that employed in the adult female.

Parasitic Vulvovaginal Infestations. Various intestinal parasites, most commonly the ubiquitous pinworm *Enterobius vermicularis* (also called the threadworm, seatworm, or *Oxyuris vermicularis*), less often the roundworm (*Ascaris lumbricoides*) or the whipworm (*Trichuris trichiura*), are transferred anteriorly into the vulvovaginal region through poor local hygiene and improper toilet habits. The intense itching and resulting scratching produces vulvar inflammation, excoriation, and secondary bacterial vulvovaginitis, and, in the case of the pinworm, actual invasion of the vaginal canal by the parasite itself. Diagnosis is best made by pressing a piece of Scotch tape against the perianal area in the early morning to recover the typical parasite ova, which can then be identified on microscopic examination. Management involves the current therapeutic programs for the elimination of these common intestinal parasites, temporary symptomatic treatment for the local inflammation and secondary bacterial infection, and attention to general hygienic measures to prevent recurrence.

Cyclic "Leukorrhea" in Premenarchal Girls

Cyclic "leukorrhea" is similar in nature to the neonatal leukorrhea previously mentioned but is frequently a source of concern to both the young girl and her mother. It is entirely physiologic, is rarely accompanied by symptoms of irritation, and is simply the earliest manifestation of beginning cyclic ovarian activity and estrogen secretion.

ABNORMAL VAGINAL BLEEDING IN INFANCY AND CHILDHOOD

Many of the childhood vulvovaginal disorders just discussed are accompanied by abnormal bleeding as well as discharge, so it is convenient as well as pertinent to note this fact here and to outline briefly the most common causes of vaginal bleeding that must be considered in any infant or young child with this symptom.

Neonatal Bleeding

Neonatal vaginal bleeding occurs only once, though it may last for several days, and is due to the sudden withdrawal of maternal estrogens in infants in whom these estrogens have produced some degree of fetal endometrial proliferation.

Foreign Bodies

The presence of foreign bodies within the vaginal canal is the most common cause of abnormal vaginal bleeding in infancy and childhood. Their presence should always be suspected and sought in the face of this symptom.

Vaginal Erosions and Ulcerations

Bleeding from vaginal erosions and ulcerations in the absence of foreign bodies is also occasionally encountered in the presence of severe vaginitis.

Endocrine Causes

Endocrine causes, which will be discussed in other sections, include precocious puberty and functioning ovarian tumors (most commonly, granulosa cell tumor). At puberty, functional menstrual disorders of early adolescence are the most common cause.

Tumors

Although rare in infancy and childhood, the possibility of tumor must be considered. Examples include the extremely rare benign vaginal, cervical, or endometrial polyps and the uncommon, highly malignant sarcoma botryoides.

Synthetic Estrogen Administration and Withdrawal

Although infrequently encountered, a few instances of bleeding induced by the accidental ingestion of estrogenic medication have been reported.

VULVAR TRAUMA

Because of the highly protected location of the vulvovaginal soft tissues, traumatic injuries might be expected to be uncommon, and in fact are rare in adult females. However, in young girls, a specific type of vulvar trauma is encountered with relative frequency. This invariably occurs as the result of a straddle-type fall while bicycling, climbing fences, walls, or jungle gyms, or sliding down banisters, and the like, the vulva often absorbing almost the entire force of impact as the child lands astride the various objects. Actual soft-tissue lacerations of varying severity may occur, usually bleed profusely, and will require suture if extensive. The more common and equally troublesome result, however, is the development of a massive vulvar and perineal hematoma, an almost inevitable phenomenon in view of the great vascularity, rich lymphatic supply, and dependency of the soft tissues of this area. This usually results in excruciating pain and often leads to acute urinary retention due to occlusion of the urethral meatus. When the young child with this type of injury is seen early, bed rest with the foot of the bed elevated and applications of ice packs to the vulva and perineum may minimize the pain and swelling. It is frequently also very important to anticipate the development of urinary retention by placement of an inlying bladder catheter for 48 to 72 hours until the edema has begun to subside.

Pelvic Tumors in Infancy and Childhood

The usual benign and malignant tumors of the pelvis occurring so frequently in adult women are seldom encountered in the younger age groups. Only rarely have the common types of malignant tumors of the cervix, endometrium, or vulva been reported, and the typical types of ovarian neoplasms seen later in life are equally uncommon. However, a special group of ovarian tumors and cysts do occur occasionally, and a specific type of highly malignant uterovaginal sarcoma characteristically arises most often during infancy. Finally — and perhaps of greatest interest —

a group of benign and malignant lesions developing in young women whose mothers took diethylstilbestrol (DES) during their pregnancies have recently been encountered with increasing frequency.

OVARIAN CYSTS AND TUMORS

As might be predicted, dermoid cysts or the less common benign solid teratomas constitute about half the ovarian neoplasms occurring in infancy and childhood. They are usually benign and, especially in infancy, are frequently asymptomatic except for the obvious presence of a mass. In older children, abdominal pain due to intermittent torsion may be the chief clinical manifestation, and an acute episode involving a cyst of the right ovary may simulate appendicitis. Usually, these benign cysts can be locally resected, preserving the remaining normal ovarian tissue of the same side. Malignant teratoid tumors such as embryonal carcinomas are rare, but a few have been reported in children.

It should also be mentioned that torsion with infarction and necrosis of a previously entirely normal ovary and tube can and does occur occasionally. It is seen most frequently in young girls between the ages of 7 and 15 and most probably is the result of a congenital excessive mobility of the adnexal supports. The typical clinical picture includes a history of repeated attacks of crampy lower abdominal pain, culminating in a final acute episode characterized by severe itching and vomiting, an enlarging pelvic mass, leukocytosis with or without fever, and signs of peritonitis. Treatment usually involves salpingo-oophorectomy on the affected side, though if the possibility is borne in mind and the diagnosis made early, conservative surgery with reduction of the torsion and fixation of the excessively mobile adnexa may be successful.

A less common group of cystic ovarian lesions may be equally dramatic with respect to the size they attain, even in newborn infants. These include (1) the giant follicle cysts, which are the most frequent ovarian lesion in neonates and account for 15 percent of all ovarian cysts during infancy and childhood, and (2) the rarer theca-lutein and corpus luteum cysts, also most commonly seen in neonates. These neonatal cysts are believed to arise as a result of stimulation of the infant ovaries by maternal gonadotropic hormones. They are occasionally also seen in the older child; in a few cases, actual function and estrogen secretion by the cyst lining has produced the picture of sexual precocity. In the majority, however, no endocrine disturbance is present, and the clinical symptomatology is entirely similar to that accompanying the dermoid cysts and teratomas. Surgical treatment can again be of the conservative variety.

Other types of germ cell tumors are also encountered, many of them malignant. The principles of management of ovarian cancer in children are similar to those employed in adults (see Chap. 15), except that in the Stage Ia lesions, a real effort should be made to employ conservative therapy (unilateral salpingo-oophorectomy).

Finally, granulosa cell tumors of the ovary should be mentioned, since they are by far the most frequently occurring true ovarian neoplasm in children. In addition to the presence of a mass, these tumors are invariably accompanied by vaginal bleeding, often periodic in nature, and by the premature development of secondary sex characteristics, since the tumor cells produce considerable amounts of estrogen, although ovulation never occurs. They are thus one of the causes of the clinical picture of precocious puberty (see p. 132). They tend to be benign in children and can generally be treated by unilateral salpingo-oophorectomy, though local recurrences following removal do occur. Following removal, all signs and symptoms of precocious sexual maturation will disappear.

Although ovarian lesions are uncommon in childhood, the presence of a pelvic or abdominal mass (the ovaries of infants are essentially abdominal in location) in an infant or young child should raise the suspicion of the presence of one of the types just discussed. This is particularly the case if urologic study, including pyelography, reveals normal findings and essentially rules out the possibility of a Wilms' tumor, the commonest childhood neoplasm. Similarly, the possible existence of a granulosa cell tumor or follicle or theca-lutein cyst must be kept in mind in the prepubertal child exhibiting evidences of sexual prococity. Finally, ovarian cysts of the dermoid or follicle variety must be considered in the differential diagnosis of chronic, recurring abdominal pain or acute episodes suggesting appendicitis in any female infant or child.

SARCOMA BOTRYOIDES (EMBRYONAL RHABDOMYOSARCOMA)

Sarcoma botryoides, a fortunately rare but highly malignant sarcoma, is actually a mixed mesenchymal tumor whose cellular components appear to be derived from the more primitive tissue types of the urogenital ridge. Although these tumors have been observed at various sites in the male urogenital tract, they occur predominantly in females. Furthermore, although they are occasionally encountered in adults, approximately 75 percent of these neoplasms appear during the first two years of life. They are usually primary in the vagina or cervix but occasionally arise in the uterus or even the bladder. Histologically, they are composed of varying mixtures of spindle, stellate, and round cells interspersed with striated muscle fibers, all frequently enmeshed in a myxomatous stroma that occasionally contains cartilaginous structures or even bone. The mixed histologic nature of the tumor suggests a relationship to the teratomatous cancers and strongly supports the concept that they are derived from embryonic rests. However, they are usually classified as embryonal rhabdomyosarcomas (botryoid type), since the characteristic cells are striated or nonstriated embryonal rhabdomyoblasts.

Grossly, these tumors usually arise in the lower two-thirds of the anterior vaginal wall and appear as clusters of soft, bulky, polypoid masses that are moist, extremely friable, and brownish-pink in color. Pfannenstiel first called attention to their grapelike appearance in 1892, and subsequently the descriptive term *botryoid* (from the Greek *botrys,* meaning "bunch of grapes") was applied and has been retained over the years. Because of their friability and tendency to necrosis, bleeding and a malodorous discharge are common early symptoms, and frequently a "grapelike" piece of tissue may actually break away and be noted by the mother. Growth is extremely rapid and often of multicentric origin, the vagina soon becoming filled with masses of tumor. At this point, recognition by the physician should be instantaneous, and biopsy confirmation is easily obtained. Since bleeding occurs early, however, it should be possible to establish a correct diagnosis much sooner in the course of the disease if one considers the possibility in any case of vaginal bleeding during infancy, and if a small "fleshy polyp" is never considered a "benign hymeneal or vaginal tab" until it has been excised and examined microscopically. (Benign polyps or other lesions of the vagina or cervix are extremely rare in childhood.) Eventually, local extension into the bladder or out to the pelvic walls, spread to regional lymph nodes, and metastases to the liver and lungs are extremely common.

Although radiation therapy has been attempted many times in the past to treat these tumors, they are not very radiosensitive, and no cures have been reported following the use of radiation treatment alone. The treatment of choice is an aggressive surgical attack, which involves a radical Wertheim hysterectomy and total vaginectomy, often with vulvectomy, at a minimum; more often, an anterior or total pelvic exenteration with en bloc vulvectomy is required to encompass all the disease. Only a few apparent cures have followed radical surgical removal, but surgery may be expected to be even more successful if the diagnosis is correctly made early, before the primary lesion becomes extensive. The prognosis at best will probably remain poor, however, with few long-term survivals, because of the highly malignant nature of the tumor and its early and rapid dissemination, both locally as well as occasionally via bloodstream and lymphatic metastasis, with death sometimes occurring within 3 to 12 months from the onset of symptoms. Although even to consider undertaking such a radical surgical approach in these tiny patients may prove difficult for both the parents and the physician, it is in reality the only possible lifesaving measure currently available. Recently, somewhat better results seem to have been achieved by combining radical surgery with preoperative and/or postoperative radiation and/or chemotherapy than had formerly been achieved by radical surgery alone, especially when the tumor had spread beyond the vaginal wall. The chemotherapy may involve double or triple combination therapy with agents such as cyclophosphamide, vincristine, and actinomycin D.

An even rarer vaginal malignant tumor most often occurring in infants under the age of 2 (occasionally seen in young adults also) is the endodermal sinus tumor, a variant of embryonal carcinoma of germ cell origin (this tumor arises far more commonly in the ovary than in the vagina). Its gross appearance and clinical course are similar to that of sarcoma botryoides, and the general plan of treatment is identical.

Clear Cell Adenocarcinomas and Congenital Disorders of the Genital Tract (Vagina and Cervix) Secondary to Prenatal Diethylstilbestrol Exposure

A cluster of 8 cases of an unusual type of clear cell adenocarcinoma of the vagina, all occurring in adolescent females, was encountered over a three year period from 1966 to 1969 at the Massachusetts General Hospital. Since this represented more than the total number of cases of this rare lesion reported in the world literature to have appeared in patients born before 1945, the possibility that a specific etiologic agent of recent origin might be responsible was immediately raised. Subsequently, a thorough epidemiologic study was carried out employing 4 carefully matched controls for each cancer patient, and it was discovered that the mothers of 7 of these 8 patients had received diethylstilbestrol (DES) or a similar synthetic nonsteroidal estrogen during the first trimester of the pregnancy. In each case the medication was given because of a history of repeated previous abortions or actual bleeding suggestive of threatened abortion during the current pregnancy; no other associated potential etiologic factors could be demonstrated. This association between maternal ingestion of DES during the first trimester and before the eighteenth week of pregnancy and subsequent vaginal and cervical abnormalities, including clear cell adenocarcinomas of both vagina and cervix, in the female offspring has subsequently been confirmed in a much larger and continuing worldwide study of the problem, the data being accumulated and analyzed in the Registry of Clear Cell Adenocarcinomas of the Genital Tract in Young Women established for this tumor at the Massachusetts General Hospital in Boston. Information on over 200 such cases has now been collected.

Furthermore, in many centers throughout this country and abroad, vigorous follow-up of daughters of women to whom DES had been administered during their pregnancies has brought to light the fact that the vast majority of these young women exhibit a variety of benign congenital anomalies and epithelial disorders of the vagina and cervix, with the clear cell adenocarcinomas actually relatively uncommon sequelae. For example, benign vaginal adenosis, though often found in association with clear cell adenocarcinoma, is actually far more commonly present in the absence of carcinoma, occurring in 35 to 40 percent (as high as 90 percent in some reported series) of these prenatally DES-exposed young women.

Thus, although the lesion of vaginal adenosis may serve as a precursor of clear cell adenocarcinoma in some cases, the incidence of such malignant transformation is low, and its occurrence has never actually been observed. Based on the available data concerning the estimated several million women who received DES in the first trimester of pregnancy during the period 1945–1960 when such a program was widely employed, the chances that clear cell adenocarcinoma of the vagina or cervix will develop in a daughter born following such a pregnancy are no more than 4 in 1000 and probably are considerably less than 1 in 1000.

Some physicians have speculated that as this exposed group of young females at risk grows older, the squamous metaplasia occurring in these areas of vaginal adenosis and in the related large cervical "erosions" (both are composed of exposed columnar epithelium created by failure of the normal squamous epithelial surface to develop at these sites) may possibly predispose them to an increased incidence of epidermoid carcinoma of the cervix and vagina. Although this possibility still lies in the realm of speculation, there have been reports from some clinics that atypical squamous cell lesions, including dysplasia and even a few instances of carcinoma in situ, have already been observed in a number of these young women.

In any case, daughters of women known to have taken DES during their pregnancies should begin a regular program of surveillance once they have begun to menstruate or when they reach the age of 14 and should, of course, be examined immediately if they experience abnormal bleeding or discharge. Such regular examinations should include careful palpation (often there is roughening or slight nodularity in involved areas), inspection of the cervix and vagina, cytologic study (keeping in mind that vaginal smears have been negative in 20 percent of the cases of proved clear cell carcinomas of the vagina), Schiller's test, and colposcopy, with biopsy of any visible abnormality, any area that fails to stain with Schiller's solution, or any suspicious area detected colposcopically.

Congenital Anomalies

A variety of congenital developmental errors has been noted in these young women exposed to DES prenatally: cervical erosions (exposed glandular epithelium on the cervical portio) in 60 to 70 percent; transverse fibrous ridges in the vagina in 20 percent; and, less frequently, transverse cervical ridges that may give the cervix an unusual "cockscomb," hooded, or polypoid appearance. These abnormalities are also all presumed to be secondary to DES exposure in utero, since similar anomalies are rarely, if ever, seen in females who have not been prenatally exposed to DES. Diethylstilbestrol apparently acts as a teratogen rather than as a direct carcinogen and interferes with the normal development of the embryonic vagina, so that the müllerian columnar epithelium fails to undergo permanent transformation and replacement by normal squamous epithelium. The vaginal ridges and the cervical hoods are probably of no clinical significance other than as clear-cut signals that the young girl was probably exposed to DES in utero. The large congenital cervical erosions need to be observed at regular intervals, employing colposcopy if at all possible, to detect the development of the uncommon clear cell adenocarcinoma of the cervix in the younger age groups and possibly to permit early recognition of an increased incidence of squamous cell neoplasia as this group at risk grows older.

Vaginal Adenosis

When glandular epithelium is present on or just beneath the surface of the vagina, the mucosa appears bright red and granular and does not stain with Schiller's solution. These areas of adenosis may be focal, with multiple punctate lesions, or they may be extensive and diffuse. Biopsy and microscopic examination will reveal that the normal squamous epithelium has been replaced or covered by a columnar glandular epithelium. These areas also exhibit a very characteristic appearance on colposcopic examination, and this is probably the most effective and reliable way of performing periodic follow-up observation to detect any transition to clear cell adenocarcinoma, which theoretically may occur in a small percentage of these young women. Such regular follow-up observations are mandatory, preferably with frequent colposcopic examination, since vaginal cytologic examination has not proved as reliable in the detection of early malignant change as might have been hoped.

There have been efforts made to hasten the normal process of squamous metaplasia in these areas of adenosis by the topical application of progesterone creams or acidi-fying jellies. Others have attempted to excise or destroy the areas of adenosis by multiple, colposcopically controlled, excision biopsies or by partial vaginectomy. However, a conservative approach, with emphasis on careful follow-up rather than removal of these lesions, is probably indicated in the majority of these young patients.

Clear Cell Adenocarcinomas of the Vagina and Cervix

Roughly 60 to 70 percent of clear cell adenocarcinomas in DES-exposed patients have arisen in the vagina, with the remaining 30 to 40 percent arising in the cervix. The patients have ranged in age from 7 to 27, but for the most part these are tumors predominately of adolescent girls; 90 percent were 14 years of age or older, and the average age was about 17½. In approximately two-thirds of the cases there was a documented exposure in utero to DES or similar synthetic nonsteroidal estrogen. Abnormal bleeding or discharge in an adolescent female, often initially felt to be due to dysfunctional bleeding or vaginitis, was the usual presenting symptom.

The tumors usually present as superficial, papillary, nodular, or polypoid masses that are reddish in color, friable, and bleed easily. Most commonly, they arise in the upper third of the anterior vaginal wall. The microscopic picture consists of cystic and tubular spaces lined by characteristic glycogen-rich clear cells or hobnail cells (the nuclei protrude into the gland lumens, giving a hobnail appearance); solid nests of clear cells also occur occasionally.

Although radiation therapy has been used as primary therapy in early and advanced lesions, in the management of patients with positive lymph nodes, and in dealing with recurrences, tumors arising in the vagina are not easily treated by radiotherapy without the risk of severe damage to the nearby bladder, bowel, ovaries, and impor-tant bony epiphyses — complications to be avoided if at all possible in these young patients. Furthermore, there is some evidence that these tumors may be somewhat less radiosensitive than the more common epidermoid carcinomas encountered in this region.

Therefore, radical surgery has been the treatment of choice in the majority of these cases. With tumors originating in the cervix, a radical Wertheim procedure with bilateral pelvic lymphadenectomies is usually carried out for the Stage I and II lesions, with an occasional pelvic exenteration for more advanced but still operable tumors; one or both ovaries can usually be preserved. In the case of primary vaginal tumors, although local excision has occasionally been successful for very small tumors, a more radical operation is usually required. Depending on the location and extent of the lesion, a radical Wertheim hysterectomy and total vaginectomy with bilateral pelvic lymphadenectomies, preserving one or both ovaries if feasible, may be ade-quate, replacing the vagina with a split-thickness skin graft at a second procedure 7 to 10 days later. For more extensive lesions, some form of pelvic exenteration (usually anterior, because the anterior vaginal wall is the most common site) with ileal loop urinary tract diversion will be required; creation of a very satisfactory artificial vagina is often also possible by employing a second ileal segment and trans-locating it with its blood supply intact to the area formerly occupied by the vaginal tube. Again, bilateral pelvic lymphadenectomies are important, because roughly 20 percent of the Stage I and 50 percent of the Stage II patients have involved pelvic lymph nodes on microscopic examination.

These tumors behave in an aggressive and lethal fashion, as indicated in the latest report from the Registry. Among 65 patients, many followed for less than two years, 24 are already dead of disease, and 13 others are living but have had recurrences. If it takes place, recurrence usually occurs within two years, most commonly in the pelvis. But in contrast to the relatively uncommon occurrence of remote metastases in patients with epidermoid carcinoma of the cervix or vagina, a high percentage (35 percent) of young women with clear cell adenocarcinomas have manifested pulmonary, supraclavicular, and even cerebral metastases, sometimes four or five years later and in the absence of local recurrence, indicating that bloodstream dissemination occurs all too readily. In the face of advanced or recurrent local disease or remote metastases, chemotherapy with agents such as 5-fluorouracil or vinblastine has been used, alone or in combination with radiotherapy. Although like endometrial cancer, these tumors are of müllerian origin, attempts to treat metastatic disease with progestational agents have been unsuccessful.

Precocious Puberty

Congenital adrenal hyperplasia and the problems it poses in the management of neonates and young infants have already been discussed in Chapter 3. The only other endocrinologic disturbance of the female reproductive tract seen in childhood is the clinical syndrome of precocious puberty, which is ordinarily defined as the occurrence of menstrual function and the appearance of secondary female sexual characteristics before the age of 9 years. On the average, these early manifestations of a normal female puberty appear most frequently between the ages of 11 to 14, although the normal range is certainly to be considered as extending from 9 to 17 years of age. Although uncommon, sexual precocity is seen far more frequently in girls than in boys, the differential ratio approaching 30:1. In females, the precocious reproductive tract maturation and function may be either isosexual (along feminine lines only) or heterosexual (accompanied by signs and symptoms of virilization or other evidence of heterosexual development); as will be seen, the distinction is of fundamental significance in arriving at a correct diagnosis. The most likely causes, the principal points in their recognition, and the general plans of treatment will now be considered.

ISOSEXUAL FEMALE PRECOCIOUS PUBERTY

Constitutional (Unknown Etiology)
In constitutional isosexual female precocious puberty, a primary disturbance in the hypothalamic-pituitary-ovarian axis apparently occurs in the absence of any organic pathologic condition, resulting in the onset of an apparently normal, although often rapidly progressing, female puberty in a child between the ages of 5 to 8 years.

(Isolated instances of this syndrome in children from 1 to 5 years of age have also been recorded in the literature, but in view of their rarity, the other, more common causes of isosexual precocity in children under the age of 5 years should always be more seriously considered first in this age group.) In addition to regular cyclic menstruation there is a marked increase in growth rate, with the development of adult-type breasts and external genitalia and the appearance of axillary and pubic hair. A skeletal x-ray survey may be of diagnostic help by demonstrating the advanced bone age and premature epiphyseal closure that are invariably evident; unfortunately, occurrence of the latter usually results in subnormal adult height. Because ovulation actually occurs (this fact has been demonstrated repeatedly by the usual tests of ovulation as well as by ovarian biopsy), pregnancy is possible in these young girls and has in fact been reported; in one widely publicized case, a 5½-year-old girl in Lima, Peru, gave birth by cesarean section to a 6-pound infant.

Once organic brain disease has been excluded (see Pituitary Disorders), treatment consists primarily of explanation and reassurance to parents and child, with continued, sympathetic supervision throughout childhood and anticipation and avoidance of as many as possible of the obvious psychological problems that may arise. This requires both the confidence of the child and the intelligent cooperation of properly informed parents. The ultimate prognosis, except for the slightly retarded height, is excellent, and the problem solves itself as adolescence is reached.

What appears to be a constitutional type of precocious puberty is also seen as a fundamental feature of the well-known but relatively uncommon Albright's syndrome. Here, multiple areas of fibrous dysplasia and cystic degeneration are seen in the long bones in association with numerous flat areas of brownish pigmentation of the skin (café au lait spots), both usually involving only one side of the body. This disorder, so-called polyostotic fibrous dysplasia, is accompanied by sexual precocity in roughly half the patients. Whether the premature hypothalamic and pituitary activity is really idiopathic or may be the result of bony overgrowth at the base of the skull is not clear. At any rate, there is definite gonadotropin secretion, with increased urinary follicle-stimulating hormone (FSH) excretion levels and normal ovarian hormonal activity, including ovulation, just as occurs in the pure, uncomplicated form of constitutional precocious puberty.

Pituitary Disorders

Pituitary disorders that may cause precocious puberty include not only primary pituitary cysts, tumors, and dysfunctions but also a variety of cerebral diseases that may secondarily affect pituitary function, such as meningitis, encephalitis, skull injuries, and brain tumors, the latter unfortunately often highly malignant. Presumably, the resulting abnormal activity of the hypothalamic-pituitary pathway results in production of pituitary gonadotropins and premature gonadal stimulation. Pituitary disturbances of this type may simulate constitutional precocity, and the former should always be excluded by thorough study before assuming the latter. This can usually be done on the basis of the associated neurologic findings and the results of complete neurologic studies (e.g., skull films, encephalography, cerebral arteriography) and the often considerably elevated pituitary gonadotropin urinary excretion. Treatment is of course directed at the primary neurologic disorder.

Ovarian Lesions

In approximately 5 percent of young girls with isosexual precocity, the condition will be secondary to an ovarian tumor or cyst, and in 30 to 40 percent of these patients, the ovarian lesion will be malignant. The association of a pseudosexual precocity with granulosa cell tumors and certain types of apparently estrogen-secreting ovarian cysts has already been discussed. These patients show normal female pubertal changes of varying degrees and rates of progression. They invariably have a palpable ovarian tumor and will demonstrate an elevated urinary estrogen excretion at least at normal pubertal levels, sometimes well above them; the urinary 17-ketosteroid and pituitary gonadotropin levels are normal or low. Since ovulation does not occur, pregnancy is impossible in this group.

Less commonly, a large theca-lutein type of follicle-cyst, apparently developing independently in the absence of any cerebral or constitutional factor and in otherwise normal ovaries, may produce the same clinical picture. In either case, all signs and symptoms of the estrogen-induced precocious state will disappear on removal of the tumor.

Even more rarely, an embryonal ovarian carcinoma containing functioning chorionepitheliomatous elements that produce chorionic gonadotropin may induce an entirely similar sexual precocity. In these cases, in addition to increased urinary estrogen excretion, a positive Aschheim-Zondek test due to the marked elevation of chorionic gonadotropin levels will also be obtained and is diagnostic. Since these tumors are highly malignant, radical surgery, with removal of uterus, tubes, and ovaries, should be done, but recurrence is unfortunately common.

Miscellaneous Causes

Children with primary hypothyroidism may occasionally have breast growth, galactorrhea (secondary to hyperprolactinemia due to stimulation of prolactin secretion by excess thyrotropin releasing factor), and menstrual activity, all of which are reversed when the euthyroid state is reestablished. Even more rarely, tumors of nonendocrine tissue origin (e.g., hepatoblastomas, bronchial adenomas, carcinoids, and teratomas) may secrete gonadotropins, with resulting premature stimulation of the pituitary-ovarian axis and precocious puberty.

HETEROSEXUAL FEMALE PRECOCIOUS PUBERTY

If virilization or other heterosexual manifestations occur in association with sexual precocity, an adrenal lesion is invariably present. Only infrequently, in the case of certain unusual adrenal tumors secreting primarily steroids with estrogenic activity, or in the equally rare instances of ovarian tumors that may produce abnormal steroids possessing androgenic or corticoid properties, are there exceptions to this general rule.

The adrenal disorders that may be encountered in this age group include the following:

1. A previously unrecognized, mild form of congenital adrenal cortical hyperplasia (diagnosis and treatment as in Chap. 3).
2. Acquired adrenocortical hyperplasia (acquired adrenogenital syndrome) (diagnosis and treatment essentially the same as for the congenital form).
3. Adrenocortical adenomas or carcinomas may also be accompanied by a marked increase in growth rate and occasionally by precocious menstruation. Obesity, hirsutism, and clitoral enlargement are invariably associated with these tumors. Laboratory findings include an elevation of the 17-ketosteroids and other adrenocorticoid levels and a normal or low pituitary gonadotropin urinary excretion. The steroid excretion pattern, particularly its response to ACTH adrenal stimulation or cortisone adrenal suppression tests, may be of help in distinguishing an adrenal tumor from hyperplasia; if a tumor is suspected, intravenous pyelography or periadrenal pneumograms may aid in localization. Treatment will involve adrenal exploration and excision of an adenoma or extensive resection if carcinoma is present. Unfortunately, the latter is often highly malignant, and its tendency to local and distant dissemination frequently renders it incurable at the outset.

COMMON GYNECOLOGIC PROBLEMS DURING ADOLESCENCE

The principal gynecologic problems more or less specifically, or at least characteristically and frequently, encountered in adolescent girls involve either (1) failure of, or marked delay in, the development of normal reproductive tract anatomy and function or (2) functional irregularities occurring after the appearance of hypothalamic-pituitary-ovarian-uterine activity at the normal pubertal age. Although by a rigid definition the former are not strictly disorders of adolescence, they are considered under this heading, because they are most frequently first discovered during adolescence.

Normal Puberty and Adolescence

Norms for the age of menarche have already been noted, the average age being 13 to 14 years. However, pituitary gonadotropin secretion with ovarian stimulation and estrogen production usually begins several years before the first menses. This normally becomes evident with the appearance of pubic hair and budding of the breasts at age 10 to 11. From age 11 to 12 there is definite growth of the uterus and external genitalia, both tending toward a more adult size and anatomic configuration. The vaginal mucosa cornifies and assumes a more mature appearance, and there is further progression in breast development to the final adolescent or primary mamma stage. By age 13 to 14, and roughly coinciding with the onset of cyclic menstrual function, axillary hair first makes its appearance.

It is well established that in the first year or two, normal adolescent menstrual function may consist almost entirely of anovulatory cycles, with irregular or even regular periodic uterine bleeding resulting only from estrogen stimulation and withdrawal. However, by age 14 to 15, regular or fairly regular ovulation and normal corpus luteum function and progesterone production have ordinarily been established, and the menses assume the typical characteristics of ovulatory periods — a more consistently identical type, amount, and duration of flow, as well as a fairly constant intermenstrual interval — and uterine cramps, the hallmark of the ovulating female, usually appear. At this point, then, normal pregnancy is possible (though hardly desirable). Finally, by age 16 to 17, the effect of estrogen on bone metabolism, and ultimately on epiphyseal closure, culminates in completion of skeletal growth and final attainment of the height that genetic and constitutional factors determine. During this same four- to five-year period, the effects of estrogen are normally also apparent in terms of distribution of fat and other soft-tissue elements and the assumption of the characteristic feminine body contours.

With due allowance of a year or two on either side of these norms for individual variations induced by such factors as heredity, body build, and climate, the brief outline of the chronological sequence and timing of the key events of normal puberty and adolescence just given may be used as a rough gauge by which to judge whether the development of reproductive tract function and the appearance of secondary sex characteristics in any individual is normal, premature, or abnormally delayed. A less obvious instance of the usefulness of such a guide is in the evaluation of the significance of hirsutism, either in the adolescent phase or in the adult female. If the excessive growth of hair began at the normal time for the appearance of pubic or axillary hair, it is probably unassociated with any fundamental endocrine disturbance and is more likely of familial or racial origin. On the other hand, the sudden development of obvious hirsutism in an 8-year-old girl or in a 20-year-old woman in whom other female sexual characteristics appeared at approximately the right age and in the correct order would be highly significant and should raise the strong suspicion of an underlying adrenal or ovarian endocrine disorder of fundamental importance.

The detailed mechanisms responsible for the automatic initiation of the pubertal process at a consistently similar time in the life of most young females are as yet unknown. There is evidence, however, that the initial release of gonadotropins at the start of puberty is triggered by a built-in, genetically transmitted neural or neurohormonal mechanism that up to this point has been actively inhibited. The implications of this concept with respect to the common types of sexual precocity are obvious. By the same token, a simple failure of release of this inhibiting influence, whatever its nature, which normally operates during infancy and early childhood but which should disappear at the appropriate prepubertal moment, is probably involved in many of the functional types of menarchal delay and adolescent menstrual disorders. More will be said on this point in subsequent sections.

The work of Wurtman [22] and that of others suggests that the pineal gland, acting as a neuroendocrine transducer in response to rhythmic changes in environmental light, may be involved in the initiation and regulation of gonadal growth and cyclic activity. The regulating mechanism appears to operate through the inhibiting effects of the rhythmic secretion of the "pineal hormone" melatonin on the hypothalamic centers responsible for triggering the release of pituitary gonadotropins.

In any case, under normal circumstances, the inhibition is released, the hypothalamic "sexual center" stimulates the adjacent anterior lobe of the pituitary to secrete gonadotropins (initially only FSH), and the ovaries eventually respond in turn by producing estrogens. Estrogen secretion in increasing amounts is ultimately responsible for the typical pubertal changes in skeletal growth, for the appearance of generalized secondary sexual characteristics, and for the maturation of the various special target organs (breasts, uterus, vagina, and external genitalia). As the endometrium begins to proliferate sufficiently, and when estrogen levels have risen to the point at which the pituitary inhibiting effect becomes manifest for the first time, a sudden fall in estrogen occurs and induces the first actual period, which is a simple estrogen-withdrawal or anovulatory flow, to be sure, but a period, nevertheless. Thus the reciprocal pituitary-ovarian relationship based on the gonadotropin-inhibiting properties of estrogen comes into play for the first time, and although the adolescent anovulatory pattern may persist for two to three years, the groundwork has been laid for the introduction of the other principal gonadotropin, luteinizing hormone (LH), into the cyclic scheme, with corpus luteum function, ovulation, and progesterone production leading gradually to the more regular, ovulatory adult menstrual pattern.

Delayed Puberty

A sharp distinction should be made between delayed puberty and the simple delay in onset of the menarche in an otherwise normally maturing adolescent girl. Perhaps this point needs little emphasis, because the difference in the significance of the two phenomena is not only obvious but fundamental. The former represents a true state of sexual infantilism and usually is secondary either to a profound generalized endocrine disturbance involving lesions in the hypothalamus or pituitary or is due to primary gonadal failure such as is encountered in Turner's syndrome (gonadal dysgenesis) and the related genetic disorders presented in Chapter 3. The latter, however, represents only a delay in the appearance of menstrual function in a young girl who has otherwise undergone the normal sexual maturation of puberty and early adolescence. The delay is most often due to some temporary functional disturbance.

Delayed puberty is really only one symptom or manifestation of a serious disorder or defect affecting the entire body in multiple ways and accompanied by widespread neurologic, metabolic, hormonal, and developmental abnormalities. Thus it is more a problem for the pediatrician or internist than for the gynecologist. It is essential only that the gynecologist bear in mind the need to differentiate between simple delayed menarche and true sexual infantilism or delayed puberty. A detailed discussion of delayed puberty therefore does not seem warranted here. Let it suffice to list the common causes as enumerated and discussed by McArthur [16].

CAUSES OF DELAYED PUBERTY*
(SEXUAL AND USUALLY GENERALIZED INFANTILISM)

1. Primary hypothalamic infantilism:
   a. Destructive lesions (intracerebral tumors or cysts, infection, or hemorrhage): Froehlich's syndrome.
   b. Congenital hypothalamic defect (etiology unknown): Laurence-Moon-Biedl syndrome.
2. Primary pituitary infantilism:
   a. Pituitary disorders.
      (1) Lesions such as tumors or cysts, or a generalized congenital defect leading to panhypopituitarism.
      (2) Fractional pituitary deficiency (etiology unknown): a congenital defect, the so-called idiopathic gonadotropin (FSH) defect.
   b. Factors inducing functional hypopituitarism.
      (1) Specific disorders of the thyroid, pancreatic islets, and adrenal cortex.
      (2) Chronic infections and other debilitating systemic diseases.
      (3) Nutritional disturbances: obesity and malnutrition.
3. Primary ovarian infantilism:
   a. Gonadal dysgenesis, etc.
   b. Castration before puberty: oophoritis (e.g., mumps or tuberculosis), radiation, or surgery for bilateral tumors, etc.

It should be noted that from the standpoint of differential diagnosis, the urinary gonadotropin excretion (FSH) will be absent or extremely low in the entities of hypothalamic or pituitary origin but considerably elevated in patients exhibiting delayed puberty on the basis of primary ovarian failure.

Delayed Menarche

Delayed menarche is ordinarily defined as a failure of menstruation to appear in a young woman over age 17 whose degree of sexual maturation otherwise corresponds with her age. The phrase as it is used with reference to adolescent females is in many instances completely synonymous with the term **primary amenorrhea** as ordinarily applied to the same problem persisting into early maturity or adulthood, and the major serious causes are identical, inasmuch as the two abnormal "conditions" or symptoms are essentially one and the same. Obviously, the congenital gonadal anomalies are excluded from this category because they are usually also accompanied by a generalized sexual infantilism. However, one must always consider the possibility that a congenital uterovaginal anomaly is responsible for failure of menstrual flow to appear; congenital absence of the uterus is a cause of true delayed menarche or primary amenorrhea, and imperforate hymen produces pseudoamenorrhea, since it represents only an apparent delay, not an actual delay, in the occurrence of menstrual bleeding.

*Modified from McArthur [16].

There is, however, a physiologic or constitutional type of menarchal delay in which menstrual activity may not begin until age 16 to 18, but thereafter, without treatment of any kind, both the menstrual cycle and subsequent fertility are entirely normal. Although this situation may be the source of considerable anxiety for both the young woman and her parents, it is actually of no fundamental significance and is most probably based on minor variations in heredity, body build, climate, and general level of physical, mental, and emotional development. The apprehension it arouses will require that the physician evaluate the problem to exclude a fundamental disorder and effectively reassure both patient and parents. Usually, a careful history, general physical examination, and simple laboratory studies will serve to exclude any psychological disorders, metabolic or obvious endocrine disturbance, or systemic disease (e.g., childhood schizophrenia, diabetes, pituitary or thyroid deficiency, tuberculosis, malnutrition). Vulvovaginal inspection, a vaginal smear for determination of estrogen effect, a buccal smear for nuclear sex chromatin determination, and a bimanual vaginal or rectoabdominal examination or both should be done to rule out obvious gross anatomic or developmental anomalies, such as gonadal dysgenesis, testicular feminization, absent uterus, or imperforate hymen and to establish whether or not some ovarian functional activity is present in the form of estrogen secretion. (Vaginal examination, if anatomically possible, is definitely indicated and proper in this and most other situations in which the adolescent female has a potentially significant pelvic problem. It is usually readily and painlessly done if a gentle, matter-of-fact, reassuring approach is used and if the proper instruments are available; only occasionally will a general anesthetic be required.) Often, these maneuvers are all that are necessary to offer a reassuring prognosis. Only rarely, if doubt still exists, will studies of thyroid function, determinations of pituitary gonadotropin and 17-ketosteroid urinary excretion levels, skull x-ray films to detect pituitary lesions and skeletal x-rays to determine actual bone age, and other complicated diagnostic procedures be necessary to rule out a significant endocrine disorder or abnormality of general development.

True Primary Amenorrhea

In essence, as previously suggested, true primary amenorrhea is the form of menarchal delay that persists into maturity and is caused by some fundamental and serious underlying developmental, endocrine, metabolic, systemic, or psychological disorder. Although by definition it is associated with an otherwise normal puberty, it also may be the result of dysfunction or disease in the hypothalamus, pituitary, or ovary, as well as of uterovaginal or gonadal anomalies or a variety of other, more generalized somatic, nutritional, and emotional disorders. It is more conveniently discussed in Chapter 6, where its various causes and its management are presented in detail along with the other fundamental endocrinologic disorders affecting the reproductive tract.

Secondary Amenorrhea

Obviously prolonged amenorrhea (at least 6 to 12 months in duration) occurring after an apparently normal menarche, with several months or even years of seemingly normal cyclic menstrual function, is often the result of the postmenarchal development of any of the conditions producing primary amenorrhea. In the adolescent, however, it is fair to state that the majority of instances of secondary amenorrhea are functional in nature and not due to organic disease or serious permanent dysfunction in the hypothalamic-pituitary-ovarian axis. Perhaps the commonest cause is to be found in minor emotional disturbances such as those occurring when the young woman goes to college and is away from home and family for the first time, or is having school problems or difficult interpersonal relationships. Such psychological upsets are frequently accompanied by a secondary nutritional disturbance (either weight loss, as in the anorexia nervosa type of syndrome, or obesity acquired when overeating is unconsciously employed as a means of relief from the tensions and anxieties of real or fancied emotional or social problems and inadequacies), contributing to the persistence of this hypothalamic or psychogenic type of amenorrhea, which may sometimes last for several years. Minor, often transient thyroid disturbances are also fairly frequent causes of secondary amenorrhea in adolescents. Less commonly, certain more fundamental ovarian disorders may begin to manifest themselves during late adolescence; the Stein-Leventhal (polycystic ovary) syndrome is an example.

As in the case of delayed menarche, amenorrhea is a frequent cause for alarm in the young girl and her parents, so that a similar, careful but restrained investigative survey should be undertaken. Once the possibility of pregnancy has been excluded, unless obvious evidence of a potential fundamental endocrine disease is uncovered, liberal reassurance should be given and a policy of watchful waiting adopted. In most cases, this will be rewarded by spontaneous return of normal menstrual activity, without the need for any active therapy or costly exhaustive diagnostic studies. Detailed consideration of the causes, diagnostic approach to, and treatment of secondary amenorrhea due to more specific and fundamental disorders will be found in Chapter 6.

Adolescent Menstrual Disorders

DYSFUNCTIONAL UTERINE BLEEDING

As is by now apparent, functional irregularities in the hypothalamic-pituitary-ovarian relationships are characteristic of adolescent reproductive tract physiology, and it is therefore not surprising that anovulatory cycles with accompanying irregularity of the periods, oligomenorrhea, polymenorrhea, menorrhagia, "intermenstrual" bleeding, and so on, are among some of the more common pelvic symptoms encountered and account for 95 percent of the cases of abnormal bleeding in this age group. Aside from their increased frequency at this time of life, the abnormal physiology, clinical picture, and management of adolescent functional menstrual disorders are the same as for the identical functional menstrual disorders encountered in the adult woman (see Chap. 5).

Obviously, minor early manifestations of more fundamental disorders and diseases of the pituitary, thyroid, adrenal, and ovary may in their early phases simulate simple temporary adolescent ovarian dysfunction. This possibility must therefore be borne in mind, particularly if there are other suggestive clues in the history and physical findings and if response to conservative management is not satisfactory. Usually, however, the diagnostic workup can safely be considerably less extensive than in the case of an adult woman, and if any treatment at all is indicated, supplemental cyclic hormone therapy for a brief time is usually all that is necessary. Only rarely will curettage be needed, either for diagnostic purposes or to control unusually prolonged, heavy uterine bleeding.

HEMORRHAGIC DISORDERS

One specific aspect of the problem of excessive menstrual bleeding as encountered in adolescents does warrant emphasis, however. This concerns the fact that a number of the various generalized hemorrhagic disorders not only occur predominantly in females but also often are first manifested during adolescence. Heavy, prolonged menstrual flow at this time may indicate the presence of such a disorder in the absence of any other suggestive symptoms or signs. Idiopathic thrombocytopenic purpura and the so-called idiopathic bleeding-time defect, the latter perhaps inaccurately often termed **pseudohemophilia**, are the two notable examples encountered most frequently in this clinical setting. There may or may not be an obvious history suggesting prior evidence of a bleeding tendency in the patient or her family, but these important historical clues should always be sought. And certainly in any young girl whose principal complaint is menorrhagia, but who has regular cycles that do not suggest a functional disturbance of ovarian origin, a complete hematologic evaluation of the type presented in Chapter 2 is definitely indicated before any therapeutic measures are invoked. In the absence of ovarian endocrine dysfunction, cyclic supplemental estrogen, progesterone, or both will be of no benefit whatsoever, and curettage is frequently followed by increased and sometimes alarming hemorrhage. A correct diagnosis is imperative, because steroid therapy directed at either of these two most commonly encountered hemorrhagic disorders is frequently highly successful in controlling both the generalized bleeding tendency and its major manifestation, the menorrhagia. Rarer causes of an abnormal bleeding tendency in females of any age will either be obvious, as in the case of profound systemic diseases or toxic states with secondary hematologic manifestations, or will also be discovered during the course of a careful hematologic investigation, as in the case of the more unusual primary hemorrhagic disorders.

ABNORMAL BLEEDING SECONDARY TO LOCAL ORGANIC DISEASE

Although extremely uncommon in adolescence, benign or malignant lesions of the uterus, cervix, and vagina may be the source of abnormal vaginal bleeding in this age group as well as in older women. As already noted, the possibility of vaginal adenosis or clear cell adenocarcinoma of the vagina or cervix must always be considered when abnormal vaginal bleeding occurs in childhood and especially in adolescence. The presence of lesions is usually readily excluded or confirmed by pelvic examination; only rarely, if none of the other more likely causes for the abnormal bleeding already discussed is discovered and no satisfactory response to treatment is obtained, will a diagnostic curettage be necessary or indicated. If such a lesion is found, treatment will be based on the same general principles that apply to the management of similar pathologic conditions in the older woman.

Dysmenorrhea

Of the entire group of functional menstrual disorders, dysmenorrhea of the primary or "essential" type is the one other problem appearing frequently — in fact, characteristically — during adolescence. Since the first few years of menstrual function are often anovulatory in nature, it usually does not become manifest until age 15 or 16. Actually, it is the most common menstrual disturbance of all in the adolescent age group; an estimated 30 to 50 percent of all young women suffer appreciably from it. Only rarely is it secondary to local pelvic disease, although the presence of an organic basis for menstrual pain must always be excluded and usually readily is. Although essentially a physiologic, almost normal phenomenon (the sign of the young, normally ovulating female), it frequently has fundamental psychological overtones, both from the standpoint of the basic etiology of pain and disability of sufficient magnitude to prompt a physically healthy, physiologically normal girl to seek medical attention, as well as from the standpoint of secondary anxieties and vague fears of serious disease aroused in the minds of both the young woman and her parents by the periodic discomfort. Because it is often allowed to produce a significant disruption in the normal activities of the young girl, it should be viewed as the real, potentially serious problem that it actually is and dealt with promptly and sympathetically. No elaborate investigation is needed, but a thorough history and physical examination must be done — in part to exclude organic disease, but primarily so that it will be obvious to both the girl and her parents that the thorough explanation and reassurance so vital to effective management is based on fact, not fancy. Since the problem is not limited to adolescence, a more detailed discussion of differential diagnosis and therapy is more appropriately presented in Chapter 5. Fortunately, the condition is usually self-limited, tending to decrease in significance as psychological or emotional maturity catches up with physical and physiologic maturity in the late teens and early twenties.

MISCELLANEOUS PELVIC DISORDERS OF ADOLESCENCE

The rare occurrence of benign and malignant pelvic neoplasms in adolescent girls has already been mentioned, including DES-induced vaginal adenosis and clear cell adenocarcinomas of the vagina and cervix. Since these adolescents are for the most part now sexually mature, pregnancy and its complications, as well as venereal diseases and pelvic inflammatory disorders, will also be seen occasionally. Clinical manifestations of pelvic endometriosis are uncommon, although the pathologic process undoubtedly has its earliest beginnings in late adolescence in many instances. As in the childhood years, vulvovaginitis is also seen occasionally and is diagnosed and treated as in childhood. In this connection, the retained tampon, its presence unknown and forgotten by the young woman, becomes one of the more common causes of vaginal discharge.

The premenstrual tension syndrome in its full-blown form is only infrequently seen in adolescence, and significant cyclic breast symptoms and chronic cystic mastitis are even less frequent, although the appearance and often rapid growth of benign fibroadenomas of the breast are not uncommon in the late teens and early twenties. Thyroid disturbances are also frequent in this age group. Hence physical examination of the older adolescent with pelvic complaints should always include careful palpation of the thyroid and breasts, as well as the abdomen, before surveying the pelvis. With regard to the latter, vaginal examination is usually possible, often helpful, and no longer likely to be associated with the risk of any psychic trauma if carefully done.

From a general feminine hygiene standpoint, the young woman should be helped to accept the point of view that an internal examination is simply a natural and important aspect of a complete health survey and as such is merely good medical practice; that the use of menstrual tampons is perfectly proper, safe, and often extremely convenient in her busy, active life; and that routine douching, regardless of ancient female traditions and former beliefs on the part of the medical profession, is entirely unnecessary in the healthy female of any age. She should be acquainted with the value and importance of premarital examination at the proper time. Above all, it should be stressed at all times when dealing with the adolescent female that the manifestations of her cyclic reproductive tract function are entirely normal and that she can be certain that menstruation is not in actuality the "curse" her mother or grandmother often felt had been inflicted on women. Reassurance along these lines is immeasurably aided by dispelling what to her mind seem to be mysteries and vagaries of this cyclic function through careful explanation in whatever simple physiologic terms seem appropriate. This is a time when the gynecologist has an opportunity not only to instruct the adolescent female in the normal anatomy and physiology of the female but also to help her begin to achieve a better understanding of the even more important psychological and emotional aspects of normal sexuality.

REFERENCES

1. Acosta, A., Kaplan, A. L., and Kaufman, R. H. Gynecologic cancer in children. *Am. J. Obstet. Gynecol.* 112:944, 1972.
2. Adelman, S., Benson, C. D., and Hertzler, J. H. Surgical lesions of the ovary in infancy and childhood. *Surg. Gynecol. Obstet.* 141:219, 1975.

3. Albright, F., Butler, A. M., Hampton, A. O., and Smith, P. Syndrome characterized by osteitis fibrosa disseminata, areas of pigmentation and endocrine dysfunction, with precocious puberty in females. *N. Engl. J. Med.* 216:727, 1937.

4. Capraro, V. J., Dillon, W. P., and Gallego, M. B. Microperforate hymen: A distinct clinical entity. *Obstet. Gynecol.* 44:903, 1974.

5. Capraro, V. J., and Greenberg, H. Adhesions of the labia minora: A study of 50 patients. *Obstet. Gynecol.* 39:65, 1972.

6. Fetherston, W. C. Squamous metaplasia of vagina related to DES syndrome. *Am. J. Obstet. Gynecol.* 122:176, 1975.

7. Forsberg, J. G. Estrogen, vaginal cancer, and vaginal development. *Am. J. Obstet. Gynecol.* 113:83, 1972.

8. Heald, F. P., Daugela, M., and Brunschuyler, P. Physiology of adolescence. *N. Engl. J. Med.* 268:192, 1963.

9. Herbst, A. L., Kurman, R. J., and Scully, R. E. Vaginal and cervical abnormalities after exposure to stilbestrol in utero. *Obstet. Gynecol.* 40:287, 1972.

10. Herbst, A. L., Poskanzer, D. C., Robboy, S. J., Friedlander, L., and Scully, R. E. Prenatal exposure to stilbestrol. *N. Engl. J. Med.* 292:334, 1975.

11. Herbst, A. L., Robboy, S. J., Scully, R. E., and Poskanzer, D. C. Clear-cell adenocarcinoma of the vagina and cervix in girls: Analysis of 170 Registry cases. *Am. J. Obstet. Gynecol.* 119:713, 1974.

12. Herbst, A. L., Ulfelder, H., and Poskanzer, D. C. Adenocarcinoma of the vagina: Association of maternal stilbestrol therapy with tumor appearance in young women. *N. Engl. J. Med.* 284:878, 1971.

13. Hilgers, R. D. Pelvic exenteration for vaginal embryonal rhabdomyosarcoma: A review. *Obstet. Gynecol.* 45:175, 1975.

14. James, D. F., Barber, H. R. K., and Graber, E. A. Torsion of normal uterine adnexa in children. *Obstet. Gynecol.* 35:226, 1970.

15. Lang, W. R. Pediatric vaginitis. *N. Engl. J. Med.* 253:1153, 1955.

16. McArthur, J. M. Functional disorders of menstruation in adolescence. *N. Engl. J. Med.* 249:361, 1953.

17. Schauffler, G. C. *Pediatric Gynecology* (4th ed.). Chicago: Year Book, 1958.

18. Smith, J. P., Rutledge, F. N., and Sutow, W. W. Malignant gynecologic tumors in children: Current approaches to treatment. *Am. J. Obstet. Gynecol.* 116:261, 1973.

19. Stafl, A., and Mattingly, R. F. Vaginal adenosis: A precancerous lesion? *Am. J. Obstet. Gynecol.* 120:666, 1974.

20. Stafl, A., Mattingly, R. F., Foley, D. V., and Fetherston, W. C. Clinical diagnosis of vaginal adenosis. *Obstet. Gynecol.* 43:118, 1974.

21. Wharton, J. T., Rutledge, F. N., Gallager, H. S., and Fletcher, G. Treatment of clear-cell adenocarcinoma in young females. *Obstet. Gynecol.* 45:365, 1975.

22. Wurtman, R. J. The pineal gland in relation to reproduction. *Am. J. Obstet. Gynecol.* 104:320, 1969.

5
Functional Menstrual Disorders

Throughout the period of reproductive tract activity, from menarche to menopause, functional disturbances in normal physiology and the closely related symptomatic manifestations of even essentially normal cyclic ovarian function constitute the single most common type of clinical problem with which the gynecologist is confronted. These disorders are often, though by no means always, transient, their symptoms being actually of no basic importance. When persistent, however, they frequently lead to excessive blood loss and secondary anemia, may cause serious disability, and, most important, may be accompanied by undesirable infertility. Finally, ever present is the need to establish the definite diagnosis of a functional disturbance and to exclude or, equally important, to avoid overlooking the concomitant presence of potentially more serious organic disease, either local uterovaginal or adnexal lesions or more generalized, fundamental endocrine disorders of ovarian, thyroid, adrenal, or pituitary origin. A preliminary review of the basic physiology involved in normal cyclic menstrual function seems essential to a better understanding of the mechanisms at work when abnormal function occurs and symptoms appear. Thereafter, the principal types of functional menstrual disorders will be discussed in some detail, with particular emphasis on specific features of the deranged physiology, the diagnostic approach, and the principles of management and types of therapy that have proved most successful in each.

BASIC PHYSIOLOGY OF THE NORMAL MENSTRUAL CYCLE

No attempt will be made to survey even briefly all the presently available information concerning the elaborate cytochemical and enzymatic details or the extremely complex and interrelated steroid-hormone synthesis and metabolism involved in the regulation of the normal menstrual cycle. Such information is available in more exhaustive textbooks or obtainable in complete form in monographs or papers reporting the original fundamental biochemical observations and discoveries. Although it is obviously of great biologic significance, it is not essential to a comprehensive, basic working knowledge of the key facts of cyclic female reproductive tract function. To this extent, this review is perhaps an oversimplification, but it is presented in the belief that a somewhat simplified or streamlined conceptual scheme can be more readily applied in a useful way to a correct understanding and management of the various clinical problems that arise in connection with disturbances of this normally regular cyclic activity.

The Hypothalamic-Pituitary-Ovarian Axis

The initiation of cyclic menstrual function at puberty has already been briefly summarized in Chapter 4. As soon as regular periodic flow has become established in a completely mature, adult pattern, the regulation of the normal cycle is under the control of the reciprocally related neurohormonal mechanism inherently present in the hypothalamic-pituitary-ovarian axis. The fundamental features of this regulatory system and the endometrial response patterns are graphically illustrated in Figure 24 but require some additional verbal elaboration.

It has now been well established that neurohormones produced by a network of neurons in the hypothalamus, namely, the luteinizing hormone (LH) releasing factor LH-RH and possibly a follicle-stimulating hormone (FSH) releasing factor FSH-RH (the two may actually be one and the same, with LH-RH serving to cause the release of both FSH and LH), are carried to the adenohypophysis via the pituitary portal circulation. There, in a complex interaction with gonadal steroids, they are responsible for the control of the pituitary secretion of FSH and LH. In essence, these releasing factors are the chemical messengers between the cerebral cortex and the secretory cells of the pituitary gland. There are similar releasing factors for the thyroid-stimulating hormone (TSH), and pituitary corticotropin (adrenocorticotropin, or ACTH); these are respectively TSH-RH and CRF, or corticotropin releasing factor. And there are releasing factors for both growth hormone secretion (somatotropin releasing factor) and growth hormone inhibition (somatostatin, growth hormone inhibiting factor).

In the first few days of each new cycle (i.e., immediately following the onset of menstruation) in response to the withdrawal of the inhibiting effect of the high premenstrual levels of estrogen and progesterone (occasioned by their sudden fall to extremely low levels coincident with corpus luteum deterioration and subsequent menstrual flow), the basophilic or "beta" cells of the anterior lobe of the pituitary are once again stimulated by the hypothalamic releasing factor to secrete increasing amounts of the pituitary gonadotropin FSH. The ovary normally responds – or more correctly, the primordial ovarian follicles respond – by secretory activity on the part of the follicular cells and stroma. In the human female a single follicle ordinarily is destined to become the dominant one, and this dominant follicle is usually the only one to continue to respond and progress in maturation and function. (Occasionally more than one follicle is stimulated to the point of ovulation and corpus luteum function, thus accounting for biovular twinning.)

During the very earliest phases of ovarian follicle response, while some growth is occurring in a number of follicles, these same anterior pituitary cells begin also to elaborate LH (identical with ICSH, or interstitial cell–stimulating hormone, in the male), and under the combined stimulation of a small amount of LH and the by now larger amounts of FSH, the follicle cells, specifically those of the granulosa and theca interna layers, begin to secrete estrogens. At first, this consists of low levels of both estrone and estradiol, but by midcycle the levels are increasing rapidly, and the ratio of estradiol (the most biologically active estrogen) to estrone is also markedly increased. (The overall level of the gonadotropins is attained through the combined effects of a constant or tonic secretion and an intermittent or pulsatile secretion.) As circulating estrogen levels rise, a reciprocal inhibition or braking effect on the pituitary output of FSH comes into play (initial negative feedback effect of estrogen

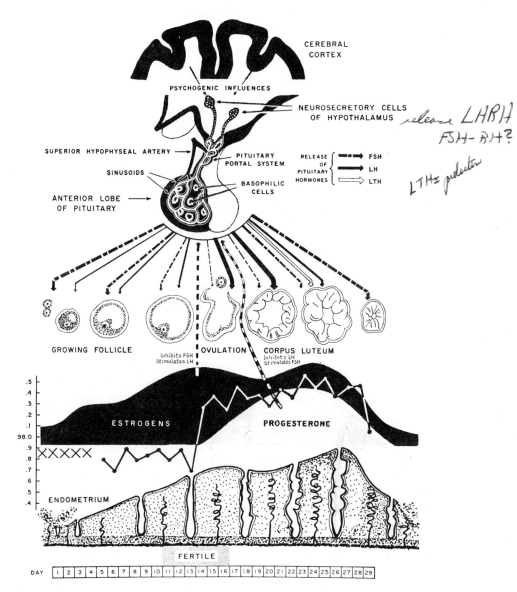

Figure 24
Diagram of the physiology of the normal menstrual cycle. Cerebral, hypothalamic, pituitary, ovarian, and endometrial interrelationships. (From L. Parsons and S. C. Sommers, *Gynecology*. Philadelphia: Saunders, 1962, p. 152, where it appeared as a modification of a drawing from *The Ciba Collection of Medical Illustrations* by F. H. Netter. Copyright CIBA Pharmaceutical Co.)

on pituitary secretion of FSH and LH), but although FSH secretion begins to decline, the pituitary continues to produce more LH (subsequent positive feedback effect of estrogen on pituitary secretion of LH alone). At a crucial point, approximately at or shortly before midcycle, with both estrogen and LH levels on the rise and already approaching a maximum, and with FSH well on the decline but still present in a small, but critical amount, the one dominant follicle undergoes characteristic vascular, cellular, and secretory changes and moves to a position near the surface of the ovary. Thereafter, ovulation is climactically stimulated to occur, probably by a sudden surge in pituitary LH production (and possibly FSH as well) initiated by the outpouring of LH releasing factor elaborated by the hypothalamus. The mechanism by which a single follicle is selected for the "final ascent to the top" is unknown; the remaining partially stimulated follicles simply persist in a resting state or ultimately become atretic but continue to secrete variable amounts of estrogen throughout the rest of the cycle.

Following ovulation, the pituitary continues to secrete increasing amounts of LH, but, in addition, the acidophilic cells ("alpha" cells) of the anterior lobe also appear to come into action and begin the release of a third gonadotropin, formerly referred to as the luteotropic hormone (LTH), but now known to be a lactogenic hormone, prolactin. Prolactin (HPRL) is chemically similar to, but definitely not identical with, human growth hormone (HGH). The mechanism by which prolactin production is triggered is again apparently based on a critical balance among the levels of the two other gonadotropins and estrogen (and possibly small amounts of progesterone as well), mediated by neurohormonal stimuli from the hypothalamus. Although HPRL is probably not absolutely essential for maintenance of the corpus luteum in man, the combined effects of LH and HPRL produce additional cytochemical changes in the granulosa and theca interna cells, and under this dual influence they become luteinized and elaborate increasing amounts of progesterone. Once again, a reciprocal inhibition effect comes strongly into play toward the end of the cycle, or premenstrual phase. At this point, rising progesterone levels have progressively suppressed the output of LH and HPRL, and the corpus luteum, increasingly deprived of their stimulating support, begins to decline. Simultaneously, with falling LH and HPRL levels, the return of active production of FSH is favored, and the beginning stimulation of new follicles that will take part in the succeeding menstrual cycle occurs before the current one has quite been terminated. With final corpus luteum deterioration, estrogen and progesterone levels suddenly fall dramatically, and the resulting rapid withdrawal of adequate hormone support for the further growth and anatomic and physiologic integrity of the endometrium and its vascular bed leads to the necrosis, sloughing or desquamation, and bleeding characteristic of the menstrual flow. By now, as already noted, the early events that will result in repetition of the same sequence of balanced, reciprocally related neurohormonal and cytochemical phenomena in the next and all subsequent normal cycles are well under way.

It should be noted that it is really the hypothalamus that exerts the controlling influence on the cyclic pituitary activity by virtue of its elaboration of the neurohormones LH-RH and (?) FSH-RH (it is still possible that LH-RH may be responsible for the release of both FSH and LH), as well as a prolactin releasing factor, HPRL-RH, and a prolactin inhibiting factor, HPRL-IF. These hormone releasing factors produced in the hypothalamus are carried directly to the pituitary via the hypothalamic-pituitary portal system of blood vessels traveling along the pituitary stalk to the gland below. This better understanding of the hypothalamic-pituitary relationships has helped to clarify the underlying mechanism involved in the several clinical entities in which both amenorrhea and persistent lactation are seen (e.g., Chiari-Frommel syndrome, discussed in Chapter 6).

If, however, ovulation should be followed by conception and proper implantation of the fertilized ovum, placental formation will proceed, and the early chorionic villi will attain a functional capacity adequate for the elaboration of sufficient chorionic gonadotropin as well as a placental lactogen (HPL) to continue to maintain the corpus luteum in a high state of secretory activity, even in the face of falling pituitary LH and HPRL. This in turn will prevent the onset of the expected menstruation and will preserve and rapidly further modify the endometrium (decidual change) in a manner even more favorable to the maintenance and subsequent normal development of the pregnancy. Placental gonadotropin secretion is adequate to this end within the first week of implantation, and the levels of chorionic gonadotropin are high enough to be detectable as a positive index of pregnancy by the radioimmunoassay pregnancy test approximately one week after the first missed period.

Cerebral, Thyroid, and Adrenal Factors

What has been presented thus far concerns only the basic regulatory physiology of the normal menstrual cycle and the modification introduced when pregnancy intervenes. In addition, three other influences on the otherwise self-contained mechanism must be acknowledged and also borne in mind as potential factors when disturbances arise.

CEREBRAL CORTICAL CENTERS

The anatomic proximity and functional connections between the higher cortical centers and the hypothalamus are also shown in Figure 24. Although the exact nature of whatever may be the neural equilibrium between cortex and hypothalamus essential for normal cycle regulations is unknown, disturbances in this equilibrium are an extremely common cause of functional menstrual disorders. Thus psychogenic influences of great variety and apparently mediated via this cortical-hypothalamic pathway often profoundly affect a previously (and subsequently) perfectly normal, regular menstrual pattern. The frequent, often prolonged, so-called hypothalamic amenorrhea of college women away from home for the first time is a familiar example, as is the delayed period in the young single woman who fears she may have recently conceived, though ultimately her fear proves to be without foundation. Grief reactions, acute or chronic anxiety states, too frantic a pace of living, periods of high excitement, and a multitude of mental problems or emotional difficulties are often wholly or in part responsible for the alterations in normal cyclic menstrual function that are so commonly encountered. (The recently elucidated, potential role of the pineal gland in regulating the hypothalamic control of pituitary gonadotropin secretion is also mentioned in Chapter 4.) Natural and synthetic hormone releasing factor preparations are now available and offer a means for the accurate diagnosis of hypothalamic menstrual disorders and the ability to differentiate them from menstrual disorders of pituitary origin; they may also provide a potential method of treatment.

In similar fashion, variations in steroid hormone levels and balance may in turn affect various areas of the central nervous system, including cortical function. One may thus account for the various emotional changes and disturbances that may sometimes be encountered in relation to the menstrual cycle, pregnancy and parturition, and oral contraceptive programs. Since the so-called mood changes often parallel a weight increase and fluid retention, it is possible that they are caused by activation of the renin-angiotensin-aldosterone system as the levels of ovarian hormones fluctuate. There is also evidence that the migraine headaches that occur regularly in association with the menstrual cycle are probably specifically related to the sharp premenstrual drop in estradiol and are not due to the equally abrupt simultaneous fall in progesterone, as had once been thought.

THYROID FUNCTION

Normal thyroid function is an essential feature of the general background for normal cyclic female reproductive tract activity. This is not surprising, because the same anterior lobe area of the pituitary also elaborates TSH, and there may well be interrelationships between gonadotropin and TSH secretion that link the menstrual cycle and thyroid function together at the hypothalamic-pituitary level. Furthermore, the general effect of thyroid hormone on tissue metabolism is obviously of importance to the proper functioning of the entire neurohormonal regulatory mechanism, as well as to the cellular-metabolic and cytochemical events that must take place in the ovary and subsequently in the rest of the target organs in the reproductive tract for the estrogen and progesterone produced by the properly maturing follicle. In view of these facts, it is obvious why thyroid disorders, either hyperthyroidism or hypothyroidism, characteristically are accompanied by functional menstrual disorders. In fact, in the case of mild degrees of hypothyroidism, menstrual dysfunction may be the sole or principal clinical manifestation prompting the patient to seek medical advice.

ADRENAL FUNCTION

In the case of adrenal function, the relationship to hypothalamic-pituitary-ovarian activity is even more complex and intimate. The ACTH elaborated by the pituitary, though normally stimulating primarily the adrenal production of corticosteroids, may, particularly in excess amounts, elicit the production of androgens and estrogens by the adrenal. Rising levels of these hormones, though of adrenal rather than ovarian origin, will inhibit pituitary secretion of FSH and LH and drastically interfere with normal gonadal function (as in congenital adrenal hyperplasia). Furthermore, both LH and HPRL, in addition to their normal effects on ovarian function, also stimulate the adrenals to produce androgens and probably aldosterone as well, and these steroids of adrenal origin are also essential to the normal hormonal, metabolic, and fluid and electrolyte alterations that occur during the normal menstrual cycle. Obviously, deficient or excessive adrenal stimulation or adrenal hypofunction or hyperactivity will be accompanied by fundamental disturbances of cyclic menstrual function; this is illustrated clinically in the menstrual disorders commonly associated with Cushing's disease, Addison's disease, and the adrenogenital syndrome, whether due to adrenocortical hyperplasia or tumor.

Finally, the inherent biochemical similarities between adrenocortical cells and ovarian cortical and stromal cells in terms of the potential ability of each to synthesize a wide variety of steroids of both androgenic and estrogenic activity are sometimes reflected in the apparent production of androgens and even adrenal-like steroids by the ovary itself in certain pathologic states.

Endometrial and Myometrial Responses in the Normal Cycle

In the first half of the cycle, when the uterus and the other target organs that are responsive to hormones of ovarian origin are primarily under the influence of estrogen, growth or proliferation is the keynote of their response. This preovulatory phase is hence often referred to as the proliferative, follicular, or estrogenic phase or half of the cycle. Estrogen activity is initiated in the target organs by the linkage of estradiol to specific estrogen receptor-binding proteins in the cells. (Such specific cellular estrogen receptors are present not only in the endometrium but also in the hypothalamus, vagina, and breast, all of which are loci of estrogen activity.) Similar specific progesterone-binding proteins and cell receptors are also present in the uterus. Proliferation on the part of the endometrial glands and stroma is extremely active and rapidly results in a complete reepithelialization of the functioning layer and a threefold increase in its thickness by midcycle. An endometrial biopsy taken during this portion of the cycle exhibits the typical histologic changes characterized by the pathologist's term, **proliferative endometrium** (Fig. 25A). The myometrial cells also enlarge and elongate, and the spiral arteriolar capillary bed of the functioning endometrial layer also proliferates to afford an adequate blood supply for the growing endometrial lining.

On the other hand, in the second half of the cycle that follows ovulation, the ovarian production of progesterone dominates the scene, and the response of the target organs is essentially one of functional change or activity rather than significant further growth. Since this involves secretory activity for the most part, and since the proper secretory response is primarily dependent on the presence of adequate amounts of progesterone, this second or postovulatory phase of the cycle is usually called the

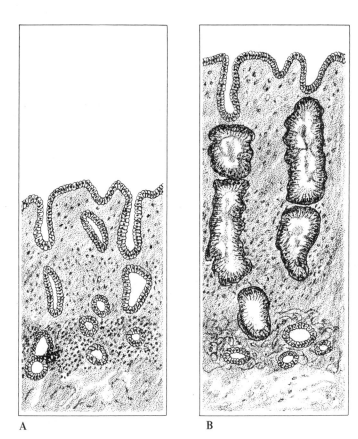

Figure 25
Endometrial histology. A. Proliferative endometrium. B. Secretory endometrium.

secretory, luteal, or progestational phase. Again, an endometrial biopsy taken well along in the second half of the cycle will show the typical histologic features of a normal response, which the pathologist has come to designate as **secretory endo-metrium** (Fig. 25B). The endometrial glands will have assumed their familiar, coiled, elongated, tortuous, sawtooth appearance, the cells showing secretory vacuoles and the tubular lumina bulging with secretion. The endometrial stroma becomes adematous, and the stromal cells begin to show predecidual changes. The spiral arteriolar network also becomes increasingly prominent and tortuous.

With the cycle nearing completion, one of two things must happen: If pregnancy has occurred, the corpus luteum will continue to be supported by the chorionic gonadotropin of the early placenta, and with the continued production of estrogen and progesterone in increasing amounts, the endometrium and myometrium will undergo further anatomic and functional changes, with the resulting decidual transformation that favors maintenance and further development of the pregnancy. If pregnancy does not occur, a rapidly increasing rate of decline in estrogen and progesterone levels accompanying normal corpus luteum degeneration will produce the typical sequence of events in the uterus that leads to menstruation. The endometrium itself shrinks in thickness in the days immediately preceding menstruation; in addition to actual loss of substance in this way, the arterioles begin to collapse and ooze beneath the outer, functional layer, forming blood "lakes" that cause further endometrial ischemic and pressure necrosis. There is evidence that a vasoconstrictor substance may be released as a result of this beginning endometrial disintegration. This appears to be locally active on the spiral arteriolar network during the 24 hours prior to the actual onset of menstrual flow, and it is probably this more profound and more generalized vasoconstriction and consequent intense endometrial ischemia that result in the actual sloughing away of the superficial, functioning endometrial layer. Because of this vasoconstrictive effect, and also because myometrial tone is increased by the premenstrual hormonal and neurovascular phenomena occurring in the normal cycle, permitting the myometrial layer to have an additional tourniquetlike constrictive effect on the more proximal portion of the spiral arterioles, excessive blood loss during the menstrual period is ordinarily neatly avoided. These same two hemostatic mechanisms are probably also largely responsible for the premenstrual and early menstrual uterine cramps so characteristic of the normal ovulatory menstrual flow. By the end of four to seven days, the old functioning endometrial layer has been completely shed, and a new growth cycle is already under way.

Important Physiologic Changes in Other Parts of the Reproductive Tract During the Normal Cycle

FALLOPIAN TUBES

Increases in the number and activity of the ciliated cells of the tubal epithelium, in tubal peristaltic activity, and in tubal secretions are all clearly evident just before and for some days following ovulation. In addition, slow contraction of the tubal musculature and shortening of the ovarian ligament at ovulation time tend to draw the fimbriated end of the tube into closer apposition with the ovary. All these mechanisms facilitate the reception of the ovum by the fimbriated end and its further passage and nourishment in transit through the length of the fallopian tube. Each mechanism in turn is brought into play as a result of the stimulus of estrogen and progesterone applied to the cellular activity of the tissues involved in the proper sequence and in the correct total and relative amounts. During this same critical time of ovum transport, these changes in the volume and composition of tubal secretions are equally important in facilitating the passage of sperm in the opposite direction, since normally they are favorable to both sperm motility and survival. It has also been established that an appropriate biochemical environment within the tube is necessary to prepare both ovum and sperm for the fertilization process and to provide a life-support system for the morula (fertilized egg) during the early days prior to the implantation.

CERVIX

In a similar fashion, alterations in the amount and chemical constitution of the cervical secretions occur during the critical few days around ovulation time and are also dependent on the proper amounts and relative balance of estrogen and progesterone. As a result of change in volume and in protein and electrolyte composition, the normally thick, gelatinous, opaque cervical secretions become thin, abundant, stringy, clear, and rich in nutrient materials, and the pH shifts from an acid range of about 4.0 to a decidedly alkaline range of 7.0 to 8.0. Thus the cervical mucus plug, ordinarily a complete barrier both to bacteria and spermatozoa, is converted into a liquid medium of entry entirely favorable to sperm penetration, motility, and survival by virtue of its altered physical characteristics, its alkalinity, and its glucose, electrolyte, and protein composition. These important physiologic changes are reflected in the various measurable items utilized clinically both as tests of the adequacy of cervical response as well as indirect evidence of the status of ovarian function and the presence or absence of ovulation. The fern test, measurement of cervical pH, quantitative determination of spinnbarkeit (or the ability of normal cervical mucus to be drawn out into long threads only at ovulation time), and the Sims-Huhner test of actual sperm penetration of the cervical mucus at ovulation time are all valuable clinical indexes of the normality of the ovarian cycle and cervical response. (Obviously, inadequate cervical response may also be seen in the presence of significant local disease such as severe chronic endocervicitis, even though ovarian function is normal.)

VAGINA

The cyclic hormonal changes accompanying normal ovarian function are also reflected in the vaginal epithelium. Proliferation as well as changes in the relative proportions of the various cell types or stages in cell maturation are involved, and, as the time of ovulation is approached, a shift from the acid pH of 4.0 to an alkaline range of 7.0 to 8.0 and an increase in the glycogen content of the now abundantly desquamating "cornified" superficial cells also occur. These preovulatory and ovulatory alterations in vaginal physiology parallel those in the cervix and also facilitate sperm survival and motility. The resulting cyclic changes in the vaginal mucosa can also be utilized clinically (by means of serial vaginal cytologic smears as described in Chapter 2) as an index of the status of ovarian function with respect to both ovulation and hormone output.

BREASTS

Mammary tissue is an integral part of the female reproductive tract and is also responsive to the monthly stimulus of estrogen and progesterone elaborated by the ovary during the normal cycle. During the estrogenic phase of the ovarian cycle, there appears to be some ductal and glandular proliferation, and during the progestational phase, this epithelial activity may be enhanced and may be accompanied by edema and vascular congestion of the supporting stroma. Clinically, these changes are manifested by the typical breast symptoms (discomfort, tenderness, and swelling) experienced by the vast majority of women during the premenstrual phase of the cycle. As might be expected, as the hormonal stimulus is removed at the onset of menstruation, these breast symptoms usually promptly subside.

General Body Changes During the Normal Cycle

BASAL BODY TEMPERATURE CHANGES

Certainly the most obvious and most readily verified and quantitated of all the systemic changes in the reproductive cycle is the abrupt shift in the level of the basal body temperature that occurs at or shortly before ovulation as a result of the thermogenic effect of progesterone. Its purpose, if any, is unknown, but this thermal shift is of course the basis for the use of the basal body temperature chart as an indicator of ovulation and adequate progesterone production by the corpus luteum.

CHANGES IN ELECTROLYTE AND FLUID BALANCE

There are numerous other cyclic fluctuations in general body physiology, with the majority most pronounced during the premenstrual or early menstrual phase. However, many of these fluctuations are as yet neither well defined nor clearly understood. One deserving of mention because of its frequent clinical significance when exaggerated is the tendency toward salt and fluid retention manifest during the late progestational and premenstrual phase. This change in electrolyte and fluid balance is apparently a reflection of the steroid hormone pattern characteristic of the last week or so of the normal cycle. It becomes more pronounced when estrogens (perhaps aldosterone or similar compounds of ovarian or adrenal origin may also be involved, at least under certain circumstances) are in relative excess, as they may be when corpus luteum function is not entirely adequate and progesterone deficiency of varying degree is present. At any rate, many of the systemic premenstrual molimina of the normal cycle are probably the result of this change in fluid and electrolyte metabolism. At least one of the symptomatic functional menstrual disorders not accompanied by failure of ovulation, namely, the premenstrual tension syndrome, is perhaps best explained on the basis of an exaggeration of this normal physiologic phenomenon.

VICARIOUS MENSTRUATION

In addition to its effects on the genital tract, elevation of the serum estrogen level near the end of each cycle produces congestion and hyperemia in a number of other tissues, most notably the nasal, gastric, and bladder mucosa, less often in the conjunctiva and in the skin. Such changes may produce so-called **vicarious menstruation** in the form of cyclic bleeding from these mucous membranes coinciding with the menses and may also be responsible for the cyclic purpura or easy bruising of the skin noted by some women just before and during the early days of each menstrual period.

RECURRING CATAMENIAL PNEUMOTHORAX

Finally, another episodic phenomenon occurring occasionally but only in women having regular ovulatory cycles, is the syndrome of **recurring catamenial pneumothorax**. Although an occasional case occurring in relation to pleural or diaphragmatic endometriosis has been reported, it almost invariably occurs as a result of the spontaneous rupture of pulmonary alvcoli (actual pulmonary blebs are usually absent and only rarely is there any demonstrable underlying pulmonary pathologic change). Apparently, alveolar rupture is triggered by some alteration in pulmonary physiology produced by exaggeration of the normal physiologic changes occurring in ovulatory cycles just before or just after the onset of menstruation. Perhaps the increased levels of prostaglandin F at this time are responsible, for this compound is known to cause bronchospasm as well as pulmonary arteriolar vasoconstriction. Invariably, the pneumothorax occurs on the right side, never occurs at any other time in the cycle, and it can be prevented by ovulation-suppressant drugs. Immediate treatment consists of prompt reexpansion of the lung by appropriate intercostal needle aspiration or tube drainage. If the pneumothorax persists despite drainage, or if it continues to recur, thoracotomy and operative pleurodesis may be necessary.

ABNORMAL PHYSIOLOGY OF THE ANOVULATORY CYCLE: THE BASIS FOR ALL DYSFUNCTIONAL OR ACYCLIC MENSTRUAL DISORDERS

Having reviewed the events and physiology of the normal menstrual cycle in some detail, it is now important to consider the fundamental disturbance in this normal cyclic physiologic mechanism that is common to all disorders involving irregular menstrual function.

Periodic uterine bleeding from an endometrium stimulated to grow by estrogen alone, sometimes occurring at regular but more often at totally irregular intervals and produced by either an absolute or a relative decline in estrogens below the critical level for continued endometrial growth and hormonal support, is called estrogen withdrawal (or anovulatory) bleeding. Such bleeding is also typically irregular in amount and duration, the flow varying in accordance with the length of time and degree of prior estrogenic stimulation, as well as with the degree and duration of the estrogen withdrawal. The absence of progesterone results from failure of any of the active ovarian follicles to mature to the point of ovulation and subsequent corpus luteum transformation and function, and hence such cycles are termed **anovulatory** (Fig. 26). The fluctuating estrogen levels that lead to periodic bleeding episodes alternating with intervals of amenorrhea of varying duration are due to intermittent

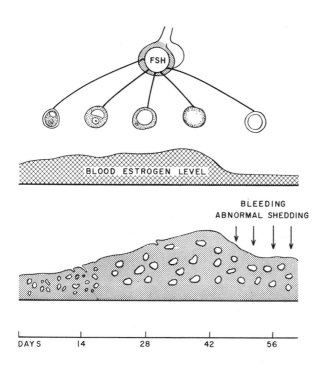

Figure 26
Pathophysiology of the anovulatory cycle.

variations in the number and functional status of the active ovarian follicles present at any particular time. If a number of follicles are present and active, and if new ones promptly assume functional capacity as some degenerate, high or even increasing levels of estrogen will be present, and the endometrium may continue to proliferate for weeks or months, even to the point of undergoing simple glandular hyperplasia (the so-called cystic or "Swiss cheese" hyperplasia) and ultimately gross, polypoid change if the stimulus to growth is sufficiently protracted (Fig. 27). If proliferation continues, though estrogen levels remain constant, a relative estrogen inadequacy will ultimately occur and lead to bleeding; one or more follicles may simultaneously deteriorate, and if these are not replaced promptly by actively functioning new ones, absolute estrogen withdrawal will result and endometrial bleeding will ensue.

As already noted, in an anovulatory cycle, the endometrium is stimulated to proliferate only, so that a specimen obtained by endometrial biopsy of curettage done at any time during such a cycle or during the bleeding phase will reveal either simple proliferative endometrium or cystic hyperplasia, with or without polypoid change, on histologic examination. Thus a biopsy performed at a time when a secretory endometrium would chronologically be expected were ovarian function normal is frequently absolutely diagnostic of the anovulatory nature of the cycle.

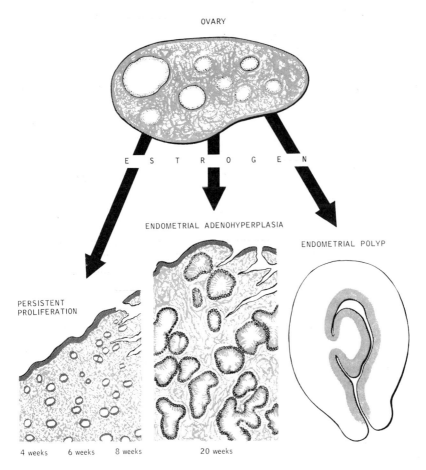

OVARY

E S T R O G E N

ENDOMETRIAL ADENOHYPERPLASIA

ENDOMETRIAL POLYP

PERSISTENT
PROLIFERATION

4 weeks   6 weeks   8 weeks   20 weeks

Figure 27
Mechanisms of anovulatory bleeding. (From L. Parsons and S. C. Sommers, *Gynecology*. Philadelphia: Saunders, 1962, p. 208.)

Because the progesterone-induced vasoconstrictive and myometrial contractive phenomena characteristic of normal ovulatory menstruation are absent, anovulatory bleeding is rarely, if ever, accompanied by cramps and is frequently excessively heavy due to the absence of these two normal hemostatic mechanisms. Excessive and prolonged flow is also due to the usual presence of a much thicker superficial endometrial layer and the accompanying richer blood supply and to the inefficiency with which it is desquamated in the absence of progesterone priming.

Abnormal responses are also forthcoming in the other ovarian hormone target areas as well, all due to the abnormal, continued estrogen stimulation in the absence of progesterone. As an example, prolonged, uninterrupted breast glandular activity induced by estrogen alone may lead to severe mastalgia and even to gross cystic changes. Similar unphysiologic responses are elicited in the fallopian tubes, cervix, vagina, and general body economy (including the monophasic basal body temperature curve, the usual ovulatory or preovulatory upward thermal shift failing to occur in the absence of progesterone), but these need not be detailed here. It is sufficient to point out that such a pattern of reproductive tract function is an infertile one, not only absolutely and primarily because of the obvious failure of ovulation but also secondarily because of the inadequacy of all the other mechanisms designed to promote ovum pickup and safe transfer, sperm penetration, survival, and transport, and a proper uterine environment favorable to the implantation and further growth of the early embryo — i.e., all the additional physiologic changes so vital to assure conception and continuation of a normal pregnancy. Thus, even were it somehow possible to supply at the proper time the ovum missing from an anovulatory cycle, conception would be most unlikely, and implantation and further development of even a hypothetically fertilized ovum would be impossible.

This concept of the more broadly viewed, overall infertility of the anovulatory type of menstrual "cycle" is not sheer academic nonsense but is important from the standpoint of the recognition, understanding, and treatment of a common and related disturbance, the so-called **inadequate luteal phase**, in which, although ovulation occurs, corpus luteum function and progesterone production are deficient. Although irregularities of menstruation may occur, they tend to be "regular irregularities," with temporary shifts in the intermenstrual intervals, transient variations in the amount, character, and duration of flow, and occasionally an almost cyclic intermenstrual or premenstrual staining. Most often the only manifestation is infertility, and since ovulation is occurring regularly, and since pregnancy frequently follows supplemental progesterone in the appropriate dosage at the proper time in the cycle, it is apparent that a broader concept of a fertile cycle than that implied by ovulation alone is valid and has practical significance.

The preceding partial digression is also intended to emphasize that it is not the lack of ovulation per se that is responsible for the various types of menstrual dysfunction that may accompany the anovulatory cycle, but the failure of normal follicle maturation and corpus luteum function (specifically, progesterone production), of which failure of ovulation is just one manifestation, although an important one in its own right.

It has already been mentioned that anovulatory menstrual function is characteristic of the first year or two following puberty. Ordinarily, the resulting irregularities are of minor importance, and excessive bleeding does not occur. However, persistence of an anovulatory type of ovarian function further along in adolescence, or its reappearance later on in adult life, is responsible for most of the clinically significant functional menstrual disorders encountered.

ACYCLIC MENSTRUAL DYSFUNCTION (DYSFUNCTIONAL OR ANOVULATORY UTERINE BLEEDING AND FUNCTIONAL AMENORRHEA)

With the underlying physiology of both normal and abnormal menstrual function clearly in mind, the groundwork has now been laid for a discussion of the various causes of menstrual dysfunction, the clinical manifestations, the diagnostic approach, the general principles of management, and some of the types and details of therapy in specific situations. Although many acyclic functional menstrual disturbances are accompanied by short intervals of amenorrhea or involve oligomenorrhea, the most prominent clinical feature is the occurrence, sooner or later, of excessive bleeding — too frequent flow, too heavy flow, too prolonged flow. Hence, this entire spectrum of functional menstrual irregularities is often considered under the term *dysfunctional uterine bleeding* or *anovulatory uterine bleeding.* (A decade or two ago, the term *metropathia hemorrhagica* was popular.)

Dysfunctional uterine bleeding is responsible for the largest single group of clinical problems that confronts the gynecologist. In a small percentage of women, the anovulatory cycles and associated irregular bleeding are in reality the result of some more fundamental endocrine disorder, the list of possibilities including the following:

1. Thyroid disease, either hyperthyroidism or hypothyroidism.
2. Adrenal disease, hyperplasia or benign or malignant tumors.
3. Pituitary disease, pituitary failure or neoplasms.
4. Diabetes mellitus, with its generalized metabolic and steroid hormonal disturbances.

Or the anovulatory type of ovarian function leading to irregular uterine bleeding may be due to a specific primary ovarian lesion, of which the following are the principal ones encountered:

1. Stein-Leventhal syndrome; ovarian hyperthecosis.
2. Functioning ovarian tumors: arrhenoblastoma, granulosa or theca cell tumors, hilus cell tumors.
3. Chronic pelvic inflammatory disease (or, more rarely, extensive pelvic endometriosis), in which there are severe pathologic changes in the ovaries leading to disturbances of follicle function.

Any of the conditions in the preceding general categories may lead to a disturbance in the normal pituitary-ovarian axis, an anovulatory type of ovarian function, and resulting irregular cycles characterized by amenorrhea, oligomenorrhea, or dysfunctional uterine bleeding ("functional menometrorrhagia"). These more fundamental endocrine disorders are discussed in Chapter 6.

Certain other generalized metabolic disturbances also seem to predispose to the development of an anovulatory type of menstrual function:

1. Marked obesity (even in the absence of diabetes or thyroid disease).
2. Severe malnutrition, e.g., the anorexia nervosa syndrome.
3. Chronic, debilitating, systemic diseases, e.g., tuberculosis.

In these conditions, the major therapeutic effort should be directed at the underlying systemic abnormality, although treatment aimed at restoring ovulatory cycles will usually be of considerable symptomatic value and should be attempted simultaneously.

In some patients the temporary development of an anovulatory type of ovarian function leads to a functional type of amenorrhea, in which there is no basic underlying impairment or abnormality of reproductive tract potential. Here, the problem is invariably one of a temporary, reversible disturbance in the hypothalamic-pituitary regulating mechanism, and hence this type of functional amenorrhea is often referred to as hypothalamic amenorrhea. These patients have no organic lesion at any point in the reproductive tract or its regulatory apparatus, and their anovulatory state and associated oligomenorrhea or functional amenorrhea has usually been initiated by (1) emotional stress at some point in their total life situation; or (2) marked variations in weight, either an abrupt loss induced by crash dieting or a sudden gain (conversion of a variety of ovarian and adrenal steroids to estrone in the peripheral adipose tissue compartment may account for the frequent occurrence of anovulatory cycles and functional amenorrhea in obese women); or, less often, (3) nonspecific metabolic and endocrine effects of a chronic systemic illness. The history, physical findings, and response to a test dose of progesterone are often sufficient to confirm the presence of a functional hypothalamic amenorrhea, without the need for a more elaborate endocrine workup; however, the latter may be necessary in some cases and is discussed in detail in Chapter 6. Treatment of simple functional amenorrhea is usually expectant, first explaining the situation to the patient and reassuring her that spontaneous recovery is the rule. Ordinarily, one should avoid using oral contraceptives or cyclic estrogen-progesterone therapy to produce an artificial menstrual cycle in these patients, since this type of therapy only perpetuates hypothalamic-pituitary inhibition and prevents spontaneous return of the normal regulatory mechanism. A cyclic program of an oral progesterone alone for five days can be given every month or two to produce withdrawal bleeding without interfering with spontaneous resumption of ovulatory function, but this is rarely necessary. In the case of women with hypothalamic amenorrhea who desire to begin childbearing without any further delay, ovulation induction with clomiphene as described in Chapter 6 can be employed.

In the vast majority of patients with dysfunctional bleeding, the problem is usually of short duration, is frequently prone to spontaneous correction, and is nearly always temporary if handled properly. Furthermore — and most important — no basic underlying endocrine or metabolic disorder is present. However, certain contributing or precipitating factors invariably lurk in the background, of which the following are the most common examples:

1. Transient, acute, physical or psychic stresses such as:
    a. The temporary emotional influences leading to the menstrual irregularities (occasionally even to the so-called hypothalamic amenorrhea) of college freshmen or first-year student nurses.
    b. Emotional upsets that may affect any woman in the prime of reproductive life; e.g., family illness or death, marital discord, problem children, pressure of outside activities, social or occupational personality clashes.
    c. A febrile illness that leads to a delayed or missed period followed by dysfunctional bleeding (the high fever interfering with normal follicular development

and resulting in failure of ovulation, or inadequate progesterone production, or both).

    d. Prolonged administration of substantial amounts of certain tranquilizers may produce anovulatory cycles with associated menstrual disturbances.

2. Moderate fluctuations in body weight; chronic physical, mental, or emotional fatigue.

3. Seasonal variations. For reasons that are not entirely clear, anovulatory cycles with short periods of amenorrhea or episodes of dysfunctional bleeding are more common in the summer months, particularly in July and August.

Finally, as already noted, dysfunctional bleeding is definitely more common at the beginning and at the end of active menstrual life, i.e., in adolescence and in the premenopausal and menopausal phase, since, as might be expected, the ovarian cycle is apparently more unstable and more subject and vulnerable to disruptive influences early and late in life.

Diagnostic Approach

The probability that abnormal menstrual bleeding is dysfunctional in origin is nearly always suggested by the history, if it is carefully elicited and accurate in detail. The various clinical manifestations of the anovulatory type of ovarian function include: a premature or delayed period that is then prolonged; oligomenorrhea or polymenorrhea, with the episodes of bleeding irregular in duration and amount; and amenorrhea of short duration followed by the onset of a continuous type of bleeding that may vary in amount from day to day. The bleeding itself, though highly variable in amount, is at some time or another usually extremely profuse but invariably painless. Careful questioning may also bring forth possible factors that have precipitated the change in what was previously a perfectly normal, regular menstrual pattern. Finally, the general physical survey and pelvic examination will usually reveal no evidence of any underlying endocrine or metabolic disturbance and no sign of any local pelvic disease. (The presence of incidental but asymptomatic local pelvic disease must be carefully evaluated and integrated with the overall clinical picture in arriving at a correct explanation for the abnormal bleeding.) With regard to the consideration of possible local disease in the differential diagnosis, it is particularly important to exclude disorders of early pregnancy, since the history accompanying an early tubal pregnancy or a threatened, incomplete, or missed abortion may be entirely similar. Obviously, it is essential also to exclude the presence of cancer of the cervix or fundus, submucous fibroids, symptomatic uterine adenomyosis, or endometrial polyps. An endometrial biopsy or a curettage that reveals a secretory rather than a proliferative or hyperplastic endometrium is often a clue to the presence of primary uterine disease as the source for the abnormal bleeding.

One other group of disorders that may at times simulate dysfunctional uterine bleeding and actually represent a type of "functional bleeding" (because again no local uterine disease is present) are the hematologic diseases with prolonged bleeding or clotting times or increased capillary fragility, previously discussed in Chapter 4. (Also see Chapter 2 for a simplified diagnostic screening program for a rapid check on the possibility of a generalized hemorrhagic disorder in a patient with excessive uterine bleeding.) For example, easy bruising, menorrhagia, and even significant mid-cycle hemorrhage are common first manifestations of von Willebrand's disease, a coagulopathy characterized by a prolonged bleeding time in association with a reduced plasma Factor VIII level, a capillary defect, and probably deficient platelet adhesiveness as well. A correct diagnosis can often be made on the basis of an accurate history (there is a strong familial tendency, since this is an autosomal dominant hereditary disorder) and a simple bleeding time determination, thus avoiding the need for diagnostic curettage, which carries the risk of provoking even more excessive hemorrhage. The immediate arrest of any major bleeding episode can nearly always be achieved by intravenous infusions of plasma or Factor VIII preparations (cryoprecipitate) and platelet transfusions if indicated.

The complexity of the diagnostic workup will also vary considerably with the age of the patient, and the general principles that follow are of some help.

1. **Adolescents and young women in their early twenties.** A detailed history, a careful general physical examination, and a pelvic or rectal examination or both in a patient with suspected dysfunctional bleeding are usually sufficient to exclude other conditions and establish the diagnosis of a functional menstrual disorder. Thyroid function studies may frequently be indicated and helpful, and a complete endocrinologic survey will be required if there are symptoms or findings suggestive of some more basic underlying endocrine disturbance, or if there is failure of response to adequate therapy. It is particularly important to rule out the presence of blood dyscrasias and abnormal bleeding tendencies in this age group. As discussed more fully in Chapter 6, the possible existence of the Stein-Leventhal syndrome should also be carefully considered. Curettage or endometrial biopsy is rarely necessary, either as a diagnostic or therapeutic maneuver.

2. **Women in the prime of menstrual life (age 25 to 40).** Early pregnancy disorders are the most important conditions to be differentiated in this age group; pregnancy tests and, in acute situations, laparoscopy or culdoscopy to rule out an ectopic gestation may be indicated. Curettage may occasionally be necessary, either to exclude the presence of submucous fibroids or endometrial polyps or to control excessive bleeding if the response to conservative management is unsatisfactory. Obviously, pelvic malignant disease must also be excluded by thorough examination cytologic studies, and biopsies if indicated. Except for thyroid disturbances, endocrine disorders or blood dyscrasias seldom manifest themselves for the first time in women of this age group, but thyroid function studies again may be important.

3. **Premenopausal and menopausal women.** Although the same general principle apply to these women, curettage is almost always necessary to be certain of ruling out endometrial or endocervical cancer.

Therapy of Anovulatory Bleeding

In patients in whom dysfunctional bleeding is merely a secondary symptom of some fundamental endocrine disorder, treatment should be directed at the primary cause, although symptomatic control of the anovulatory bleeding may be temporarily achieved by some of the methods to be described. In the vast majority of cases, however, the dysfunctional bleeding is temporary and the disturbance in ovarian function completely reversible by simple therapeutic measures. Since the underlying feature is failure of normal follicular maturation and hence inadequate progesterone production, these patients bleed abnormally and irregularly from a proliferative or hyperplastic (occasionally atrophic) endometrium. It is the lack of progestational change in the endometrium that results in the irregularity of the onset of flow and in the frequently excessive and prolonged bleeding. The various therapeutic programs therefore aim to supply progesterone in some form to promote normal endometrial maturation artificially and ultimately to achieve complete shedding of the secretory type of endometrial lining so produced, in place of the prolonged and incomplete sloughing and accompanying abnormal bleeding of the proliferative and hyperplastic endometrium. Examples of specific types of treatment regimens commonly employed will now be presented.

SINGLE COURSE OF PROGESTERONE

A single course of progesterone is particularly useful if the dysfunctional bleeding is of short duration (perhaps involving only one or two cycles) in women in the prime of menstrual life with little or no history of previous irregularities. The progesterone can conveniently be given as a single intramuscular injection; e.g., progesterone in oil (short-acting), 25 to 50 mg, or one of the newer, more potent progestational preparations such as Delalutin (long-acting), 250 mg. The current bleeding will usually cease within a few days of the injection as the progestational response occurs in the endometrium, to be followed at an interval of a few days to as long as one or two weeks by the artificially produced "normal period" or flow from the resulting secretory type of endometrium. This form of therapy is sometimes referred to as a "medical curettage." The patient should be warned that during the first 48 hours of this "normal period" the flow may be excessive (because of the varying degrees of endometrial overproliferation prior to the administration of progesterone), but she can be reassured that the flow will thereafter be more normal and will ordinarily cease in the usual five to seven days.

A single, short course of treatment can also be administered orally with similar beneficial effect, using any of the variety of progestational compounds now available; e.g., Enovid (5 to 10 mg), Norlutate (5 to 10 mg), Provera (5 to 10 mg), or Duphaston (10 to 20 mg), each given daily for 10 to 14 days. Whether given by injection or by mouth, this single course of progesterone results in return of normal ovulatory ovarian function in the following cycles in approximately 85 percent of patients in whom the functional disturbance has been an isolated event. As can be surmised

from the drugs listed, progesterone itself is rarely used nowadays for oral administration. Although formerly available commercially in several drug forms, it was
poorly absorbed and to a large extent metabolized by the liver before it could be
effectively utilized. A great number of synthetic steroids with potent progestational
activity are now available. The principal chemical groups are (1) the 19-norsteroid
compounds, including Enovid (norethynodrel, plus ethinylestradiol 3-methyl ether),
Norlutate (norethindrone acetate), and Ortho-Novum (norethindrone, plus ethinylestradiol 3-methyl ether), and (2) the 17-hydroxyprogesterone compounds, including
Provera (medroxyprogesterone acetate) and Delalutin (hydroxyprogesterone
caproate). Another addition to the list of compounds now in use is Duphaston
(dydrogesterone [6-dehydroretroprogesterone]), which is closely related structurally
to natural progesterone. However, it is over 30 times as potent pharmacologically,
does not inhibit ovulation, and has no thermogenic or androgenic effects. Presumably, it possesses the endometrium-stimulating properties of progesterone but because
of slight chemical differences does not have its antigonadotropic effects with respect
to the pituitary-hypothalamic regulatory centers.

It is of some clinical importance to note that most of these synthetic progestogens
produce their most beneficial effects as far as improvement in the secretory pattern
of endometrium is concerned when administered only in the latter half of the cycle.
When therapy is begun in the first half of the cycle, normal proliferation is somewhat
inhibited and final maturation less complete. (This may account for the frequent
occurrence of breakthrough bleeding when they are used as oral contraceptives
throughout the cycle.)

CYCLIC PROGESTERONE THERAPY

Supplemental progesterone therapy more prolonged than single-course therapy will
invariably be required in the following patients: those who fail to respond to a single
course of therapy; those whose irregularities are of considerable duration; those
whose "periods" remain fairly regular but who suffer from increasing menorrhagia
(excessive and prolonged flow, the so-called inadequate luteal phase type of abnormal
bleeding); and those who required curettage to control the original bleeding episode
and in whom anovulatory cycles promptly recur. Such therapy is most effectively
given during the latter half of the cycle and in an appropriate physiologic amount,
so that the normal progestational phase is simulated as closely as possible. Any of
the current oral progestational compounds in the dosages previously indicated can
be employed and are usually begun on the fifteenth or twentieth day of the cycle
and continued for 10 or 5 days respectively (e.g., Provera, 5 to 10 mg for 5 to 10
days; or Norlutate, 5 to 10 mg for 5 to 10 days). Ordinarily, cyclic therapy should
be continued for three or four cycles, and then a trial off therapy should be given.
In the vast majority of patients, return to spontaneous normal ovarian function and
ovulatory cycles will follow such a program. Presumably, the artificially created,
relatively normal estrogen-progesterone balance aids in reestablishing the normal
reciprocally related pituitary-ovarian regulatory mechanism, and normal follicle

stimulation and subsequent maturation, ovulation, and corpus luteum function are restored. If a satisfactory response is not obtained, further investigation is definitely indicated to rule out a more fundamental endocrine disturbance or a local organic cause for irregular bleeding.

CYCLIC ESTROGEN-PROGESTERONE THERAPY

The addition of estrogen to the cyclic program of supplemental progesterone therapy may be required in adolescents and in premenopausal women, because in both age groups an estrogen as well as a progesterone deficiency is commonly present. Endometrial biopsies that show an atrophic type of proliferative endometrium, or vaginal cytologic smears revealing a low estrogen effect, are helpful in determining whether or not the patient will require estrogen as well as progesterone in the program of therapy. Estrogen in the form of diethylstilbestrol (1.0 mg) or Premarin (1.25 mg) once or twice daily is begun on day 1 and continued for 25 days, adding the progestational agent as usual on the fifteenth or twentieth day and continuing it also until the twenty-fifth treatment day, when both drugs are discontinued. (Since oral contraceptives contain both an estrogen and a progestational agent, the addition of estrogen will not be necessary when they are used.) Bleeding usually ensues two to three days later, and the course is repeated for three or four cycles, beginning medication with estrogen again on the first day of each withdrawal flow. If withdrawal flow is substantially delayed beyond the usual two to three days, it usually indicates that the patient has ovulated spontaneously. A trial off therapy is then in order, and return of normal ovulatory cycles will frequently be observed thereafter.

Management of Acute Bleeding Episodes

Dysfunctional bleeding can at times be extremely heavy, and an acute episode of profuse hemorrhage with a fall in hemoglobin and blood volume sufficient to require transfusions is not uncommon. In this situation, a prompt arrest of the bleeding is obviously desirable, and curettage is often the most rapidly effective way of achieving control. As an alternative, or in cases in which for any of a number of reasons it may not be safe or advisable to proceed with immediate curettage, short-term hormone therapy can also be of assistance in the emergency arrest of excessive dysfunctional bleeding. Estrogens are usually more rapid than progestational compounds in this respect and can be given as a single intravenous injection (e.g., Premarin Intravenous, 20 mg) or orally (e.g., Premarin, 2.5 mg, or diethylstilbestrol, 2.0 mg) every 2 hours until bleeding ceases or abates considerably. Although hemostasis is usually rapidly obtained, the use of estrogens rather than progestational drugs is often less satisfactory in the long run, because both the tendency to endometrial hyperplasia and the relative progesterone insufficiency are accentuated, and subsequent management may therefore be rendered more difficult. If estrogens are used for rapid arrest of hemorrhage, a maintenance dose should be continued for 20 to 25 days and progesterone added during the last two weeks in an attempt to create a more normal secretory endometrium when withdrawal bleeding is allowed to occur at the end of that time. Cyclic therapy will then be advisable for another three to four months. Perhaps an even simpler alternative, when the oral medication route is feasible, is the use of one of the combination oral contraceptive agents, selecting a higher-than-usual dosage for more prompt response (e.g., Enovid, 5 mg, or Ortho-Novum, 2 mg), administering it two to four times daily to arrest the hemorrhage and then allowing a more normal withdrawal menstrual flow to occur. Thereafter, cyclic therapy may be wise for three to four months to minimize the chances of recurrent dysfunctional bleeding.

If curettage has become necessary, it may be followed in 40 to 60 percent of cases by return to a normal ovulatory pattern without further maneuvers — or at least by a remission of months or years — and is often sufficient to tide the premenopausal patient over completion of the menopause. At the same time, it has served to exclude any organic lesions. If abnormal bleeding should recur within a few months of the curettage, cyclic hormonal management can then be undertaken.

Additional Measures

Attention to more general factors may also be indicated and prove extremely helpful in the correction of the anovulatory pattern with its associated dysfunctional bleeding. Reassurance, a thorough explanation of the mechanism involved, and efforts to ferret out and modify, when possible, any underlying psychogenic or general health factors should be a routine part of the general management of all patients. Regulation of the body weight and the administration of thyroid when a hypometabolic state seems to exist may be important.

If repeated curettages and adequate attempts to control recurrent refractory dysfunctional bleeding by supplemental hormone therapy fail and excessive bleeding persists, hysterectomy may ultimately prove necessary in a small minority of patients.

CYCLIC FUNCTIONAL MENSTRUAL DISORDERS

Abnormal Bleeding Associated with Ovulatory Cycles

In considering abnormal bleeding associated with ovulatory cycles we are still concerned with "functional bleeding" occurring in the absence of local organic disease anywhere in the reproductive tract. Obviously, the hemorrhagic disorders result in a type of cyclic "functional bleeding" associated with normal ovarian function, and the importance of their recognition has already been emphasized. There are, however, a number of other situations in which abnormal bleeding not due to a local pathologic condition may occur in association with otherwise regular ovulatory cycles.

MINOR CYCLIC BLEEDING EPISODES

The category of minor cyclic bleeding episodes includes intermenstrual staining, or at times moderate flow for a day or two, experienced on occasion by many women around midcycle at ovulation time. The climactic events within the ripening dominant follicle and the regressing partially stimulated follicles that precede and accompany ovulation simply result in a temporary fall in estrogen levels for a short interval. Similarly, premenstrual and postmenstrual staining appearing during ovulatory cycles is due to disorderly corpus luteum regression in the case of the former, and delayed or irregular early follicular response and function in the case of the latter. All these minor irregularities are usually transient, relatively infrequent, and of no consequence. Therapy consists only of reassurance and explanation, once the possibility of local disease has been ruled out.

INADEQUATE LUTEAL PHASE

Mention has already been made of the occurrence of inadequate corpus luteum function and progesterone output in what are otherwise regular ovulatory cycles. This inadequate luteal phase may well be due to low preovulatory FSH levels with resulting abnormal follicle development and subsequent inadequate LH levels. Although infertility or repeated spontaneous abortions are the principal manifestations of this functional disorder, variations in cycle length and in the duration and amount of flow are also encountered. The basic regularity of the cycle persists, however, even though excessive bleeding may occur, and this typical clinical picture, together with the characteristic histologic features of a premenstrual endometrial biopsy, enables the physician to make the correct diagnosis. Cyclic supplemental progesterone therapy will be effective in controlling the excessive flow and often in restoring normal corpus luteum function and fertility. It should be noted that the short luteal phase, manifested by a short menstrual cycle length (around 21 days), is probably a variation of this disorder.

IRREGULAR RIPENING AND SHEDDING SYNDROME

The irregular ripening and shedding syndrome is a relatively uncommon dysfunctional type of bleeding characterized by prolonged (e.g., 10 to 14 days), frequently heavy, but otherwise very regular periods. It is associated with ovulation and normal (at least initially) progesterone secretion by the corpus luteum. This syndrome derives its descriptive name from the fact that the prolonged flow is due to a disorganized maturation response produced in the endometrium and the resulting irregular shedding from this heterogeneous type of uterine lining made up of both proliferative and secretory elements (the latter predominating) of varying degrees of maturity. A definite diagnosis is best established by performing curettage on the fourth or fifth day of flow, at which time the typical histologic features are invariably present. There is some evidence that the unusual microscopic picture in the endometrium may be secondary to a faulty, retarded, and irregular regression of the corpus luteum, because in many patients the basal body temperature and pregnanediol excretion levels remain elevated for a number of days after the onset of flow, paralleling the persistent secretory glandular changes in the endometrium; in a few patients, actual corpus luteum cysts or persistent, apparently active corpora lutea have been demonstrated. It is also possible that the dysfunction is primarily in the endometrium rather than in the pituitary-ovarian axis, however, since the irregular ripening and shedding pattern, once established, tends to persist unless surgical curettage is done, the curettage resulting in an immediate and permanent cure in most instances. Occasionally, the syndrome will respond to a "medical" (hormonal) curettage as well.

IRON DEFICIENCY MENORRHAGIA

Taymor and associates [36] have drawn attention to a type of functional menorrhagia occurring in the presence of chronic iron deficiency but in the absence of any uterine disease or ovarian dysfunction, although in some instances excessive blood loss accompanying a prior period of anovulatory bleeding may have been responsible for the initial depletion of total body iron stores. In many cases, however, the initial chronic iron lack is on a dietary basis and is of course subsequently aggravated by the ensuing secondary menorrhagia. Diagnosis depends not so much on the finding of an associated secondary anemia (the hemoglobin is often normal) but on the presence of a markedly decreased serum iron level, in turn a direct reflection of the depleted tissue and total body iron reserves. Obviously, organic lesions and endocrine dysfunction must also be excluded. A possible explanation advanced for the phenomenon is based on the importance of iron to the cytochrome oxidase enzyme systems, which are vital to normal muscle metabolism; iron deficiency leads to inadequate contraction of both the myometrium and the muscular coats of the spiral arterioles, with a resulting prolonged, heavy loss of blood during the period of endometrial slough. Adequate iron-replacement therapy is curative and can usually be given orally, although intramuscular iron may be employed for more rapid effects or in the occasional case of faulty iron absorption from the gastrointestinal tract. It is important to be aware of this entity, and it is also obvious that iron-replacement therapy should be a useful adjunct in the management of all other types of functional uterine bleeding as well.

Mittelschmerz: Ovulation and Postovulation Pain

Mittelschmerz, or ovulation discomfort, is extremely common and is probably due to ovarian capsular distention, the result of the final peak of intrafollicular pressure just prior to ovulation, as well as to the slight intraperitoneal leakage of fluid during the event itself. It is ordinarily transient and dull and aching in character, occurring almost exactly at midcycle, and is more frequently felt in the right lower quadrant than on the left side. Many women experience it each month to a mild degree, some only when they ovulate from the right (or left) ovary, some never. Physical examination ordinarily reveals only minimal lower quadrant abdominal tenderness and a slightly tender, perhaps slightly enlarged ovary on the affected side. There should never be any real difficulty in distinguishing this normal physiologic event from truly significant intraperitoneal disorders.

RUPTURED CORPUS HEMORRHAGICUM

Ruptured corpus hemorrhagicum is somewhat similar in many of its clinical features to simple follicle rupture. However, it may occur at any time during the luteal phase of the cycle (typically about one week before the period), and the pain is more severe, more generalized, and of longer duration. Considerable bleeding from the site of rupture of the ripening corpus luteum results in peritoneal irritation of varying extent and degree and, depending on the amount of blood accumulating, may result in generalized abdominal pain and tenderness, radiation of pain to the back, shoulder, or leg, and rectal or bladder discomfort. If bleeding is massive, as it occasionally may be, actual surgical shock will develop and require emergency laparotomy to control hemorrhage by suture of the bleeding site. When bleeding is moderate, the findings may suggest the possibility of any of a number of other acute intraabdominal disorders, e.g., appendicitis, mesenteric adenitis, acute salpingitis, ureteral colic, and pyelonephritis. In the vast majority of cases, however, a carefully elicited history of the sudden nature of the onset of the acute episode and its chronological relationship to the menstrual cycle, the usual absence of associated symptoms suggestive of gastrointestinal or urinary tract disease (there may be nausea and vomiting, however), and clinical and laboratory findings pointing to simple, chemical peritoneal irritation rather than infection or inflammation (relatively little if any elevation of temperature, pulse, or white count) should permit a correct diagnosis. In doubtful cases, culdoscopy or laparoscopy will easily resolve the problem of differential diagnosis; exploratory laparotomy, except to control massive hemorrhage, should rarely be necessary. The symptoms usually subside spontaneously in a day or two, and no specific treatment is required once the diagnosis is established.

RUPTURED CORPUS LUTEUM CYST

A related entity with somewhat similar manifestations is ruptured corpus luteum cyst. The cyst may develop during the current cycle or in some instances may have originated in a previous cycle. Development of a corpus luteum cyst is initiated by excessive hemorrhage into the center of a corpus luteum, with resulting hematoma formation and ultimately a cystic cavity lined by luteinized granulosa and theca cells. Actual rupture may be preceded by an interval of several days of increasing adnexal discomfort caused by slow bleeding within the cyst capsule and a steadily rising intracystic pressure. Because roughly two-thirds of these luteal cysts may have some functional activity, the preceding period may have been scanty, the present expected period may be delayed, sometimes for three to four weeks (rarely, for as long as four to six months), and the endometrium may show a pseudodecidual change histologically. Actual rupture usually occurs either late in the cycle or during or after the delayed period, and bleeding is often extensive. Because of the sudden, often massive hemoperitoneum, and in the face of the described menstrual irregularities and endometrial abnormalities, this entity may almost precisely simulate ruptured ectopic pregnancy. In its milder forms, the ruptured corpus luteum cyst may suggest a ruptured endometrioma, acute salpingitis, twisted ovarian cyst, or any of the other previously mentioned acute abdominal disorders. In fact, the corpus luteum cyst is the greatest masquerader of all and is a frequent cause of either acute or chronic pelvic pain and menstrual irregularities. Diagnosis is again frequently facilitated by laparoscopy or culdoscopy. When massive bleeding has occurred, laparotomy with resection of the cyst will be necessary; this can nearly always be accomplished with preservation of the ovary. Although many corpus luteum cysts undoubtedly are spontaneously resorbed, either with or without rupture, a significant number will persist and will be manifested as tender ovarian enlargements producing chronic intermittent pelvic pain and menstrual irregularities. The latter most commonly consist of menorrhagia or metrorrhagia due to excessive secretion by the cyst of both estrogen and progesterone, but occasionally there will be oligomenorrhea or secondary amenorrhea if the cyst persists for more than a few months. These cysts, too, will usually ultimately require surgical removal for relief of symptoms, even when rupture never occurs.

Primary or Essential Dysmenorrhea

By definition, primary dysmenorrhea is the development, usually within a few years of the menarche, of painful menstruation in the absence of any organic pelvic disease, the menstrual discomfort being severe enough to cause the patient to consult a physician. It is thus completely distinguished from so-called secondary, or acquired, dysmenorrhea, which invariably has its onset later on in life and which is secondary to some specific pelvic pathologic process such as endometriosis, chronic pelvic inflammatory disease, ovarian cysts, intramural or submucous fibroids, adenomyosis of the uterus, or endometrial polyps. One type of acquired dysmenorrhea in which the crampy menstrual pain is almost identical with that of essential dysmenorrhea, except that it is most often seen in somewhat older women, is **membranous dysmenorrhea**. In this case, the endometrium is shed in large fragments or in the form of an endometrial or decidual-like cast that causes cervical obstruction, thus initiating exceedingly painful tetanic uterine contractions. (A six-months' course of cyclic progestogen therapy to induce anovulatory cycles will usually correct this disorder.) Another type of acquired, cyclic type of menstrual pain is seen in the **right ovarian vein syndrome**. This consists of cyclic recurring right flank pain, often with associated recurrent right pyelonephritis, occurring in the premenstrual and early menstrual phase and caused by cyclic ureteral obstruction resulting from dilatation of the right ovarian vein during the premenstrual phase of pelvic venous congestion and increased blood flow; sometimes there is an associated periureteral fibrosis. In most patients the syndrome appears after one or more pregnancies, the latter possibly producing incompetency of the ovarian vein valves and a greater tendency to dilatation. If the recurring pain and urinary tract infection do not respond to conservative treatment with diuretics and urinary antibiotic therapy, surgery with excision of the right ovarian vein and ureterolysis may be necessary.

Finally, an equally uncommon cause of acute menstrual pain in the category of secondary dysmenorrhea is the infrequently encountered phenomenon of **acute**

retrograde menstruation. The patient experiences the sudden onset of severe pelvic and lower abdominal pain shortly before or just after the onset of menstruation (the period may be a particularly heavy one), and shortly thereafter there may be signs and symptoms resembling peritonitis due to chemical irritation by the sudden tubal reflux of several ounces of menstrual blood into the cul-de-sac. The cause for this event is unknown, and fortunately there is little if any tendency to recurrence.

Where secondary dysmenorrhea due to organic disease is concerned, the diagnosis is usually obvious from the history and positive pelvic findings, and treatment is directed at the underlying disease.

The typical appearance of essential dysmenorrhea a few years (three to five) after the menarche coincides with the usual delay in assumption of the regular ovulatory cycles characteristic of normal adolescent females. Essential dysmenorrhea is never seen in the absence of ovulation, since the crampy discomfort is the direct result of the effects of progesterone, which produces the increased myometrial contractility and intense arteriolar vasospasm, both of which contribute to the painful cramps. As might be predicted, mild cramps may precede the actual onset of flow by 12 to 24 hours, but the most severe pain commences approximately with the flow and usually lasts only 12 to 24 hours thereafter. The pain itself is midline, lower abdominal, and crampy, resembling a labor pain. In its severe forms, the dysmenorrhea may be accompanied by nausea, vomiting, headache, irritability, and low backache.

Although not a serious medical disorder, essential dysmenorrhea does have considerable socioeconomic significance, because it produces monthly disability for a day or two in a significant proportion of the female population. It is estimated that approximately 35 percent of all older adolescent girls, 25 percent of female college students, and an astounding 60 to 70 percent of older, single women in their thirties and forties experience monthly distress sufficient to interfere with their normal activities to the point that they are invalided and lost to society for a day or two.

Older theories of origin attempted to explain the pain on an anatomic (e.g., cervical stenosis, hypoplastic uterus), but none of these theories is tenable when examined critically. Although there is no question that women who experience truly significant functional dysmenorrhea have a different (probably of degree) neuromuscular and neurovascular pattern at work in the uterus than other women do, in the majority of the sufferers the disorder is basically a temporary one and spontaneously ceases to be a problem within a few years, suggesting that the difference is not fundamental or permanent.

ETIOLOGY

Modern concepts of the etiologic mechanisms involved and applicable in varying degrees to each individual patient include the following:

1. The basic physiologic mechanism: Ovulation and the production of progesterone with its myotonic and vasospastic effects on the myometrium and endometrial arterioles.

2. In some cases: A constitutional predisposition consisting not of a low pain threshold but of a hyperreactivity or overresponsiveness to potentially painful stimuli.
3. In many instances: Psychological factors.
   a. Immaturity and dependency, or rejection of becoming an adult female.
   b. Manifestation of general anxieties and tensions, which are all too common during adolescence.
   c. Maternal and environmental conditioning (e.g., if the mother "suffers," so will the daughter).

In some patients in whom the psychological factors appear to be prominent, their severe dysmenorrhea meets all the criteria of a psychosomatic illness.

DIAGNOSIS

The typical history and the finding of normal pelvic viscera on vaginal and/or rectal examination are usually all that is required to assess the situation correctly. If the pain and related symptoms are suspected to be entirely on a psychogenic basis, the differentiation from simple essential dysmenorrhea may be made by the **estrogen test**: Diethylstilbestrol, 1.0 mg, or Premarin, 1.25 mg, is administered daily from day 1 through day 25 of the cycle. This will produce an anovulatory period three to five days later, and the bleeding from a purely proliferative endometrium in the absence of any progesterone effect will be painless if the symptoms are due to true, essential dysmenorrhea. However, if discomfort is entirely on a psychogenic basis, the estrogen withdrawal flow will continue to be accompanied by severe distress.

TREATMENT

The most important aspect of treatment is thorough and sympathetic reassurance after careful examination to rule out organic disease, accompanied by an explanation of the mechanism producing the cramps (its hemostatic purpose as well as its significance as an index of normal reproductive tract function should be expressly noted), with emphasis on the benign and self-limited nature of the symptoms. It is equally important to offer this explanation and reassurance to the mother, who often accompanies the young patient. It should not be implied that the pain is imaginary, for it is not, but that it is functional or physiologic and can be relieved by simple measures once worry and fear over its possible significance are dispelled through correct understanding. It is helpful to stress that normal sexual function and fertility can be anticipated and that the symptoms usually subside in a few more years or with regular sexual activity and childbearing and in the meantime can easily be alleviated. The physician should be aware, however, that it is not primarily any anatomic or physiologic change accompanying intercourse or childbearing that causes the symptoms to disappear. Rather, it is the attainment of the physical, physiologic, and emotional maturity of a normal adult female, able to take on adult responsibilities and to establish a normal relationship with a member of the opposite sex.

Symptomatic relief of the discomfort can almost always be provided by various combinations of the following simple maneuvers:

1. The patient should be urged to carry on normal activities (including physical exercise) as much as possible; there is a real neurophysiologic basis for what in effect is "taking her mind off her troubles."

2. Simple analgesics usually suffice, but the importance of taking them early, in anticipation of the more severe cramps, should be stressed. She must have her own supply of pills (college or student-nurse dormitory rules notwithstanding): aspirin, Empirin, Edrisal with or without codeine (2 tablets every 4 hours as needed for two to three doses and beginning with the first sign of discomfort may be prescribed). An even more specific antispasmodic effect is claimed for lututrin (Lutrexin), given in a dose of 2 to 3 tablets every 4 hours. Occasionally, antiemetics and mild tranquilizers may also prove helpful.

3. When dysmenorrhea is severe, reassurance and subsequent benefit from simple analgesics may be made more effective by first producing an anovulatory cycle or two by estrogen administration in the same fashion as for the estrogen test.

4. Oral contraceptives have been used to produce anovulatory cycles for the purpose of relieving dysmenorrhea. One of the newer synthetic progestogens, dydrogesterone (Duphaston), has been moderately successful in this respect, and in the dosage employed (10 mg twice daily from day 5 to day 25 of each cycle) does not inhibit ovulation.

5. Dilatation and curettage is mentioned only to emphasize that it seldom is of lasting benefit and is never indicated as a method of therapy.

6. Psychiatric evaluation and treatment may occasionally be necessary if the problem seems to be essentially a psychosomatic one, or if a more serious psychiatric disturbance is suspected.

PRESACRAL NEURECTOMY

Presacral neurectomy (sometimes with uterosacral ligament division, interrupting also the parasympathetic nerve supply to the uterus) has a limited role to play in the overall management of essential dysmenorrhea. It is rarely if ever necessary in the simple case but is occasionally warranted in the management of the single working woman in her late twenties or thirties in whom severe, incapacitating dysmenorrhea has persisted, has failed to respond to conservative measures, and is a definite handicap in her business or professional life. An estrogen test is again of considerable value in screening out those patients who are unlikely to benefit from the operation. Favorable results can be expected in 80 to 90 percent of patients if they are properly selected and the surgery correctly performed.

Premenstrual Tension

Premenstrual tension represents a marked exaggeration of the normal minimal premenstrual distress (the so-called menstrual molimina) that accompanies the hormonal, metabolic, and fluid and electrolyte changes characteristic of the secretory and premenstrual phases of the normal cycle. When these changes are pronounced, a symptom complex that is exceedingly troublesome to the patient develops, usually 3 to 7 days, but occasionally as long as 10 to 14 days, before the period is due, reaches a peak 24 to 48 hours premenstrually, and ordinarily subsides 24 to 48 hours after the onset of menstruation. The oppressive feeling of physical, mental, and emotional tension is the most disturbing symptom of all from the patients' standpoint and can be a real source of disability as well as impaired interpersonal relationships within the family and community. In its severest forms the syndrome may include inability to concentrate and impaired mental acuity, anxiety, depression, emotional instability and irritability, as well as physical complaints such as the following: headaches, visual disturbances, and increased tendency to migraine attacks (if a migraine tendency exists); insomnia; fatigue; marked breast swelling and tenderness (mastalgia); abdominal distention; abdominal and pelvic pain; functional gastrointestinal and urinary tract disturbances, including anorexia, nausea with occasional vomiting, constipation, and urinary frequency and urgency; back and thigh pain; tachycardia; weight gain; and often overt peripheral edema. Although the syndrome may be encountered at any age between the menarche and the menopause, it is usually mild in the adolescent or early adult years, the severe and full-blown picture appearing most often after the age of 35.

ETIOLOGY

The exact etiologic mechanisms that result in the appearance of these distressing symptoms are not absolutely clear, but the vast majority appear to be secondary to a generalized, excessive sodium and fluid retention, probably in turn secondary to a slightly altered estrogen-progesterone balance. Since most of the distress is subjective in nature, it is not surprising that psychogenic factors can also frequently be incriminated. These involve a variety of social, family, marital, and sexual problems, as well as intrinsic personality disorders and emotional maladjustments. Current concepts concerning etiology of the symptoms can perhaps be summarized as follows:

1. **Psychic factors:** Always present; often obviously the most prominent feature.
2. **Endocrine-metabolic factors:**
    a. There is definite evidence for an estrogen-progesterone imbalance, with a relative excess of the former. Since the sodium-retention effect of estrogen is well known and documented (progesterone tends to promote the renal excretion of sodium) this in turn results in:
    b. Sodium and water retention with weight gain and a generalized form of edema, an obvious source of many of the somatic symptoms and signs and a potent

factor in producing many of the central nervous system manifestations as well, since some degree of cerebral edema must also be assumed. Since the symptoms rarely, if ever, occur during an anovulatory cycle, it is the abnormal estrogen-progesterone balance, not estrogen alone, that is responsible.

c. Some degree of corpus luteum insufficiency is undoubtedly present in many instances, and in certain cases an underlying, subclinical form of hypothyroidism (hypometabolic state) has been shown to be responsible for the luteal deficiency and inadequate progesterone production.

d. The tendency to premenstrual hypoglycemia may be a contributing factor.

e. Occasionally, 17-ketosteroid excretion has been observed to be abnormal. The significance of this is not yet clear, but it could conceivably be associated with increased excretion of aldosterone, known to occur when progesterone levels are sufficiently high to inhibit the renal action of aldosterone. Rising aldosterone levels in turn might also predispose to sodium and fluid retention.

TREATMENT

Explanation and reassurance are again important, and the psychological aspects of the problem should be thoroughly explored. General health measures, including adequate diet, rest, exercise, and opportunities for mental and emotional relaxation, all too often lacking in the world of the "tired housewife," may be absolutely essential for adequate relief of symptoms. Subclinical hypothyroidism must be ruled out, and supplemental thyroid should be administered if a hypometabolic state is demonstrated.

The principal and most effective specific forms of therapy, however, are the following:

1. Measures aimed primarily at directly minimizing sodium and water retention:
   a. Limited salt intake and moderate fluid restriction during the 7 to 10 premenstrual days.
   b. Use of diuretics to facilitate salt and water excretion: e.g., ammonium chloride, 1.0 to 2.0 gm four times daily; chlormerodrin (Neohydrin), 1 to 2 tablets daily; furosemide (Lasix), 20 to 40 mg daily; chlorothiazide (Diuril), 250 to 500 mg daily. Whichever diuretic is chosen, the dosage is given for 7 to 10 days premenstrually.
2. Attempts at opposing the relative excess of estrogen and/or correcting the estrogen-progesterone imbalance:
   a. Testosterone, in the form of methyltestosterone, 10 mg two to three times weekly throughout the cycle, or 10 mg daily from the fifteenth to the twenty-fifth day, with a view to suppressing the effects of the estrogen excess. This appears to be particularly effective against premenstrual mastalgia.
   b. Progesterone: Small doses of any of the synthetic progestogens, or progesterone, 25 mg, every other day, given during the last 8 to 10 days of the cycle, with a view to correcting the theoretical progesterone insufficiency. A useful combination

medication now available and quite effective is Cytran, which contains the progestin, Provera, as well as a mild diuretic and a mild tranquilizer. It is administered orally once or twice daily during the last 7 to 10 days of the cycle.

Other maneuvers that may be helpful in some cases include dietary regulation to minimize hypoglycemia, and the use of mild sedatives and tranquilizers. Rarely, in extremely severe and refractory cases, psychiatric evaluation and therapy may be necessary.

The Pelvic Congestion Syndrome

The pelvic congestion syndrome is a vague disorder characterized by chronic but often intermittent pelvic and lower abdominal pain, acquired dysmenorrhea, low backache, and dyspareunia. It invariably increases in severity during the premenstrual and menstrual phases of the cycle but is often symptomatic throughout the cycle. There is sometimes an associated menorrhagia that fails to respond to the usual conservative management. Although not encountered frequently, it appears to be a real entity, the associated symptoms and some of the etiologic mechanisms involved resembling in part those of the premenstrual tension syndrome, but with the addition of a local pelvic vascular and autonomic nervous system disorder that produces grossly visible vascular congestion, tissue edema, hypersecretion, and muscle spasm throughout the pelvis and pelvic viscera.

A frequent, almost pathognomonic sign is extreme tenderness and pain on motion of the boggy pelvic organs and supporting structures. Since clinically significant and recognizable instances of this particular entity seem to be relatively infrequent, it will not be considered further here, but the reader is referred to Taylor's thoughtful and authoritative discussion [35], based on his lengthy study of its etiology, clinical features, and therapy, and to several more recent contributions to our current understanding of this functional disorder [1, 2, 4, 13, 33].

An even more specific variant of the pelvic congestion symptom complex, the **Allen-Masters syndrome** (or **"universal joint syndrome"**), was described by Allen and Masters [1, 2] as a common cause of the pelvic congestion syndrome and as due to obstetric trauma. In some patients with the symptom complex they were able to demonstrate a laceration of the broad ligament resulting in a very unstable, cervico-fundal junction resembling a universal joint and a characteristically retroflexed, retroverted uterus with excessive and independent mobility of the fundus and cervix. Dilatation of the venous system with the appearance of huge pelvic varicosities occurs as a result of poor support and torsion of the veins, and continued engorgement further softens the lower uterine segment and weakens its supports. The symptoms are definitely acquired ones and can usually be shown to have developed after a traumatic delivery. In the experience of Allen and Masters, operative repair of the broad ligament fascial defects ("Masters windows") with uterine suspension was highly successful in alleviating the condition in patients who desired to preserve their childbearing potential; in those not desiring further pregnancies, hysterectomy is probably the procedure of choice when the diagnosis is firmly established.

Great care should always be taken in arriving at the diagnosis of chronic pelvic congestion, with or without the associated Allen-Masters syndrome, because many patients are encountered with somewhat similar symptoms occurring purely on a psychosomatic basis, without any underlying vascular congestion, and these patients are best managed symptomatically. Nevertheless, in a small number of patients with well-documented pelvic congestion, hysterectomy may be indicated and will completely obliterate the symptoms. If the patient desires sterilization as well as relief from her disabling symptoms, abdominal hysterectomy is clearly the treatment of choice.

Cyclic Breast Disorders

The normal mild premenstrual breast discomfort (often attended by slight swelling and tenderness) that accompanies the physiologic interstitial edema and increased glandular activity produced by the hormonal stimuli present at this phase of the cycle has already been noted. The exaggerated form of this phenomenon invariably associated with the premenstrual-tension symptom complex has also been discussed.

Not infrequently, repeated occurrence of these cyclic breast changes leads to palpable anatomic abnormalities that may either be transient, subsiding postmenstrually, or may ultimately become chronic. In either case, symptoms usually continue to be most prominent during the 7 to 10 premenstrual days. Such significantly symptomatic and more permanent histologic and often grossly palpable structural alterations of breast tissue appear to occur more often in women in whom there is a tendency to progesterone-estrogen imbalance, with a relative excess of the latter. Thus, they are most likely to occur in women approaching the menopause and menopausal women receiving estrogens. It may well be, however, that in many women, the cause is not an abnormal hormone balance but rather an abnormal breast tissue response.

This general type of breast change is frequently classified under the broad, descriptive term **chronic cystic mastitis.** In addition to cystic dilatation of breast glands and ducts, on histologic examination one finds varying degrees of inflammatory cellular infiltrates, interstitial fibrosis, actual intraductal epithelial hyperplasia, and even intraductal papilloma formation. Thus subtypes of chronic cystic change, many of which can only be recognized on microscopic examination, include the following: macroscopic cysts – the so-called blue-domed cysts, (often solitary) – as well as multiple, smaller ones; periductal mastitis; adenofibrosis (this is an entirely different entity from the fibroadenoma, a localized, benign neoplasm appearing most often in adolescents or women in their early twenties); intraductal epithelial hyperplasia; and intraductal papillomas (the latter characteristically produce a nipple discharge that is usually dark black or bloody; their location, usually just outside the areolar margin, can be accurately determined, since pressure at the site invariably produces the discharge). Macroscopic cysts are readily palpable as discrete, rounded, movable cystic masses, whereas adenofibrosis results in a typical diffuse involvement of the breasts (usually both, though it may be more extensive in one) by multiple, shotty nodules. The other histologic types, including the less common variants, blunt duct adenosis and sclerosing adenosis, usually present as firm, discrete masses.

These cyclic breast disorders present two problems for the physician: diagnosis and relief of discomfort. In the case of adenofibrosis, the diffuse, finely granular or shotty nodularity without a truly discrete mass is usually sufficiently characteristic to eliminate any concern over possible malignancy. A macroscopic cyst is also usually readily recognizable. Furthermore, such cysts can be easily aspirated in the office or clinic, thus absolutely confirming the presumptive diagnosis of cyst, as well as removing it, and they rarely recur. No local anesthetic is required, and only an ordinary syringe and a No. 20 needle need be at hand. This valuable minor procedure should be used far more often than it is, since, in a few minutes' time, the patient's inevitable fear of cancer can be immediately dispelled, saving the time and expense that hospitalization and excision biopsy require.

When a discrete mass is present that is either obviously noncystic or does not yield fluid on attempted aspiration, hospitalization for excision and immediate frozen-section histologic examination is mandatory, lest breast carcinoma fail to be detected at the earliest possible moment. There has been increasingly widespread use of mammography and a resulting increased skill in performing and interpreting mammograms and xeromammograms (soft-tissue x-ray techniques for the visualization of breast tissue and any contained masses). Mammograms and xeromammograms have proved to be extremely helpful in resolving some of the diagnostic dilemmas posed by many of the hormonally related breast changes, avoiding the need for surgical biopsy in some cases.

The same general plan of management applies to the problem of bloody nipple discharge. Here, the approximate location of the lesion can usually be determined (pressure over it reproducing the discharge) even though the lesion itself is usually not palpable, and excision of the area involved should be done to remove the duct papilloma and exclude the possibility that it is in fact an intraductal carcinoma.

With regard to relief of troublesome cyclic breast symptoms, the use of testosterone (presumably for its antiestrogenic effect) as well as diuretics and other medications has already been mentioned in the section on premenstrual tension. Since breast cysts are also often painful, aspiration is effective therapy in this situation. Finally, in women who have suffered from any of the manifestations of the cyclic breast disorders during their active menstrual life, estrogens should probably be avoided in the management of any menopausal symptoms, since the breast discomfort and cystic changes will frequently recur and be troublesome if estrogenic drugs are used.

REFERENCES

1. Allen, W. M. Chronic pelvic congestion and pelvic pain. *Am. J. Obstet. Gynecol.* 109:198, 1971.

2. Allen, W. M., and Masters, W. H. Traumatic laceration of uterine support. *Am. J. Obstet. Gynecol.* 70:500, 1955.
3. Askell, S., and Jones, G. S. Etiology and treatment of dysfunctional uterine bleeding. *Obstet. Gynecol.* 44:1, 1974.
4. Atkinson, S. M., Jr. The universal joint syndrome. *Obstet. Gynecol.* 36:510, 1970.
5. Baulieu, E. Steroid receptors and hormone receptivity. *J.A.M.A.* 234:404, 1975.
6. Berger, M. J., and Taymor, L. L. The role of luteinizing hormone in human follicular maturation and function. *Am. J. Obstet. Gynecol.* 111:708, 1971.
7. DeCosta, E. J. Menstrual problems — dysfunctional uterine bleeding. *J.A.M.A.* 193:950, 1965.
8. Dingman, J. F. Current concepts: Pituitary function. *N. Engl. J. Med.* 285:617, 1971.
9. Dunn, J. M. Vicarious menstruation. *Am. J. Obstet. Gynecol.* 114:568, 1972.
10. Dykhuisen, R. F., and Roberts, J. A. The ovarian vein syndrome. *Surg. Gynecol. Obstet.* 130:443, 1970.
11. Fournier, P. J. R., Desjardins, P. D., and Friesen, H. G. Current understanding of human prolactin physiology and its diagnostic and therapeutic applications: A review. *Am. J. Obstet. Gynecol.* 118:337, 1974.
12. Gay, V. L. The hypothalamus: Physiology and clinical use of releasing factors. *Fertil. Steril.* 23:50, 1972.
13. Hartnett, L. J., Edwards, D., Knight, W. A., and Woods, R. Broad ligament laceration and pelvic congestive disease syndrome. *Obstet. Gynecol.* 36:16, 1970.
14. Holmstrom, E. G., and McLennan, C. E. Menorrhagia associated with irregular shedding of the endometrium. *Am. J. Obstet. Gynecol.* 53:727, 1947.
15. Jones, S. G., Askell, S., and Wentz, A. C. Serum progesterone values in the luteal phase defect. *Obstet. Gynecol.* 44:26, 1974.
16. Lundy, L. E., Lee, S. G., Levy, W., Woodruff, J. D., Wu, C. H., and Abdalla, M. The ovulatory cycle: A histologic thermal, steroid, and gonadotropin correlation. *Obstet. Gynecol.* 44:14, 1974.
17. McSweeney, D. J., and Fallon, R. F. Ovulation and postovulation pain. *Am. J. Obstet. Gynecol.* 59:419, 1950.
18. Moghissi, K. S., Syner, F. N., and Evans, T. N. A composite picture of the menstrual cycle. *Am. J. Obstet. Gynecol.* 114:405, 1972.
19. Morton, J. H. Premenstrual tension. *Am. J. Obstet. Gynecol.* 60:343, 1950.
20. Piver, M. S., Williams, L. J., and Marcuse, P. M. Influence of luteal cysts on menstrual function. *Obstet. Gynecol.* 35:740, 1970.
21. Porges, R. F. Acute retrograde menstruation. *Obstet. Gynecol.* 35:524, 1970.
22. Pugh, M. von Willebrand's disease in gynecologic and obstetric practice. *Int. J. Gynecol. Obstet.* 10:137, 1972.
23. Reifenstein, E. C., Jr. Psychogenic or "hypothalamic" amenorrhea. *Med. Clin. North Am.* 30:1103, 1946.
24. Rodgers, C. H. Neuroendocrine mechanisms responsible for gonadotropin release. *J. Reprod. Med.* 14:1, 1975.
25. Rogers, J. Menstruation and systemic disease. *N. Engl. J. Med.* 259:676, 721, 770, 1958.
26. Rossi, N. P., and Goplerud, C. P. Recurrent catamenial pneumothorax. *Arch. Surg.* 109:173, 1974.
27. Rothchild, I. The central nervous system and disorders of ovulation in women. *Am. J. Obstet. Gynecol.* 98:719, 1967.

28. Schally, A. V., Kastin, A. J., and Arimura, A. The hypothalamus and reproduction. *Am. J. Obstet. Gynecol.* 114:423, 1972.
29. Schally, A. V., Kastin, A. J., and Arimura, A. The hypothalamus and reproduction. *Am. J. Obstet. Gynecol.* 122:857, 1975.
30. Shane, J. M., Naftolin, F., and Newmark, S. R. Gynecologic endocrine emergencies. *J.A.M.A.* 231:393, 1975.
31. Sherwood, L. M. Current concepts: Human prolactin. *N. Engl. J. Med.* 284:774, 1971.
32. Speroff, L., and van de Wiele, R. L. Regulation of the human menstrual cycle. *Am. J. Obstet. Gynecol.* 109:234, 1971.
33. Stearns, H. C., and Sneeden, V. D. Observations on the clinical and pathologic aspects of the pelvic congestion syndrome. *Am. J. Obstet. Gynecol.* 94:718, 1966.
34. Strott, C. A., Cargille, C. M., Ross, G. T., and Lipsett, M. B. The short luteal phase. *J. Clin. Endocrinol.* 30:246, 1970.
35. Taylor, H. C. Pelvic pain based on a vascular and autonomic nervous system disorder. *Am. J. Obstet. Gynecol.* 67:1177, 1954.
36. Taymor, M. L., Sturgis, S. H., Goodale, W. T., and Ashbaugh, D. Menorrhagia due to chronic iron deficiency. *Obstet. Gynecol.* 16:571, 1960.
37. Yen, S. S. C., Vela, P., Rankin, J., and Littell, A. S. Hormonal relationships during the menstrual cycle. *J.A.M.A.* 211:1513, 1970.

6
Fundamental Endocrinologic Disorders

Fundamental disturbances in the endocrine function of the female reproductive tract may arise in connection with basic structural or biochemical defects or both in any of the hormone-producing glands normally involved in its regulation and normal physiologic nature or which, if not functioning normally, may interfere with reproductive tract physiology. These true endocrine disorders may be of primary ovarian origin or may be the result of a more generalized endocrine-metabolic disturbance primary in one of the other endocrine glands (pituitary, thyroid, or adrenal) or in the hypothalamic regulatory centers, with secondary gynecologic manifestations due to the associated disturbance of function in otherwise normal ovaries. Although some of the clinical aspects of many of these fundamental endocrinologic disorders are discussed in other chapters, they are discussed individually as specific entities in the first portion of this chapter. In the last section of this chapter, the approach to differential diagnosis and general management of patients with the two most common symptomatic manifestations of a basic endocrinologic disturbance will be considered: (1) amenorrhea and (2) hirsutism with or without virilization.

PRIMARY OVARIAN DISORDERS

Functioning Ovarian Tumors

Functioning ovarian tumors are derived from the cortical cells and stromal elements of the ovary, cell types that originally arose from the undifferentiated mesenchymal tissues of the primitive gonad. Such cell types might therefore be expected to retain the potential for the biochemical elaboration of either estrogens or androgens when assuming more undifferentiated, neoplastic characteristics. This is indeed the case. Accordingly, for a long time, these tumors have been classified as either primarily estrogen-secreting or androgen-secreting, as indicated both by the resulting clinical picture of increased feminization or of masculinization (virilism), or defeminization, and by actual laboratory observations of increased estrogen or androgen excretion. (Hence the terms **feminizing** or **masculinizing mesenchymomas** or **mesenchymal tumors of the ovary**, and **estrogenic** or **androgenic tumors of the ovary**, frequently appear in the literature.) Furthermore, on microscopic examination, the tumors not infrequently present the histologic appearance appropriate to their hormonal and clinical manifestations. Thus tumors composed primarily of granulosa cell and theca cell types and hence strongly resembling normal ovarian estrogen-secreting elements are most commonly associated with the clinical picture of feminization. On the other hand, the arrhenoblastomas, made up principally of Sertoli cells and Leydig cells, often with well-developed testiclelike tubules and thus highly reminiscent of normal testicular androgen-secreting elements, are nearly always associated with the

183

clinical picture of masculinization. An even rarer third type of functioning ovarian tumor exhibiting both ovarian-estrogenic and testicular-androgenic histologic features, the gynandroblastoma, containing both granulosa-theca cell and arrhenoblastoma (Sertoli-Leydig cell) elements, is often associated with a clinical and endocrinologic picture that combines features of both masculinization and feminization. Not all pathologists are agreed on the validity of the existence of this mixed type of functioning tumor, however. Morris and Scully [32], for example, prefer to classify such lesions in the category of "sex cord mesenchyme tumors of indeterminate or mixed cell types."

However, it is becoming more apparent that none of these histologic-hormonal-clinical correlations invariably holds true, and numerous instances have been reported in which tumors presenting testicular-androgenic histologic features were accompanied by feminization, while others exhibiting the granulosa cell or the theca cell microscopic ovarian-estrogenic characteristics were associated with the clinical picture of masculinization. For this reason, an absolutely rigid classification of these tumors in accordance with their associated hormonal patterns and clinical manifestations is certainly not valid. From the pathologist's perspective, a classification based on the histologic picture would be more correct; but here, too, the microscopic features are not always clear-cut. In general, it can be said that granulosa cells, theca cells, stroma cells, and Sertoli cells may and usually do produce estrogens and have a feminizing effect, whereas lutein cells, luteinized theca cells, Leydig cells, and ovarian hilus cells may and usually do produce androgens and have a masculinizing effect. That there are exceptions is perhaps not surprising when one considers that all these cell types are descended from the originally sexually indifferent gonadal mesenchyme and — even more important — when one considers the actual chemical transformations involved in the synthesis of estrogens and androgens (and adrenal steroids), with testosterone, for example, being an important intermediate-stage compound in the formation of estradiol, the presumed ovarian estrogen. Apparently, the most frequent exceptions actually do involve the granulosa and theca cells, which under certain circumstances may change more or less permanently into lipoid producers of androgens or androgenlike substances, or in which there may exist a shifting balance between estrogen and androgen production. It must also be remembered that tumors of these various histologic types occasionally have no apparent associated endocrine function whatsoever. This is particularly true of the more malignant variants of these tumors, of which the most common example is the granulosa cell carcinoma or, perhaps more accurately, the sarcomatoid type of granulosa cell tumor. Finally, the dysgerminomas, derived from an even more primitive but histogenetically related cell type, are not hormonally active, nor are the rarer, highly undifferentiated, extremely malignant solid ovarian tumors taking origin from ovarian cortical and stromal cell elements, though both groups of tumors appear to be histogenetically related in the same fashion to the group of functioning ovarian neoplasms.

From the clinician's viewpoint, the matter of histologic classification is not of fundamental importance in the management of the patient. The matter of greatest significance is whether the functioning tumors of this group are estrogenic or androgenic; in the case of the former, diagnosis of the site of the abnormal function is readily apparent — it must be in the ovary — while in the masculinized patient the site of abnormal androgens may be either ovarian or adrenal. Thus it is important to bear in mind, for the reasons mentioned, that the clinical picture in the patient does not always correspond completely to a certain histologic picture in the tumor itself. Nevertheless, it usually does, and from a practical standpoint the framework of the old classification is useful.

GRANULOSA CELL TUMORS

Although occasionally mildly androgenic or without any hormonal effects, the vast majority of granulosa cell tumors are associated with estrogen production on the part of the tumor cells. Approximately 5 percent occur before puberty and are hence accompanied by a pseudosexual precocity due to the premature presence of excessive amounts of estrogen in the absence of ovulation. The "precocity" is completely reversible on removal of the tumor, which terminates the abnormal estrogenic stimulation. The majority of granulosa cell tumors (55 percent) appear during active reproductive life, and the continuous, uncontrolled, and often excessive estrogen production results in total interference with normal cyclic function and fertility, irregular and excessive bleeding, and often complete amenorrhea. However, the amenorrhea may ultimately give way to irregular and excessive bleeding again as endometrial hyperplasia eventually develops, which is a common sequence of events.

A significant number of cases (40 percent) occur after the menopause, the ensuing estrogenic stimulation leading to endometrial proliferation, hyperplasia, and polyp formation, with resulting postmenopausal bleeding, as well as to obvious, more generalized manifestations of hyperestrinism; e.g., renewed breast glandular stimulation, nipple and areolar pigmentation, uterine growth (also renewed growth of fibroids if present), stimulation of vaginal and cervical epithelial growth and secretion, and cessation of hot flashes if present — that is, a "refeminization" to the young adult stage as far as certain secondary sex characteristics are concerned. A potentially far more serious result of this prolonged, unopposed endometrial stimulation is the development of atypical glandular hyperplasia, carcinoma in situ, and, ultimately, frank endometrial carcinoma. In fact, roughly 10 to 20 percent of patients with granulosa cell tumors, most of them postmenopausal women, will have an associated carcinoma of the endometrium.

Pathologic Features

From the standpoint of their gross pathologic characteristics, granulosa cell tumors are usually partially solid, partially cystic tumors, solid yellow or grayish-yellow in color, and they occur bilaterally in 5 to 10 percent of cases. Because of their relatively rapid growth, extreme cellularity and vascularity, and relatively scanty stroma, they are frequently complicated by necrosis and hemorrhage into either or both of the solid or cystic portions, and sudden rupture is not uncommon, particularly in the sarcomatoid type. In fact, approximately 10 percent present as acute surgical emergencies, the rupture, bleeding, and resulting massive and sometimes fatal hemo-peritoneum completely overshadowing what may have been only mild manifestations of the accompanying endocrine disturbance. They sometimes attain considerable size, and several weighing close to 35 pounds have been reported, although the diag-nosis is usually made before the tumor reaches these proportions.

Microscopically, there are usually solid cords and nests of typical granulosa cells, sometimes arranged in a follicular or cylindroid pattern. Degeneration and lique-faction within large masses of granulosa cells often produce clear spaces with a central body of degeneration products, the Call-Exner bodies. The masses of gran-ulosa cells are separated by clusters and strands of cells resembling theca cells, en-meshed in an abundant stromal reticulum. The cytoplasm of the theca cells usually contains large amounts of lipoids, whereas the granulosa cells are usually lipid-free, and this and other evidence suggest that the theca cells are the actual source of the accompanying estrogen secretion. Although it is frequently difficult to say definitely on histologic grounds alone whether a given granulosa-theca cell tumor is benign or malignant, the sarcomatoid or frankly malignant type occurs in from 15 to 25 per-cent of patients (almost always in the postmenopausal group) and is more often bilateral (in 10 to 25 percent). Microscopically, solid masses of granulosa cells with almost no stroma are seen, but again there are usually areas of theca cells accompa-nied by an abundant reticulum. The frequently associated benign and malignant pathologic changes in the endometrium have already been commented on.

Diagnosis

The typical clinical manifestations already described, especially in the presence of a palpable ovarian tumor, should suggest the diagnosis. Laboratory confirmation of hyperestrinism may be obtained, particularly in the postmenopausal group, by finding increased urinary or blood estrogen levels or by noting the typical changes of exces-sive estrogen stimulation in vaginal cytologic smears. One other diagnostic clue, provided the patient has not received any estrogenic medication, may be found in the uterine scrapings; the presence of numerous mitotic figures in the endometrium removed at curettage for the frequently associated endometrial hyperplasia is strongly suggestive of the presence of an estrogen-producing tumor, even though no ovarian enlargement is palpable.

Treatment

Treatment is by surgical removal, and since the tumors are usually benign and uni-lateral in the younger age group, unilateral salpingo-oophorectomy is proper in women in whom preservation of childbearing function is desirable, provided that the opposite ovary is shown to be normal by means of wedging and biopsy with frozen section examination of any suspicious areas, there is no gross evidence of spread at operation, and final histologic examination does not disclose frank malig-nancy. In such cases, the five-year survival is 90 percent or more, though there are recurrences, even in the cases that appear benign on microscopic examination; such recurrences often do not appear until after 5 to 10 or more years. Reoperation and removal of a recurrent tumor, if still localized and resectable, may still result in cure in many of these patients. In the older age group, where childbearing potential is no longer a factor and where the incidence of frank malignancy as well as bilaterality is considerably higher, total hysterectomy and bilateral salpingo-oophorectomy is the operation of choice. The overall five-year survival rate for all types and age groups is 80 percent, but if there is extension beyond one ovary, the figure falls to 60 percent; again, late recurrences are frequent. Furthermore, the highly undifferentiated tumors have a very poor prognosis. These tumors are not as radiosensitive as a rule as are the ovarian dysgerminomas, but some do respond favorably. Therefore, x-ray therapy should be given postoperatively if known disease was left behind, or if a recurrent tumor not amenable to further surgery should develop later.

THECA CELL TUMORS (THECOMAS AND SOME OVARIAN FIBROMAS)

Morris and Scully [32] state that thecomas are only one-third as common as granulosa cell tumors. However, in some reported series of estrogen-secreting ovarian neoplasms, the thecoma-fibroma group of functioning tumors was encountered one-and-a-half times more frequently than the granulosa cell lesions. Theca cell tumors grossly resemble simple ovarian fibromas. In some cases, histologic differentiation is difficult even though the presence of clinical manifestations of hyperestrinism may be made known to the pathologist. Theca cell tumors are firm, solid, fibrous, and slightly yellowish or white in color. Microscopic sections reveal varying numbers of plump, pale, lipoid-filled cells resembling theca-lutein cells and interspersed among bundles of broad spindle cells and dense bands of connective tissue. They are often heavily hyalinized, and cystic degeneration is common. They are invariably benign (no more than 5 percent exhibit malignant change) and unilateral, rare before puberty, and usually attain only a moderate size. They have essentially the same clinical manifestations as the granulosa cell tumors.

The treatment is surgical removal. Unilateral salpingo-oophorectomy suffices, although in the older woman, total hysterectomy with removal of both adnexa is usually the procedure of choice. In the case of younger women, there is usually a rapid return to normal, cyclic reproductive tract function following removal of the tumor.

ARRHENOBLASTOMAS (COMBINED SERTOLI CELL AND LEYDIG CELL TUMORS)

Arrhenoblastomas are the most common of the androgen-secreting tumors of the ovary, although tumors of this histologic type may occasionally have estrogenic activity. Typically, they occur during the active reproductive years, but occasionally they are encountered at or just before puberty or following the menopause. The characteristic clinical picture, which is the result of the associated excretion of androgens that inhibit both ovulation and estrogen production, is one of menstrual irregularities and infertility, usually rapidly leading to amenorrhea and then progressive virilization, with increasing hirsutism in a masculine distribution, temporal baldness, acne, oily skin, clitoral enlargement, atrophy of the breasts, deepening of the voice, and even a masculine type of muscular development and weight distribution. The tumors are invariably unilateral and most often benign, varying in size from a few centimeters or less to 25 to 30 cm in diameter. If the tumor is large enough, the patient may have abdominal pain or be aware of a mass.

Grossly, arrhenoblastomas are solid, smooth, often encapsulated tumors, frequently bright yellow in color and with occasional cystic degeneration, necrosis, or hemorrhage, especially in the larger or more malignant tumors. The cellular features seen on microscopic examination are highly variable, but nearly always both Sertoli cell types (often forming tubular structures after the pattern of the testicular tubular adenoma of Pick variant) and Leydig cell types (the large, lipoid-containing mature Leydig cells showing the diagnostic crystalloids of Reinke) can be identified. In some instances the cellular pattern is highly undifferentiated and may assume a sarcomatoid, embryonal carcinomalike, or teratomalike appearance. Such tumors are usually highly malignant and rapidly pursue a fatal course. Both the uninvolved ovarian tissue and the endometrium are usually atrophic and do not sustain permanent ill effects if the tumor is benign and is resected.

Diagnosis

The dramatic clinical manifestations of the abnormal androgenic effects and the presence of a palpable ovarian tumor nearly always are sufficient to establish a definite diagnosis. It is important to exclude the possibility of adrenal disease, but this is usually readily done. The 17-ketosteroid excretion levels in patients with arrhenoblastomas are usually normal or only slightly elevated, presumably because the tumor secretes only small amounts of testosterone, the very potent, true male androgen. However, plasma testosterone levels will usually be elevated and suggest an ovarian source for the excess androgen.

Treatment

Surgical removal is indicated, and although small, benign variants may be well encapsulated and have on numerous occasions been locally excised or shelled out with preservation of the remaining normal ovarian tissue on that side, it is perhaps wiser in most instances to perform unilateral salpingo-oophorectomy, particularly in view of the highly variable cellular characteristics and growth pattern of these neoplasms. If the tumor is grossly or histologically malignant, then total hysterectomy and bilateral salpingo-oophorectomy should be done (many of the malignant forms are bilateral, although 95 percent or more of the group as a whole are unilateral). If known extension of disease has been left behind, postoperative x-ray therapy should be given. The reported incidence of malignancy varies from 3 percent to as high as 20 to 25 percent in different series, and the malignant types may exhibit rapid and prompt fatal termination at one extreme or be associated with late recurrence after a symptomless interval of many years at the other. The vast majority are cured by surgical removal, however, and in younger patients in whom local resection is possible, normal reproductive tract function with return of regular menstruation usually follows within a month or two. Hirsutism may only partially improve, however, and voice changes and clitoral enlargement often persist, the latter sometimes requiring plastic surgery.

SCLEROSING STROMAL TUMOR OF THE OVARY

Sclerosing stromal tumors of the ovary are relatively uncommon and benign functional tumors that usually occur in young women. Menstrual irregularities secondary to the hormone output of the tumor represent their most frequent clinical manifestation. Microscopically, they are seen to be composed of the entire spectrum of ovarian stromal cells, including cortical cells, granulosa and theca cells, Sertoli-Leydig cells, and fibroblasts and containing abundant lipid material; an abundance of collagen among the cells accounts for their sclerotic appearance. As might be expected from their histologic appearance, these tumors may secrete estrogens, androgens, and at times a mixture of both. They are most often unilateral, and simple salpingo-oophorectomy is the indicated treatment and invariably results in resumption of a normal menstrual pattern.

GYNANDROBLASTOMA

The controversial nature of the gynandroblastoma, a rare, possibly separate variety of functioning ovarian tumor that appears to contain both granulosa-theca cell and arrhenoblastoma elements has already received comment. This histologic type, though infrequent, has most often been reported to be accompanied by a clinical picture that is a variable mixture of signs and symptoms of both abnormal androgenic and estrogenic excretion. Treatment of gynandroma consists of surgical removal of the tumor, usually by oophorectomy.

GONADOBLASTOMA

Gonadoblastomas are extremely rare tumors composed not only of cells of sex cord type and cells of mesenchymal origin but also of germ cells. The few reported cases have occurred almost without exception in intersex patients with gonadal dysgenesis, nearly all of them with chromatin-negative nuclear patterns and virilization but with a female internal genital tract. They are therefore frequently termed *dysgenetic gonadomas,* and obviously they secrete androgens in most instances. Their most characteristic pathologic feature is the invariable presence of both gross and microscopic calcification, which is almost diagnostic of this tumor, since the other tumors of this histogenetic type (e.g., dysgerminoma, arrhenoblastoma) rarely if ever calcify. Although some have been highly malignant, the majority are benign, and removal usually results in disappearance of the manifestations of excessive androgen production. These tumors are often bilateral, though the tumor in the opposite gonad may be microscopic. Therefore, removal by bilateral adnexectomy is the treatment of choice, and the cure rate approaches 100 percent, since they rarely recur or metastasize. Because germ cell tumors such as the gonadoblastoma so commonly arise in dysgenetic gonads in patients whose chromosome complement includes the Y chromosome, removal of both gonads is strongly recommended once it is established that a Y chromosome is present in any patient with gonadal dysgenesis.

HILUS CELL TUMOR (PURE LEYDIG CELL TUMOR)

Although abundant Leydig cells are a prominent (sometimes the predominant) feature of most of the arrhenoblastoma group of functioning ovarian tumors, they presumably arise from the primitive mesenchymal element of this basically mixed tumor of both Sertoli and Leydig cell types. In contrast, the much less common, true Leydig cell tumors probably most often arise directly from the mature type of ovarian hilus cell. In fact, they are often found in association with — and perhaps actually develop from — what was originally a simple hilus cell hyperplasia. They are usually small, unilateral, yellowish-brown or reddish-brown tumors (they may occasionally attain a clinically palpable size, however), that are composed of nodular masses of pure Leydig cells, identifiable by the characteristic intracellular eosinophilic rods, or crystalloids of Reinke. The presence of the latter and the gross anatomic location of the tumor within the hilus of the ovary serve to establish the diagnosis definitely. They are invariably virilizing, producing a masculine type of hirsutism, clitoral enlargement, and so on, but as is the case in arrhenoblastomas with androgenic activity, the 17-ketosteroid excretion levels are usually normal or only slightly elevated, and the 17-hydroxycorticoid levels are of course always normal. However, as in the case of arrhenoblastomas, plasma testosterone levels are often elevated and indicative of the ovarian origin for the excess androgen. Although these tumors may occasionally develop in the younger age group, they are more prone to appear in menopausal or, even more often, postmenopausal women, in contrast to arrhenoblastomas, which are far more frequent during active reproductive life. In addition to virilization, the clinical picture accompanying hilus cell tumors may also include postmenopausal bleeding, the result of associated endometrial hyperplasia, polyps, and growing fibroids, which may in turn be secondary to the frequent coexistence of ovarian cortical stromal hyperplasia and luteinization. These tumors are invariably benign, treatment is oophorectomy, and the virilism usually regresses more or less completely following removal of the tumor.

ADRENAL-LIKE TUMORS

Adrenal-like tumors, which are rare and poorly understood, are variously designated as adrenal rest tumors, masculinovoblastomas, luteomas, or lipoid cell tumors, because on microscopic examination they are seen to be composed of large, clear, fat-filled cells resembling adrenocortical cells or, at times, even Leydig or thecalutein cells. In the more undifferentiated types, the typical histologic pattern and appearance may be lost. Those arising in the ovarian hilus may actually be variants of true Leydig cell tumors. Most of them are located in the ovarian cortex, however, and may have arisen from ovarian stromal cells of the lutein type or even from adrenal cell rests. Clinical features suggesting the latter origin have been the not infrequent association of Cushing's syndrome with this histologic type of tumor (20 percent of cases), although the majority are masculinizing and produce an acquired adrenogenital syndrome type of clinical picture. Furthermore, the 17-ketosteroid excretion is nearly always elevated in patients with these tumors, and chemical fractionation studies not infrequently reveal an adrenal steroid pattern.

These essentially solid tumors are yellowish to reddish-brown in color, are usually small (less than 5 cm in diameter, although they may occasionally attain a fair size), are rare after the menopause, and may be either benign or malignant. Because of the associated typical clinical features and 17-ketosteroid elevation, it is essential to exclude the possibility of primary adrenocortical hyperplasia or tumor unless an obvious ovarian tumor is palpable. The 17-hydroxycorticosteroid levels are usually normal, and ACTH and cortisone tests have no effect on the 17-ketosteroid levels, as would be the case with primary adrenal hyperplasia. On the other hand, when stimulated by human chorionic gonadotropin (HCG), the response observed in patients with virilizing lipoid cell tumors of the ovary is one of further elevation in the 17-ketosteroid excretion levels. If the technique for their determination is readily available, both peripheral blood and ovarian vein blood testosterone levels will be found to be elevated; FSH and LH levels are low due to the secondary pituitary suppression by the elevated testosterone. Other helpful diagnostic maneuvers would include culdoscopy or laparoscopy, to attempt to demonstrate a small, nonpalpable ovarian tumor, and presacral pneumoretroperitoneal adrenal studies, to evaluate the possibility of a primary adrenal tumor. Treatment is resection of the tumor by oophorectomy. The malignant varieties are only rarely cured, however, since they are often highly undifferentiated and usually metastasize widely.

MISCELLANEOUS OVARIAN TUMORS WITH ENDOCRINE SIGNIFICANCE

A **struma ovarii**, a benign dermoid cyst or teratoma of the ovary composed chiefly of ectopic thyroid tissue, may rarely produce sufficient amounts of thyroxine to cause clinical hyperthyroidism. If the thyroid gland is normal (it, too, is occasionally simultaneously overactive) and an ovarian tumor is palpable, the diagnosis may be obvious, but radioactive iodine studies with actual pelvic radioactive counts may confirm the suspicion in equivocal cases. If the thyroid itself is normal, removal of the ovarian struma completely cures the hyperthyroidism. Some of these tumors are accompanied by a benign type of ascites and occasionally by hydrothorax as well (Meigs' syndrome) (see Chap. 15). Although they are usually entirely benign histologically and in their clinical behavior, 4 to 5 percent of these "ovarian goiters" prove to be thyroid carcinomas.

Stromal luteinization of certain benign and malignant ovarian tumors, both primary and metastatic in origin, has been shown to occur and to be associated with steroid production (either estrogens or androgens) on the part of these luteinized stromal cells. This phenomenon has been observed in the case of a few Brenner tumors, a few benign cystadenomas, an occasional primary cystadenocarcinoma, and perhaps most often in association with ovarian metastases from primary gastrointestinal tract cancer, notably of the colon and stomach. The numerous fat-containing stromal cells of these tumors show a striking resemblance to luteinized theca cells of the normal ovary, and a number of the patients with this histologic picture have exhibited androgenic or estrogenic effects (e.g., mild virilism, uterine bleeding due to endometrial hyperplasia), with regression in many instances after removal of the tumor. **Luteoma of pregnancy** is a related but benign disorder, with large, luteinized cystic ovaries within which is found a mass of solid, tumorlike tissue. Sometimes the lesion is accompanied by maternal or fetal virilization or both. Both the ovarian enlargement, which may be either bilateral or unilateral, and the virilization disappear spontaneously when the pregnancy terminates, suggesting that a continuous and excessive stimulation by, or overreaction to, HCG is responsible for the excessive theca cell and stromal luteinization that produces these functioning pseudotumors.

Finally, exceedingly rare **endocrine effects** observed with certain ovarian tumors include the **carcinoid syndrome** secondary to small carcinoid neoplasms arising in the wall of an ovarian dermoid or teratoma; **hypercalcemia** in association with a few otherwise unremarkable ovarian cancers suspected of producing a parathyroid-stimulating substance; and at least one reported tumor of the arrhenoblastoma group that appeared to be producing a corticotropinlike substance, resulting in massive adrenal hyperplasia and a **secondary Cushing's syndrome.**

Nonneoplastic Ovarian Endocrinopathies

STEIN-LEVENTHAL (POLYCYSTIC OVARY) SYNDROME

Stein and Leventhal first described the syndrome that bears their names in 1935. They included in their original group of cases only women with the classic form of the disease (or what would now be considered unmistakable, flagrant examples of what is probably a somewhat broader clinical entity than they initially envisioned), all of whom had bilaterally pale, smooth, markedly (three to five times) enlarged polycystic ovaries and varying combinations of the typical symptom complex of amenorrhea, infertility, obesity, and hirsutism. They also demonstrated nearly 30 years ago that bilateral ovarian wedge resections, with excision of the bulk of the multiple follicular microcysts and surrounding luteinized theca interna and with reduction of the total ovarian mass approximately to normal, were highly successful in restoring normal cyclic ovarian function and normal fertility. Although the method of surgical treatment they described remains essentially unchanged and just as eminently successful today, a great deal more is now known about the abnormal endocrine physiology involved. As a direct result of this better understanding of the underlying pathophysiology as well as the recent availability of drugs capable of inducing ovulation, there is now some hope for the ultimate development of an effective medical therapy that will permanently correct this disorder.

It has also become apparent that the clinical picture may be considerably more varied than was set forth in Stein and Leventhal's original description, and hence

[handwritten margin notes: menometrorrhagia — excessive menstrual bleeding during flow & unpredictable interval]

that the actual pathologic entity occurs more frequently than the original classic syndrome but may have somewhat different clinical manifestations. It should be emphasized at the outset, however, that this disorder is still relatively uncommon in comparison with the very frequent, simple, temporary dysfunctional menstrual irregularities seen in women of the same age group; further, most of the clinical features are also common to many of the other endocrine disorders. Since ovarian wedge resection is neither required nor helpful in the management of simple ovarian dysfunction or in the treatment of the other endocrine disorders affecting ovarian function, the importance of strict criteria for the diagnosis of the polycystic ovary syndrome and the performance of ovarian wedge resections is obvious.

Clinical Features

The typical patient is a young woman in her late teens or twenties in whom, following a menarche at the normal age and after a few years of somewhat irregular and invariably anovulatory cycles, either oligomenorrhea (perhaps one to three, often scanty periods yearly) or secondary complete amenorrhea develops, either of which may be of long duration before medical attention is sought. However, roughly 10 to 15 percent of patients will complain instead of menometrorrhagia, with episodes of prolonged and sometimes profuse bleeding alternating with intervals of amenorrhea. There is a tendency to obesity in many patients, and definite hirsutism is present in 50 to 60 percent; actual virilization is rare, although slight clitoral enlargement has occasionally been noted. In most cases the patients are otherwise normally female in appearance, though many will give evidence of an immature feminine development with small breasts (50 percent) and a small, infantile type of uterus (75 percent).

The symptom complex mirrors the fact that, with few exceptions, there is complete failure of ovulation as a result of the basic disturbance in ovarian function. Hence infertility, the other chief feature of the syndrome and often the one that finally prompts the patient to seek medical advice, is usually absolute. However, pregnancy has been known to occur, and evidence of occasional ovulation is seen in a small percentage of patients at the time of laparotomy. That ovulation might occasionally occur is perhaps not surprising, since the usual excellent response to wedge resection is proof that the basic disturbance in ovarian endocrine physiology is a potentially reversible one and might sporadically undergo spontaneous, if only transient, correction.

Pathologic Features

There is always bilateral ovarian involvement, both ovaries often being grossly and usually symmetrically enlarged, sometimes approaching three to five times the size of normal ovaries. However, it is now clear that this degree of enlargement is not necessarily always present. Perhaps due to increasing awareness of the existence of the disorder and its consequent earlier diagnosis, it is currently being recognized clinically, confirmed histologically, and successfully treated by bilateral wedge resections in many patients whose ovaries are found to be only one and one-half to two times enlarged, or in some cases even essentially normal in size, but who otherwise present the typical clinical and biochemical features. The ovarian surface is usually smooth and pearly white with prominent surface vessels, in contrast to its normal, pale-yellowish, wrinkled appearance, and although the ovarian capsule is characteristically thick and fibrous, often the more superficial follicle microcysts can be seen shining through. On sectioning the ovary, the increased capsular thickness is apparent, and the many small cysts, usually 5 to 10 mm in diameter, are seen lying within a dense, fibrous stroma.

On microscopical examination the markedly thickened capsule (tunica albuginea) is again noted, the ovary being literally surrounded by a dense layer of collagenous tissue. Multiple subcapsular follicle cysts are seen in all stages of development or atresia, many with a normal granulosa cell layer and an active, at times hyperplastic, theca interna, the latter showing a characteristic, often excessive luteinization. The degree to which luteinization of the theca cells of the cysts themselves is present varies considerably but appears to be most marked in patients with hirsutism and other evidences of an androgenic effect. Occasionally, there is some hyperplasia of the stroma in the central portion of the ovary as well. The final typical feature is the virtual absence of any corpora lutea or corpora albicantia except in an occasional instance, which is histologic verification that, as suggested by the clinical picture, ovulation never or only rarely has occurred.

Pathogenesis

Although the basic cause remains unknown, the older theory, that a (perhaps congenitally) thick ovarian capsule, by mechanically preventing ovulation, interfered with normal ovarian function and pituitary-ovarian cyclic regulatory mechanisms, became untenable long ago in the light of modern biochemical and hormonal studies in patients with the disease. This evidence, which will not be summarized here (key references are given at the end of this chapter, however), suggests rather that the original and basic disturbance may be in the hypothalamic-pituitary regulatory mechanism and may consist of an abnormal, almost continuous (instead of periodic and appropriately synchronized and sequential) stimulation of the ovaries by both FSH and LH. Neither gonadotropin is presumed to be excreted at abnormally high levels at any time, so that 24-hour urine gonadotropin assays are and would be expected to be within the normal range; the difficulty lies in the fact that they are secreted more or less continuously at a fairly constant level, and so fail to trigger ovulation and corpus luteum maturation. Newer, more sophisticated hormonal studies made possible by radioimmunoassays for measuring serum gonadotropins (both FSH and LH) and by the availability of synthetic LH releasing factor (LH-RH) suggest that a steady, at times erratic, LH secretion, coupled with a deficient FSH secretion, may be the fundamental problem in the polycystic ovary syndrome. Thus there are more or less constant levels of LH and estrogen (both elevated), as well as deficient FSH (low-normal or slightly decreased) and no midcycle surge of LH to trigger ovulation. This in turn would explain the failure of ovulation and the development of follicle cysts and subsequent luteinization of the theca interna of these cysts. There is much biochemical work in support of the probable excretion of abnormal steroids, notably androstenedione, testosterone, and other androgens, by these luteinized theca cells, and the presence of these substances would readily account for both the hirsutism and the endometrial atrophy leading to amenorrhea. Because androstenedione and the other androgens are known to be intermediate compounds normally produced during the synthesis of estradiol from progesterone in the ovary, only a potentially reversible disturbance in ovarian function need be postulated. On the other hand, a variable pattern of steroid production would be expected, and if compounds with predominantly estrogenic activity were continuously, though irregularly, secreted instead, the endometrial hyperplasia and clinical picture of menometrorrhagia encountered in 10 to 15 percent of patients could also be explained.

It is also obvious that once sufficient pathologic change has occurred in the ovaries, spontaneous correction of what may have been only a potentially reversible pubertal dysfunction at the hypothalamic-pituitary level is blocked by the accumulated collection of actively (though abnormally and irregularly) functioning follicle cysts and their excessively luteinized theca cells. (The occasional onset of the disorder after one pregnancy may perhaps be viewed in a similar light, because from the standpoint of both the ovary and hypothalamic-pituitary regulatory control, the need for resumption of cyclic function after a rest period imposed by pregnancy represents in a partial sense a repetition of the pubertal process.) Thus the high degree of success of bilateral ovarian wedge resection in correcting the disorder need not be completely incomprehensible if one postulates that by removal of most of the accumulated follicle cysts and abnormally luteinized theca cells, abnormal ovarian function, with the constant production of estrogens as well as androgens, is halted in many cases. In this way an opportunity is created for the return of normal hypothalamic-pituitary activity, with restoration of the normal, reciprocal pituitary-ovarian relationships and the development of a dominant follicle that proceeds to ovulation, normal corpus luteum maturation, and normal estrogen and progesterone production rather than an abnormal steroid excretion pattern that includes the presence of significant amounts of androstenedione.

Some have attempted to involve the adrenals in the pathophysiology of the Stein-Leventhal syndrome, but for a number of reasons it appears doubtful that they play any role. First, it seems highly unlikely that a primary adrenal disorder would respond so successfully to ovarian surgery. Second, 17-ketosteroid, 17-hydroxysteroid, and other adrenal steroid excretion parameters are usually normal in the polycystic ovary syndrome. Furthermore, as previously discussed, an ovarian mechanism for which there is considerable laboratory evidence readily explains the androgenic effects seen in 50 percent of cases. In occasional patients with moderately elevated 17-ketosteroids who nevertheless respond to ovarian wedge resections (but not to adrenal suppression with oral cortisone medication), one need only assume a somewhat greater ovarian production of abnormal androgens. On the other hand, there is a small group of women with a similar clinical picture, including elevated 17-ketosteroids and "polycystic ovaries," who respond to adrenal suppression with cortisone but not to ovarian wedge resections. These cases would seem actually to be instances of a mild adrenal hyperplasia, with secondary ovarian changes due to interference with normal pituitary-ovarian endocrine relationships by the elevated level of androgens of adrenal origin. That the secondary ovarian changes are not a specific feature of adrenal disease is borne out by the fact that the ovaries in patients with Cushing's disease rarely, if ever, even remotely resemble the polycystic ovaries of the Stein-Leventhal syndrome, being instead usually small and atrophic. It is important to bear in mind, however, that many clinical similarities are shared by patients with the Stein-Leventhal syndrome and women with a mild form of adrenal hyperplasia of the adrenogenital type. Thus the latter must definitely be excluded before considering ovarian wedge resections, particularly when the 17-ketosteroid levels are slightly to moderately elevated.

Diagnosis

The finding of bilaterally grossly enlarged ovaries on pelvic examination in a patient with a typical history is strongly suggestive of the disorder. However, pelvic examination findings are often inconclusive, because the frequently associated obesity makes ovarian palpation and size evaluation difficult. Stein therefore routinely employs gynecography (see Chap. 2) to detect ovarian enlargement. Since the ovaries may not be significantly enlarged in some cases, however, the diagnosis can never be made or excluded on the basis of the pelvic findings alone. The diagnostic plan in all suspected cases is as follows:

1. Basal body temperature recordings, endometrial biopsy, pregnanediol excretion studies, vaginal cytologic studies, fern test, and so on, for proof of ovulation failure.

2. Pituitary gonadotropin assay; if abnormal, a lateral skull film to detect possible enlargement of the sella turcica, to rule out pituitary disorder. (Random, baseline FSH levels are invariably normal in Stein-Leventhal syndrome.) If LH and FSH radioimmunoassay studies are available, urinary excretion and/or serum LH and FSH measurements can be obtained; FSH levels are normal or slightly low and LH levels are usually somewhat elevated. Furthermore, patients with the Stein-Leventhal syndrome show an exaggerated LH response and a diminished FSH response to the administration of synthetic luteinizing hormone releasing factor (LH-RH).

3. 17-Ketosteroid determinations; if elevated, other adrenal steroid determinations, including an adrenal suppression test with dexamethasone (if no fall in 17-ketosteroids is obtained, an ovarian suppression test with an estrogen-progestin combination agent should also be done) and presacral pneumoretroperitoneal adrenal studies to rule out an obvious adrenal hyperplasia or tumor. As previously noted, 17-ketosteroid excretion is usually normal in the Stein-Leventhal syndrome. Therefore, if the level is found elevated, a six-months' trial of oral corticosteroid therapy (e.g., prednisone, 5 mg daily or 2.5 mg twice a day) is indicated. If normal ovulatory menses result and the 17-ketosteroid excretion falls to normal, the diagnosis of a mild form of adrenal hyperplasia is established, and cortisone therapy should be continued on a

permanent basis. If there is no response, then a diagnosis of the Stein-Leventhal syndrome with elevated 17-ketosteroid excretion pattern is most likely. Plasma testosterone levels are often mildly to moderately elevated in patients with an associated hirsutism. If available, retrograde femoral vein catheterization and differential measurements of adrenal vein and ovarian vein blood androgen levels coupled with laparoscopy and ovarian biopsies will often facilitate the distinction between an ovarian or an adrenal disorder as the cause of the hirsutism.

4. Thyroid studies (e.g., basal metabolic rate, protein-bound iodine) may be indicated in some cases to rule out hypothyroidism.

5. Also to be considered in the differential diagnosis are androgenic tumors of the ovary, ovarian hyperthecosis, and precocious menopause. The ovarian tumors rarely present diagnostic problems, since the history and findings are usually totally different; they are only one-tenth as common as the polycystic ovary syndrome in women with a masculine type of hirsutism. An elevated pituitary gonadotropin excretion rate and decreased urinary estrogen levels will serve to distinguish the patient with precocious menopause, with culdoscopy or laparoscopy also of diagnostic value, although again, the history is usually different, and an associated hirsutism is rare. Finally, as will be discussed, the clinical picture and findings in patients with ovarian hyperthecosis may be almost identical; in fact, it may represent a different phase of the same basic disorder. Since the therapy to be tried is also the same, the frequent inability to make an absolute distinction between the two conditions except on pathologic examination of resected ovarian tissue causes no serious difficulties in clinical management.

6. Laparoscopy or culdoscopy should ideally be the final diagnostic maneuver in all cases and is easily done immediately prior to laparotomy for wedge resections. The characteristic gross appearance of Stein-Leventhal ovaries is readily recognized and the diagnosis firmly established.

Surgical Treatment

As already described, the standard treatment prior to the availability of drugs capable of inducing ovulation has been bilateral ovarian wedge resections, removing from one-third to one-half or more of each ovary to reduce the total mass to normal size, puncturing any remaining follicle microcysts and then resuturing the ovary (Fig. 28). If accurate diagnostic criteria are utilized and proper indications for wedge resections are strictly maintained, restoration of normal ovulatory menses will follow in 80 to 90 percent of patients, and essentially normal fertility with subsequent pregnancies will result in 60 to 80 percent. Hirsutism will only occasionally undergo significant regression, but its further progress is usually halted. Recurrences are rare and are usually secondary to inadequate resection; some failures to restore normal menses and fertility are probably due to too extensive a resection of each ovary. In some postoperative failures with moderately elevated 17-ketosteroids not initially responding to cortisone adrenal suppression, a second trial of cortisone postoperatively is indicated and sometimes yields a favorable response.

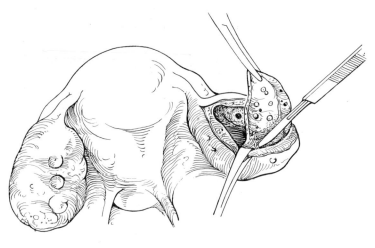

A

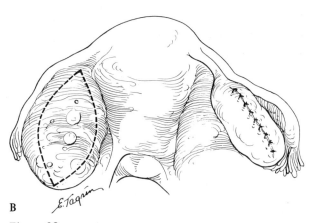

B   *E. Tagrin*

Figure 28
Technique of bilateral ovarian wedge resections in the Stein-Leventhal syndrome.
A. Wedge resection of right ovary under way, exposing thickened capsule and multiple microfollicular cysts. B. Right ovary resutured; wedge-shaped area to be resected from left ovary shown by dotted line.

Medical Treatment

Ovulation, with resulting pregnancy in a number of cases, has been induced in some patients with the Stein-Leventhal syndrome by administering the hypothalamic-pituitary stimulating drug clomiphene (Clomid), sometimes supplemented by HCG or LH-RH administration or by the use of human menopausal gonadotropins (HMG) to stimulate the ovaries directly (see section on induction of ovulation on page 214).

The unpredictable response and the occasional significant side effects (multiple ovulations with increased incidence of multiple births, and the production of giant ovarian cysts accompanied by acute abdominal symptoms) are obvious drawbacks to this type of medical therapy. Furthermore, permanent cure does not result; and the treatment program with either clomiphene or HMG, which is time-consuming, expensive, and requires careful supervision at frequent intervals throughout each monthly cycle, has to be repeated each time an attempt to induce ovulation is desired. However, medical therapy undoubtedly can and should be utilized in selected cases and probably should be given an initial trial in all patients with Stein-Leventhal syndrome whose main problem is infertility and who are currently anxious to achieve pregnancy. For the single woman or the married woman who is not immediately concerned with achieving pregnancy, performance of ovarian wedge resections seems a more rational and feasible approach than an expensive and time-consuming program of continuing, monthly medical therapy. If ovulation cannot be induced, if pregnancy does not occur after a six-months' trial, or if the complication of significant and symptomatic cystic ovarian enlargement is regularly encountered with each course of treatment, bilateral ovarian wedge resections should certainly be done.

One other aspect of the medical treatment of patients with polycystic ovarian disease concerns the management of the recurring endometrial hyperplasia that may develop. As previously noted, in 15 percent of patients with Stein-Leventhal syndrome, recurring and prolonged dysfunctional bleeding is the chief problem. Adenomatous hyperplasia of the endometrium may develop in a significant number of these patients if permanent correction of the underlying disorder of ovulation by wedge resection of the ovaries is not elected. In this age group, this potentially premalignant lesion of atypical endometrial hyperplasia is often reversible by the use of cyclic progestin therapy. Such patients should be followed closely and carefully, however, because the atypical adenomatous hyperplasia sometimes persists, or recurs, or progresses to carcinoma in situ and ultimately to invasive carcinoma of the endometrium, despite an adequate and prolonged program of medication. A long-term (1 to 30 years) follow-up study of a group of 97 such patients was reported by Chamlian and Taylor [9]. In 14 of these women, all of whom were less than 36 years old when the diagnosis of recurring endometrial hyperplasia was first made, adenocarcinoma had developed in from 1 to 14 years after the initial diagnosis of endometrial hyperplasia had been made. A total of 40 patients ultimately required hysterectomy. It is hoped that the proper drug or combination of drugs may eventually be found that can effect a permanent restoration of normal spontaneous ovulatory function in these patients.

*Relationship Between Stein-Leventhal Syndrome
and Endometrial Carcinoma in Young Women*

There have been numerous case reports and collected small series of instances in which carcinoma of the endometrium has developed in young women (below the age of 40 and often below the age of 25) in association with a clinically and pathologically documented Stein-Leventhal syndrome. In fact, when carcinoma of the endometrium does occur in young women, it appears that in from 20 to 25 percent of cases there has been a coexisting polycystic ovary syndrome. In view of the high probability that an abnormal, relatively unopposed type of estrogenic stimulation acting over a prolonged period of time is etiologically related to the development of endometrial carcinoma at any age (see Chap. 14), it is perhaps not surprising that patients with Stein-Leventhal syndrome, some of whom certainly exhibit signs and symptoms of just this type of prolonged, unphysiologic estrogen excretion, are predisposed to endometrial hyperplasia, atypicalities, and ultimately malignant change. Although it is not common, the possibility must be borne in mind, particularly in the group with menometrorrhagia (the so-called estrogenic form of the disorder), and perhaps it is another indication for reasonably prompt therapy by ovarian wedge resections once the diagnosis of Stein-Leventhal syndrome has been firmly established.

OVARIAN HYPERTHECOSIS (DIFFUSE OVARIAN STROMAL LUTEINIZATION)

Some researchers feel that ovarian hyperthecosis is an independent entity and should be separated completely from the Stein-Leventhal syndrome, whereas others consider it a variant or different phase of the same basic disorder. In any event, although in some instances there may be marked differences between the two disorders both in symptomatology and ovarian anatomy, there is more often an obvious general resemblance and a frequent overlap in the clinical features as well as in the gross and microscopic changes in the ovaries.

From a clinical standpoint, the symptoms may appear shortly after the menarche and progress slowly; less often, they may appear abruptly in an older woman, not infrequently developing after one or more pregnancies. At times, the clinical picture may be indistinguishable from that of the Stein-Leventhal syndrome, and it invariably includes amenorrhea or oligomenorrhea (less often, endometrial hyperplasia and dysfunctional bleeding) and sterility. However, there is nearly always an associated, often pronounced hirsutism and even an actual virilization with clitoral enlargement, temporal balding, and so on. Manifestations suggesting a hyperadrenal state are also frequently present and include obesity, hypertension, disturbances in carbohydrate metabolism as indicated by an abnormal glucose tolerance test of the pattern seen in Cushing's disease, and often a decidedly elevated 17-ketosteroid excretion. Rarely, an associated endometrial carcinoma has been found present. As in the case of the Stein-Leventhal syndrome, the evidence favors an ovarian rather than an adrenal origin for these androgenic and adrenogenic effects.

Grossly, the ovaries may be somewhat enlarged (they are perhaps as often normal in size) and may resemble Stein-Leventhal ovaries externally by virtue of a smooth, pale-white capsule showing no evidence of ovulation. They tend, however, to be firm and solid, often sclerotic, rather than soft and cystic, and the small follicle cysts so typical of the polycystic ovary syndrome are frequently absent or few in number.

As the term **hyperthecosis** suggests, the characteristic microscopic feature is the presence of nests of lipoid-laden, theca-lutein cells in the ovarian stroma, the latter being decidedly hyperplastic and usually forming a dense, tumorlike mass in the central portion of each ovary. When the ovaries are enlarged and polycystic, the stroma is nevertheless extensively luteinized, permitting differentiation from the Stein-Leventhal type of ovarian histologic appearance. Presumably, the abnormal presence of the abundant lipoid-laden theca-lutein cells is the result of a prolonged fundamental disturbance in the normal pituitary-ovarian relationship similar to that associated with the polycystic ovary disorder, and the heavily luteinized stroma secretes abnormal steroids with androgenic and, at times, adrenogenic activity.

The problem of differential diagnosis is entirely similar to that presented by the Stein-Leventhal syndrome, although the clinical picture is often even more suggestive of an adrenal disorder or a masculinizing ovarian tumor, and both must be carefully excluded. The same diagnostic plan of study is employed. With regard to therapy, bilateral ovarian wedge resections will sometimes restore normal ovulatory menses and fertility as well as halt the further progression of androgenic manifestations. However, the results have not been nearly so successful as is the case with the Stein-Leventhal disorder, and failures are particularly likely to occur in patients with pronounced virilism. Furthermore, patients with hyperthecosis usually fail to respond to clomiphene therapy, whereas ovulation can be induced by treatment with clomiphene in a significant percentage of patients with Stein-Leventhal syndrome.

PRECOCIOUS MENOPAUSE

The development of secondary amenorrhea and hot flashes (not all patients with premature menopause have hot flashes, however), often preceded by an interval of gradually increasing menstrual irregularities, in a woman under the age of 40 (frequently in her late twenties or early thirties) with a prior history of a normal menarche at the usual time and previously perfectly normal and regular ovulatory cycles strongly suggests the possibility of premature menopause. These patients are often, but by no means always, nulliparous; some are multiparous. There will be no other symptoms or signs suggestive of an underlying endocrine or local pelvic disorder (the breasts and external genitalia are normal, but the uterus and ovaries may be slightly smaller than normal), and all laboratory studies will show normal findings, with the exception of a considerably elevated 24-hour pituitary gonadotropin (FSH) excretion that will be in the correct range for women in the normal menopause and is essentially diagnostic for this entity. If culdoscopy or laparoscopy, either of which is frequently of value in definitely establishing the diagnosis, is performed, the ovaries will present the typical atrophic appearance of the normal menopausal state, and this together with the menopausal type of pituitary response, not only confirms the diagnosis but is further evidence that the basic cause lies within the ovaries rather than in the hypothalamic-pituitary regulatory mechanism.

Presumably, the original primordial ovarian follicles are deficient in quantity (or they migrated in inadequate numbers from the primitive streak to the genital ridges during the stage of fetal gonad differentiation) in these patients, possibly on a genetic basis, for in some instances a familial tendency has been noted. A few patients have been reported to have X chromosomal abnormalities, e.g., mosaicism (XO/XX/XXX/XXXXX), and an occasional patient will be found to have unilateral or bilateral streak gonads; the majority of these patients have a normal chromosomal pattern, however. There is no known curative treatment for this disorder, but it does represent one of the most valid and definite indications for prolonged substitution therapy with estrogens to prevent the various manifestations of a premature deficiency of the basic ovarian hormone.

CORTICAL STROMAL HYPERPLASIA

Hyperplasia of the ovarian cortical stroma, which contains abundant lipoid matter and thus exhibits an associated thecomatosis not unlike that occurring in the more specific entity of ovarian hyperthecosis previously described, is common in women approaching the menopause and is seen with increasing frequency and degree after the menopause. The presence of this change is ordinarily detected only on microscopic examination, and in many cases it is of no apparent clinical significance. However, the incidence of cortical stromal hyperplasia has been reported by some to be twice as great in patients with endometrial carcinoma, and the concept has been advanced that the ovarian stromal hyperplasia is responsible for the continuous secretion of abnormal amounts of estrogen, which in turn leads to endometrial hyperplasia, atypical changes, and ultimately carcinoma. This is an attractive but controversial theory, for unfortunately there is as yet no concrete evidence that cortical stromal hyperplasia is in fact the source of abnormal estrogen production. Furthermore, ovarian hyperplasia has been found present in no more and often less than 50 percent of patients with endometrial carcinoma in various reported series. An increased incidence of uterine myomas and adenomyosis, breast disease (including both fibrocystic disease and carcinoma), and diabetes has also been noted in several reported series of patients with proved ovarian stromal hyperplasia. Again, the fact that all these disorders are generally felt to be related to or dependent on estrogen metabolism suggests that abnormal estrogen excretion may be linked with corticostromal ovarian changes.

HILUS CELL HYPERPLASIA

The presence of abnormally large numbers of ovarian hilus cells (hilar Leydig cells) is sometimes a coexisting histologic feature of cortical stromal hyperplasia and hyperthecosis, and it may also be noted in association with true hilus cell tumors. Although exceedingly rare, a pure hilus cell hyperplasia has seemed to be the sole ovarian abnormality present in a few virilized women.

GENERALIZED ENDOCRINE AND METABOLIC DISORDERS WITH SECONDARY GYNECOLOGIC MANIFESTATIONS

Generalized endocrine and metabolic disorders with secondary effects on the reproductive system are many and varied and, in most instances, relatively uncommon. Since they are extrapelvic in origin and not primarily gynecologic in nature, no attempt will be made here to consider them in great detail. However, insofar as possible, they will be completely enumerated, and, where indicated, the highlights of their clinical features and their diagnosis and treatment will be presented in outline form.

Thyroid Gland Disorders

Either hypothyroidism or hyperthyroidism may ultimately lead to anovulatory cycles and menstrual irregularities, including hypomenorrhea, menorrhagia, menometrorrhagia, oligomenorrhea, or complete amenorrhea. Obesity is often associated with hypothyroidism. In mild cases, menstrual abnormalities may be minimal or absent, with infertility or repeated abortion representing the principal gynecologic symptom. The diagnosis is often apparent on the basis of the rest of the clinical picture, but studies of thyroid function are obviously needed for confirmation (see Chap. 2) and should be part of any evaluation of patients with persistent menstrual disorders of this type, since mild thyroid disorders (so-called subclinical hypothyroidism or hypometabolic state) are common and often not recognizable on clinical grounds alone. The primary treatment is aimed at correcting the thyroid disease, although cyclic progesterone, with or without supplemental estrogen, together with weight reduction if the patient is obese, may be of help in managing the dysfunctional bleeding while a euthyroid state is being restored. As emphasized by Skelton [46], the obstetrician-gynecologist is the physician who most often encounters the symptomatic "relatively hypothyroid" woman. The objective and subjective responses to thyroid medication in these patients are often very dramatic.

Adrenal Disease

ADRENOGENITAL SYNDROME

Adrenogenital syndrome is produced by an acquired form of adrenal hyperplasia limited to the androgenic zone of the adrenal cortex. It is characterized by hirsutism of the male type, usually progressing to actual virilization, without accompanying hypertension or alterations in glucose or electrolyte metabolism and with inhibition of ovarian function and failure of ovulation resulting in oligomenorrhea and eventually amenorrhea secondary to the pituitary inhibition induced by rising androgen levels. Signs of virilization in addition to amenorrhea and masculine hirsutism may include acne, breast atrophy, clitoral hypertrophy, deepening of the voice, and a male type of muscular development and weight distribution. It is important to remember that, in its mildest forms, the only manifestation may be anovulatory menstrual disturbances, with or without moderate elevation of the 17-ketosteroids. The syndrome may be caused either by a tumor (adenoma or carcinoma) or diffuse, bilateral hyperplasia. The latter is due to a congenital or acquired deficiency in the hydroxylating enzymes (most commonly, 21-hydroxylase) necessary for the synthesis of cortisone.

Diagnosis

In addition to the frequently characteristic clinical features of adrenogenital syndrome, a number of laboratory determinations and other studies may be diagnostic: moderate elevation of 17-ketosteroids; normal 17-hydroxycorticosteroids and 11-oxycorticosteroids; usually, normal pituitary gonadotropins. ACTH stimulation (40 units in an 8-hour intravenous infusion) and dexamethasone suppression (2 mg daily for three days) tests may help to distinguish between adrenal tumor and adrenal hyperplasia. Thus 150 mg of cortisone daily will produce a fall in the 17-ketosteroids in adrenal hyperplasia, but no effect will be observed if the disorder is due to adrenal tumor. A stimulatory dose of ACTH may produce elevation of the 17-ketosteroids in either hyperplasia or tumor, but this response is more likely with the former. Culdoscopy or laparoscopy will show normal or atrophic-appearing ovaries; presacral pneumoretroperitoneal periadrenal studies will usually reveal or exclude the presence of any but the smallest adrenal tumor.

Treatment

Treatment consists of resection of the adrenal tumor or cortisone treatment for hyperplasia (e.g., cortisone, 25 to 50 mg daily, or equivalent dosages of other corticosteroid drugs).

CONGENITAL ADRENAL HYPERPLASIA

For a discussion of congenital adrenal hyperplasia (female pseudohermaphroditism), see Chapter 3.

MILD ADRENAL HYPERPLASIA

Mild adrenal hyperplasia presents a Stein-Leventhal type of clinical picture except for moderately elevated 17-ketosteroids. The differential diagnosis is the same as in adrenogenital syndrome and as discussed in the section on the Stein-Leventhal syndrome.

Treatment

Treatment consists of 15 to 50 mg of cortisone daily in divided doses, or 5 mg of prednisone daily.

CUSHING'S DISEASE

In Cushing's disease, the abnormality in overproduction of adrenal steroids primarily involves the corticoid compounds having to do with carbohydrate, protein, and electrolyte metabolism; the androgenic or 17-ketosteroid substances are involved only to a slight extent. Again, the hyperadrenal state may develop either as the result of diffuse, bilateral adrenal hyperplasia (50 to 60 percent of cases), sometimes in association with and possibly secondary to a basophilic adenoma or diffuse "basophilism" of the pituitary, or as the result of an adrenal adenoma (30 to 40 percent of cases) or adrenal carcinoma (5 to 10 percent of cases). The characteristic clinical features of classic Cushing's disease include the following: obesity of the trunk, with associated "buffalo hump" and moon face; amenorrhea; hirsutism; acne; osteoporosis; hypertension; purple striae of the skin (particularly of the abdominal wall, the so-called skin fractures); polycythemia; a plethoric appearance; and, rarely, true virilization. Again, it is important to remember that mild forms of the disease frequently are accompanied by only a portion of the usual clinical symptoms and signs, many of which may be atypical and equivocal, and also that in many hyperadrenal states, whether due to tumor or hyperplasia, one sees a wide spectrum of clinical and biochemical abnormalities that include features of both Cushing's syndrome and the adrenogenital syndrome and reflect the varying cytochemical disturbances present in the particular type of tumor or hyperplastic glandular tissue.

Laboratory Studies

The following are the laboratory findings in Cushing's disease: the 17-ketosteroids are inconstant (normal to slight elevation); the 11-oxysteroids are markedly elevated; the 17-hydroxycorticosteroids are usually markedly elevated; the glucose tolerance test results are diabetic in type; the skeletal x-ray films show osteoporosis. Culdoscopy or laparoscopy again shows normal, though atrophic, ovaries. The ACTH test will show elevation of 11-oxysteroids if the condition is due to hyperplasia and no change if it is due to tumor. A presacral pneumoretroperitoneal adrenogram may show tumor, if present.

Treatment

The treatment is resection if a tumor is present and bilateral total adrenalectomy for hyperplasia, with subsequent adrenal steroid replacement therapy.

ADDISON'S DISEASE

Addison's disease (adrenal failure) will invariably lead to amenorrhea and ordinarily should not pose any diagnostic problem.

Hypothalamic-Pituitary Disorders

PITUITARY INSUFFICIENCY OR FAILURE

Pituitary insufficiency or failure is usually secondary to severe postpartum hemorrhage with thrombosis and necrosis or infarction of the pituitary (Sheehan's syndrome). Occasionally, it may be due to a chromophobe adenoma or a suprasellar cyst.

Symptoms include amenorrhea, occasionally persistent galactorrhea, progressive atrophy of the uterus and vagina, muscular weakness, and an initial weight gain followed by progressive cachexia (Simmonds' disease) as thyroid and adrenal function also becomes depressed.

Laboratory Studies

Laboratory studies show low basal metabolic rate, protein-bound iodine and FSH, and depressed 17-ketosteroids and 11-oxysteroids. Failure of response to LH-RH administration or to clomiphene or human menopausal gonadotropin stimulation is to be expected.

Treatment

Treatment is by replacement therapy for thyroid, adrenal, and gonadal insufficiency.

PITUITARY TUMORS

Pituitary tumors include eosinophilic adenomas (acromegaly) and basophilic adenomas (Cushing's disease), which lead to amenorrhea with or without galactorrhea, with associated headaches, visual disturbances, and other symptoms.

Diagnosis

Diagnostic techniques include lateral skull x-ray films to detect enlargement of the sella turcica, FSH and LH assays, a serum prolactin assay, and special neurologic studies, including visual fields.

Note: An unusual and uncommon condition of unknown cause referred to as the empty sella syndrome is seen most often in obese adult women, many of whom also have hypertension and diabetes. The pituitary gland is actually present but is severely compressed and flattened against the sella floor, the sella being filled primarily with cerebrospinal fluid and appearing empty on x-ray examination. Levels of pituitary, adrenal, and ovarian hormones as well as plasma testosterone levels are usually normal, although some of these patients have been reported to have had an associated hirsutism and menstrual irregularities. This entity is important only from the standpoint of differential diagnosis and the need to distinguish it from abnormalities of the sella accompanying pituitary tumors or cysts.

Treatment

Treatment is by surgical removal or radiation.

Amenorrhea-Galactorrhea Syndromes

Amenorrhea-galactorrhea syndromes result from a specific type of endocrine disturbance of pituitary or hypothalamic origin and are characterized by amenorrhea accompanied by the excretion of milky fluid from the breast as in lactation. It is now clear that these disorders are the result of an inappropriate hypersecretion of prolactin, either by a prolactin-secreting tumor of the pituitary or by a hypothalamic-pituitary disturbance that results in deficient production of prolactin inhibiting factor. The excessive prolactin is directly responsible for the galactorrhea and indirectly responsible for the amenorrhea as a result of interference with the elaboration by the hypothalamus of LH releasing factor. Formerly, it was encountered most often following delivery in otherwise normal postpartum women (Chiari-Frommel syndrome). It is also known to occur occasionally without relation to pregnancy in women with prolactin-secreting pituitary tumors (Forbes-Albright syndrome). In a few patients the syndrome has been observed in the absence of either pregnancy or pituitary adenoma, and presumably some form of specific pituitary or hypothalamic dysfunction resulting in excessive prolactin or inadequate prolactin inhibiting factor secretion is involved in these cases. (In the case of amenorrhea and persistent lactation not related to pregnancy or pituitary tumor, the disorder has been termed the *Ahumada-Argonz-del Castillo syndrome.*)

Far more common nowadays is a similar, physiologic type of amenorrhea-galactorrhea encountered in patients receiving antihypertensives and tranquilizers (e.g., reserpine, the phenothiazines, or tricyclic antidepressants), as well as in patients who have discontinued an oral contraceptive program of some duration and then not only failed to resume normal, spontaneous menstrual cycles but also noted the onset of persistent lactation ("post-pill galactorrhea-amenorrhea syndrome," or the "oversuppression syndrome"). It seems obvious that a functional disturbance of hypothalamic-pituitary activity has been induced by the medication in both instances. The typical, almost diagnostic clinical features include amenorrhea, which is often permanent, a constant milky breast discharge, or galactorrhea, that is usually chronic and persistent, often lasting for years in association with large, engorged breasts and a profound atrophy of the ovaries, uterus, and vagina. The diagnosis is confirmed by finding a markedly reduced pituitary gonadotropin (FSH and LH) excretion and low or undetectable estrogen levels. Both the endometrium and vaginal mucosa are atrophic. As indicated by clinical and laboratory evidence of normal thyroid, adrenal, and pancreatic function, no other fundamental pituitary dysfunction is present. Thyroid function particularly should be carefully evaluated in all patients with the Chiari-Frommel variant of the syndrome, since hypothyroidism, especially when it develops post partum, can cause amenorrhea-galactorrhea and is easily treated by administration of thyroid hormone.

Treatment

Only occasional spontaneous recovery with return of normal menses and cessation of lactation has been observed. For the most part, these patients have been refractory to all previous forms of therapy, including cyclic estrogen and progesterone. However, a better understanding of normal hypothalamic-pituitary physiology has recently led to a more effective therapeutic approach. It is now believed that the pituitary is deficient in its production of FSH and LH, while at the same time it is secreting excessive amounts of prolactin. The pituitary dysfunction is in turn second-ary to failure on the part of the hypothalamus to elaborate FSH and LH releasing factors as well as the prolactin inhibiting factor. Based on this hypothesis, treatment with clomiphene, the synthetic hypothalamic-pituitary stimulating agent, has recently been employed in patients with amenorrhea-lactation disorders, and resumption of normal menses along with cessation of the abnormal galactorrhea has been reported in a number of instances. Good results have also been achieved in some patients treated with L-dopa and a specific ergot alkaloid, 2-alpha bromergocryptine (CB-154), both of which inhibit the pituitary secretion of prolactin. Equally good responses to the familiar and readily available drug ergonovine maleate in a dosage of 0.2 mg three times daily have also been reported.

It is obviously also very important to discover and treat the roughly 25 percent of patients with this syndrome in whom a pituitary tumor is present. The amenorrhea and abnormal lactation usually respond promptly following removal or irradiation of the pituitary tumor or cyst that has been secreting excessive amounts of prolactin or, rarely, interfering with the normal production of prolactin inhibiting factor. A helpful differential diagnostic point is the fact that most patients with pituitary tumors have high serum prolactin levels (this diagnostic abnormality will be detectable long before the sella turcica enlargement or visual field abnormalities become apparent), whereas in the other forms of the syndrome the plasma prolactin level is normal.

PITUITARY "DYSFUNCTION"

The "diagnosis" of pituitary "dysfunction" is made on the basis of a depressed FSH and an apparent pituitary insufficiency in the absence of any obvious cause (e.g., absence of pituitary tumor or possibility of postpartum necrosis and lack of any apparent underlying psychosomatic factors, nutritional factors, or associated chronic disease such as tuberculosis or nephritis.

Diabetes Mellitus

Frequently, the various metabolic disturbances occurring in diabetic women are reflected in an increased incidence of anovulatory menstrual irregularities, including dysfunctional bleeding, oligomenorrhea, amenorrhea, infertility, and premature menopause.

Treatment

Dietary and insulin management of the diabetes will be of the greatest benefit, but other routine diagnostic and therapeutic measures such as are used in the management of any kind of menstrual dysfunction or infertility problem may be of additional help.

DIAGNOSTIC APPROACH TO HIRSUTISM AND AMENORRHEA DUE TO A BASIC ENDOCRINOLOGIC DISORDER

The two most frequent symptomatic manifestations of a basic endocrine disorder that is affecting or has its origin in the reproductive tract are (1) hirsutism (sometimes also accompanied by virilization) with or without obesity (often) and menstrual irregularities (usually) and (2) amenorrhea (or oligomenorrhea). By way of summarizing and consolidating in one place the essence of the material already presented, the differential diagnosis of each of these two symptomatic features is now presented in outline form. The actual diagnostic study plan to be employed in patients with hirsutism has been covered in the preceding sections and will not be reviewed again, but a suggested diagnostic approach that can be utilized in the evaluation of patients with amenorrhea is set forth.

Differential Diagnosis of Hirsutism (with or without Virilization, Obesity, and Menstrual Irregularities)

1. **Idiopathic**: congenital, familial, racial. (Normal, ovulatory menses and normal 17-ketosteroids, etc., but plasma testosterone levels are elevated in a significant number of these patients.) Perhaps due to an as yet unknown type of adrenocortical dysfunction, or more likely due to a familial tendency to excessive hormone sensitivity of the hair follicles and sebaceous glands (pilosebaceous apparatus) at certain times, especially during puberty, menopause, or pregnancy.
2. **Adrenal disease**
   a. Mild congenital hyperplasia, unrecognized until primary amenorrhea and hirsutism with virilization appear.
   b. Adrenal tumors (adenoma or carcinoma) or hyperplasia — acquired adrenogenital syndrome.
   c. Cushing's disease (hyperplasia or tumor).
   d. Mild hyperplasia with a syndrome resembling Stein-Leventhal syndrome ("adrenal dysfunction").
3. **Ovarian disorders** (the most common cause of female hirsutism)
   a. Stein-Leventhal syndrome.
   b. Ovarian hyperthecosis.
   c. Ovarian tumors:
      (1) Arrhenoblastomas (Sertoli-Leydig cell tumors).
      (2) Hilus cell (pure Leydig cell) tumors or hyperplasia.
      (3) Adrenal rest (lipoid cell) tumors.
      (4) Gynandroblastomas (mixed granulosa-theca cell and Sertoli-Leydig cell tumors).
4. **Pituitary disorders**
   a. Nonfunctioning tumors and cysts with pituitary destruction.
   b. Acromegaly (eosinophilic adenoma).
   c. Cushing's disease with basophilic adenoma.

5. **Miscellaneous**
   a. Postmenopausal hirsutism.
   b. Androgen therapy.
   c. Diphenylhydantoin (Dilantin) therapy.
   d. Some epileptic patients and some types of insanity and mental deficiency.
   e. Morgagni-Stewart-Morel syndrome: hyperostosis frontalis interna, obesity, mental retardation, and hirsutism of unknown cause (no abnormality of androgenic hormone levels demonstrable). Diabetes mellitus, thyroid dysfunction, menstrual disorders, and hypertension are often present as well. There is usually no demonstrable disease in either the pituitary or hypothalamus, despite the many similarities to acromegaly and Cushing's disease.

Differential Diagnosis of Amenorrhea (or Oligomenorrhea)

(See also Etiologic Mechanisms in Amenorrhea.)

PRIMARY AMENORRHEA

1. **Uterovaginal.** In approximately 20 percent of patients with primary amenorrhea the cause will prove to be a congenital müllerian duct anomaly of some type:
   a. Congenital anomalies (absent or hypoplastic uterus).
   b. Imperforate hymen or congenital absence of the vagina (not true amenorrheas but must be considered in the differential diagnosis).
2. **Ovarian**
   a. Primary gonadal disorder (gonadal dysgenesis, testicular feminization, etc). Actually, 40 to 50 percent of apparent females with primary amenorrhea have a sex chromosomal disorder, roughly 75 percent with Turner's syndrome or mosaic forms of gonadal agenesis, the other 25 percent with a 46-XY chromosome constitution and either the testicular feminization syndrome or, less often, pure gonadal dysgenesis, mixed gonadal dysgenesis, or dysgenetic male pseudohermaphroditism.
   b. Congenital absence of the ovaries.
   c. Hypogonadotropic hypogonadism associated with anosmia (Tagatz-Fialkow syndrome), a distinct entity that is probably of central nervous system origin. The hypogonadism responds to clomiphene or gonadotropin administration and most likely is due to hypothalamic dysfunction with a gonadotropin releasing factor defect.
3. **Hypothalamic**
   a. Generalized hypothalamic defect, with deficiency of thyrotropic, adrenotropic, and gonadotropic releasing factors.
   b. Isolated gonadotropin deficiency (low-to-absent LH, FSH, and estradiol) with normal TSH, ACTH, and growth hormone secretion. Again, the defect resides in the hypothalamus (lack of the gonadotropic releasing factor LH-RH).
4. **Pituitary insufficiency (pituitary dwarfs)**

5. **Premenarchal occurrence of any of the disorders ordinarily producing secondary amenorrhea.** (See the following section.)

In roughly 25 to 40 percent of patients with primary amenorrhea, the problem will lie in the hypothalamic-pituitary-ovarian axis, 40 to 50 percent will be secondary to sex chromosomal disorders, and in the remaining 15 percent, miscellaneous systemic, nutritional, and psychological factors will be responsible.

SECONDARY AMENORRHEA

1. **Physiologic**
   a. Pregnancy (signs and symptoms of pregnancy and positive test for HCG).
   b. Postpartum (failure of menses to return within 18 months of delivery); usually responds to a three-months' course of cyclic estrogen-progesterone. Rule out postpartum pituitary necrosis (Sheehan's syndrome), or Chiari-Frommel syndrome.
   c. Menopause (elevated FSH is diagnostic).
2. **Pituitary** (depressed FSH is diagnostic) or **Hypothalamic**
   a. Insufficiency or failure: Sheehan's syndrome, Simmonds' disease.
   b. Tumors (adenomas, cysts) of the pituitary gland, or stalk, or suprasellar space.
   c. Chiari-Frommel syndrome and related amenorrhea-galactorrhea disorders.
3. **Ovarian**
   a. Dysfunction (anovulatory cycles in the phase of oligomenorrhea or amenorrhea). (See Chap. 5.)
   b. Neoplasms:
      (1) Granulosa cell or theca cell tumors.
      (2) Arrhenoblastoma or hilus cell tumors.
      (3) Adrenal cell rest (lipoid cell) tumors.
   c. Stein-Leventhal syndrome.
   d. Ovarian hyperthecosis.
   e. Precocious menopause (ovarian failure).
   f. Severe pelvic inflammatory disease or mumps oophoritis with bilateral ovarian destruction.
4. **Adrenal**
   a. Adrenogenital syndrome and related disorders.
   b. Cushing's disease.
   c. Addison's disease.
5. **Thyroid**
   a. Hyperthyroidism.
   b. Hypothyroidism.
6. **Diabetes mellitus**
7. **Nutritional**
   a. Severe malnutrition.
   b. Marked obesity.

8. **Chronic disease**, e.g., tuberculosis, nephritis, rheumatoid arthritis.
9. **Psychosomatic and neurogenic (hypothalamic)**, e.g., major psychoses, anorexia nervosa, pseudocyesis, emotional shock, organic brain disease.
10. **Artificial**, e.g., hysterectomy and/or bilateral oophorectomy, radiation therapy, excessively traumatic curettage, severe endometritis, Asherman's syndrome (intrauterine adhesions).

ETIOLOGIC MECHANISMS IN AMENORRHEA

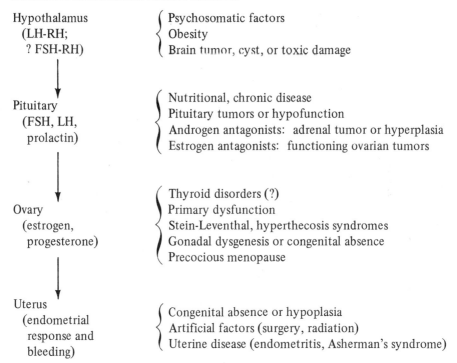

Hypothalamus (LH-RH; ? FSH-RH)
- Psychosomatic factors
- Obesity
- Brain tumor, cyst, or toxic damage

Pituitary (FSH, LH, prolactin)
- Nutritional, chronic disease
- Pituitary tumors or hypofunction
- Androgen antagonists: adrenal tumor or hyperplasia
- Estrogen antagonists: functioning ovarian tumors

Ovary (estrogen, progesterone)
- Thyroid disorders (?)
- Primary dysfunction
- Stein-Leventhal, hyperthecosis syndromes
- Gonadal dysgenesis or congenital absence
- Precocious menopause

Uterus (endometrial response and bleeding)
- Congenital absence or hypoplasia
- Artificial factors (surgery, radiation)
- Uterine disease (endometritis, Asherman's syndrome)

PROGRAM OF STUDY OF AMENORRHEA

A useful program of study that will avoid unnecessary tests in the vast majority of patients suffering from amenorrhea is shown in Figure 29. The treatment procedure is then as follows:

After a careful history, general physical examination, and pelvic and rectal examinations, which may already suggest the most likely possibilities, and assuming that pregnancy and obvious congenital uterovaginal anomalies have been ruled out and that a buccal smear to evaluate the nuclear sex chromatin pattern and chromosomal karyotyping have been done to eliminate the possibility of gonadal dysgenesis or testicular feminization in cases of primary amenorrhea or of XX/XO mosaicism in patients with secondary amenorrhea or oligomenorrhea:

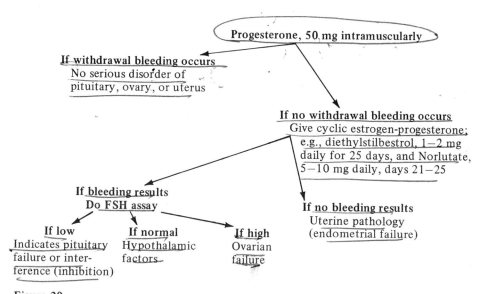

Figure 29
Simple, initial diagnostic approach to amenorrhea. (From T. H. Green, Jr. Gynecology. In G. L. Nardi and G. D. Zuidema [Eds.], *Surgery: A Concise Guide to Clinical Practice* [3rd ed.]. Boston: Little, Brown, 1972, Chap. 39.)

1. Progesterone, 50 mg, is given intramuscularly in a single dose.
   a. If withdrawal bleeding occurs, the presence of an adequate amount of estrogen, and hence basically normal pituitary, ovaries, and uterus, is indicated. Thus simple lack of ovulation is suggested, and any serious disturbance of the normal pituitary-ovarian-uterine axis is excluded. (Miscellaneous tests that may be used to establish this same point include a vaginal smear, a cervical mucus fern test, or an endometrial biopsy for estrogen effect, as well as estrogen and pregnanediol excretion studies.) Further studies would then be in order to rule out thyroid disease, the Stein-Leventhal syndrome, or any of the other conditions that may produce temporary and reversible failure of ovulation with normal estrogen production.
   b. If no withdrawal bleeding occurs, the absence either of estrogen or of a normal endometrial response to estrogen is indicated (e.g., pituitary or ovarian disease, or functional interference, or a basic uterine disorder).
2. Then a course of estrogen and progesterone is given in cyclic fashion:
   a. If no bleeding occurs, endometrial failure is indicated, e.g., absent uterus.
   b. If bleeding occurs, do 24-hour pituitary gonadotropin (FSH) urinary excretion studies. High levels indicate primary ovarian failure (menopause). Low levels indicate pituitary failure. If levels are normal, the amenorrhea is the hypothalamic type.

Further tests will be indicated if serious endocrine disease is suggested: e.g., lateral skull x-ray films; 17-ketosteroid, 17-hydroxycorticosteroid, 11-oxycorticosteroid, and plasma testosterone studies; serum FSH and LH radioimmunossays; thyroid studies (BMR, PBI, RAI uptake); culdoscopy or laparoscopy with ovarian biopsy; presacral pneumoretroperitoneal adrenal pneumograms; administration of LH releasing hormone to differentiate between hypothalamic and pituitary disorders.

GENERAL REMARKS ON THE TREATMENT OF AMENORRHEA

It is obvious that amenorrhea is simply a symptom of a wide variety of disorders, and proper therapy should be directed at the specific disorder responsible once an exact diagnosis has been established. In most instances, the plan of treatment for the various underlying disorders is discussed in the previous section.

Two well-established methods and a third, relatively new therapeutic approach to the problem of anovulation and secondary amenorrhea as encountered in a number of these underlying conditions, particularly those that are primarily functional in nature, are now under trial. Since they are essentially nonspecific in their application, it seems most convenient to mention them briefly at this point. These therapeutic approaches are often helpful because in most anovulatory disorders the ovary itself is not at fault, but rather the hypothalamic-pituitary regulatory mechanism.

Induction of Ovulation with Purified Human Pituitary Gonadotropins

Previous attempts to simulate normal pituitary function in amenorrheic women by the sequential administration of pregnant-mare serum gonadotropins (PMS) having largely FSH activity, followed at an appropriate interval by HCG isolated from the urine of pregnant women and having largely LH activity, have not been particularly successful in producing ovulation or restoring normal menstrual function. However, following the preparation of relatively pure human pituitary gonadotropin extracts, which possess primarily FSH activity (HP-FSH), Gemzell [17] and others have had some success in both primary and secondary amenorrhea using either HP-FSH alone or in combination with HCG at the appropriate intervals. Not only were ovulation and normal menstruation produced, but in several instances pregnancy resulted, and many of the patients treated had been amenorrheic for years.

The chief indications for the use of human gonadotropin preparations are secondary amenorrhea and anovulatory oligomenorrhea in women with deficient gonadotropin and hence secondarily decreased estrogen activity. Patients with primary amenorrhea or premature menopause who have associated elevation of endogenous gonadotropin levels never respond, as would be predicted; in both instances the problem is one of either primary or secondary gonadal failure or a fundamental abnormality of the pituitary itself that has permanently rendered it incapable of responding. Ovulation has resulted in as high as 80 to 90 percent of properly selected patients, with pregnancy following in roughly 35 to 50 percent. Two significant complications of this type of therapy have been encountered: massive cystic enlargement (in 15 to 20 percent of patients) and a markedly increased frequency of multiple births (in 15 to 30 percent). Both of these undesirable side effects are due to the use of excessive amounts of gonadotropin and a resulting overstimulation of the ovaries. In several reported series, the frequency of multiple births equaled that of single births, and 20 percent of the patients had triplets. For these reasons the dosage levels must be extremely carefully controlled, and it is equally important that therapy with pituitary gonadotropins be restricted to patients with proved low or absent endogenous pituitary gonadotropins.

Pooled urine from menopausal females has now been concentrated and purified sufficiently to serve as another potent and useful source of human FSH (Pergonal, Cutter Laboratories). This preparation (HMG), in combination with HCG (the latter serves as the principal source of LH), is now also undergoing clinical trials, with the indications for, potential complications, and apparent results of its administration entirely similar to those of the purified human pituitary product. In the case of patients who initially fail to respond, both preparations have also been tried in combination with the drug clomiphene citrate, described in the next section. It should be borne in mind that this type of therapy is expensive; the total cost of a single course of Pergonal, or Humegon (Organon), or Pregova (Ortho Research Foundation) treatment in 1975 was $400 to $500.

Induction of Ovulation with Clomiphene Citrate

Clomiphene citrate (Clomid), which has no estrogenic, progestational, or androgenic properties (it is actually an estrogen antagonist), is closely related to chlorotrianisene (TACE), a nonsteroid substance with potent estrogenic activity. Clomiphene apparently acts on the pituitary or hypothalamus (probably the latter) to permit or stimulate the release of the woman's own pituitary LH, which in turn stimulates the ovary, with resulting follicle maturation, ovulation, and corpus luteum development. When given in proper dosage for an optimal length of time (the proper dosage has proved highly variable so far), normal ovulation and menstruation as well as pregnancy have resulted in a number of patients treated for secondary amenorrhea and in some patients with the Stein-Leventhal syndrome. The usual dose range employed has been 50 to 100 mg daily for five days, starting on day 5 of the cycle if the patient is having any spontaneous menstrual activity, with ovulation tending to occur 2 to 10 days later. In some cases this daily dose may have to be increased to 200 to 250 mg, and when even this dose fails to produce ovulation, success will be achieved in some patients if HCG is also administered at midcycle following the five-day course of clomiphene. When the optimal dosage has been exceeded, massive bilateral ovarian enlargement produced by multiple enlarging follicles and corpora lutea has been observed, sometimes accompanied by ascites (rarely, hydrothorax also) and marked ileus, with a few patients requiring laparotomy to control massive bleeding from hemorrhagic follicles. In most cases the bilateral ovarian enlargement disappears following the withdrawal of the drug. Multiple pregnancies have also occurred in 10 to 12 percent of patients.

Not infrequently, repeated courses have been necessary before normal regular cycles would continue spontaneously, though in many instances only one treatment cycle has been followed by permanent restoration of a regular ovulatory pattern. Obviously, basically normal pituitary and ovaries are necessary if a favorable response is to be obtained, and the drug is therefore of no value in the management of amenorrhea due to fundamental organic disease of either gland. Preliminary studies that include x-ray films of the sella turcica, thyroid function tests, and 24-hour assays of endogenous gonadotropin, 17-ketosteroids, and 17-hydroxycorticoids should be done to exclude serious pituitary, ovarian, or adrenal disease. The drug is excreted by the liver and is therefore contraindicated in patients with hepatic disease. Clomiphene seems to be a very useful agent on the basis of fairly extensive experimental and clinical trials. It appears possible to induce ovulation in approximately 50 to 80 percent and to achieve pregnancies in roughly 30 to 40 percent of the patients receiving therapy with clomiphene (the complication rate has been 15 to 20 percent). Some believe that the low pregnancy rate achieved by clomiphene (only half the apparent rate of ovulation following clomiphene therapy) is because many of the ovulations are intraovarian, with failure of extrusion of the ovum because of an inadequate LH surge. Furthermore, because of its antiestrogen effects, clomiphene therapy may impair the quality of cervical mucus, thus interfering with conception despite its production of ovulation. So when treating anovulatory infertile patients, it may be necessary to supplement the overall drug program by giving very small doses of estrogen during the preovulatory phase of the cycle.

The chief indications for the use of clomiphene have been in infertile patients with marked oligomenorrhea or secondary amenorrhea, but with normal estrogen levels (i.e., good FSH, probably poor LH). In other words, it should be effective in patients with potentially competent pituitary and ovaries but with presumed anovulation due to hypothalamic dysfunction and failure of adequate LH production. Women with the Stein-Leventhal syndrome and those with the Chiari-Frommel and related amenorrhea-galactorrhea syndromes fulfill these criteria, as do a much larger number of women with less specific forms of anovulatory ovarian function.

In the face of a fundamental endocrinologic disturbance, clomiphene will not permanently restore regular ovulation. For this reason, it is not necessarily a long-term substitute for a wedge resection in the treatment of patients with the Stein-Leventhal syndrome, even for those who show an ovulatory response each time the drug is administered. Most patients who can be successfully induced to ovulate with clomiphene will do so with the first treatment cycle, and a total of three courses is considered adequate to determine whether or not a response can be obtained. In a few patients, to be certain the corpus luteum is stimulated sufficiently to produce enough progesterone for an adequate luteal phase, it will be necessary to add HCG in sequence shortly following the five-day course of clomiphene.

The occurrence of the ovarian hyperstimulation syndrome (in 10 to 20 percent) and of multiple births (in 5 to 10 percent) is observed with considerably less frequency during therapy with clomiphene than with Pergonal or any of the other preparations of pituitary gonadotropins. Clomiphene therapy is also considerably less expensive; in 1975, one course cost $5 to $15, depending on the daily dosage.

Potential Role of LH—Releasing Hormone in Therapy of Anovulatory Disorders

Several years ago, the decapeptide hypothalamic neurohormone LH-RH that is responsible for initiating the pituitary release of LH (and possibly of FSH also) was identified and then prepared synthetically. Since then, its potential role in the diagnosis and therapy of anovulatory disorders continues to be widely explored. For example, in a useful test to distinguish between hypothalamic and pituitary dysfunction in women with secondary amenorrhea, 100 μg of synthetic LH-RH is administered intravenously, and if appropriate increases in serum LH and FSH are detected, pituitary function is thereby shown to be normal, and the hypothalamic origin of the secondary amenorrhea is established. The LH-RH test is of limited value in the differential diagnostic evaluation of patients with primary amenorrhea, however.

Attempts to utilize LH-RH alone to induce ovulation have been less rewarding, although a number of women with a variety of anovulatory disorders have received this type of therapy. It has definitely been shown that the intravenous, intramuscular, subcutaneous, or intranasal administration of either natural or synthetic LH-RH is capable of causing release from the pituitary of both LH and FSH in the human subject, but it has only occasionally been possible to trigger ovulation by this means, presumably because it does not result in the LH surge known to be essential for induction of ovulation, and there has been a correspondingly low pregnancy rate. However, in one study [29], the synthetic decapeptide LH-RH did seem to be more effective when given in daily doses of 50 to 200 μg after the administration of either clomiphene or HMG, even in women who had previously failed to ovulate with either of the other drugs alone.

REFERENCES

1. Anderson, W. R., Levine, A. J., and MacMillan, D. Granulosa theca cell tumors: Clinical and pathologic study. *Am. J. Obstet. Gynecol.* 110:32, 1971.
2. Andrews, W. C., and Andrews, M. C. Stein-Leventhal syndrome with associated adenocarcinoma of the endometrium. *Am. J. Obstet. Gynecol.* 80:632, 1960.
3. Arrata, W. S. M., and deAlvarez, R. R. The oversuppression syndrome. *Am. J. Obstet. Gynecol.* 112:1025, 1972.
4. Berger, M. J., Taymor, M. L., and Patton, W. C. Gonadotropin levels and secretory patterns in patients with typical and atypical polycystic ovarian disease. *Fertil. Steril.* 26:619, 1975.
5. Board, J. A., and Bhatnagar, A. S. Serum prolactin levels in galactorrhea. *Am. J. Obstet. Gynecol.* 123:41, 1975.
6. Boyar, R. M., Katz, J., Finkelstein, J. W., Kapen, S., Weiner, H., Weitzman, E. D., and Hellman, L. Anorexia nervosa: Immaturity of the 24 hour luteinizing hormone secretory pattern. *N. Engl. J. Med.* 291:861, 1974.
7. Brown, E., and Barglow, P. Pseudocyesis. *Arch. Gen. Psychiatry* 24:221, 1971.
8. Chalvardjian, A., and Scully, R. E. Sclerosing stromal tumors of the ovary. *Cancer* 31:664, 1973.
9. Chamlian, D. L., and Taylor, H. B. Endometrial hyperplasia in young women. *Obstet. Gynecol.* 36:659, 1970.

10. Damjanov, I., Drobnjak, P., Grizelj, V., and Longhino, N. Sclerosing stromal tumor of the ovary. *Obstet. Gynecol.* 45:675, 1975.

11. DeAlvarez, R. R., Mendelson, E. G., Castellanos, H., and Lundy, L. E. Virilizing lipoid tumors of the ovary. *Obstet. Gynecol.* 35:956, 1970.

12. DeVane, G. W., Czekala, N. M., Judd, H. L., and Yen, S. S. C. Circulating gonadotropins, estrogens, and androgens in polycystic ovarian disease. *Am. J. Obstet. Gynecol.* 121:496, 1975.

13. Emperaire, J. C., Audebert, A., and Greenblatt, R. B. Premature ovarian failure. *Am. J. Obstet. Gynecol.* 108:445, 1970.

14. Farber, M., Daoust, P. R., and Rogers, J. Hyperthecosis syndrome. *Obstet. Gynecol.* 44:35, 1974.

15. Gambrell, R. D., Greenblatt, R. B., and Mahesh, V. B. Post-pill and pill-related amenorrhea-galactorrhea. *Am. J. Obstet. Gynecol.* 110:838, 1971.

16. Gambrell, R. D., Greenblatt, R. B., and Mahesh, V. B. Inappropriate secretion of LH in the Stein-Leventhal syndrome. *Obstet. Gynecol.* 42:429, 1973.

17. Gemzell, C. Induction of ovulation with human gonadotropins. *Int. J. Gynecol. Obstet.* 8:593, 1970.

18. Goldfarb, A. F., and Crawford, R. Polycystic ovarian disease, clomiphene, and multiple pregnancies. *Obstet. Gynecol.* 34:307, 1969.

19. Goldston, W. R., Johnston, W. W., Fetter, B. F., Parker, R. T., and Wilbanks, G. D. Clinicopathologic studies in feminizing tumors of the ovary. *Am. J. Obstet. Gynecol.* 112:422, 1972.

20. Greenblatt, R. B., and Mahesh, V. B. Some new thoughts on the Stein-Leventhal syndrome. *J. Reprod. Med.* 13:85, 1974.

21. Greenblatt, R. B., and Stahl, N. L. Constitutional hirsutism: Endocrinopathy or genetic curse. *J. Reprod. Med.* 11:96, 1973.

22. Hughes, P., Gillespie, A., and Dewhurst, C. J. Amenorrhea and galactorrhea. *Obstet. Gynecol.* 40:147, 1972.

23. Ingersoll, F. M., and McArthur, J. W. Longitudinal studies of gonadotropin excretion in the Stein-Leventhal syndrome. *Am. J. Obstet. Gynecol.* 77:795, 1959.

24. Jackson, R. L., and Dockerty, M. B. Stein-Leventhal syndrome: Analysis of 43 cases with special reference to association with endometrial carcinoma. *Am. J. Obstet. Gynecol.* 73:161, 1957.

25. Jewelewicz, R. Management of infertility resulting from anovulation. *Am. J. Obstet. Gynecol.* 122:909, 1975.

26. Jones, H. W., and Jones, G. E. S. The gynecological aspects of adrenal hyperplasia and allied disorders. *Am. J. Obstet. Gynecol.* 68:1330, 1954.

27. Karp, L., and Herrman, W. L. Diagnosis and treatment of hirsutism in women. *Obstet. Gynecol.* 41:283, 1973.

28. Kase, N., Andriole, J. P., and Sobrinho, L. Endocrine diagnosis of pituitary tumor in galactorrhea syndromes. *Am. J. Obstet. Gynecol.* 114:321, 1972.

29. Keller, P. J. Treatment of anovulation with synthetic luteinizing hormone-releasing hormone. *Am. J. Obstet. Gynecol.* 116:698, 1973.

30. Kletzky, O. A., Davajan, V., Nakamura, R. M., Thornycroft, I. H., and Mishell, D. R., Jr. Clinical categorization of patients with secondary amenorrhea using progesterone-induced uterine bleeding and measurement of serum gonadotropin levels. *Am. J. Obstet. Gynecol.* 121:695, 1975.

31. Mahesh, V. B. Current status of luteinizing hormone-releasing hormone in diagnosis and treatment of disorders in reproductive function. *J. Reprod. Med.* 15:145, 1975.

32. Morris, J. M., and Scully, R. E. *Endocrine Pathology in the Ovary.* St. Louis: Mosby, 1958.

33. Norris, H. J., and Taylor, H. B. Prognosis of granulosa-theca tumors of the ovary. *Cancer* 21:255, 1968.
34. Northrop, G., Archie, J. T., Patel, S. K., and Wilbanks, G. D. Adrenal and ovarian vein androgen levels and laparoscopic findings in hirsute women. *Am. J. Obstet. Gynecol.* 122:192, 1975.
35. Novak, E. R., Kutchmeshgi, J., Mupas, R. S., and Woodruff, J. D. Feminizing gonadal stromal tumors: Analysis of the granulosa-theca cell tumors of the Ovarian Tumor Registry. *Obstet. Gynecol.* 38:701, 1971.
36. Parker, C. R., Jr., Servy, E., McDonough, P. G., and Mahesh, V. B. In vivo endocrine studies in adrenal rest tumor of ovary. *Obstet. Gynecol.* 44:327, 1974.
37. Polansky, S., DePapp, E. W., and Ogden, E. B. Virilization associated with bilateral luteomas of pregnancy. *Obstet. Gynecol.* 45:516, 1975.
38. Poliak, A., Smith, J. J., and Romney, S. L. Clinical evaluation of clomiphene. *Fertil. Steril.* 24:921, 1973.
39. Rifkin, I., Nachtigall, L. E., and Beckman, E. M. Amenorrhea following use of oral contraceptives. *Am. J. Obstet. Gynecol.* 113:420, 1972.
40. Rosenfield, R. L. Relationship of androgens to female hirsutism and infertility. *J. Reprod. Med.* 11:87, 1973.
41. Rust, L. A., Israel, R., and Mishell, D. R., Jr. An individualized graduated therapeutic regimen for clomiphene citrate. *Am. J. Obstet. Gynecol.* 120:785, 1971.
42. Sarto, G. E. Cytogenetics of 50 patients with primary amenorrhea. *Am. J. Obstet. Gynecol.* 119:14, 1974.
43. Schenker, J. G., and Polishuk, W. Z. Ovarian hyperstimulation syndrome. *Obstet. Gynecol.* 46:23, 1975.
44. Scully, R. E. Gonadoblastoma: A review of 74 cases. *Cancer* 25:1340, 1970.
45. Shippel, S. The ovarian theca cell: Part IV. The hyperthecosis syndrome. *J. Obstet. Gynaecol. Br. Commonw.* 63:321, 1955.
46. Skelton, J. B. The relative hypothyroid woman. *Obstet. Gynecol.* 39:823, 1972.
47. Sobrinho, L. G., and Kase, N. G. Adrenal rest cell tumor of the ovary. *Obstet. Gynecol.* 36:895, 1970.
48. Spadoni, L. R., Cox, D. W., and Smith, D. C. Use of human menopausal gonadotropin for the induction of ovulation. *Am. J. Obstet. Gynecol.* 120:988, 1974.
49. Spitz, I. M., Diamant, Y., Rosen, E., Bell, J., David, M. B., Polishuk, W., and Rabinowitz, D. Isolated gonadotropin deficiency. *N. Engl. J. Med.* 290:10, 1974.
50. Stearns, H. C., Sneeden, V. D., and Fearl, J. D. A clinical and pathologic review of ovarian stromal hyperplasia and its possible relationship to common diseases of the female reproductive system. *Am. J. Obstet. Gynecol.* 119:375, 1974.
51. Stein, I. F. The Stein-Leventhal syndrome. *N. Engl. J. Med.* 259:420, 1958.
52. Stein, I. F., and Leventhal, M. L. Amenorrhea associated with bilateral polycystic ovaries. *Am. J. Obstet. Gynecol.* 29:181, 1935.
53. Taymor, M. L. The use of luteinizing hormone-releasing hormone in gynecologic endocrinology. *Fertil. Steril.* 25:992, 1974.
54. Taymor, M. L., Thompson, I. E., Berger, M. J., and Patton, W. Luteinizing hormone—releasing hormone (LH-RH) as a diagnostic and research tool in gynecologic endocrinology. *Am. J. Obstet. Gynecol.* 120:721, 1974.
55. Tyson, J. E., Andreasson, B., Huth, J., Smith, B., and Zacur, H. Neuroendocrine dysfunction in galactorrhea-amenorrhea after oral contraceptive use. *Obstet. Gynecol.* 46:1, 1975.
56. Warren, M. P., and Vande Wiele, R. L. Clinical and metabolic features of anorexia nervosa. *Am. J. Obstet. Gynecol.* 117:435, 1973.

57. Zarate, A., Karchmer, S., Gomez, E., and Castelazo-Ayala, L. Premature meno-
    pause: A clinical, histologic, and cytogenetic study. *Am. J. Obstet. Gynecol.*
    106:110, 1970.
58. Zourlas, P. A., and Jones, H. W., Jr. The gynecologic aspects of adrenal tumors.
    Obstet. Gynecol. 41:234, 1973.

7
Infections and Benign Disorders of the Vulva, Vagina, and Cervix

THE VULVA

Detailed knowledge of the specialized physiology and cytochemistry of vulvar skin is scanty, but it is important to bear in mind that there are unquestionably significant differences and special features and that the vulva actually represents a skin organ, not just another area of general body integument. The following are three obvious gross anatomic peculiarities:

1. The vulvar skin and subcutaneous tissues are highly vascular, being supplied by the dorsal artery and vein of the clitoris and by the bilateral internal pudendal arterial and venous systems, and the organ is, at least in part, an erectile one.

2. The vulvar structures are extremely heavily innervated, receiving a bilateral somatic sensory and motor supply from the pudendal nerves and another sensory supply, largely to the skin of the labia majora and mons veneris from the femoral, genitofemoral, and ilioinguinal nerves bilaterally. There is also an extensive autonomic nerve supply, the so-called plexus cavernosus, with sympathetic components derived from the sympathetic trunk and the inferior mesenteric ganglion and with parasympathetic components originating in the second, third, and fourth sacral nerve roots and the sacral ganglia. Undoubtedly, the rich cutaneous sensory innervation explains why itching is an extremely prominent symptom of almost all vulvar diseases and why, even in the absence of local organic disease, severe pruritus of the vulvar skin may also accompany a variety of psychosomatic disturbances as well as certain generalized metabolic disorders with cutaneous manifestations.

3. The lymphatic supply to the vulva is one of the most extensive of any of the surface areas of the body. There is an extremely rich, delicate network of local lymphatics, many cross-pathways between the two sides of the vulva via anterior and posterior "commissure" anastomotic channels or via the communicating network of channels in the mons veneris, and abundant collecting trunks passing anteriorly within the boundaries of the labiocrural folds and draining into the regional nodes of the inguinofemoral region. This extensive lymphatic supply is responsible for many of the gross pathologic characteristics of local vulvar diseases and is, of course, extremely important in connection with the natural history and proper treatment of vulvar carcinomas (see Chap. 16).

The functions of the vulva are largely supportive and protective. The skin and subcutaneous structures, including the secretory glands and hair-bearing appendages, serve the twofold purpose of adequately supporting and protecting this sensitive and delicate area, much of the time sealing it off from a potentially injurious external environment, while at the same time permitting (and in some ways facilitating) normal sexual and reproductive function, including delivery of offspring. In this

221

regard, both its lubricative function and its mating function — the latter is particularly obvious in lower animals — suggest that vulvar physiology is probably to some extent linked to the female steroid hormone cycle and that the vulvar skin and its appendages may be responsive to variations in steroid metabolism.

An awareness of the specialized anatomy of the vulva and its specific histologic components is most helpful both in understanding the nature and origin of the various vulvar disorders as well as in their clinical recognition. This information is shown in the following outlines:

Specialized Anatomy of the Vulva

1. **Gross anatomic components:** mons veneris, labia majora, labia minora, clitoris, vestibule, accessory glands (Bartholin's, Skene's).
2. **Histologic components of the vulvar skin organ**
   a. Epidermis.
   b. Dermis.
   c. Glandular elements
      (1) Hair follicles.
      (2) Sebaceous glands.
      (3) Sweat glands
         (a) Eccrine glands.
         (b) Apocrine glands.
3. **Normal underlying tissues:** fat, muscle, fibrous tissue, lymphatics, blood vessels, nerves.
4. **Aberrant tissues:** accessory breast tissue, paramesonephric (müllerian) and mesonephric (wolffian) duct remnants, endometriosis.
5. **Gross anatomic abnormalities:** pudendal and inguinal hernias.

Histologic Origin of Certain Vulvar Diseases

1. **Epidermis-dermis:** epidermoid carcinoma, malignant melanoma, leukoplakia, lichen sclerosus et atrophicus, and many other common dermatologic disorders.
2. **Glandular elements**
   a. Hair follicles: folliculitis.
   b. Sebaceous glands: wens, seborrheic dermatitis; rarely, carcinoma.
   c. Sweat glands
      (1) Eccrine: benign hidradenoma, malignant hidradenoma.
      (2) Apocrine: hidradenitis suppurativa, Paget's disease, Fox-Fordyce disease.
3. **Normal underlying tissues:** lipoma, fibroma, sarcomas, hemangiomas, lymphangiomas, lymphoma, myoblastoma, etc.
4. **Aberrant tissues:** ectopic breast tissue (rarely, adenocarcinoma), vulvar cysts, endometriosis (rare cancers arising in the latter two entities).

Vulvitis and Common Dermatologic Disorders of the Vulva

Vulvitis is not a specific disease or even group of diseases. Rather, vulvar inflammation may arise in connection with a number of underlying disorders, both local and generalized in nature:

1. It may be the first manifestation of a systemic disease (e.g., the specific type of vulvitis seen in diabetes) or part of a generalized dermatologic disorder.
2. It may be entirely secondary to a specific vaginitis, the irritating discharge from the latter producing vulvar inflammation (vulvovaginitis), as seen in trichomonal or candidal vaginitis.
3. It may represent a secondary inflammatory reaction arising in a potentially far more serious vulvar lesion (e.g., leukoplakia or any of the vulvar epithelial dystrophies, carcinoma in situ, Paget's disease, or even early invasive carcinoma).
4. It may be an accompanying manifestation of a specific local dermatologic condition or a venereal disease.

It is therefore obvious that a thorough, detailed history, a complete physical examination and careful pelvic evaluation, and appropriate laboratory studies, including vaginal smears and cultures and urine and blood tests to investigate the possibility of an underlying diabetes, are essential to accurate diagnosis and proper management. If the possible presence of a malignant or premalignant vulvar lesion is suggested, a vulvar biopsy should also be done.

The common entities to be considered in the differential diagnosis of vulvar infections and inflammatory processes include the following:

1. Simple intertrigo due to poor local hygiene and lack of cleanliness.
2. Folliculitis and furunculosis.
3. Vulvovaginitis: e.g., *Candida, Trichomonas* (see The Vagina).
4. Diabetic vulvitis.
5. Venereal diseases: syphilis, gonorrhea, chancroid, lymphogranuloma venereum, granuloma inguinale, and including condyloma acuminatum and herpes progenitalis (see Chap. 8).
6. Parasitic diseases such as scabies and pediculosis pubis, with or without secondary infection.
7. Specific dermatologic disorders: psoriasis, lichen planus, lichen sclerosus et atrophicus, herpes simplex, hidradenitis suppurativa, Fox-Fordyce disease, contact or allergic dermatitis, etc.
8. Leukoplakia and related epithelial dystrophies (see Chap. 16).
9. Neoplastic disorders: Bowen's disease (carcinoma in situ), Paget's disease, and malignant tumors (see Chap. 16).
10. Simple atrophy (often with associated symptomatic atrophic vaginitis; see The Vagina).
11. Neurodermatitis or "idiopathic pruritus vulvae" (frequently encountered in the absence of any obvious vulvar or vaginal lesions).

The essential features of some of the more frequently encountered lesions that are not discussed elsewhere are now briefly summarized in the following paragraphs.

DIABETIC VULVITIS

Diabetic vulvitis presents as a diffuse, pinkish or bright-red, slightly edematous inflammatory change of the vulva proper, the surrounding skin appearing relatively normal. There may be intense local discomfort, with burning and itching. The condition is most commonly seen in women with unsuspected diabetes or in patients in whom a known diabetes is poorly controlled. Often — but by no means always — a monilial vaginitis, which is also common in diabetics, will also be present. Diabetic vulvitis usually responds rapidly to proper regulation of the diabetes, but local symptomatic measures are helpful, and if monilial vaginitis is also present, this should of course receive specific therapy.

LICHEN SCLEROSUS ET ATROPHICUS

Lichen sclerosus et atrophicus is often mistaken for leukoplakia, since there is a superficial gross resemblance, but is an entirely different disorder from both a clinical and histologic standpoint. It is seen in all age groups. Not only is the vulvar skin as well as mucous membrane affected, but the skin of other areas of the body is also frequently involved; e.g., on the thighs, in the oral, perianal, and umbilical regions, over the shoulders, and under the breasts. Grossly discrete, very slightly raised whitish papules or macules are seen that may coalesce to form larger patches, often with polygonal margins, and the involved skin and mucosa are usually thin and wrinkled, producing an appearance similar to cigarette paper. There may be dark, comedolike plugs in the center of the whitish plaques due to hyperkeratosis of the follicular or sweat gland ducts. Histologically, it is seen to be essentially a disease of the dermis rather than the epidermis. There is marked thinning and atrophy of the epidermal layer as well as a zone of dense homogenization in the upper dermis, beneath which is a zone of heavy inflammatory cell infiltration. This histologic picture is absolutely diagnostic and, together with the characteristic gross appearance, should permit this lesion to be readily distinguished from leukoplakia. Symptoms are usually mild and are completely absent in half the cases, in sharp contrast to the essentially universal occurrence of symptoms, most especially intense pruritus, with leukoplakia. Although formerly considered not to be a premalignant condition, it is now apparent that approximately 10 percent of patients with cancer of the vulva have an associated lichen sclerosus, with or without an accompanying leukoplakia. Hence biopsy of any suspicious areas is definitely indicated, and patients with this condition should have a regular follow-up program. If symptoms are present, symptomatic management as described later usually suffices.

HIDRADENITIS SUPPURATIVA

Hidradenitis suppurativa is a deep-seated chronic or recurring suppurative bacterial infection of the apocrine glands of the vulva. (An identical process is also encountered in the axillary, perianal, and nipple areas, where again there are abundant apocrine glands.) It may present as one or more subcutaneous nodules that may resolve spontaneously or proceed to abscess formation. Typically, numerous nodules will coalesce to form thick, subcutaneous cords, and sinus tracts extending deeply into the subcutaneous tissues are common, producing extremely painful and tender areas and, ultimately, extensive scarring. The actual infection involves not only the apocrine glands, which become dilated and cystic, but also the subcutaneous soft tissues and lymphatics and eventually the skin and its other glandular appendages as well. The disease never occurs before puberty. It is important to distinguish it from simple furunculosis, cellulitis, carbuncles, or infected sebaceous cysts, because the treatment and prognosis, though similar in mild cases, are considerably different in severe cases. The latter usually require extensive surgical drainage, all sinus tracts being widely opened and the chronically infected and indurated tissues excised. In chronic cases, wide excision of all the hair-bearing (and apocrine gland—bearing) skin and involved underlying subcutaneous tissue may be necessary, followed either by primary closure, if possible, or, more often, by split-thickness skin grafting.

FOX-FORDYCE DISEASE

Fox-Fordyce disease is a less common disorder, arising, at least in part, in connection with the apocrine glands. It presents as a diffuse, intensely pruritic, pinkish-red papular eruption on the vulva and frequently in the axillary and areolar areas of the breast as well. It is almost exclusively a disease of women in the years between puberty and the early forties. Although the etiology is unknown, the process is apparently one of abnormal apocrine gland activity or ductal obstruction. There is no known specific therapy, and symptomatic measures are only partially successful in relieving the intense itching.

NEURODERMATITIS

Neurodermatitis, so-called idiopathic pruritus vulvae, is common, and relief of symptoms often proves extremely difficult. At least in its initial stages, it is essentially a psychosomatic disorder, tending to occur in the tense and insecure woman who is constantly in an adversary relationship with her total physical and social environment (she even tends to give the impression of challenging the physician to relieve her symptoms). Often, the precipitating factor or factors can be elicited by a careful history; e.g., a delayed grief reaction, marital difficulties, job frustrations, or disturbed interpersonal relationships. Frequently, the symptoms are most marked at night, though minor episodes of troublesome pruritus may also occur during the day. Examination of the vulvar skin may reveal no abnormalities whatsoever, but in more acute cases, an eczematoid picture with erythema, edema, vesiculation, and weeping, crusted, scratch lesions may be seen. Most commonly, in the chronic form, the vulvar skin is simply thickened and hyperpigmented (the so-called lichenification so characteristic of neurodermatitis) due to the constant and repeated scratching.

The keystone of proper therapy lies in a tactful, reassuring attempt to provide the patient with some insight into her underlying emotional problems. She should be urged to vary her pattern of life accordingly and slow down her pace; this may require the help of sedatives, at least at first, and formal psychotherapy in some instances. As far as local therapy is concerned, it should be kept to a minimum, and all strong medications should be discontinued. The vulvar area should be kept clean and dry, the nails cut short and nail polish forbidden, and plain cotton underwear laundered only in pure soap should be worn and changed frequently. Topical cortisone ointments or lotions are often of considerable benefit; e.g., the hydrocortisone ointment 0.5%, applied in a thin film and worked gently into the skin two to three times daily. To promote healing and achieve immediate relief in the acute eczematoid stage, or where secondary infection has occurred, warm sitz baths or boric acid compresses two to three times daily followed by thorough air drying may be used. Above all, the patient must not scratch, for the vicious circle of itch-scratch, more itch—more scratch is a formidable aspect of the overall problem in this disorder.

PEDICULOSIS PUBIS

Infestation of the hairy portions of the external genital skin by the crab louse *(Phthirus pubis)* is another common cause of itching in the pubic and groin areas of the female. Severe pruritus is the hallmark of this parasitic skin disease, and secondary infections or eczematoid skin changes often develop. The parasites themselves, as well as their eggs (nits) attached to the short pubic hairs, are visible to the naked eye, aided at times by a small magnifying glass, rendering the diagnosis relatively easy. The treatment of choice is the local application of 1% gamma benzene hexachloride (Kwell), which is available as a lotion, cream, or shampoo. All contaminated linen and clothing should be thoroughly laundered or dry-cleaned, and all patient contacts should be examined carefully if possible and treated if indicated.

GENERAL APPROACH TO MANAGEMENT OF VULVITIS OF ALL TYPES

Since many of the vulvar inflammatory processes are nonspecific in nature, certain basic types of treatment are useful in the management of nearly all of them.

Local measures of importance in the treatment of vulvitis of any type include discontinuance of all prior medication, avoidance of scratching and too frequent washing and scrubbing, particularly with harsh soaps (use detergent soaps such as pHisoHex sparingly), maintenance of clean, dry skin, using talcum powder if necessary, and avoidance of tight clothing, synthetic fabrics, and perineal pads. There is no question but that the current widespread wearing of tight-fitting panty hose, slacks, and pants suits has contributed to an increased incidence of all types of vulvitis and vaginitis. These occlusive types of clothing produce chafing, increase heat and moisture, and interfere with normal ventilation in the vulvovaginal area. All these factors promote favorable conditions for the growth of fungal, protozoal, bacterial, and viral organisms and related agents, as well as promoting chronic, nonspecific irritation.

For immediate symptomatic relief, give hydrocortisone ointment or lotions for their antiinflammatory and antipruritic properties. In general, avoid all other medication.

Institute specific therapy for an underlying cause as indicated, when an exact diagnosis has been established. It is particularly important to exclude early malignant or premalignant changes in the presence of any long-standing, chronic vulvar inflammatory process. Use of the toluidine blue staining technique, as described in Chapter 2, can be extremely helpful in indicating the sites where biopsy specimens should be taken.

Benign Tumors, Cysts, and Miscellaneous Lesions of the Vulva

Benign tumors and cysts of the vulva are relatively uncommon, and their varied nature and origin have already been indicated. The most frequently encountered are sebaceous cysts, hidradenomas, condylomas, lipomas, fibromas, leiomyomas, and hemangiomas. Therapy is usually simple excision, which also serves to confirm the presumptive diagnosis. Rare types of vulvar cysts include those derived from vestigial remnants of the müllerian (paramesonephic mucinous cysts) or wolffian (mesonephric cysts) duct systems.

BARTHOLIN'S CYST

Bartholin's cyst is not a true cyst at all but a postinflammatory pseudocyst of Bartholin's gland that forms proximal to an obstructed duct. Usually, the ductal obstruction is the end result of a prior gonorrheal infection, but it occasionally occurs in connection with atrophic vaginitis and secondary blockage of the vaginal opening of the duct. These pseudocysts attain a variable size, some becoming as large as an orange, and they are prone to undergo secondary infection and intracystic abscess formation. They occupy a characteristic location in the posterior half of the labium, with their inner wall immediately adjacent to the lower vaginal canal (Fig. 30A). When acutely inflamed, they are extremely painful and tender, and the patient finds sitting or even walking almost impossible. The ideal treatment, particularly if the cyst is discovered before infection supervenes, but even in the presence of abscess when the latter is well localized within the cyst itself, is total excision of the intact cyst, with the contained abscess, if present. If the wall is incompletely excised, the cyst may recur. If total excision is not technically possible because of the presence of cellulitis accompanying an acute abscess, the cyst should simply be incised and drained. It can then be excised four to six weeks later as a second-stage procedure when the drainage incision has completely healed and the cyst has reformed. Some advocate treatment by simple marsupialization of Bartholin's cysts; drainage is established from within the vagina, and the edges of the vaginal and cyst wall incisions are sutured together to form a new duct opening. However, it is difficult to evaluate whether the long-term results have been or will be satisfactory.

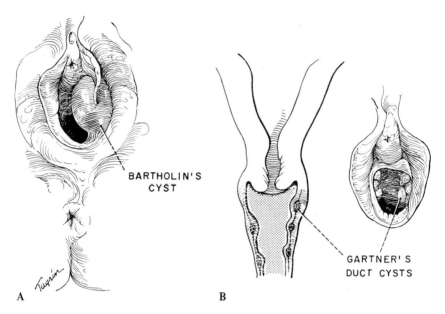

Figure 30
Common vulvar and vaginal cysts. A. Bartholin's cyst. B. Gartner's duct cysts.

A rare, but extremely serious infection that arises in Bartholin's gland abscesses and vulvar abscesses but culminates in a progressive synergistic bacterial gangrene of the adjacent soft tissues and fascial planes is most commonly seen in obese diabetic women with an associated ketoacidosis. Antibiotic therapy and simple incision and drainage are frequently inadequate, and exploration of the area under general anesthesia with wide, radical excision of all necrotic tissue may be necessary to prevent a fatal outcome.

VULVAR HERNIAS

Vulvar hernias (pudendal, or simple labial extensions of the congenital inguinal variety) are rare but are important both from the standpoint of differential diagnosis as well as approach to therapy, because proper treatment of a pudendal hernia usually involves a combined abdominal and vulvar approach. Both an inguinolabial and a pudendal hernia are seen in the labial area. However, the sac of the pudendal hernia comes down through a defect in the levator muscle sling and then courses alongside the lateral vaginal wall, whereas the sac of the inguinolabial hernia comes through an incompetent external inguinal ring. Persistence of a coelomic cavity lining below a normally obliterated inguinal ring may lead to the later development of a so-called hydrocele of the canal of Nuck, the canal lying within the labium; usually, there is no associated inguinal hernia in this situation.

THE VAGINA

Although most of the other primary vaginal disorders are relatively rare, vaginal infections and inflammatory processes are extremely common and represent the most frequently encountered diagnostic and therapeutic problem in gynecologic office practice. Since vaginal discharge is such a frequent complaint and is most often, although by no means always, indicative of an underlying vaginitis, it is well to begin by considering the most common causes of vaginal discharge:

1. Physiologic variations in normal secretion and epithelial desquamation (ovulatory, premenstrual, or related to pregnancy, stress, or sexual excitement), usually with no associated symptoms of vulvovaginal irritation.
2. Congenital cervical erosion, usually with no associated symptoms.
3. Chronic cervicitis and/or cervical polyps.
4. Trichomonal vaginitis.
5. Monilial vaginitis.
6. Atrophic vaginitis.
7. Hemophilus vaginitis.
8. Foreign bodies (a variety of objects in children; in adult women, chiefly a retained tampon).
9. Gonorrheal cervicitis, urethritis, skenitis, and bartholinitis.
10. Irritating douches; occasionally, contraceptive devices and jellies.
11. Early cervical, endocervical, endometrial, vaginal, or tubal cancers.
12. Pyometrium (secondary to a benign cervical stenosis or in association with carcinoma of the fundus or cervix).
13. Condyloma acuminatum of the cervix, vagina, and vulva.

Differential Diagnosis of Vaginal Discharge

HISTORY

The main points to be covered in the history are the following:

1. Presence or absence of associated symptoms, e.g., burning, itching. The mucoid discharge of a congenital cervical erosion or the physiologic increase in normal secretions at midcycle or premenstrually are asymptomatic, as is the pubertal monthly mucoid discharge of young girls. This is in sharp contrast to monilial (candidal) and trichomonal vaginitis, in which pruritus is intense, and to atrophic vaginitis, in which a burning discomfort is often the most prominent symptom.
2. Relation to menses. Symptoms of trichomoniasis invariably have their onset or become worse just after a period, whereas those of monilial vaginitis are often worse just before a period.
3. Relation to other features of the history. Moniliasis is common in pregnant women and in diabetic women, after therapy with broad-spectrum antibiotics, after estrogen therapy, and after therapy for trichomonal vaginitis.

LOCAL EXAMINATION

Check for an associated vulvitis or other vulvar lesion (e.g., leukoplakia or cancer) that might be responsible for the symptoms. Check for the presence of visible vaginal inflammation, cervicitis or cervical erosion, or for a retained foreign body, and determine the status of the vaginal mucosa with regard to estrogen effect. Rule out gonorrhea, malignancy (cervical, endocervical, and endometrial biopsies if necessary, as well as routine Papanicolaou smears), or pyometrium (probe the cervix or do an endometrial biopsy; if doubt still exists, formal curettage is indicated).

EXAMINATION OF DISCHARGE

1. Gross appearance, color, consistency, odor, pH. **Trichomonas:** yellow, thin, foamy, malodorous, alkaline pH (e.g., 5.0 to 6.0). **Monilia:** white, thick, flaky, cheesy, usually not malodorous, often acid pH (e.g., 3.0 to 4.0). **Atrophic:** scant, yellowish or brownish, occasionally blood-tinged. **Malignancy:** bloody, often malodorous. **Retained tampon:** often bloody and malodorous. **Chronic cervicitis:** mucoid or mucopurulent.
2. A wet smear (see Chap. 2) is usually diagnostic for trichomoniasis and of considerable help also in the diagnosis of vaginal moniliasis and atrophic vaginitis.
3. Cultures: Routine for nonspecific vaginitis, special (Nickerson's medium) for *Candida* (monilia) (see Chap. 2).
4. Cytologic smears.

Diagnosis and Therapy of Specific Types of Vaginitis

TRICHOMONAL VAGINITIS

Trichomonas vaginalis is probably a nearly universal and ordinarily innocuous inhabitant of the vaginal tract, usually appearing only in small numbers in the presence of normal secretions, normal mucosa, and normal environmental pH. It seems likely that in some instances a change in these environmental conditions favorable to the overgrowth of *Trichomonas* is responsible for the development of symptomatic vaginitis. On the other hand, there is also strong evidence for its venereal transmission, and it is frequently found present in both sexual partners, the male urethra and prostate serving as asymptomatic carrier sites. Both these etiologic mechanisms should be kept in mind when treating patients with stubbornly recurring trichomoniasis, and it probably should be considered one of the venereal disorders, although it is also encountered among women who are not sexually active.

Trichomonal vaginitis has a typical thin, yellow to yellowish-brown, very irritating, malodorous discharge, and there is marked local vulvovaginal burning and itching, often with a severe associated vulvitis. It becomes worse after a period, is prone to chronicity, and is stubborn in 15 to 20 percent of women suffering from it. Diagnosis is easily made by recognition of the motile, flagellate organisms on a simple fresh smear of the discharge.

Treatment

The medication of choice is Flagyl, an oral trichomonacide (metronidazole), and the recommended dosage schedule is 1 tablet (250 mg) by mouth two to three times daily, with meals, for 10 to 15 days. (Flagyl should probably be avoided in pregnant patients or in the presence of liver disease, and one of the local vaginal medications should be substituted.) Therapy with Flagyl has proved highly successful, with permanent cure rates of 95 to 100 percent reported in many large series and a low incidence of recurrences, most of which have responded to a repeated course of treatment. The great advantages of Flagyl are that it can be administered orally (no douches or other local therapy are required) and that an effective course of therapy takes only 10 to 15 days.

Recently, a single-dose program for both the female patient and her usually asymptomatic sexual partner has been advocated. It consists of administering 2 gm (8 tablets) of Flagyl in one dose to both, preferably under the direct observation of the physician, emphasizing that *Trichomonas* is a venereal infection and thus hopefully ensuring that the patient's consort will also receive and take his medication. When the regimen is followed exactly, it is reported to be essentially 100 percent effective, yet having the advantage of being a short and inexpensive treatment program. So far, side effects from the medication have been few and insignificant.

Flagyl is supplied also as vaginal inserts of 500 mg. In stubborn cases, treatment consists of 2 to 3 tablets orally and one vaginal insert daily for 10 days. Vaginal inserts are not given routinely, however, and are never used alone.

If recurrence follows a course of therapy, it is advisable to treat both the patient and her sexual partner simultaneously during the second 10-day course of treatment. For men, the dosage is also 1 tablet two to three times daily.

For pregnant patients or for refractory cases, some of the other drugs formerly widely used in the management of trichomonal vaginitis should be tried. The aim of most of these other therapeutic preparations or treatment programs is to restore the normal vaginal acidity and, if possible, destroy the *Trichomonas* organisms. Since none of the commonly employed medications is effective in every patient, it is well to be familiar with the use of a number of them. A few examples include:

1. Diiodohydroxyquin (Floraquin) vaginal tablets: 2 tablets in the posterior fornix nightly for 30 days, preceded by a vinegar douche.
2. Tricofuron vaginal suppositories: 1 nightly or 1 morning and night for 30 nights; douching is not necessary.
3. Aci-Jel vaginal jelly: one instillation twice daily or nightly for two to four weeks. Useful in women who do not respond to or tolerate Flagyl and for whom douching is difficult and inconvenient (e.g., college students or nurses living in dormitories) or in those who find tablets or suppositories difficult to insert (e.g., young women with intact hymens).

(**Note:** It is often difficult to clear up trichomoniasis when the cervix is chronically infected, and hence both infections may have to be treated simultaneously if the vaginitis is to be permanently controlled. Furthermore, trichomoniasis in postmenopausal women may be extremely refractory to therapy if an atrophic vaginitis co-exists, and both must therefore be treated to obtain relief of symptoms.)

Useful adjuncts to treatment, particularly in stubborn cases, include the following:

1. General measures, as noted under the management of vulvitis, such as avoidance of perineal napkins, the wearing of loose clothing, and avoidance of excessive moisture (including overbathing) and the use of soap or other irritating agents on the vulvar or perineal skin.
2. If douching is employed, instruction in proper technique, with avoidance of over-douching once the acute vaginitis subsides. (An adequate therapeutic vinegar douche involves the use of one-half cup of vinegar to 2 quarts of warm water.)
3. Instruction in, and check on, proper placement of vaginal suppositories or tablets.
4. Use of tampons during periods. (This avoids the inevitable chafing of perineal napkins and also appears to favor maintenance of normal vaginal acidity, even during the menstrual flow.)
5. Use of vaginal medication for a few days immediately prior to, during, and after the menses. (Suggestions 4 and 5 may need to be continued for three to six months after a course of treatment to avoid relapses at the time of the menses.)
6. Evaluation of the possible role of contraceptives or excessive douching.
7. If a carrier state in the husband is suspected:
   a. The husband should use a condom for six to eight weeks.
   b. Medication for the husband: Nitrofurantoin (Furadantin), 100 mg four times daily for 10 days; or Tritheon, 100-mg tablets, 1 tablet three times daily after meals for 10 days. The oral trichomonacide Flagyl is probably the drug of choice: 250-mg tablets two to three times daily for 10 to 15 days.
8. Symptomatic relief of itching: Hydrocortisone vulvar ointments (see Vulvitis) or cortisone vaginal tablets.

MONILIAL VAGINITIS

Monilial vaginitis is characteristically accompanied by intense itching, with or without typical patches of thick, white, cheesy discharge on a brightly inflamed vaginal mucosa; secondary vulvitis is often intense. It is frequently associated with diabetes, pregnancy, or broad-spectrum antibiotic therapy. The diagnosis is confirmed by culture on Nickerson's medium or by special examination of a fresh smear of the discharge (see Chap. 2).

Treatment

The following fungicidal agents have proved very effective:

1. Miconazole nitrate 2% (Monistat Cream): 1 applicator full applied intravaginally once daily at bedtime for 14 days.
2. Candicidin (Vanobid) vaginal tablets or ointment: 1 tablet or 1 applicator full of ointment applied intravaginally twice daily for 14 days.

3. Nystatin (Mycostatin) vaginal tablets: 1 or 2 tablets inserted vaginally each day for 10 to 14 days and then 1 tablet daily for a second interval of 10 to 14 days (package of 15 tablets with a handy vaginal applicator).
4. Gentia-Jel: one vaginal application nightly for 12 to 24 nights (package of 12 disposable prefilled applicators).
5. Gentersal Cream: one vaginal application nightly for 15 to 30 days (large tube with 15 disposable applicators).
6. Propion Gel: one vaginal application every morning and every night for three to four weeks (95-gm tube with applicator).
7. Sodium perborate douches for excessive monilial discharge: 1 teaspoon sodium perborate to 1 quart of water.
8. For extensive vulvar involvement, Mycolog Cream, which contains a topical steroid and antibacterial agent as well as mycostatin, may be applied locally to the skin.

It is also important to be aware of and correct all the potential factors that may be favoring the overgrowth of the monilial organisms that normally inhabit the vulvovaginal area and lower intestinal tract. These factors include broad-spectrum antibiotic therapy, pregnancy, diabetes, estrogenic or oral contraceptive medication, and excessive moisture and chafing (e.g., tight clothing, overbathing, excessive perspiration).

ATROPHIC VAGINITIS

Following the menopause, or after surgical or radiation castration, estrogen lack may ultimately result in a very atrophic type of vaginal epithelium, with loss of all but the basal cell layer (Fig. 31A). Such a thinned-out epithelium is prone to infection

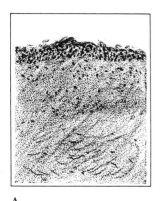 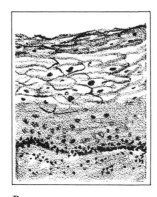

A   B

Figure 31
Characteristic histologic appearance of (A) atrophic vaginal mucosa, as contrasted with (B) normal mature vaginal epithelium.

and inflammation of the submucosal tissues, with resulting local irritation, and may tend to bleed at the slightest trauma or even spontaneously. There is usually an accompanying shrinkage of the surrounding soft tissues, and there may be an associated vulvar atrophy as well. Although this condition sometimes is referred to as senile vaginitis, the term **atrophic vaginitis** is decidedly preferable for obvious reasons. Symptoms include vaginal and vulvar burning or soreness and occasionally pruritus. Secondary symptoms often present are: vaginal discharge and bleeding (the symptom of postmenopausal bleeding invariably requires a curettage to rule out carcinoma of the endometrium); bladder irritability with frequency, urgency, and pseudoincontinence; and, not infrequently, vague lower abdominal discomfort. Once other causes have been excluded, a premenopausal type of vaginal epithelium (Fig. 31B) can usually be readily restored by administration of systemic or local estrogens, with rapid clearing of symptoms.

Treatment

Local. Local treatment consists of one of the following:

1. Dienestrol cream: vaginal application once nightly for 7 to 14 nights and then once every other night for 14 nights (large tube with applicator).
2. Premarin (0.625 mg per gram) vaginal cream (with or without hydrocortisone, 1 mg per gram): 1 to 2 gm nightly for 30 nights (large tube with applicator).
3. Diethylstilbestrol suppositories: 0.1-, 0.5-, or 1.0-mg suppositories every night for 30 nights.

Systemic (Oral). Systemic treatment consists of one of the following:

1. Chlorotrianisene (TACE): 12 to 24 mg (1 to 2 capsules) nightly for 30 to 60 nights.
2. Premarin: 1.25 mg nightly for 30 nights.
3. Diethylstilbestrol: 1.0 mg nightly for 30 nights.

Complications

Abacterial urethritis and cystitis (the urethral and trigonal mucosa share in the atrophic changes) usually respond to estrogens plus urethral dilatations. The urethra may be readily dilated in the office, using ordinary Hegar cervical dilators, proceeding from a No. 10 or No. 12 up through a No. 18 or No. 20 and employing dibucaine (Nupercaine) ointment as an anesthetic lubricant. Dilatations are usually very effective in hastening subsidence of urinary frequency, urgency, and pseudoincontinence or urgency incontinence when carried out in conjunction with a short course of estrogen.

Urethral "caruncle" and urethral mucosal prolapse, a carunclelike lesion probably produced by shrinkage of the urethral wall and a resulting protrusion of the posterior urethral mucosa at the meatus, may occur. Either may respond to estrogen therapy alone and completely disappear, but if the pseudocaruncle is large, excision and urethroplasty or electrocoagulation of the lesion may be necessary.

HEMOPHILUS VAGINALIS (CORYNEBACTERIUM VAGINALE) VAGINITIS

Formerly, a diagnosis of nonspecific bacterial vaginitis was made if fresh wet smears of vaginal discharge showed bacteria and pus cells but failed to reveal specific pathogens such as trichomonal or candidal organisms. Routine bacteriologic cultures in such cases occasionally permit identification and specific antibiotic therapy for the particular bacteria primarily responsible for the infection (e.g., streptococci or staphylococci) but primary bacterial vaginitis due to these pyogenic organisms is relatively uncommon. It is now recognized, however, that the majority (90 percent or more) of cases of what were formerly termed *nonspecific bacterial vaginitis* are due to a specific infection by *Hemophilus vaginalis,* a small, pleomorphic, gram-negative bacillus. A profuse, grayish, or sometimes creamy-yellow to grayish-green discharge with a particularly strong, disagreeable odor is characteristic of *H. vaginalis* vaginitis, and burning and pruritus are often intense.

The organism can frequently be recognized on a routine fresh wet-mount smear, which will show clumps of the bacilli, only a few pus cells, but large numbers of epithelial cells, many of which appear stippled or granulated due to the adherence and uniform spacing of *H. vaginalis* bacilli on their surfaces, the so-called clue cells. A gram-stained smear will definitely reveal the tiny, short gram-negative bacilli; it can also be definitely identified by special cultures, but the latter are rarely necessary to establish the diagnosis. The vaginal pH usually lies between 5.0 and 5.5, which, in the absence of trichomonads, is also highly suggestive of *Hemophilus* vaginitis in any woman of childbearing age with a vaginal discharge.

Treatment

The disease is venereally transmitted, and both the patient and her consort should be treated simultaneously. Oral ampicillin, 500 mg four times daily for 5 days, should be given to both partners, or oxytetracycline (Terramycin) can be used in case of penicillin allergy. Supplementary treatment with one or more of the following medications may occasionally be necessary:

1. Sultrin Triple Sulfa Cream: apply morning and night for 7 to 10 days (one large tube with applicator).
2. Sterisil Vaginal Gel: one application nightly or every other night for 6 to 12 applications, always carrying treatment through one menstrual period (package of 1½-oz tube and six applicators).
3. Nitrofurazone (Furacin) vaginal suppositories: 1 nightly for 12 to 24 nights.
4. AVC cream: one vaginal application once or twice daily for 30 days (4-oz tube with applicator).

VAGINITIS DUE TO INFECTION WITH GENITAL MYCOPLASMAS

Formerly classified as "pleuropneumonialike organisms (or L organisms), the genital mycoplasmas are now known to cause a number of genitourinary tract infections in both men and women, including vaginitis, chronic cervicitis, endometritis, urethritis, and chronic recurring cystitis in the female. Less often, they have been implicated in pelvic inflammatory disease, septic abortion, or postpartum infections. T-strain (*T* for "tiny," or small-colony organisms) mycoplasmas appear to be the ones chiefly involved, and evidence is accumulating to suggest that genital tract infections with this organism may be responsible for infertility, spontaneous abortion, and premature births in some couples. However, large-colony organisms *(Mycoplasma hominis)* are also frequently recovered at the same time, and they, too, may be pathogenic.

There are no clinical characteristics to distinguish acute, chronic, or recurring vaginitis, cervicitis, or urethritis, and in the past these infections have probably been included in the nonspecific category. Genital *Mycoplasma* infection also frequently coexists with the other more common genital infections such as *Trichomonas,* gonorrhea, *Hemophilus,* and *Candida,* and failure of symptoms to clear after successful treatment of any of these infections may be a clue to the presence of *Mycoplasma.* A diagnosis can usually be made from material obtained directly from the cervix, vagina, or urethra employing special cultural techniques developed for identification of the organism.

Infections due to the genital mycoplasmas usually respond to demeclocycline (Declomycin), tetracycline, or erythromycin. Both the woman and her sexual partner should be treated, since the organisms are probably acquired and maintained via venereal transmission.

VAGINITIS DUE TO HERPESVIRUS HOMINIS

Vaginitis resulting from herpesvirus infection is usually accompanied by cervicitis, or vulvitis, or both (see Chap. 8).

MISCELLANEOUS VAGINAL INFECTIONS

Less common causes of vaginitis, cervicitis, and urethritis include the following: the imperfect fungus *Torulopsis glabrata;* the coccoid microorganism *Chlamydia trachomatis,* the so-called genital TRIC (trachoma — inclusion conjunctivitis) agent; the cytomegalovirus; and the virus of molluscum contagiosum, a skin disease (the genital infection is called molluscum contagiosum venereum). All these infections belong in the category of venereally transmitted disease.

DESQUAMATIVE INFLAMMATORY VAGINITIS

Gardner [6] has called attention to a condition that resembles atrophic vaginitis but which is seen in women with normal estrogen levels. In the case of postmenopausal women, it even fails to respond to estrogen therapy. Characteristically, it involves only the upper third of the vagina, which presents as an acutely inflamed, irregularly denuded, fiery-red, raw surface. There is an accompanying profuse, purulent, occasionally bloody discharge with moderate local discomfort. Neither estrogens nor antibacterial, antitrichomonal, or antifungicidal agents are of benefit, and the use of intravaginal corticosteroid preparations has proved to be the most effective treatment. The etiology is unknown, but a possible viral origin is suspected.

VAGINITIS EMPHYSEMATOSA

Vaginitis emphysematosa is a relatively uncommon inflammatory lesion seen almost invariably in association with pregnancy and characterized by the diffuse appearance of multiple small, gas-filled cysts in the mucosa of the vaginal wall and portio of the cervix; there is an accompanying edema and inflammation of the vaginal mucosa. The cysts vary in diameter from a millimeter or less to several centimeters and present a characteristic x-ray appearance. They may be accompanied by vaginal discharge, but more often they are asymptomatic and disappear spontaneously following delivery. Although most of the cases have occurred during pregnancy, some have been reported in nonpregnant and even postmenopausal women. In some cases the presence of *Trichomonas* appeared to have been of possible etiologic significance, but no specific bacterial organism is usually involved. The cystic lesions appear to be dilated lymphatic channels. Treatment is symptomatic.

Vaginal Cysts and Benign Tumors

The commonest cystic lesions of the vagina are cysts of Gartner's duct. They are small (a few millimeters in diameter), usually multiple, and asymptomatic. Typically, they are found in a relatively straight line along the anterolateral section of the vaginal walls on either side and frequently are bilateral (Fig. 30B). They arise in the most caudal remnants of the mesonephric or wolffian duct system. Rarely, they achieve sufficient size to cause discomfort or interfere with intercourse or obstetric delivery and may then require excision. Much less common are the retention or inclusion cysts of müllerian duct origin.

   Benign vaginal tumors are even less frequently encountered, fibromas and leiomyomas being the most common. (Adenomyomas of the vagina or rectovaginal septum are not true tumors but instances of endometriosis.) Usually, these are best excised, even if asymptomatic, primarily for histologic confirmation that they are benign. A benign type of vaginal adenosis encountered in young females whose mothers received diethylstilbestrol during their pregnancy is discussed in Chapter 4, and also in Chapter 16 (since it occasionally can be the precursor of clear cell adenocarcinoma of the vagina).

Miscellaneous Benign Vaginal Conditions

Congenital anomalies have already been discussed in Chapter 3. The so-called vaginal relaxations (e.g., cystocele, rectocele) are not, strictly speaking, primary vaginal disorders and are more properly considered as pelvic support disorders (see Chap. 18).

THE CERVIX

Although the cervix has a similar embryologic origin and is grossly an extension of the uterine fundus, it behaves essentially as an independent anatomic and physiologic entity and from many standpoints is almost a separate organ. Although its muscular wall is continuous with that of the fundus, even this responds in a different fashion to various physiologic or abnormal stimuli (e.g., hormonal, neurogenic). It is also important to remember that the cervix contains both the columnar and glandular epithelium of the endocervical canal as well as the squamous epithelium that covers the exocervix, all of which differ considerably in behavior from the epithelium lining the endometrial cavity.

The rare congenital anomalies of the cervix have been mentioned in Chapter 3, and the relatively uncommon specific anatomic abnormality of incompetency of the internal cervical os will be discussed in Chapters 9 and 11. The more common benign diseases of the cervix will be considered here.

Congenital Cervical Erosion

Also known as cervical ectropion, congenital cervical erosion is in fact neither an erosion nor an eversion of the external os of the cervix. The "eroded" appearance of the exocervical epithelium surrounding the external os is due to the covering of the area by the thinner, more vascular columnar epithelium that ordinarily does not extend beyond the limits of the endocervical canal instead of by the squamous epithelium normally present here. The exposed area of columnar epithelium stands out as a discrete, bright-red, circumferential band of varying width against the background of the normal pale, bluish-pink color of the squamous epithelium and thus at first glance may appear eroded to the uninitiated (Fig. 32). In other words, the squamocolumnar junction is plainly visible on the surface of the exocervix in this condition, whereas under normal circumstances it is located at the lower margin of the endocervical canal and, unless the cervix is lacerated, is hidden from view.

Congenital cervical ectropion is found to be present in 15 to 20 percent of young women. Because it is usually asymptomatic and of no serious import, it is important to recognize it and be aware of its benign nature. Occasionally, exposure of this columnar, glandular type of epithelium to the irritating effects of vaginal acidity and bacterial flora may lead to hypersecretion, the patient noting a variable amount of mucoid discharge that is usually unaccompanied by pruritus or discomfort of any kind. A simple explanation and reassurance usually are sufficient, though an occasional mild vinegar douche might be advised for women in whom the mucus secretion is profuse.

Cauterization is rarely, if ever, necessary or effective, and it is indicated only if secondary infection has led to a true cervicitis. Some feel strongly that the abnormal

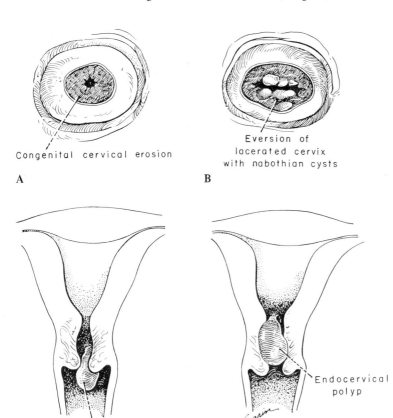

Congenital cervical erosion

A

Eversion of
lacerated cervix
with nabothian cysts

B

Exocervical
polyp

C

Endocervical
polyp

D

Figure 32
Common benign lesions of the cervix. A. Congenital cervical erosion. B. Cervical laceration with eversion and multiple nabothian cysts. C. Exocervical polyp. D. Endocervical polyp.

location of the squamocolumnar junction and its exposure to chemical and bacterial trauma predispose the epithelium to undergo atypical changes and ultimately to an increased risk of carcinoma, but this concept is controversial and unproved. In the vast majority of cases the condition either regresses spontaneously with advancing years or disappears after the first pregnancy and delivery as a result of the healing process, usually further aided by modern-day routine postpartum cauterization of the cervix.

Congenital Cervical Anomalies Associated with Fetal Diethylstilbestrol Exposure

Certain characteristic cervical erosions or ectropions, cervical and vaginal ridges (so-called vaginal hoods), cervical pseudopolyp formation, and, even more frequently, areas of so-called vaginal adenosis (islands of columnar and glandular epithelium where squamous epithelium should be) have been encountered in adolescent girls whose mothers received diethylstilbestrol (DES) during their pregnancy. Since the most serious — but fortunately far less common — lesions so far encountered in this situation have been clear cell adenocarcinomas of the vagina (less often of the cervix), this subject, including pertinent details of these benign cervical and vaginal abnormalities, is discussed in Chapter 4.

True Cervical Eversion

In true cervical eversion, exposure of the squamocolumnar junction follows an actual laceration of the exocervical os and lower endocervical canal during childbirth, subsubsequent healing resulting in a visible eversion of a portion of the endocervical epithelium (Fig. 32). In the absence of secondary infection this condition is usually either asymptomatic or is accompanied only by a slight nonirritating mucoid secretion, and it is of importance only insofar as it must be differentiated from other, more serious cervical lesions.

True Cervical Erosions or Ulcers

Actual erosion or ulceration of the surface of the cervix is relatively uncommon and may be the result of a number of local traumatic influences, including mechanical injury from pessaries or other foreign bodies, irritating chemical douches, or the constant chafing of the epithelial surface that accompanies uterine prolapse. A careful history will usually disclose the cause, but the possibility of carcinoma should be excluded by vaginal and cervical cytologic studies and adequate biopsies.

Chronic Cervicitis

Almost all parous women (perhaps 90 to 95 percent) have at least microscopic evidence (varying amounts of leukocytic infiltration) of chronic cervicitis, but this is usually minimal, asymptomatic, and not even clinically apparent. Clinically obvious and symptomatic chronic cervicitis is the result of a more extensive, chronic infection in a badly lacerated cervix, the offending organisms usually being a mixed flora of vaginal origin. The bacteria burrow deeply into partially obstructed glands and their surrounding stroma, giving rise to a mucopurulent, alkaline, irritating, and often malodorous discharge (leukorrhea). The cervix itself is grossly inflamed, edematous, and boggy, and this, together with the irregularly everted lacerations, gives an eroded appearance often entirely similar to that of carcinoma. If some of the mucus gland ducts become obstructed, as is often the case, the dilated glands filled with inspissated mucus and chronic inflammatory debris become visible on the surface of the exocervix and adjacent lower endocervix as typical yellowish or orange-colored nabothian cysts (Fig. 32). The epithelial thickening, inflammation, and edema frequently lead to the formation of mucosal polyps in either the exocervix or endocervix (Fig. 32). If the infection extends deeply enough, a low-grade pelvic cellulitis may develop and lead to pelvic and back pain, dyspareunia, and dysmenorrhea. The irritating discharge frequently produces a secondary vulvovaginitis, and occasionally a low-grade urethritis or repeated bouts of cystitis may be associated features.

It is obvious that chronic cervicitis (endocervicitis and/or exocervicitis) poses a diagnostic as well as a therapeutic problem. Before treatment is begun, it is extremely important to exclude early cervical cancer (or carcinoma in situ or any of the premalignant cervical dysplasias) by vaginal and cervical cytologic smears, by colposcopy, if available, and by adequate biopsies. In most cases these should be multiple or colposcopically guided and should adequately sample the abnormal cervical epithelium. It is important to emphasize that the final reports on both cytologic smears and tissue biopsies should be awaited before cauterization is instituted, because the latter will render further investigation difficult, if not impossible, if, for example, the vaginal or cervical smear should be reported positive, or doubtful, or if the biopsy findings are interpreted by the pathologist as "marked epithelial dysplasia, possible carcinoma in situ," with the additional note, "Believe further biopsies indicated."

Once a diagnosis of unequivocal chronic cervicitis has been definitely established, if the process is minimal and largely confined to the exocervix, and if the cervix is only moderately lacerated, simple office cauterization or cryotherapy may suffice to clear up the infection. If the endocervix is extensively involved, however, hospitalization for cervical dilatation and more thorough cauterization, cryotherapy, or actual surgical conization under anesthesia will be necessary. If an extensive cervical laceration is present (the "fish-mouth" cervix), surgical trachelorrhaphy with actual excision of the chronically infected everted anterior and posterior cervical lips may be more satisfactory than cauterization in correcting the situation.

There is little doubt that the chronically infected cervix deserves treatment to eradicate the infection and to restore a more nearly normal epithelial surface, not only to relieve symptoms but also as prophylaxis against the potential development of epithelial atypicalities that may ultimately progress to frank cervical carcinoma. Certainly, the weight of evidence strongly suggests that there is a causal relationship between chronic cervicitis of long standing and cervical cancer; the latter is much more prone to appear in the lacerated, chronically infected cervix than it is in the well-epithelialized cervix that has received proper postpartum attention for any laceration or foci of eversion, erosion, or chronic cervicitis.

CERVICITIS OF SPECIFIC ETIOLOGY

Much less commonly encountered causes of acute or chronic cervicitis include specific infections such as gonorrhea, syphilis, chancroid, granuloma venereum, herpesvirus hominis, and tuberculosis, all of which are discussed in Chapter 8. Again, the differentiation of any of these lesions from carcinoma should go hand in hand with the recognition of their specific etiology, following which appropriate specific therapy can be instituted.

Cervical Polyps

The formation of mucosal polyps in either the exocervix (the relatively broad-based, superficial type) or endocervical canal (the pedunculated type) (Fig. 32) is invariably secondary to an underlying chronic exocervicitis or endocervicitis. Polyps are frequently accompanied by vaginal discharge and sometimes by irregular vaginal bleeding, which, according to the individual circumstances, may be spontaneous and intermenstrual, postcoital, or postmenopausal. Since the majority of cervical polyps do not bleed, however, they can never be assumed to be the cause of intermenstrual or postmenopausal bleeding until cytologic smears and a careful endocervical and endometrial curettage (a formal D&C) have excluded other lesions, the polyp itself being excised at the same time. If the polyp is small and superficial, and if there is no history of abnormal bleeding, simple office excision often suffices, but the tissue should be submitted to the pathologist for histologic examination to be certain of its benign nature. Although so-called squamous metaplasia is common, malignant degeneration in simple mucosal polyps of the cervix is extremely rare. Occasionally (1 percent or less of all cervical polyps), however, superficial epidermoid or glandular carcinomatous change is encountered in an otherwise apparently benign polyp. In such cases, particularly in older women, hysterectomy may be indicated after additional studies have ruled out invasive cancer elsewhere in the cervix or endocervical canal.

Condyloma Acuminatum

Condyloma acuminatum, a warty lesion of the cervix, is identical to similar lesions occurring in the vagina and on the vulva (the process frequently involves all three areas simultaneously), is of viral origin, and is probably venereally transmitted. Although its gross appearance is usually characteristic, biopsy confirmation is desirable, following which the cervical (and vaginal) lesions are best treated by electrodesiccation. (The vulvar lesions are perhaps better treated with podophyllin applications — unless they are large, coalescent, and exceedingly numerous [see Chap. 8].)

Epithelial Dysplasia of the Cervix

Atypical abnormalities of the cervical epithelium can manifest themselves clinically in several ways: They may be grossly visible as white patches (the general clinical term **leukoplakia of the cervix** is often applied, but the histologic findings are variable) or may visibly fail to take up the iodine stain when a Schiller's test is performed. The desquamated atypical epithelial cells may give rise to a suspicious (Class III) vaginal or endocervical cytologic smear, or even occasionally a positive smear (in the case of marked atypicalities bordering on intraepithelial carcinoma). They are otherwise asymptomatic but are important because some of them probably represent various stages in a progressive spectrum of epithelial abnormalities that may advance to carcinoma in situ and ultimately to invasive cervical cancer.

In the case of visible leukoplakic patches or areas that fail to take Schiller's stain, adequate biopsy and cytologic studies, as well as colposcopy, if available, are indicated to establish definitely the histologic nature of the abnormal epithelium. The most common histologic types in this general category include squamous metaplasia and/or epidermidization of the columnar and glandular epithelium of the endocervix in the vicinity of the squamocolumnar junction (the so-called transformation zone) and leukokeratosis or leukoparakeratosis of the squamous epithelium of the ectocervix. The latter two lesions are the ones commonly grossly visible as white patches; they not infrequently give rise to suspicious cytologic smears and are often found in cervices that also harbor intraepithelial or invasive cancer. The importance of an adequate evaluation of the entire cervix is therefore obvious, and when, as is often the case, conservative therapy is elected, the need for prolonged and regular follow-up supervision of the patient is also apparent.

When suspicious or positive cytologic findings are the only clue to an epithelial abnormality, any of the preceding histologic lesions may be present, as well as grossly invisible epithelial dysplasia, which is characterized by varying degrees of hyperactivity of the basal cells and an atypical epithelial hyperplasia with loss of normal differentiation, increased mitotic activity, and varying degrees of actual cellular atypicality bordering on the histologic pattern of carcinoma in situ. The incidence of cervical dysplasia has been steadily rising, and gynecologists are encountering this lesion with increasing frequency among younger age groups, including sexually active teenagers. With an ever-larger segment of the female population being subjected to annual or more frequent cytologic screening, the need for proper investigation and treatment of the many patients with abnormal smears due to the presence of a cervical dysplasia or some other form of intraepithelial atypicality or neoplasia has now become an important problem of considerable magnitude for the specialty.

Cervical dysplasia is usually graded (cytologically as well as histologically) as mild, moderate, or severe. A general rule of thumb regarding the ultimate fate of cervical dysplasia is as follows: Roughly 40 percent will disappear spontaneously (these are usually in the mild to moderate category); 40 percent will persist indefinitely, unchanged in the degree of epithelial abnormality (again, these are usually mild to moderate in degree); and 20 percent are either initially associated with, or are ultimately destined to progress to, carcinoma in situ or invasive cervical cancer (these are usually in the moderate and severe categories).

When the patient's cytologic smear is reported abnormal, suggestive of cervical dysplasia or possibly of an even more serious lesion, although biopsy of areas of cervical epithelium that are visibly abnormal or fail to take Schiller's stain may be helpful, colposcopic examination with colposcopically guided biopsies and endocervical scrape biopsy represents the most satisfactory way to establish a definite diagnosis. If colposcopy is not available, a formal, fractional curettage, together with cold-knife cone biopsy of the cervix, will be necessary to establish a definite diagnosis and exclude the presence of carcinoma in situ or invasive cancer.

If only a cervical dysplasia is ultimately identified after detailed study, conservative management can be elected in many instances, particularly when it is desirable to preserve the childbearing function. If a conization is necessary for diagnostic purposes, this procedure alone usually will serve as the definitive conservative procedure. If the diagnosis is established by colposcopy and directed biopsies, electrocauterization, thermal cauterization, or cryotherapy may be employed as conservative therapy for the cervix harboring dysplasia. There are many who still favor electrocauterization or thermal cauterization. The equipment is inexpensive, the technique simple and quick, the healing time short and free of significant morbidity, and complications are rare. However, cryosurgical treatment is now widely used and preferred by many others who believe that it permits adequate treatment without complications to a greater depth within the substance of the cervix than can be safely carried out using thermal or electrocauterization. It is important that the need for long-term follow-up surveillance is clearly understood by both patient and physician, in order that persistence or recurrence of the lesion may be promptly detected.

When moderate or severe cervical dysplasia is found in older women no longer desirous of retaining childbearing function, definitive treatment by total hysterectomy is probably the management of choice. For as long as the cervix that has harbored dysplasia is allowed to remain, there is a significant risk of progression to carcinoma in situ and eventually to invasive cervical cancer. Additional discussion of cervical dysplasia and its management will be found in Chapter 13.

Atypical Adenomatous Hyperplasia of the Cervix Associated with Oral Contraceptives

There have been a number of reports of an atypical polypoid hyperplasia of the endocervix in women taking oral contraceptives [21]. Grossly, polypoid areas that frequently are multiple, are nearly always friable, and bleed easily are seen, often clinically suggesting carcinoma. Although there are no symptoms in some, most of the patients have noted an abnormal discharge, often with intermenstrual or postcoital bleeding. The majority of the women have been taking one of the contraceptive drugs for several years, although a few have been using them for less than six months. The lesions are usually located near the squamocolumnar junction and microscopically show a distinctive adenomatous and medullary type of atypical hyperplasia of both gland cell and reserve cell elements of the endocervical epithelium.

The real significance of this entity, now known to be benign, lies in its striking clinical and histologic resemblance to, and easy confusion with, adenocarcinoma of the cervix. However, careful interpretation of the microscopic picture — notably the uniform appearance of the hyperplastic cells and their nuclei, the tendency to orderly arrangement, the relative absence of mitotic figures, and the lack of stromal invasion — should make it possible to distinguish this entity from carcinoma, particularly when the patient is known to be on oral contraceptive medication. The dangers of an erroneous diagnosis of cancer and subsequent radical therapy for what is a perfectly benign lesion are obvious. Although most of the reported lesions have been treated by excision (usually conization), a few have been observed to regress completely following simple discontinuance of the oral progestational agents.

Benign Tumors of the Cervix

With the exception of cervical polyps, which are not true neoplasms but inflammatory proliferations of the cervical mucosa, benign tumors of the cervix are relatively uncommon. Most frequently encountered are the **leiomyomas,** which arise in the smooth muscle of the wall of the cervix in the same way that fibroids develop in the myometrium of the uterine fundus, the site in which they are far more common. As they enlarge, cervical fibroids may result in a localized tumor of the wall of the endocervix or of a segment of the margin of the exocervix; they may bulge into the paracervical area, or they may project into the cervical canal, sometimes as a pedunculated or polypoid type of fibroid. In the former two situations they may cause pelvic pain or simulate an adnexal tumor; in the latter location they frequently become ulcerated or undergo spontaneous necrosis with associated abnormal bleeding, or infection, or both. In the intracavitary site, continued enlargement usually results in a marked dilatation of the surrounding rim of normal cervix, the greatly distended cervical segment of the uterus frequently becoming wedged tightly within the pelvis. This circumstance often makes hysterectomy difficult owing to the limited exposure in the crucial areas where the ureters and the uterine vessels are even more closely approximated than usual. Hysterectomy is often indicated in the management of a symptomatic cervical fibroid in patients no longer desiring to preserve childbearing function; in younger women, myomectomy can usually be accomplished, sometimes employing the vaginal route, if the fibroid is readily accessible by this approach.

Miscellaneous, much less common benign tumors of the cervix include true fibromas and fibroadenomas, hemangiomas, and squamous papillomas, the latter sometimes grossly resembling carcinoma. All these lesions should be excised, or at least adequately examined by biopsy, to confirm their benign nature histologically and exclude the possibility of carcinoma.

Other relatively rare benign cervical lesions that may be encountered are endometriosis, adenomyosis, and small cysts and adenomas of mesonephric duct remnant origin. Again, biopsy excision is usually necessary to establish a definite diagnosis, whether or not symptoms are present.

REFERENCES

1. Chanen, W., and Hollyock, V. E. Colposcopy and electrocoagulation — diathermy for cervical dysplasia and carcinoma-in-situ. *Obstet. Gynecol.* 37:623, 1971.
2. Cockerell, E. C., and Knox, J. M. Dermatologic diseases of the vulva. *Am. J. Obstet. Gynecol.* 84:537, 1962.
3. Dickie, E. G. Herpes vulvitis. *Obstet. Gynecol.* 34:434, 1969.
4. Dykers, J. R. Single-dose metronidazole for trichomonal vaginitis. *N. Engl. J. Med.* 293:23, 1975.
5. Farrar, H. K., Jr., and Nedoss, B. R. Benign tumors of the uterine cervix. *Am. J. Obstet. Gynecol.* 81:124, 1961.
6. Gardner, H. L. Desquamative inflammatory vaginitis: A newly defined entity. *Am. J. Obstet. Gynecol.* 102:1102, 1968.

7. Gardner, H. L. The Vulvovaginitides: New Interpretations and Treatment Methods. In M. L. Taymor and T. H. Green, Jr. (Eds.), *Progress in Gynecology,* Vol. VI. New York: Grune & Stratton, 1975. Pp. 307–338.

8. Gardner, H. L., and Dukes, C. D. *Hemophilus vaginalis* vaginitis: A newly defined specific infection previously classified "nonspecific" vaginitis. *Am. J. Obstet. Gynecol.* 69:962, 1955.

9. Hermann, G. Pudendal (labial) hernia. *N. Engl. J. Med.* 265:435, 1961.

10. Janovski, N. A. Dysontogenetic cyst of the vulva: Report of a case, with reference to etiologic classification of vulvar cysts. *Obstet. Gynecol.* 20:227, 1962.

11. Knaysi, G. A., Jr., Cosman, B., and Crikelair, G. F. Hidradenitis suppurativa. *J.A.M.A.* 203:19, 1968.

12. Kundsin, R. B. Mycoplasma infections of the female genital tract. In M. L. Taymor and T. H. Green, Jr. (Eds.), *Progress in Gynecology,* Vol. VI. New York: Grune & Stratton, 1975. Pp. 291–306.

13. McCormack, W. M., Braun, P., Lee, Y. H., Klein, J. O., and Kass, E. H. The genital mycoplasmas. *N. Engl. J. Med.* 288:78, 1973.

14. McKay, D. G., Terjanian, B., Poschyachinda, D., Younge, P. A., and Hertig, A. T. Clinical and pathologic significance of anaplasia (atypical hyperplasia) of the cervix. *Obstet. Gynecol.* 13:1, 1959.

15. Richart, R. M., and Barron, B. A. A follow-up study of patients with cervical dysplasia. *Am. J. Obstet. Gynecol.* 105:386, 1969.

16. Roberts, D. B., and Hester, L. L., Jr. Progressive synergistic bacterial gangrene arising from abscesses of the vulva and Bartholin's gland duct. *Am. J. Obstet. Gynecol.* 114:285, 1972.

17. Schachter, J. S., Hanna, L., Hill, E. C., Massad, S., Sheppard, C. W., Conte, J. E., Jr., Cohen, S. N., and Meyer, K. F. Are chlamydial infections the most prevalent venereal disease? *J.A.M.A.* 231:1252, 1975.

18. Sedlis, A. Cervical dysplasia — diagnosis, prognosis, and management. In M. L. Taymor and T. H. Green, Jr. (Eds.), *Progress in Gynecology,* Vol. VI. New York: Grune & Stratton, 1975. Pp. 559–581.

19. Shaughnessey, D. M., Greminger, R. R., Margolis, I. D., and Davis, W. C. Hidradenititis suppurativa: A plea for early operative treatment. *J.A.M.A.* 222:320, 1972.

20. Shoch, E. P., Jr., and McCuistion, C. H. Diagnostic and therapeutic errors in certain dermatoses of the vulva. *J.A.M.A.* 157:1102, 1955.

21. Taylor, H. B., Ivey, N. S., and Norris, H. J. Atypical endocervical hyperplasia in women taking oral contraceptives. *J.A.M.A.* 202:637, 1967.

22. Tredway, D. R., Townsend, D. E., Howland, D. N., and Upton, P. J. Colposcopy and cryosurgery in cervical neoplasia. *Am. J. Obstet. Gynecol.* 114:1020, 1972.

8

Pelvic Inflammatory Disorders and Venereal Diseases

Infections and inflammatory processes that remain localized to the vulva, vagina, and/or cervix (the external genitalia and lower reproductive tract) are, with the exception of the specific venereal diseases, discussed in Chapter 7. The pelvic infections remaining to be considered are those that tend to spread to or involve primarily the internal genitalia or upper reproductive tract, particularly the fallopian tubes (salpingitis). However, both the uterus (endometritis) and its adjacent supporting tissues with their accompanying vascular and lymphatic channels (parametritis, pelvic cellulitis, septic pelvic thrombophlebitis, and pelvic lymphadenitis), as well as the ovaries (oophoritis, tuboovarian abscess) and the pelvic peritoneal cavity itself (pelvic peritonitis, pelvic abscess), are frequently also involved. Furthermore, in many instances a more or less generalized abdominal peritonitis may exist, particularly in the early acute phases. Despite varying etiologies, this general type of pelvic infection is usually termed **pelvic inflammatory disease**, a description that correctly connotes an infectious process within the pelvic cavity and, for the most part, outside the uterus. Initially, any of the pelvic inflammatory disorders appears as an acute process, but as this subsides, or with repeated flare-ups or reinfections, a chronic stage of the disease develops with its own symptomatology, findings, and complications, and it is the chronic stage that usually is of the greater clinical significance. With regard to specific bacterial etiology, infection with gonococci is responsible for 65 to 75 percent of all pelvic inflammatory disease. Other pyogenic organisms gaining access to the pelvis as the result of septic abortion or puerperal infection account for another 20 to 30 percent of cases. Last, tuberculous salpingitis and endometritis are present in approximately 5 percent of patients with pelvic inflammation.

GONORRHEA AND GONORRHEAL PELVIC INFLAMMATORY DISEASE

Gonorrhea (neisserian infection) is caused by the gonococcus, *Neisseria gonorrhoeae,* named after its discoverer Neisser, who in 1879 first showed it to be the specific bacterial cause. It is the most common venereal disease and is the only one to involve both the lower and the upper female reproductive tract routinely. It is estimated that there are currently over 3 million new cases of gonorrhea in the United States each year. Thus the disease has truly reached epidemic proportions. Unfortunately, the venereal disease rate has risen most sharply for the youth of the country, persons under age 25 accounting for over half the total cases of both gonorrhea and syphilis and both diseases appearing in an increasing number of juveniles. Although the organism is rarely present in the male without producing symptoms, 50 to 80 percent of women with gonococcal infections are asymptomatic carriers. Herein lies the real problem in controlling this disease. Recent development of a serologic test for gonorrhea that would permit mass screening may provide the long-awaited means for detecting and treating the disease in this large, asymptomatic female carrier population. Gonosticon Dri-Dot (Organon), a commercially prepared 2-minute agglutination slide test, is now available for this purpose for use in office or clinic.

Acute Gonorrhea

The initial or lower tract phase of gonorrhea begins as an acute infection in the urethra, cervix, and Skene's and Bartholin's glands (gonococcal urethritis, cervicitis, skenitis, and bartholinitis). Rectal involvement may also occur, the organism gaining access to the rectal crypts. Acute gonorrhea is usually readily recognized on the basis of the typical clinical features, which include the following: a history of exposure (sometimes the patient knows that the sexual partner was infected); the one-week incubation period; the characteristic profuse, creamy, rather thick, highly irritating urethral and vaginal discharge; the urethral burning, dysuria, bladder irritability, and the often accompanying vulvovaginitis; and the obvious evidence of inflammatory involvement of the urethra and cervix, and often of Skene's and Bartholin's glands as well, seen on pelvic examination. Signs and symptoms of gonorrheal pharyngitis may also be present. At this stage of the disease, prior to the phase of ascending infection, there are essentially no lower abdominal symptoms or findings.

Confirmation of the diagnosis can sometimes (in 50 to 60 percent of infected females) be obtained by identifying the gram-negative intracellular diplococci on a stained smear of the urethral, vaginal, or cervical discharge or of secretions milked from Skene's glands in the paraurethral area, or of material from rectal crypts obtained via anoscopy. However, a definite and unequivocal diagnosis of gonorrhea can best be made by culture (urethral, endocervical, anal, and, when indicated, pharyngeal), streaking the material directly and immediately on Thayer-Martin medium, which yields rapid and highly reliable results in 90 percent or more of infected females, and incubating under increased carbon dioxide tension in a candle-jar. If a laboratory is not close at hand, Transgro (Difco), a transport medium with the proper ingredients and already charged with carbon dioxide, is now on the market to facilitate the preparation and transport of cultures. Subsequent further confirmation, if necessary, can then be done by subculture on special carbohydrate media that permit even more specific identification of the gonococcus. (Additional confirmation can also be obtained by a direct fluorescent—antibody staining technique.) It is important to carry out complete bacteriologic studies in all cases, even though the diagnosis may be obvious clinically, for the disease is a reportable one in most states, and there are often medicolegal problems once the diagnosis is officially made.

Penicillin has been and remains the antibiotic of choice for the treatment of gonorrhea since it first became available in the early 1940s. For nearly 20 years there was little evidence of the development of penicillin-resistant strains of the gonococcus. Subsequently, this situation has definitely altered, and both the number and prevalence of strains of the organism with diminished susceptibility to penicillin have shown a steady and alarming increase. Fortunately, this resistance is, for the most part, not absolute. However, the recommended dosage of penicillin has been increased considerably, and the following regimen is currently advised for the treatment of acute gonorrhea in the female: 2.4 million units of procaine penicillin G (aqueous) (e.g., Wycillin) should be injected intramuscularly into each buttock, for a total dose of 4.8 million units. Oral probenecid, which blocks renal tubular reabsorption of penicillin, should be given in a 1-gm dose 30 to 60 minutes before penicillin injection to delay excretion of the penicillin and thus to achieve prolonged high blood levels. Because it is the initially high systemic level of penicillin that is important in overcoming the lessened susceptibility of an increasing number of strains of the gonococcus, this program is far superior to older programs that used lower dosages of long-acting procaine penicillin in oil or beeswax; the latter provided relatively low concentrations over long periods, and they are no longer used. Fairly effective results have also been obtained with an oral medication program of ampicillin (3.5 gm), together with probenecid (1 gm), with the total dose of both given simultaneously.

If the patient is allergic to penicillin, or if drug resistance is encountered despite adequate dosage of aqueous penicillin G (as much as 8 million units has been given), tetracycline may be used, giving 1.5 gm orally as an initial dose, followed by 0.5 gm four times daily for four days. Unfortunately, increasing numbers of tetracycline-resistant strains are now also being reported. However, equally good or better results are reported following the single-dose intramuscular injection of 4 gm of spectinomycin (Trobicin), and either spectinomycin or doxycycline (Vibramycin) may be superior agents for use in penicillin-resistant cases.

Since 2 to 3 percent of patients with gonorrhea have also been infected with syphilis, and since the antibiotic therapy for the gonorrhea may not have been adequate for the incubating syphilis (if intramuscular penicillin has been used, it is simultaneously curative for any incubating syphilis), it is important that all patients treated for gonorrhea by other than the standard intramuscular penicillin regimen have follow-up serologic tests for syphilis during the next four months to detect this possibility. Obviously, follow-up physical examination, smears, and cultures are also indicated to be certain the gonorrhea has been eradicated.

Acute Gonorrheal Pelvic Inflammatory Disease

If treatment of the primary phase is delayed or inadequate, an ascending surface spread of the organism may take place, usually occurring toward the end of or just after the next menstrual period. At this time the normal barrier of the impenetrable cervical mucus plug is temporarily absent, and the menstrual blood provides an excellent medium for bacterial growth. The end result is the development of an acute salpingitis and pelvic peritonitis. The patient then presents with an acute

abdominal complaint that must be distinguished not only from other acute gynecologic disorders (e.g., ectopic pregnancy, twisted ovarian cyst, ruptured corpus
hemorrhagicum or corpus luteum cyst, ruptured endometrioma, twisted or degenerating fibroid) but also from appendicitis, diverticulitis, or other intraabdominal
disorders associated with peritonitis; occasionally, it must be distinguished from
acute urinary tract conditions (infection and calculi).

DIAGNOSIS

Acute gonorrheal pelvic inflammatory disease is suggested if a typical history can be
elicited of vaginal discharge preceding the onset of fever and abdominal pain during
or just after the next period. Gastrointestinal symptoms are often completely absent
or minimal in spite of obvious and often diffuse peritonitis (as contrasted with such
symptoms in appendicitis, for example).

Pelvic Findings

A urethral or cervical discharge may still be present and permit identification of
gonococcal organisms by smear or culture; if antibiotics have been administered,
however, this will often be impossible. Pelvic tenderness is bilateral and exquisite,
and the cervix is extremely painful on motion. There may or may not be palpable
adnexal swelling or thickening.

Abdominal Findings

Tenderness and muscle spasm may be generalized but are usually maximal in the
lower abdomen and, again, are bilateral and diffuse. Rarely, a perihepatitis may
develop (Fitz-Hugh-Curtis syndrome) due to spread of purulent fluid above the liver,
giving rise to upper abdominal pain and tenderness, especially in the right upper
quadrant. Intestinal peristalsis is often relatively normal, and the patient may even
be hungry and thirsty in spite of considerable evidence of peritoneal irritation (in
contrast to appendicitis, for example). A high temperature (102° to 103°F) and a
marked leukocytosis (a white cell count of 20,000 to 30,000 with a shift to the left)
are often present, but in spite of this the patient rarely appears very ill (in contrast
to the patient with the peritonitis of appendicitis, diverticulitis, perforated ulcer,
pancreatitis, and so on, who usually appears toxic). The characteristically mild
clinical manifestations of gonorrheal pelvic inflammatory disease are a reflection of
the relatively noninvasive potential of the gonococcus, an organism that tends to
remain localized to mucosal and serosal surfaces and not to penetrate deeper tissues
or spread via the bloodstream or lymphatics. Thus the clinical picture contrasts
sharply with that of peritonitis due to a ruptured appendix or similar acute general
surgical conditions, as well as with that of acute pelvic inflammatory disorders caused
by highly virulent and invasive organisms such as the *Streptococcus, Staphylococcus,
Escherichia coli,* and other related gram-negative bacilli commonly present in many
cases of puerperal or postabortal sepsis.

In the other acute gynecologic situations to be distinguished, the process is usually unilateral and more localized than in gonorrhea, and the clinical picture only rarely suggests infection. Laparoscopy or culdoscopy is an extremely useful diagnostic procedure if any doubt whatsoever exists and perhaps might even be done routinely in all but the most obvious cases. Either procedure not only will establish a definite diagnosis of the current acute illness but also may avoid a meddlesome laparotomy for diagnosis only, a step that might otherwise be necessary if the possibility of appendicitis or some other acute condition requiring emergency surgery is also under consideration. Furthermore, it is important that patients never be labeled as having had pelvic inflammatory disease on equivocal clinical grounds, because further management — in particular, evaluation and therapy of future episodes of abdominal pain — will invariably become fixed and stereotyped, based on and prejudiced by what may have been an entirely erroneous clinical impression of the nature of the initial acute illness.

Although much less common than the direct contiguous spread of gonococcal salpingitis and peritonitis, **blood-borne metastatic spread** of the gonococcus is far more serious and should be looked for in any patient with acute gonorrheal disease. The most common entities that result are migratory gonococcal arthritis, usually polyarticular (e.g., wrists, knees, ankles, hands, feet), and septicemia, with fever and associated skin lesions (initially hemorrhagic bullae); meningitis and endocarditis, myocarditis, and pericarditis also occur. These remote complications of the acute disease usually require and respond well to intensive, high-dose intravenous penicillin therapy.

TREATMENT

Although mild, subacute cases of salpingitis without significant pelvic peritonitis may sometimes be treated on an outpatient basis with oral tetracycline, or oral ampicillin, or intramuscular aqueous penicillin G with probenecid, the management of acute gonorrheal pelvic inflammatory disease in which the patient is ill enough to be hospitalized includes the following:

1. **Peritonitis regimen** (and infrequent pelvic examinations once a definite diagnosis is established): Bed rest, low or medium Fowler's position; restriction of oral intake, depending on the degree of ileus (rarely, intestinal intubation), with intravenous fluids as indicated.
2. **Antibiotics:** Aqueous penicillin G, 20 million units intravenously daily for several days, shifting to oral ampicillin when clear-cut improvement has occurred; or other specific chemotherapy as indicated by the results of cultures and sensitivity studies and by the patient's response.

In the acute phase of an initial attack of the disease, the clinical response to therapy is usually rapid and dramatic, with subsidence of fever and discomfort within 24 to 48 hours. If a prompt response is not forthcoming, look for more chronic manifestations of the disease with unresolved sepsis (pyosalpinx, tuboovarian abscess, cul-de-sac abscess), or suspect some other diagnosis (e.g., appendicitis or diverticulitis with abscess; twisted, gangrenous ovarian cyst).

Good management will include hospitalization for 7 to 14 days, with gradual ambulation and maintenance of oral chemotherapy with ampicillin (0.5 gm four times daily) for 5 to 7 days after the temperature becomes normal. If an intrauterine device (IUD) is present, it probably should be removed, since its continued presence will tend to favor persistence of bacterial infection in both the fallopian tubes and the endometrium. Prolonged restriction of activities with adequate rest and nutrition and occasionally continuation of antibiotics at home are indicated for several months. Proper care and gradual return to normal activity may increase the number of patients who recover with minimal permanent tubal damage and with preservation of normal tubal function. It is a favorable sign if adnexal swelling or induration never occurs, or if it is detected only during the acute phase and rapidly subsides thereafter. If symptoms and fever clear promptly and do not recur, this, too, is encouraging. When the patient is completely asymptomatic, has a completely negative pelvic examination, and has had several subsequently normal periods, she can be considered to have completed her convalescence and can be allowed more activity. In the case of a mild, acute, first attack of salpingitis with prompt response to early treatment, subsequent fertility may run as high as 70 percent. After two or three attacks, it will be 10 to 20 percent at best; and once the chronic, recurring phase is reached, permanent sterility is the rule.

It should also be emphasized that in almost all states the physician (also the hospital, clinic, or laboratory) is required by law to report all cases of venereal disease that come to his (its) attention. This information is considered confidential, but in any case the physician is protected from suit for revealing it to the proper authorities, because not to do so would constitute violation of the law on his part. (He cannot properly or legally reveal this information to anyone else, including the patient's spouse, however, without the patient's permission.) Only by each physician's fulfilling this legal obligation to report all cases of venereal disease can adequate measures be taken to trace all contacts and treat them adequately. A vigorous public health program of this type is sorely needed if the rising venereal disease rate in this country is to be halted and reversed.

Chronic Gonorrheal Pelvic Inflammatory Disease

CLINICAL FEATURES

Typical symptoms and findings of chronic gonorrheal pelvic inflammatory disease include the following: persistent pelvic pain, usually aggravated during menstrual periods, an acquired type of dysmenorrhea; dyspareunia; recurrent bouts of acute pain and fever; infertility; often, dysfunctional uterine bleeding secondary to involvement and poor function of the ovaries; and palpable adnexal disease (e.g., dilated, tortuous hydrosalpinx or pyosalpinx, tuboovarian abscesses, periadnexal adhesions, ovarian cysts, chronic parametrial induration).

PATHOLOGIC FEATURES

Both the initial acute salpingitis and the chronic inflammatory process (Fig. 33) that so often follows are invariably bilateral. However, the severity and extent of the involvement, as well as the type of secondary chronic pathologic manifestation, may vary considerably on the two sides. In the acute phase there is marked inflammation of the tubal mucosa, with edema of the walls of the tubes and a tremendous outpouring of an abundant purulent exudate that fills the tubes and spills forth into the peritoneal cavity. The exudate and its contained organisms are highly irritating to the serosa of the parietal peritoneum, and acute peritonitis results. This is often at first confined to the pelvis, but not infrequently, with continued exudation, there is more widespread and generalized peritonitis as the exudate is dispersed more widely through visceral and body movements.

The visceral peritoneum of adjacent organs (uterus, ovaries, rectosigmoid, and small bowel) also becomes inflamed, and there is a great tendency for these structures, together with the omentum, to be drawn down to the region of the fimbriated ends of the tubes, from whence flows the noxious exudate, as the body attempts to wall off the primary sites of the infection. As body defense mechanisms, with or without the aid of antibiotics, begin to localize and ultimately to control the acute infection, it is this walling-off process, together with the organization and eventual fibrosis of the areas where the inflammatory exudate has collected, that produces the secondary complications of the chronic phase of the disease. These involve both distortion of normal anatomy, gross and microscopic, as well as the element of chronic infection due to a superimposed, secondary bacterial invasion by organisms other than the gonococcus. The latter usually survives for only a limited time during the acute phase and only rarely is present in the chronic stages of the disease.

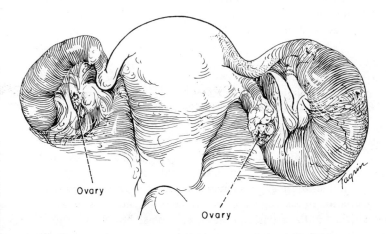

Ovary

Ovary

Figure 33
Typical gross pathologic appearance of the ovary in the chronic phase of gonorrheal pelvic inflammatory disease.

As far as the tubes themselves are concerned, by the time the acute infection has subsided, irreparable damage to the tubal mucosa has often been done, with destruction of the ciliated epithelium and narrowing or occlusion of the lumen. This is produced either by inflammatory fibrosis of the tubal walls, by localized or diffuse organization and fibrosis of the intraluminal exudate, or by peritubal and fimbrial adhesions and blockade — again either as a result of the organized, fibrotic exudate or due to adherence to the neighboring visceral surfaces, which have also become involved by the inflammatory process. Thus, even if some degree of tubal patency remains, tubal function is usually seriously impaired due to mucosal destruction, thickening and rigidity of the wall, and peritubal fixation. More often than not, however, actual tubal occlusion occurs, either at the fimbriated or cornual end or, in many instances, at both ends. (A specific type of chronic, inflammatory fibrosis of the tubal wall, nodular in gross appearance, and restricted to and producing obstruction at the cornual ends of the tubes is commonly referred to as **salpingitis isthmica nodosa**.)

Regardless of the site of block, sterility is inevitable and complete; furthermore, the damaged, obstructed tubes are not only the site of a low-grade, symptomatic, chronic infection but also are extremely susceptible to recurring secondary acute infectious flare-ups. Again, these often develop during or just after a period, when secondary bacterial invaders from the vagina (e.g., *Streptococcus, E. coli*) gain access to the cervix and ascend to the tubes, where a perfect culture medium and a local environment ideal for their further growth awaits them. Such is the pathogenesis of recurring attacks of chronic pelvic inflammatory disease.

If the tubes are blocked at both fimbrial and cornual ends, the accumulating mucus and inflammatory secretions eventually fill and distend the tubes themselves, leading either to a hydrosalpinx or, if the material is or becomes infected, to a pyosalpinx on one or both sides — the "retort tubes," so named because of their gross resemblance to the glass retorts of the chemistry laboratory (Fig. 33). At times, secondary hemorrhage may occur in a hydrosalpinx or pyosalpinx, producing a hematosalpinx.

If, as is sometimes the case, the fimbriated end of a tube and its adjacent ovary have been fused together as part of the "wall" of an artificial abscess cavity, a chronic tuboovarian abscess results and may attain a considerable size (varying from a few centimeters to 30 to 40 cm in diameter); often, the rectosigmoid, uterus, lateral pelvic wall, and loops of small bowel form other portions of the wall of such a chronic tuboovarian abscess. It is likely that the ovary becomes so extensively involved because organisms gain entrance to its deeper substance through the corpus luteum at the time of ovulation, when an actual defect in the serosal barrier is present.

As is already apparent, neighboring viscera may also be distorted by the adhesions that result from organization of the original acute exudate. The uterus is commonly drawn back into the hollow of the pelvis, and the adjacent small bowel (or even more distant loops elsewhere in the abdomen) may become fixed, or kinked, or both, often leading to intestinal obstruction years later. The classic "violin-string" adhesions that form between the upper surface of the liver and the overlying diaphragm are such frequent and characteristic sequelae of the disease as to permit a diagnosis in retrospect whenever they are found at the time of laparotomy for whatever reason.

MANAGEMENT

In a young woman suffering her first or second recurrent attack of chronic gonorrheal pelvic inflammatory disease, a conservative program should again be tried, although the chances of resolution of the disease process with return of normal function in the face of repeated acute attacks and persistently palpable adnexal involvement are increasingly slight. Carefully controlled administration of corticosteroid compounds in conjunction with appropriate antibiotic therapy appears, in some patients at least, to facilitate the resolution of chronic adnexal inflammation and particularly the woody induration of chronic pelvic cellulitis and parametritis that is frequently present. Apparently, the antiinflammatory properties of the corticoids soften and inhibit the excessive fibrous tissue reaction and allow both the normal body defenses and the antibiotic to combat the chronic infection more effectively. Disappearance of symptoms, with marked reduction in the amount of palpable induration and even successful pregnancies, has been reported to follow such a program in some instances.

If the disease fails to respond permanently after one or two attempts at conservative therapy, surgical resection (total hysterectomy and bilateral salpingectomy) is often necessary and advisable as the only means of avoiding continued and increasingly frequent acute flare-ups with repeated hospitalizations, prolonged incapacity, and serious socioeconomic handicaps. If the ovaries are extremely involved by the chronic inflammatory process, they, too, should be excised, or recurrence of symptoms will frequently develop and require reoperation later. If one or both ovaries are totally uninvolved, they can and probably should be preserved in young women, since the risk of future symptoms is then less. Neither simple bilateral salpingo-oophorectomy alone nor hysterectomy alone should ordinarily be done, ever. Actually when procedures less than total hysterectomy with bilateral salpingo-oophorectomy are performed, a calculated risk of recurrent difficulties must be accepted by both patient and physician.

A particularly serious complication of chronic pelvic inflammatory disease is the sudden, spontaneous rupture of a tuboovarian abscess, with massive flooding of the peritoneal cavity with its purulent contents. This acute abdominal emergency is rapidly fatal if not treated surgically, and even when surgical exploration is done, the mortality is high, approaching 50 percent if the correct diagnosis is not made immediately and operation carried out within 12 to 24 hours of the time rupture occurs. Therefore this diagnosis should always be entertained first whenever an acute abdominal disorder develops in a patient with known or suspected chronic pelvic inflammatory disease. Temporizing management, even with massive antibiotic therapy, invariably leads to a fatal outcome; the treatment of choice is a short (6- to 8-hour) course of large intravenous doses of several broad-spectrum antibiotics to cover potential gram-positive, gram-negative, and anaerobic organisms, followed by immediate laparotomy with excision of the tuboovarian abscess and drainage of the peritoneal cavity. This is usually best accomplished by total hysterectomy and bilateral salpingo-oophorectomy, provided laparotomy is done promptly. In situations in which there has been prolonged delay in establishing the correct diagnosis and embarking on surgery, the patient's general condition may have deteriorated to the point where only life-saving salpingo-oophorectomy can be done. (If there is widespread intraperitoneal sepsis, it may be necessary to explore and drain abscesses in various parts of the upper abdominal cavity as well as in the pelvis and lower abdomen.) In such cases, subsequent reoperation and pelvic cleanout will be necessary after recovery from the acute episode. Postoperatively, appropriate chemotherapy and other indicated supportive measures to combat shock and infection should be utilized. Because of the great danger posed by this acute complication of a chronic tuboovarian abscess, earlier elective surgical intervention when this particular type of chronic pelvic inflammatory disease is believed present should be seriously considered.

Occasionally, the inflammatory process will subside completely, but, although no longer the source of repeated flare-ups of active infection, the damaged tubes are functionally impaired, and the patient is infertile because of tubal occlusion or adherent tubes and ovaries. Although tubal malfunction can be demonstrated by Rubin's test and hysterosalpingography, culdoscopy or laparoscopy again provides an even more valuable diagnostic approach. Not only can the presence of chronic pelvic inflammatory disease be definitely confirmed in this way but also the extent and severity of the pathologic process can be accurately evaluated in terms of the chances of success of a trial of conservative management or the indications for some type of corrective surgery. If a sterility investigation of both husband and wife is otherwise normal and satisfactory, and if it is clearly understood that the chance that tuboplasty and mobilization of the adnexa will be successful in restoring fertility is at best 20 percent — perhaps only 5 percent in many instances — this type of attempt at reparative surgery may be suggested to the patient.

Special techniques for salpingostomy (fimbrioplasty), resection and tubal anastomosis, and cornual reimplantation have been developed using polyethylene or other plastic materials as stents and protective hoods and employing antibiotics, hyaluronidase preparations, heparin, and cortisone compounds to promote healing with minimal postoperative adhesions and fibrosis (see Chap. 11).

PUERPERAL AND POSTABORTAL PELVIC INFLAMMATORY DISEASE

Acute postabortal or puerperal pelvic sepsis accounts for 15 to 20 percent of all pelvic inflammatory disease. Acute pelvic sepsis following illegal or even legal abortion is becoming an increasingly serious problem, with mortality running 3 percent or higher, primarily in the group of patients in whom septic shock develops.

For a number of reasons, acute puerperal infections or acute pelvic inflammations associated with or following immediately after criminally induced, infected abortions differ considerably from the acute phases of gonorrheal pelvic inflammation in their course, complications, and clinical manifestations. Furthermore, they are potentially far more serious from the standpoint of their threat to life and require even more careful, vigorous management if extreme morbidity and high mortality are to be avoided. To begin with, the gravid or postpartum uterus and the adjacent pelvic soft tissues are extremely vulnerable to infection, the uterine contents being an excellent medium for the growth and survival of bacteria as a focus of continuing systemic contamination. Furthermore, the placental site, the edematous, congested, highly vascular uterine wall nearby, and the parametrial areas characteristic of the pregnant state offer little in the way of a barrier to bacterial invasion coming by way of both lymphatic and venous channels as well as by direct penetration of tissue planes, so that a diffuse pelvic cellulitis and a generalized septicemia are common. Finally, the nature of the bacteria usually involved has a profound influence on the course of the disease. This type of pelvic sepsis is frequently due to a mixed infection. Formerly, hemolytic streptococci and staphylococci were the chief offenders; today, in roughly two-thirds of these cases, gram-negative bacteria are the predominate organisms (*E. coli, Pseudomonas, Proteus, Klebsiella,* and allied gram-negative enteric pathogens). Occasionally, members of the *Clostridium* group, notably *Cl. welchii* — less often, *Cl. tetani* — may be the principal organisms involved, producing even more local necrosis, sepsis, and overwhelming toxemia. (As noted in the discussion of therapy, proved clostridial infection is an urgent indication for hysterectomy in the management of a septic abortion; less radical treatment in this situation invariably leads to a fatal outcome.)

Since all of the pathogens usually encountered in septic abortions are highly virulent and invasive bacteria, the rapid local invasion and more generalized septic course, in contrast to the more benign inflammatory process and clinical picture of acute gonorrheal pelvic infection, are readily understandable. In addition, the gram-negative organisms, when permitted to propagate undisturbed in degenerating, necrotic uterine contents or in the actual wall of the uterus or adjacent parametrial tissues, may produce and liberate into the general circulation massive quantities of bacterial endotoxin. This flooding of the systemic circulation (gram-negative endotoxemia) with bacterial endotoxins from a septic focus within the uterine cavity, the wall of the uterus, or in the parametrium or pelvic veins (septic thrombophlebitis) may lead to a specific, highly lethal type of circulatory failure, termed **gram-negative endotoxemic shock.** When not promptly recognized and vigorously treated, endotoxemic shock has been associated with a mortality of 50 to 80 percent in the past. With proper early treatment, however, mortality can be kept to 5 percent or less.

Pathogenesis of Septic Shock

The endotoxin present in the cell walls of gram-negative bacilli is a lipopolysaccharide or lipoprotein-carbohydrate complex. When large quantities enter the bloodstream, the most important adverse effect is a generalized intense vasoconstriction, primarily at the microcirculatory level. This leads to a marked increase in peripheral vascular resistance with a corresponding marked decrease in tissue perfusion. The intense vasospasm results in part from a direct effect on the microcapillaries and in part from the release of catecholamines from sympathetic nerve endings and the adrenal medulla, both endotoxin-induced. Even a superficial examination of the patient in the early phases of endotoxemic shock suggests the underlying vasospastic and sympathomimetic effects of endotoxin: there is cutaneous vasoconstriction and increased perspiration, and the patient's skin is pale, cold, and clammy, despite the raging fever that is often present.

The ensuing generalized hemodynamic changes produce a "stagnant anoxia" that results in direct tissue damage as well as a metabolic acidosis due to defective oxygen delivery and metabolism. Ultimately, a hypovolemic state develops because of shunting and pooling of intravascular fluid beyond the constricted portion of the microcirculation (possibly significant pooling occurs in the splanchnic bed also) as well as plasma losses into areas of capillary congestion and local tissue damage. Hypotension soon follows and increases in severity as the metabolic lactacidosis, together with decreasing venous return, begins to impair cardiac function as well. (The increasing impairment of cardiac function may even result in electrocardiographic changes suggestive of acute coronary occlusion.) Increasing hypotension, coupled with the intense vasoconstriction and impaired tissue perfusion, rapidly leads to failing renal function, with oliguria and eventually anuria. The pulmonary microcirculation is equally vulnerable to these endotoxin effects, and the impaired pulmonary oxygenating capacity is often manifested clinically by cyanosis as well as by a striking tachypnea. Ultimately, acute pulmonary edema may appear, the end result of both cardiac and pulmonary failure. The neurotoxic effects of endotoxin, together with the generalized anoxia, are reflected clinically by the appearance of mental confusion and even a semicomatose state in the late stages. Liver damage due to intense vasoconstriction of the hepatic microcirculation may occasionally lead to the appearance of jaundice in the late states. When the gram-negative endotoxemic shock syndrome has entered the irreversible phase, a complete vasomotor collapse with generalized vasodilatation may occur as a preterminal event.

With prolonged duration of endotoxic shock, especially in association with the pregnant state, disseminated intravascular thromboses in the kidneys, liver, lungs, and adrenals are prone to occur (the "generalized Shwartzman reaction"), usually leading to progressive renal, cardiac, liver, and pulmonary failure, irreversible shock, and death. The diffuse intravascular coagulation results from stagnation of blood within the microcirculation, producing intimal damage, fibrin deposition, and an initial hypercoagulability with rapid conversion of fibrinogen to fibrin and generalized thrombosis in the smaller vessels. The most devastating effect of this sequence is the deposition of fibrin in the glomeruli, resulting in acute renal cortical necrosis, irreversible kidney damage, complete anuria, and eventually death in uremia. In addition, the resulting hypofibrinogenemia, depletion of platelets and other clotting factors, and secondary fibrinolysis (generalized fibrinolytic systems are activated when disseminated intravascular thrombosis occurs) may rapidly lead to a state of hypocoagulability and abnormal bleeding of serious proportions, further complicating the clinical management of the desperately ill patient. (It is this predilection for the development of the generalized Shwartzman reaction that increases the risk of death from gram-negative endotoxemic shock in the pregnant patient.)

Septic shock may also accompany overwhelming gram-positive bacterial infection; usually, hemolytic streptococci or staphylococci are the responsible organisms, because they are among the few gram-positive bacteria that produce an exotoxin. Gram-positive toxemic shock is much less common, and the mortality is much lower. The circulatory abnormality is usually one of generalized vasodilatation. Hence the resulting shock is of the normovolemic type, and the patient is warm and flushed in appearance. (As discussed in the following section on diagnosis and management, vasoconstrictor drugs may therefore frequently be indicated in the treatment of gram-positive septic shock, whereas they are rarely beneficial and usually have deleterious effects if employed in the therapy of the much more common gram-negative endotoxemic shock.)

Clinical Features

The clinical course is entirely similar whether the infection follows a septic induced abortion, spontaneous premature rupture of the membranes with resulting chorioamnionitis and placentitis, or normal delivery (postpartum puerperal infection). It is characterized by high fever, rapid pulse, and shaking chills, and the general appearance of the patient is one of extreme toxicity. Examination reveals the typical picture of generalized peritonitis and septicemia; pelvic pain and tenderness are often extreme, and there is usually a purulent discharge from the cervix. In the presence of septic abortion there may be obvious retained placental fragments within the dilated cervical canal, and bleeding may also complicate the picture. The accompanying leukocytosis is usually marked.

Later on there may be a sudden, dramatic change in the picture, often ushered in by shaking chills, or a sudden marked rise in temperature, or both, with the rapid development of vasomotor collapse, profound hypotension, and oliguria, all of which are resistant to the usual therapy and out of all proportion to any blood loss, dehydration, or plasma depletion that may have occurred. In the initial phases of this septic, bacteremic, and gram-negative endotoxemic shock, the patient may remain alert, highly perceptive, and restless, with a feverish, flushed skin and a full, bounding pulse, in spite of marked hypotension. Her appearance at this point is deceptive, however, for within a few hours, or even minutes, she may rapidly become pulseless, have a subnormal temperature with pale, cold, clammy skin, become dyspneic and cyanotic, and exhibit mental confusion. With more prolonged duration of the endotoxemic shock phase, especially if diffuse intravascular thrombosis occurs, the patient may enter a near-moribund, totally anuric, semicomatose state that invariably implies irreversible shock and a fatal outcome. It is therefore essential that the true nature of the situation be clearly recognized and that vigorous, aggressive therapy be begun long before this preterminal phase.

Septic pelvic thrombophlebitis with the development of septic pulmonary infarcts is another complication that may lead to the appearance of a shocklike picture. These events usually occur later on in the course of the disease, however, after the septicemia has subsided and the infection has become localized, so that the danger or likelihood of septic endotoxemic shock has passed. When there is clinical and roentgenologic (chest films) evidence of septic pulmonary infarction, anticoagulant therapy is indicated; if repeated infarcts occur, then vena caval and bilateral ovarian vein ligations will usually prove necessary to prevent a fatal outcome.

Diagnosis and Management

The typical clinical features and the circumstances under which the pelvic infection arose usually render the diagnosis obvious, although other causes of peritonitis must occasionally be considered (e.g., perforated appendicitis). In the case of septic abortion, the physician should not be misled by the patient's refusal to admit that interruption of the pregnancy has been attempted, either by herself or another person, since it is common for patients to deny attempted abortion vigorously. Fever or other evidence of infection in the presence of obvious abortion can and should be accepted as almost prima facie evidence of criminal induction, and vigorous treatment should be instituted forthwith. It is important, if possible, to learn the method and agent (mechanical or chemical) employed to induce the abortion. If a chemical agent has been used (soaps, bleaches, detergents, formalin), the likelihood of extensive uterine necrosis as well as systemic chemical toxicity (hemolysis, renal tubular damage, liver and adrenal injury) is great, and the chances of an associated, serious gram-negative or clostridial infection are also markedly increased. Hence this situation is also one in which prompt hysterectomy is often indicated to prevent an otherwise uniformly fatal outcome.

From the standpoint of diagnosis, one of the most important steps, as soon as feasible, is the specific identification of the offending bacterial organisms, so that the most effective antibiotic can be employed as soon as possible. Immediate gram-stained smears of fresh cervical discharge may sometimes be helpful, particularly in the recognition of the *Cl. welchii* bacillus, which can often be identified by its characteristic capsule. Cultures and sensitivity studies of the cervical discharge and peripheral blood should be initiated immediately; they will ultimately provide the most valuable and reliable guides to antibiotic therapy.

Equally important is an immediately instituted, continuous record of frequent observations (at least every 30 to 60 minutes until the period of acute danger has passed) of the vital signs (blood pressure, pulse, and respirations) and urine output (hourly measurements are indicated at first); for the purpose of the latter, an indwelling Foley catheter is usually essential. This permits a constant appraisal of the patient's condition and response to therapy and will serve to give immediate notice of any sudden change that would indicate the need for reevaluation and alteration of the therapeutic program.

TREATMENT OF SIMPLE, UNCOMPLICATED SEPTIC ABORTION

Fortunately, in most simple, uncomplicated cases of septic abortion seen early (pregnancy of less than three months' duration, no chemical agent used, no occurrence of uterine perforation, absence of clostridial organisms), bacterial invasion of the uterine wall and beyond is either negligible or completely absent. Therefore the key to successful treatment lies in evacuation of the infected uterine contents before significant bacterial spread to the uterus itself can take place. However, this goal is best achieved and morbidity and mortality best avoided by a 6- to 12-hour delay in emptying the uterus (unless continuing severe hemorrhage forces earlier intervention) while appropriate preoperative antibiotic therapy is begun. For broad-spectrum antibiotic coverage, penicillin and chloramphenicol are currently the drugs of choice. To obtain prompt, effective blood levels, penicillin, 10 to 20 million units, and chloramphenicol, 1.0 to 2.0 gm, should be given in a continuous intravenous infusion during the preliminary 6- to 12-hour period, together with blood and fluid replacement as indicated. Thereafter, with both local and systemic control of the infection well under way and the patient preferably afebrile, the uterus should be emptied of all retained infected and necrotic tissue in as gentle and atraumatic a fashion as possible.

Cervical dilatation will ordinarily be unnecessary, and the uterus can usually be emptied manually with the finger or by the use of placental forceps. Unduly vigorous curettage is to be avoided at all costs, lest further systemic dissemination or even uterine perforation result. However, light anesthesia will be necessary, and the uterus should be completely emptied as meticulously as possible by this atraumatic technique, for the whole purpose is to remove all potential foci of infection that might serve as a source for continuing septicemia and gram-negative endotoxemia and ultimately lead to septic shock and a fatal outcome.

In this way the infection can be controlled and eradicated in most instances before it has spread beyond the confines of the uterine cavity, and parametritis, perisalpingitis and perioophoritis, pelvic and generalized peritonitis, pelvic abscesses, and septic pelvic thromboembolic complications, as well as overwhelming septicemia and endotoxemia, can be avoided. Early evacuation of the uterus after a preliminary 6- to 12-hour period of antibiotic therapy and restoration of normal blood volume and fluid and electrolyte balance appear to be the most important factors in reducing mortality and morbidity in dealing with septic abortions, particularly when the patient is seen relatively soon (within 24 hours) after the criminal induction.

TREATMENT OF SEPTIC ABORTION COMPLICATED BY
IMPENDING OR EARLY ENDOTOXEMIC SHOCK

Progression to the extremely dangerous stage of septic abortion occurs in roughly 3 percent of patients and is a medical emergency of the highest order. It usually is the result of long delay by the patient in seeking medical attention or failure on the part of her physician to recognize the existence and serious nature of the potential complications inherent in any septic abortion, premature delivery, or puerperal infection and to anticipate and prevent their development by prompt institution of proper treatment. In the past the mortality has ranged from 30 percent to as high as 80 percent in some reported series.

Once the acute process has progressed to the phase of incipient or early bacteremic shock, first heralded by the appearance of mild hypotension and a relative oliguria (hence the importance of continuous and frequent observations of blood pressure and urinary output throughout the treatment), the following additional measures should be instituted immediately:

Monitoring

A central venous pressure (CVP) catheter should be placed in the superior vena cava via the antecubital or external jugular vein for continuous monitoring of the CVP. This is the best indicator of cardiac status as well as of the **effective circulating** blood volume. (The normal CVP range is 8 to 12 cm H_2O; a CVP of 5 cm or less is indicative of hypovolemia, while a CVP of 15 cm or greater is a sign of circulatory volume overload, or impending cardiac failure, or both.) Frequent, regular observations of the CVP and the hourly or half-hourly urine output (an indwelling Foley catheter should be in place; an hourly urine volume of 25 ml is a reasonable satisfactory minimum), together with regularly recorded vital signs (blood pressure, pulse pressure, pulse, and respirations every 15 to 30 minutes) serve as the most reliable indexes of renal and cardiovascular function as well as circulating blood volume and are also the best guides both to fluid and vasoactive drug therapy. Clinical observations of the state of the peripheral circulation may also prove helpful: peripheral pulses, state of the neck veins, auscultatory chest findings (possible incipient pulmonary edema), and status of cutaneous circulation (patient's skin warm, dry, and flushed, or cold, clammy, and pale, or cyanotic).

Laboratory and Diagnostic Studies

Laboratory and diagnostic studies to be initiated as treatment gets under way include:

1. A complete blood cell count and hematocrit. (These may indicate the need for administering blood or plasma.)

2. Serum electrolytes (Na, K, Cl, CO_2) and blood urea nitrogen. (These will guide fluid and electrolyte replacement as well as correction of the metabolic acidosis frequently present due to the increased anaerobic cellular metabolism accompanying endotoxemic shock.)

3. Cultures (both aerobic and anaerobic) and sensitivity studies on cervical discharge, placental tissue, and peripheral blood if not already done.

4. Gram-stained smears of the cervical discharge if not already done. (These are primarily intended for the immediate identification of *Clostridia,* if present, but sometimes help to distinguish between the more frequent predominantly gram-negative and the less common primarily gram-positive mixed infections.)

5. X-ray studies: Abdominal scout film (KUB) to detect foreign bodies or free peritoneal air, indicating uterine perforation; chest films, in search of signs of septic pulmonary emboli.

6. Confirmatory cul-de-sac aspiration may be indicated if the findings on vaginal and rectal examinations raise the suspicion of a pelvic abscess.

Rapid Institution of Massive Intravenous Antibiotic Therapy
Rapid institution of massive intravenous antibiotic therapy is best done intermittently rather than continuously, giving one-fourth of the total 24-hour dose of each agent every 6 hours in a 300- to 500-ml infusion of 5% D/W run in over a period of 2 to 3 hours. Such an intermittent ("piggyback") intravenous antibiotic program achieves effective blood levels and helps to avoid the problem of fluid overload in the presence of impaired cardiovascular function and oliguria. Initial antibiotic programs of choice, pending the results of culture-sensitivity studies of the specific organisms present in the individual case, are:

1. Penicillin, 40 to 60 million units (total 24-hour dosage), in combination with chloramphenicol, 3.0 to 6.0 gm (total 24-hour dosage), both given by the intermittent intravenous infusion technique. This can be supplemented by streptomycin, 250 to 500 mg given intramuscularly every 6 hours. Crystalline sodium penicillin G should be used, avoiding potassium penicillin G in these often oliguric patients. If the patient is allergic to penicillin, large doses of cephalexin monohydrate (Keflex) can be used instead.

2. If the urine output is satisfactory, 250 mg of kanamycin (Kantrex) can be given intramuscularly every 6 hours in place of chloramphenicol and streptomycin. Kanamycin is particularly effective in *Proteus* infections, but the *Pseudomonas* organism has proved to be resistant to it. Furthermore, it is nephrotoxic (the dosage should never exceed 1 gm daily even under ideal circumstances), so that its use is probably best avoided, particularly if oliguria is present.

3. A shift to another antibiotic program may be indicated if a favorable clinical response is not obtained or if sensitivity studies reveal the organisms to be more sensitive to other agents. One of the newer antibiotics, gentamicin sulfate (Garamycin) administered intramuscularly or intravenously (60 to 80 mg every 8 hours), may prove extremely useful, because it is active against both *Pseudomonas* and *Proteus* as well as against virtually all other gram-negative pathogens including *E. coli* and *Klebsiella-Aerobacter* species. However, it, too, has potential nephrotoxicity as well as ototoxicity (hence it should never be used in combination with kanamycin, streptomycin, polymyxin, or colistin) and should be employed with caution in the presence of oliguria and impaired renal function and then only if the infection has failed to respond to the usual agents. If sensitivity studies indicate that a favorable response can be expected, tetracycline can be safely used intravenously in a total daily dosage of 2 gm, even in the presence of impaired renal function. Other antibiotics known to be effective against gram-negative organisms (e.g., ampicillin, colistin, neomycin, polymyxin, paromomycin) may be indicated by sensitivity studies in individual cases. If *Bacteroides* organisms (*B. fragilis* is the most common anaerobe in this group) are detected, or if their presence is suspected on the basis of delayed clinical response or a particularly foul-smelling, effusive purulent drainage, chloramphenicol or clindamycin should definitely be administered,

since they appear to be the most effective antibiotics against these anaerobic species, with tetracycline and lincomycin somewhat less so.

A booster dose of tetanus toxoid and/or tetanus antitoxin (100,000 units) should also be given, and if clostridial infection has been proved or is suspected, polyvalent gas gangrene antitoxin (100,000 units) should probably also be given intravenously, although its value is questionable.

In the initial phases of antibiotic therapy one must be on the alert for a possible increase in the severity of signs and symptoms of septic shock that may follow the rapid lysis of gram-negative organisms with release of more endotoxin.

Intravenous Fluid Therapy

Electrolyte and fluid replacement should include sodium bicarbonate solutions and should preferably be lactate-free (Ringer's solution with added sodium bicarbonate is probably ideal) to correct more effectively the metabolic lactoacidosis (the end result of the anaerobic cellular metabolism induced by stagnant anoxia in the micro-circulation); correction of dehydration also helps by reducing the abnormally elevated viscosity of the blood pooling in the constricted microcapillaries. Plasma may be needed to restore a normal circulating extracellular fluid volume, because the previously discussed generalized plasma losses occurring in the early endotoxemic shock phase may be large. Some advocate the use of dextran 40 as a volume expander because of its potential beneficial attribute of lowering blood viscosity. Whole blood is less often indicated because it may further aggravate the problem of increased blood viscosity, but it may be needed if there have been external blood losses as a result of continued uterine bleeding. The best guides to the total volume as well as to the rate of fluid replacement will be the CVP, hourly urine output, and hematocrit, together with the regular blood pressure and pulse observations. It is important to avoid overloading the circulation. On the other hand, it is necessary at times to increase the rate of fluid replacement, especially if vasodilator drugs are employed, as discussed in the next section.

Specific Drug Therapy in Support of the Circulation

Before administering the vasoactive drugs as described in this section, restoration of circulating blood volume and correction of acidosis should be well under way or nearly complete.

1. **Corticosteroids** should be given in so-called pharmacologic doses to all patients, regardless of the degree of hypotension and oliguria. They are not given for their usual physiologic effects, because there is no evidence that an adrenal insufficiency per se develops during septic shock. In large doses, however, corticosteroids have an effect resembling that of alpha adrenergic blocking agents in that they diminish vasospasm and thus tend to reverse the abnormal circulatory dynamics in endo-toxemic shock by decreasing peripheral vascular resistance and increasing cardiac output. There is also evidence that corticosteroids exert a direct protective effect against endotoxin at the cellular level, possibly preventing damage to the cell mem-

brane and thus avoiding increased capillary membrane permeability. Finally, it is also possible that corticosteroids provide specific protection against the development of bacterial hypersensitivity and subsequent anaphylactic reaction after the sudden release of endotoxic antigen triggered by the antibiotic treatment of the bacteremia.

Intravenous hydrocortisone, 1 gm, or its equivalent (e.g., Solu-Medrol, 250 mg every 4 to 6 hours), is given immediately, and depending on the clinical response, the same dose may have to be repeated in a few hours. A daily dosage of 2.0 to 5.0 gm may be necessary for as long as five days in some patients.

2. When hypotension and oliguria persist after a few hours of the previously outlined therapeutic program, trial of a **vasoactive drug** is indicated. The question as to whether vasoconstrictor or vasodilator drugs should be used was at one time highly controversial and the subject of heated debate. Because there may be alternating periods of vasoconstriction and vasodilatation in the early phases of endotoxemic shock, both may be useful in individual cases. Nevertheless, since the fundamental and ultimately the principal deleterious effect of endotoxin is widespread vasospasm, and the typical patient is cold and clammy despite an adequate CVP and increasing hypotension, a **vasodilator** is usually the agent of choice:

Isoproterenol (Isuprel) has both a vasodilating and cardiac stimulant action, thus increasing tissue perfusion as well as tending to elevate cardiac output and blood pressure. It therefore would seem to be ideal for correcting the hemodynamic alterations of endotoxemic shock and far more appropriate than a vasoconstrictor drug in the cold, clammy, hypotensive, oliguric patient in whom intense vasoconstriction is obviously already present. It is administered intravenously in a solution of 2.5 to 5.0 mg of isoproterenol dissolved in 500 ml of 5% D/W, adjusting the rate of infusion at 0.5 to 1.0 ml per minute, depending on the response as evaluated by the effects on blood pressure, urine output, CVP, and general condition of the patient. If necessary, either the concentration or the rate of flow may be doubled. When vasodilators are used, the CVP must be watched closely, a significant decrease indicating that fluid replacement with blood, plasma, and electrolyte solution has been inadequate and that the volume and rate of fluid therapy will need to be increased. It is also important to watch for the possible development of significant tachycardia or cardiac arrhythmias with isoproterenol because of its positive inotropic effect on the myocardium. A heart rate of 120 beats per minute or more or the appearance of a cardiac arrhythmia (in both cases cardiac output will decrease rather than increase) contraindicates the initial or continued use of isoproterenol. In this situation, other vasodilating drugs should be used instead: e.g., intravenous chlorpromazine (Thorazine), 5 mg or 10 to 15 mg if necessary, given at intervals, in accordance with the effects on the CVP and skin temperature; or phenoxybenzamine (Dibenzyline), 1 mg per kilogram of body weight, also given intravenously at intervals, depending on the response.

Much less often in gram-negative septic shock, but fairly characteristically in the occasional patient with gram-positive bacterial shock, the clinical picture (hypotension, low CVP, adequate urine output, warm and dry skin) will suggest a generalized decrease in vascular tone, and a **vasoconstrictor** may be tried instead.

Metaraminol bitartrate (Aramine) affects both the myocardium and peripheral arterioles directly, producing an elevation of both systolic and diastolic blood pressure and increasing the blood flow through the cerebral, renal, and coronary vasculature. It is administered intravenously in a solution of 100 mg dissolved in 1000 ml of 5% D/W at a rate of roughly 20 mg per hour, adjusting this as necessary to maintain the systolic blood pressure in the 90 to 100 mm Hg range. If the amount of drug required increases, if the CVP rises abnormally, or if oliguria develops, a prompt switch to a vasodilator is indicated.

3. General cardiovascular (and pulmonary) supportive measures include oxygen therapy (and endotracheal intubation or tracheotomy if maintenance of an adequate airway is in doubt), and rapid digitalization if the CVP rises above 15 cm H_2O or if signs of congestive failure appear.

Removal of the Source of Infection

The previously enumerated measures in support of the circulation in shock, together with massive antibiotic therapy of the systemic infection, are all important, but eradication of the source of the continuing infection is ultimately the keystone of successful treatment.

In the majority of cases this can be accomplished by careful and complete evacuation of the uterus. In the presence of endotoxemic shock, this should be done reasonably soon after the preceding supportive measures have been taken, usually within 4 to 6 hours. (As will be noted, an exception to this plan should be made in the presence of clostridial infection, in which case hysterectomy without a preliminary D&C is indicated.) Occasionally, if the pregnancy is of three to four months' duration, the D&C can be facilitated by administering oxytocics beforehand to aid in evacuating the uterus. Oxytocics should be used cautiously, however, for there is some evidence that the resulting increase in uterine contractions may, in the presence of significant myometrial necrosis and/or infection, lead to flooding of the circulation with large numbers of bacteria and additional endotoxin. If effective support of the circulation and adequate antibiotic therapy have been given preoperatively and are continued as long as necessary postoperatively, the favorable clinical response after removal of all retained necrotic and infected uterine contents by a D&C is often dramatic.

However, in roughly 10 percent of cases, the infection will have spread beyond the confines of the uterine cavity and its contents, and a D&C will not adequately deal with the local source of infection. This situation should be recognized as early as possible, because an aggressive approach involving emergency hysterectomy may be the only hope of saving life. As the patients are usually young women in whom preservation of childbearing function, if possible, is often a vital concern, and because the majority will recover on a proper medical program in combination with early evacuation of the uterus, the decision as to whether or not hysterectomy will be necessary to save life, and precisely when in the course of the disease this decision should be made and the operation performed, is always a difficult one. In the presence of endotoxemic shock, hysterectomy is nearly always indicated under the following circumstances:

1. *Clostridium perfringens* infection. Although clostridial organisms are responsible for only 1 to 2 percent of all septic abortions (3 to 5 percent of those involving gram-negative bacteria), the infection is highly lethal unless promptly and properly treated, in which case the mortality can be held to 5 to 10 percent or lower. These anaerobic organisms produce tissue-necrotizing and hemolyzing toxins, as well as large amounts of hyalouronidase, which permits rapid tissue invasion, and a copious amount of gas that permeates the tissues and is characteristic of these "gas gangrene" infections. As emphasized by Decker and Hall [7], clostridial infection can often be suspected on the basis of the following clinical picture: extreme toxicity, high fever, rapid pulse, and marked leukocytosis; a very tender, boggy uterus; occasionally, palpable soft-tissue crepitus or x-ray evidence of gas in the tissues; early oliguria; occasionally, hemoglobinuria, hemoglobinemia, and jaundice due to hemolysis; and a strikingly euphoric, placid appearance of the patient despite her grave condition. The diagnosis can be rapidly established by gram-stained smear of the purulent discharge taken directly from the cervix, revealing large gram-positive encapsulated rods; there should be no delay for confirmation by culture. Prompt hysterectomy with bilateral salpingo-oophorectomy, *without* a preliminary D&C, should be done; if an attempt at medical management supplemented by D&C alone is made, mortality approaches 100 percent.

2. History of induction of abortion, by corrosive, chemical, or toxic douches (formalin, soaps, Lysol, detergents, bleaches). Uterine necrosis with secondary infection of the uterine wall is invariably present, so that simple evacuation of the uterus cannot possibly eradicate the septic focus. The overwhelming infection and chemical injury that almost invariably accompany septic abortions induced by chemical solutions should usually be treated in the same fashion as a clostridial infection (i.e., by adequate initial medical therapy followed by prompt hysterectomy) if the almost universally fatal course that otherwise usually follows in this situation is to be prevented. Only occasionally will conservative management by intensive antibiotic therapy and simple evacuation of the uterus suffice and permit hysterectomy to be avoided. If an initial conservative approach is adopted, the patient must be followed extremely closely and carefully, so that hysterectomy can be done immediately at the first sign of deterioration of her condition.

3. Evidence of intraabdominal foreign body, uterine perforation, pelvic abscess. (Cul-de-sac aspiration will yield pus under these circumstances.)

4. Uterus larger than three to four months' size. Here again, a D&C is usually inadequate to the task of completely eliminating the source of the infection, which is vital to prevent mortality in the face of established endotoxemic shock.

5. Palpable adnexal abscess (also indicating clearly that sepsis has spread beyond the uterine cavity).

6. Assuming that adequate preliminary supportive therapy has been given, additional indications for prompt hysterectomy are as follows: (1) failure of the patient to improve within 4 to 6 hours after a D&C; (2) sudden deterioration of the patient's condition during or immediately following a D&C; (3) the finding of little or no retained products of conception at the time of curettage; or (4) progressive oliguria.

In other, less specific situations, only constant, close supervision of the patient's course and response to medical therapy as indicated by changes in the vital signs, the local findings, the urine output, and so on, will enable the physician to make the timely decision that hysterectomy is indicated as an emergency lifesaving measure. It is extremely important to make the decision and act on it promptly (preferably within 6 to 12 hours of the onset of shock) before the preterminal stage of irreversible shock has developed. As is so often the case in medicine, there is no substitute for experience and sound judgment in arriving at the correct choice of management in critical situations, and each case must be considered individually.

Hysterectomy should nearly always be accompanied by bilateral salpingo-oophorectomy, since microabscesses of the ovaries are often present despite a normal external appearance.

Prophylactic vena caval ligation and high ligation of both ovarian veins should also be considered at the time the hysterectomy is performed and should definitely be done if recurrent septic pulmonary embolism has already occurred. Ovarian vein and vena caval ligations, not anticoagulants, represent the treatment of choice for septic thrombophlebitis in this situation.

Other Supportive Measures

Other supportive measures include the following:

1. Hypothermia (reduction of body temperature to as low as 90°F) has been employed by some, partly to control the frequent raging fever (103° to 105°F is not uncommon in the early stages of septic shock) but primarily to reduce tissue oxygen requirements in the face of prolonged hypotension in a desperately ill patient. Hyperbaric oxygen chambers have also been utilized by some for this same purpose.

2. Hemodialysis may be indicated and may have to be repeated several times during the recovery period in patients who have experienced acute temporary renal failure and who may be essentially anuric for as long as 7 to 10 days.

Prevention or Treatment of Disseminated Intravascular Coagulation

Although the generalized Shwartzman reaction with the formation of diffuse intravascular thrombi throughout the microcirculation can be one of the most serious, life-threatening complications of endotoxemic shock, whether or not prophylactic therapy should be given remains controversial. Intravenous heparin would be the appropriate drug, given in a dosage of 60 mg every 6 hours to maintain the clotting time at roughly twice normal until the infection is completely controlled. However, where there is definite evidence that disseminated intravascular coagulation (DIC) is occurring, there is no question but that heparin therapy should be instituted promptly and may prove lifesaving.

Clinically, the first manifestation of DIC may be the appearance of an abnormal bleeding tendency (the so-called consumption coagulopathy). The onset of DIC can also be recognized by simple laboratory tests, since it is accompanied by an obvious fall in platelet count and serum fibrinogen level and an increase in both prothrombin and partial thromboplastin times. Examination of a thin blood smear is very helpful not only in estimating the platelet count but also in finding malformed red cells ("helmet cells," "comma cells," and "burr cells," misshapen because they have been stripped away from partially thrombosed capillary walls), which are essentially diagnostic of DIC.

Heparin can either be given by continuous intravenous infusion, 8 to 12 mg per hour, or intermittently in a dosage of 50 to 100 mg every 4 to 6 hours. It prevents further progress of the intravascular coagulation process, and only occasionally is it necessary to give platelet transfusions, fibrinogen, and fresh frozen plasma or whole blood, since both platelets and fibrinogen as well as other depleted coagulation factors (e.g., V, VIII) are rapidly replaced once the pathologic clotting process is halted. In any case, heparin should definitely be administered first, and unless a severe hemorrhagic problem is encountered, platelets should be given only if the platelet count remains depressed for more than 12 hours and fibrinogen replacement considered only if the fibrinogen level persists at less than 100 mg per 100 ml. Although secondary fibrinolysis usually occurs in the presence of DIC, in this situation it is a valuable protective mechanism that, it is hoped, will result in widespread lysis of the potentially lethal thrombi, especially those in the renal capillaries. Therefore the use of antifibrinolytic drugs such as aminocaproic acid is definitely contraindicated, because DIC is not a primary fibrinolytic disorder, and it is highly undesirable and inadvisable to inhibit this beneficial secondary lysis of thrombi already present in the microcirculation.

Chronic Postabortal or Puerperal Pelvic Inflammatory Disease

The course and features of the chronic phase and the principles of management in chronic postabortal or puerperal pelvic inflammatory disease are in general similar to those in chronic pelvic inflammation following gonorrheal salpingitis. However, because of the deeply invasive propensities of the usual original causative bacterial organisms, a chronic woody, or "ligneous," pelvic cellulitis and parametritis are frequently encountered, with the result that the uterus and adnexa are literally frozen in place by the extensive chronic inflammatory reaction and fibrosis that surround them. On the other hand, pyosalpinx, hydrosalpinx, and tuboovarian abscess are somewhat less common, since the initial acute adnexal infection is usually in the nature of a perisalpingitis and perioophoritis, and the resulting peritonitis, though intense, is not accompanied by the profuse, thick exudate so characteristic of acute gonorrheal salpingitis, the latter being primarily an ascending, surface infection of the tubal endothelium.

TUBERCULOUS PELVIC INFLAMMATION

Tuberculous salpingitis, with or without an accompanying secondary involvement of the endometrium, constitutes 5 to 10 percent of the total of all types of pelvic inflammatory disease. Between 40 and 50 percent of patients suffering from pelvic tuberculosis are asymptomatic except for "unexplained" infertility. (Tuberculosis is found to be responsible for approximately 5 percent of all cases of female infertility in the United States. In other areas of the world, the percentages are higher [e.g., India, 20 percent; Europe, 10 percent].) The remaining 50 to 60 percent of patients have one or more of the following symptoms and signs: pelvic and abdominal pain and dysmenorrhea; a low-grade fever; fatigue and weight loss; occasional menstrual irregularity (less common than with other forms of chronic pelvic inflammation); slightly tender adnexal masses; and, rarely, ascites secondary to tuberculous peritonitis, or ulcerations and sinus tracts involving the external genitalia. The tuberculin skin test is usually strongly positive.

Pathologic Features

The fallopian tubes are the primary site of pelvic tuberculosis in all cases, the disease is nearly always bilateral, and spontaneous healing is rare. The endometrium is only involved secondarily, and endometrial tuberculosis (tuberculous endometritis) occurs in less than half the patients with tuberculous salpingitis and associated pelvic inflammatory disease. The tubal lesion always develops as the result of spread via the bloodstream from a primary focus elsewhere, usually the lung. In this respect, tuberculosis of the reproductive tract is entirely similar to urinary tract tuberculosis, which is also invariably a blood-borne infection; not infrequently, both develop in the same patient.

In the early phases of the disease the tubes may appear grossly normal, or only slightly injected and imperceptibly swollen and edematous, even though definite histologic evidence of tuberculosis is already present and smears and cultures will readily reveal the presence of acid-fast bacilli. It is this deceptively normal gross appearance in the early stages and the lack of symptoms, even when moderately advanced lesions are present, that often makes the disease difficult to recognize. However, even in the early, microscopic stage, infertility may already have resulted due to the mucosal damage and impaired tubal function. In fact, in well over half the cases it is the complaint of sterility that prompts the patient to seek medical advice and ultimately leads to establishing the presence of pelvic tuberculosis. The occasional occurrence of ectopic pregnancy is probably also a complication of minimal, early disease, or of disease arrested by therapy, for in either case tubal function is often impaired.

As the pathologic process advances, the typical gross lesions of tuberculosis make their appearance, and the tubes often become filled with and distended by caseous material, resembling the "retort tubes" of chronic gonorrheal salpingitis with pyosalpinx. Peritubal adhesions, which are characteristically dense, form and encase the tube and ovary together in a solid mass of fibrocaseous reaction. The tubal fimbriae become agglutinated, and eventually complete fimbrial occlusion occurs. Often, tubercles are visible on the serosal surfaces of the tubes as well as on the adjacent parietal and cul-de-sac peritoneum, rectosigmoid, and nearby loops of ileum; adhesions between these structures and the adnexa may also form.

Occasionally, in advanced pelvic tuberculosis, before tubal occlusion has occurred, the outpouring of caseous exudate may result in a generalized tuberculous peritonitis, with both tubercles and intense serosal inflammation present over a widespread area of the general peritoneal cavity. There is often an accompanying ascites, the peritoneal fluid having a characteristic "ground-glass" appearance and yielding a positive diagnostic result when submitted for culture and guinea pig inoculations.

A similar discharge of infected material into the endometrial cavity is presumably the cause of the usually superficial infection of the endometrium that is present in less than half the cases.

The ovaries are involved in 10 to 15 percent of cases, and this, together with the debilitating systemic effects of the infection, may lead to menstrual irregularities and amenorrhea.

Although fortunately rare, one of the most serious complications of the disease is the occurrence of pregnancy in untreated patients, for the possibility of acute, fatal miliary dissemination is great, occurring in approximately one-third of such patients.

Diagnosis and Evaluation

In patients with minimal pelvic tuberculosis who are asymptomatic except for infertility and who have essentially negative pelvic examinations, the diagnosis may be suggested unexpectedly by the findings on hysterosalpingography, at culdoscopy, or on a routine endometrial biopsy (typical tubercles noted on microscopic examination), all of which are procedures frequently done during the course of a routine sterility investigation. Diagnosis can and should be confirmed by bacteriologic studies performed on menstrual discharge (acid-fast-stained smear, tuberculosis cultures, and guinea pig inoculations).

In patients with a suggestive history, as well as with positive physical findings (e.g., tuboovarian masses), or in other words, **advanced pelvic tuberculosis,** the diagnosis can be made and confirmed by any or all of the preceding studies. If the diagnosis is suspected, curettage or hysterosalpingography should be avoided, since an acute flare-up of the usually low-grade tuberculous salpingitis frequently occurs following either procedure and is due to secondary pyogenic bacterial invasion.

All patients should have chest roentgenograms and sputum cultures and smears (pelvic tuberculosis invariably is the result of blood-borne spread from a primary pulmonary focus, usually currently inactive), as well as an intravenous pyelogram, cystoscopy, and acid-fast smears, cultures, and guinea pig studies of the urine, to rule out concomitant tuberculosis of the urinary tract.

Treatment

MINIMAL PELVIC TUBERCULOSIS

In addition to assurance of adequate diet and rest and the initiation of other general health measures, specific chemotherapy for tuberculosis should be given: isoniazid,

100 mg orally three times daily for 12 months, with dihydrostreptomycin, 1 gm intramuscularly twice weekly for three to six months. It is important to use two or more antituberculosis drugs or antibiotics because of the frequency and rapidity with which drug-resistant strains develop when only one chemotherapeutic agent is employed. There should be a careful and prolonged follow-up period with premenstrual endometrial biopsies and menstrual cultures at intervals of four to six months for several years following cessation of treatment. Complete, permanent cures and occasionally even normal pregnancies and deliveries have been reported following the use of this type of program in women with minimal disease. The chances for restoration of fertility are in reality poor, however, because even though the infection may be completely arrested and tubal patency maintained, impairment of tubal function is often unrelieved and ovum pickup and transfer remain unsatisfactory. For this reason the incidence of subsequent tubal pregnancy has also been high.

If the disease recurs at any time, as indicated by positive menstrual cultures or endometrial biopsies or by the development of clinical symptoms or palpable adnexal disease, the patient should receive another course of chemotherapy followed by surgical removal of the uterus, tubes, and ovaries, for the process has now reached the stage of advanced disease. Today, with adequate and specific systemic chemotherapy available, hysterectomy and bilateral salpingo-oophorectomy are necessary in only about 20 percent of patients, provided the disease is discovered and drug treatment instituted in the early phases.

ADVANCED PELVIC TUBERCULOSIS

In advanced pelvic tuberculosis, the institution of general measures, including bed rest, are even more important than in the earlier phases. Specific chemotherapy, as follows, is indicated for even longer periods: isoniazid, 100 mg by mouth, three times daily for 12 to 18 months, with dihydrostreptomycin, 1 gm intramuscularly two to three times weekly (or if there is sensitivity to streptomycin, aminosalicylic acid [PAS], 3 gm four times daily) for 6 to 12 months. The course of treatment should be longer if a pronounced systemic reaction (e.g., fever, weight loss) was present initially. Adnexal masses may become temporarily smaller, though they rarely disappear, but the patient usually shows a favorable general response. At the end of this time, total hysterectomy and bilateral salpingo-oophorectomy are carried out, and then the antituberculosis chemotherapy is continued postoperatively for another 9 to 12 months.

The diagnosis of pelvic tuberculosis is sometimes first made at laparotomy. When this occurs, total hysterectomy with bilateral salpingo-oophorectomy should be done, if feasible, and the operation followed by chemotherapy for 9 to 12 months. Occasionally, the diagnosis is totally unsuspected even at laparotomy and is not apparent until after histologic examination of part or all of the pelvic organs resected for what was believed to be chronic pelvic inflammatory disease of gonococcal or postabortal origin. If the operation was a complete one (total hysterectomy and bilateral salpingo-oophorectomy), postoperative chemotherapy should be given according to the preceding schedule. If the operation was incomplete, the patient should have specific chemotherapy for three to four months and then reoperation with removal of the remaining potentially involved pelvic structures.

OTHER CAUSES OF SALPINGITIS AND PELVIC INFLAMMATORY DISEASE

Nonspecific Infections

Although considerably less common than the infections discussed thus far, nonspecific pelvic infections sometimes occur and may be caused by other pyogenic organisms (e.g., streptococcus, staphylococcus) or by the mixed bacterial flora present in the vagina and anogenital region. The organisms may ascend superficially through the endometrial cavity to produce an endometritis, salpingitis, and pelvic peritonitis. Or they may gain direct access to the deeper parametrial areas by invading venous and lymphatic channels in the wall of the cervix or fundus to produce a diffuse pelvic cellulitis and, ultimately, often a peritonitis, perisalpingitis, and perioophoritis. These nonspecific pyogenic infections are invariably secondary to some form of local trauma, either acute or chronic, that disturbs the normal barrier or resistance of the vaginal mucosa and endocervix to ascending or invasive infection. Circumstances under which this may occur include the following:

1. **Operative trauma**, e.g., curettage, cervical biopsy or cauterization, and various local diagnostic or therapeutic procedures such as endometrial biopsy, a Rubin's test, and hysterosalpingography; fortunately, such complications are rare. (Pelvic sepsis following major pelvic surgery is discussed in Chapter 21.)
2. **Abnormal uterine drainage situations**, with retained secretions acting as a nidus for ascending infection, e.g., cervical stenosis, usually secondary to previous surgery or improper cauterization, or congenital anomalies of the uterus, particularly the various duplications.
3. **Trauma and chronic infection** associated with the old-fashioned cervical contraceptive stem pessary, less often in connection with improperly fitted or neglected vaginal pessaries.
4. **Improper (high-pressure) douching,** particularly if chemically irritating solutions are used.
5. **Infected tumors**, e.g., cervical or endometrial carcinoma, carcinosarcoma of the uterus, necrotic polyps, or fibroids.

The course and symptomatology of these nonspecific pyogenic infections are much the same as are encountered in postabortal pelvic inflammatory disease, although in the absence of pregnancy the process is more likely to be mild, and fulminating septicemia and toxemia are only rarely encountered. Conservative treatment with antibiotics and general supportive measures will usually rapidly bring these secondary infections under control, although occasionally they will progress to the formation of a pelvic abscess requiring drainage. Even rarer causes of acute or chronic salpingitis and associated diffuse pelvic inflammation and peritonitis include infection with the typhoid-paratyphoid group of organisms, actinomycosis, and parasitic infestations such as *Enterobius vermicularis* (pinworms) and schistosomiasis (common in Caribbean waters as well as in Egypt and South Africa).

Intrauterine Contraceptive Devices

Intrauterine contraceptive devices are now widely employed, and their use has been accompanied by the occurrence of acute and chronic pelvic inflammatory disease (endometritis, salpingitis, parametritis, and pelvic peritonitis) in a significant number of patients. The usual pyogenic organisms are the ones commonly involved, but, interestingly enough, a few cases of actinomycosis infections occurring in association with intrauterine devices have also been reported.

Pelvic and Ovarian Vein Thrombophlebitis

Pelvic and ovarian vein thrombophlebitis should also be mentioned, not only as inflammatory disorders in their own right but also because they tend to simulate pelvic or lower abdominal inflammatory processes of a purely infectious type. Flagrant septic pelvic thrombophlebitis with or without septic embolization may occur as a complication of any of the acute pelvic infections previously described and is usually easily recognized, especially if pulmonary emboli occur. Such a septic thrombophlebitis should be treated with both antibiotics and anticoagulants, together with eradication of the primary septic focus within the pelvis, and usually by ovarian vein and vena caval ligations as well, especially if septic emboli are occurring. However, a more benign type of pelvic phlebitis may develop in a postpartum or postoperative gynecologic patient and present diagnostic difficulties. Pelvic pain and a febrile course with absence of any positive findings other than tenderness on physical examination are characteristic and suggest low-grade pelvic inflammatory disease. The sudden occurrence of a small pulmonary infarct may be the first clue to the real nature of the pelvic disorder. In the case of ovarian vein thrombophlebitis, which also occurs most frequently in postpartum patients (presumably because of the pelvic venous stasis and hypercoagulability present at term), the pain is unilateral and most often in the right lower quadrant (the venous flow on the right is often antegrade, hence more prone to stasis, whereas it is always retrograde in the left ovarian vein), thus frequently raising the question of appendicitis or twisted ovarian cyst. If thrombosis of the ovarian veins is extensive, the dilated mass of clotted veins and the swollen ovary, congested by venous obstruction, may present as a palpable, ropelike, tender pelvic or lower abdominal mass.

In spite of the febrile course and occasionally positive blood cultures, antibiotic therapy invariably has no effect on the clinical course of the disease. However, if the diagnosis is suspected on the basis of the typical sequence of events, and there is no obvious indication for exploratory laparotomy, institution of anticoagulant therapy will usually produce a prompt response, with disappearance of pain, fever, and leukocytosis in a few days. Frequently, laparotomy does prove necessary before a definite diagnosis can be established, particularly in the case of ovarian vein thrombophlebitis. In this situation, the thrombosed veins should be resected, preserving the adnexa when possible but otherwise carrying out unilateral salpingo-oophorectomy; anticoagulant therapy is then given postoperatively. If an episode of embolization occurs, anticoagulation should be instituted and maintained for an adequate length of time. If there are recurring small pulmonary infarcts, ligation or plication of the inferior vena cava, as well as bilateral high ovarian vein ligation, is indicated.

OTHER VENEREAL DISEASES

In addition to gonorrhea, there are four other major specific venereal infections involving the reproductive tract: syphilis, chancroid, lymphogranuloma (lymphopathia) venereum, and granuloma inguinale. Several minor diseases of the lower genital tract, including trichomoniasis, condyloma acuminatum, herpes progenitalis, *Hemophilus vaginalis* infections, and several others, are also of venereal origin, and some even feel that pediculosis pubis should be considered a venereally transmitted disorder. (These minor venereal diseases are discussed in Chapter 7.) The various venereal diseases will be considered only briefly, since they are less frequently encountered nowadays, and the major ones, with the exception of gonorrhea, are not customarily treated by the gynecologist. However, from the standpoint of the differential diagnostic problems they sometimes pose, as well as the importance of their prompt recognition and, if indicated, referral for treatment, it is well to have the basic facts concerning them clearly in mind.

Syphilis

Infection with the spirochetal organism *Treponema pallidum* invariably occurs by direct genital (occasionally by oral-genital) contact with an actively infected sexual partner. Rarely, accidental direct bloodstream infection can occur following transfusion with blood from an infected donor (hence the vital necessity for routine serologic tests for syphilis in all prospective blood donors); or, in the female only, the disease is occasionally transmitted through impregnation by a male in the tertiary phase of the disease, the maternal bloodstream ultimately becoming infected via the fetal-placental-maternal circulatory pathways. (The child of such a union will frequently be born with congenital syphilis.) For some years, syphilis was erroneously believed to be declining in incidence and importance. That such is unfortunately not the case was revealed by a 1970 national survey indicating that 1 out of every 81 marriage applicants and 1 out of every 99 pregnant women had a positive blood test for syphilis.

The reproductive tract is involved for the most part only during the initial or primary stage of the disease, serving essentially as the portal of entry. Thereafter, and following the brief secondary phase, the very prolonged (usually lifelong, unless discovered and successfully treated) tertiary stage of the disease is a generalized systemic infection that may be latent or silent or have widespread and highly protean manifestations throughout the body.

In the female the primary lesion is a chancre, which appears three or four weeks after exposure and most often is located on the labia majora. It may also develop elsewhere on the external genitalia or occasionally on the cervix, where it often resembles a simple "erosion" and frequently passes completely unnoticed. Even the vulvar lesions may be tiny, presenting only as small "abrasions" or superficial erosions or fissures that easily escape detection or go unrecognized. The classic lesion, however, is a deeper ulceration surrounded by a painless zone of induration. A few weeks later, a nontender, nonsuppurating, rubbery-firm inguinal lymphadenopathy appears and is usually bilateral. In addition to the primary chancre and associated lymphadenopathy, other symptoms and signs include a leukorrheal discharge and abnormal bleeding, particularly if the cervix is involved, and moist, ulcerating, coalescing, papular lesions of the vulva and adjacent skin of the perineum and thighs, the condylomata lata, which are probably manifestations of the secondary stage. Tertiary lesions of the reproductive tract are uncommon, although gummas of the cervix have been reported.

DIAGNOSIS

Recognition of syphilis in the acute early primary stage is accomplished by dark-field examination of the clear serum that can be expressed from the ulcerated surface of the lesion, with direct microscopic visualization of the spirochetes. The organisms can usually also be identified in the discharge from condylomata lata, and biopsy excision of a condyloma can also be done and a histologic diagnosis of syphilis made. Finally, the serologic tests for syphilis (e.g., Wassermann, Hinton) are usually strongly positive by the end of five or six weeks. It is therefore important that any patient who has not received the standard penicillin treatment for acute gonorrhea be recalled in six weeks to have a serologic test for syphilis and be followed at intervals for another three to four months to be certain that any masked incubating syphilis is detected. The two diseases are not infrequently transmitted simultaneously, but unless penicillin has been used, the drug therapy for the gonorrhea may mask or prevent the development of the primary luetic lesion, even though it is inadequate treatment for syphilis, and the latter could therefore easily go unrecognized and progress silently into the tertiary phase. A fluorescent treponemal antibody-absorption test is now available and is of considerable value in eliminating the possibility of a false-positive test in all patients with reactive serologic tests for syphilis. All these diagnostic maneuvers will be helpful, often essential, in the differential diagnosis of suspicious ulcerated or papular lesions of the external genitalia that may be caused by any of the venereal diseases as well as by various other infectious processes or by certain neoplasms.

TREATMENT

Penicillin therapy remains the treatment of choice, and treponemal resistance has not been observed. For acute infectious syphilis, the recommended therapy is 2.4 million units (1.2 million units in each buttock) of long-acting benzathine penicillin G (e.g., Bicillin) in a single session. Thus the standard treatment for gonorrhea is also curative for incubating syphilis. The standard course of treatment for late syphilis consists of a total of 6 to 9 million units of procaine penicillin given in divided doses of 3 million units once every seven days over a period of 14 to 21 days. The patient must be carefully followed up, and at least a year should elapse with maintenance of negative serologic tests before she can be pronounced cured. If the patient is allergic to penicillin, treatment with large doses of tetracycline, erythromycin, or cephaloridine will have to be employed. As is true for all venereal diseases, every potential contact should be traced, investigated, and treated when indicated.

Chancroid (Soft Chancre)

Chancroid is a highly contagious infection caused by Ducrey's bacillus (*Hemophilus ducreyi*), a small, gram-negative, coccuslike bacillus. The principal manifestation is the development of a painful, tender, ulcerated, maculopapular lesion of the external genitalia, usually 3 to 10 days after sexual exposure (there is often considerable surrounding inflammation, but never the hard induration that nearly always accompanies the primary chancre of syphilis), usually followed shortly thereafter by the unilateral or bilateral appearance of enlarged inguinal nodes that frequently suppurate. The ulcerated lesion is accompanied by a profuse, purulent, malodorous discharge.

Diagnosis is ordinarily readily made by gram-stained smears and cultures carried out on the discharge from the ulcerated lesion or — perhaps more reliably — on material aspirated from the swollen inguinal glands; an antigen skin test is also available but is rarely required. Dark-field examination should also be done to exclude the possibility of syphilis, and the specific diagnostic tests for the other granulomatous venereal diseases to be discussed are also in order.

Treatment consists of a two-week course of sulfonamides or streptomycin, either of which is specific and highly curative. With regard to management of the suppurative lymphadenitis, simple aspiration is highly preferable to open incision and drainage, for the latter usually lead to troublesome secondary infection with extensive ulceration and prolongation of healing.

Lymphogranuloma Venereum

Lymphogranuloma venereum, which is caused by a filterable virus, is essentially a disease of tropical or subtropical climates and is perhaps more common in blacks, although whites are by no means immune. An increased incidence of lymphogranuloma venereum has been noted in the United States, due in large part to dissemination of the disease by American soliders returning from Southeast Asia. The infection and associated inflammatory process involve primarily the lymph channels and lymph nodes in the genital, inguinal, perianal, and anal regions — hence the name.

The clinical manifestations begin with a transient and inconspicuous initial external genital lesion, which usually appears as a small vesicle 7 to 21 days after exposure to an infected sexual partner and then rapidly fades away. Initially, there may be symptoms of systemic infection, including fever, malaise, headache, and arthralgia. A low-grade, invariably unilateral inguinal adenitis appears two to three weeks later, the inflammatory process in the groin then steadily progressing until all the inguinal lymph nodes and surrounding soft tissues are involved, and a firm, tender, bulging inguinal mass, the bubo, is produced. Necrosis frequently occurs, leading to multiple fistulas and extensive ulceration and scarring in the groin. Further extension along lymphatic channels typically leads to involvement of the deeper nodes and lymph trunks of the pelvic wall, parametrium, and broad ligaments and particularly of the lymphatic tissues in the region of the perineum, anus, rectum, and sigmoid. As a result of the latter, chronic rectal and anal strictures and mucosal ulcerations are common sequelae of the disease. Vulvar elephantiasis due to chronic lymphatic blockade is also a frequent and exceedingly troublesome manifestation.

DIAGNOSIS

Diagnosis can usually be made by means of a specific antigen skin test, the Frei test, which becomes positive 10 to 14 days after the appearance of the initial lesion and remains positive for the life of the patient. A complement-fixation test is also available. Again, the gamut of procedures to exclude the possibility of one or more of the other venereal diseases is in order. Where chronic anorectal lesions are concerned, proctoscopy and biopsy are essential to rule out carcinoma.

TREATMENT

Treatment involves a 21-day course of either a sulfonamide, chlortetracycline, or chloramphenicol, all of which are effective in the early phases of the disease even though the disease is of viral origin. The inguinal buboes should be aspirated in preference to surgical drainage if suppuration occurs and breakdown seems imminent. Colostomy may ultimately prove necessary in the management of extensive anal or rectal strictures with complete or nearly complete obstruction, although sometimes repeated dilatations suffice.

Granuloma Inguinale

Unlike the situation in lymphogranuloma venereum, the inflammatory process accompanying granuloma inguinale spreads through the skin rather than via lymphatic channels. This chronic, ulcerating, granulomatous infection is caused by the microorganisms of *Donovania granulomatis,* which can be identified on the basis of their appearance as encapsulated inclusion bodies, the characteristic Donovan bodies, which are visible in the large mononuclear cells accompanying the chronic inflammatory process. The disease tends to be limited exclusively to blacks.

Following sexual contact with an infected person, the initial lesion usually appears on the vulva, perineum, or vagina (less commonly in the groin and rarely on the cervix) as a small circumscribed, elevated area of soft granulation tissue. Ulceration and secondary infection rapidly follow, and there is an accompanying profuse and malodorous discharge. Thereafter, there is a chronic and progressive spread of the ulcerated area and a tremendous proliferation of masses of granulation tissue. The process tends to be limited to the skin and immediate subcutaneous tissues of the external genitalia and inguinal areas, although in the presence of severe secondary infection, deep, penetrating ulcers may form, and a secondary bacterial lymphadenitis may result in lymph node enlargement in the groins and elephantiasis of the vulva. In the absence of secondary infection, pseudobuboes may form in the groin that actually represent a perilymphadenitis due to involvement of the soft tissues surrounding the nodes by the granulomatous process itself. There is little tendency to spontaneous healing; rather, the lesion slowly enlarges and advances peripherally to involve the groins (by direct extension, not by lymphatic spread), vagina, urethra, anus, and perineum. Local discomfort is often severe, and intercourse, urination, defecation, and even sitting or walking may become extremely painful, if not impossible.

DIAGNOSIS

Diagnosis is made by obtaining smears or biopsies directly from the ulcerating surface, staining with Wright's or hematoxylin-eosin stain, and identifying the pathognomonic Donovan bodies within the huge, phagocytic mononuclear cells that are the most outstanding histologic feature of this chronic granulomatous process. The various clinical and laboratory tests for all the other venereal diseases should also be done, not only as a means of differential diagnosis but also because one or more of the venereal disorders frequently coexist.

TREATMENT

Treatment with streptomycin, tetracycline, or chloramphenicol has proved reasonably effective. Streptomycin is the only specific therapy that has proved at all successful in clearing up moderately advanced lesions. It is usually administered in a dosage of 4 gm daily for two to four weeks. For lesions that fail to respond to antibiotic therapy, resection by electrosurgical excision with wide margins and coagulation of the underlying base has given good results.

Condyloma Acuminatum

Condyloma acuminatum, an infection of viral origin, which was mentioned briefly in Chapter 7, results in multiple papillary proliferations on the vulva, vagina, and, less frequently, the cervix. It is also probably subject to venereal transmission. There is usually an associated profuse, irritating vaginal discharge and secondary vulvitis, and the lesions multiply rapidly over an ever-increasing area of the vulva, perineum, and perianal region.

DIAGNOSIS

The diagnosis is usually obvious on clinical grounds, the typical narrow-based, pedun-culated growths being readily distinguished from the more sessile, broad-based, flat condylomata lata of syphilis or from other benign tumors. However, a biopsy should always be submitted for histologic confirmation, and routine as well as gonococcal cultures and dark-field examination of the accompanying discharge should be done to exclude the presence or coexistence of other venereal diseases whenever any doubt exists.

TREATMENT

The most effective treatment of the externally situated condylomata, provided that they are small and not too numerous, has been the application of a solution of 25% podophyllum in tincture of benzoin directly to each individual growth, coating the surrounding normal skin with petrolatum. For large, coalescing lesions, actual sur-gical excision, or, more often, electrocoagulation followed by curettage, is usually preferable. For recalcitrant lesions, topical applications of 5% 5-fluorouracil in a cream base (Efudex) may be tried. When there are lesions involving the vagina and cervix, surgical electrocoagulation or excision is absolutely necessary and will require general anesthesia. Cryosurgical therapy, though feasible and effective, is more elaborate treatment than is really necessary to rid the patient of the lesions, and the postcryotherapy healing is prolonged and may result in excessive scarring.

Herpesvirus Type 2 Infections
(Herpes Progenitalis, Herpes Genitalis, Herpes Preputialis)

Type 2 herpesvirus hominis is closely related to herpes labialis (type 1 herpes simplex) It causes herpetic lesions on the cervix, vagina, and external genitalia, and the disease is considered to be the result of venereal transmission. Symptoms generally appear within three to seven days, occasionally in less than 24 hours. The majority of patients afflicted are teenagers or young unmarried adults. For a number of reasons, herpetic infections of the genital tract occasionally involve the type 1 virus (in 5 to 10 percent), and herpesvirus type 2 is the occasional etiologic agent for lesions about the mouth (in 5 to 10 percent). The characteristic appearance on the vulva is that of a group of multiple vesicles surrounded by a diffuse area of inflammation and edema; the lesions are usually located on the clitoral prepuce, the labia minora, and the medial aspects of the labia majora. There is usually intense itching and an asso-ciated burning sensation (often preceding the appearance of the vesicles), and erosion and secondary infection of the vesicles by scratching is common and may create difficulties in diagnosis. There may also be multiple small superficial ulcers, with or without vesicles, on the vulva, vagina, or cervix. Although the symptoms of herpes vulvovaginitis are usually more dramatic, cervical involvement is actually more common and is present in 75 percent of cases. The cervix may be diffusely edem-atous and inflamed, bleeding easily when touched; there may be a large punched-out ulceration, or there may be a granulomatous-appearing tumorlike mass, covered with gray exudate. There is often a profuse, watery discharge. However, a significant number of patients with the primary herpetic infection are completely asymptomatic, and a previous type 1 infection elsewhere in the body probably modifies a subsequent type 2 genital tract infection and minimizes its signs and symptoms. Herpes genitalis is frequently associated with hemophilus vaginalis, or *Trichomonas* vaginitis, or both, as well as with gonorrhea and condyloma acuminatum, and it is important to look for all these possibilities in each patient.

The possible significance of type 2 herpesvirus infection in the etiology of cervical cancer is discussed in Chapter 13. During pregnancy, herpes genitalis poses a special problem, for in early pregnancy it is responsible for an increased incidence of spontaneous abortion. Late in pregnancy, especially at delivery, there is the danger of transmission of the infection to the infant, with significant fetal morbidity and mortality.

With the initial or primary herpes infection there may be a prodromal period of several days with constitutional symptoms such as fever, malaise, and headache. The disease tends to be recurrent and unaccompanied by systemic reaction in 75 percent of cases, however, and some patients have repeated flare-ups for years, often related to the menses. These recurrent attacks probably represent reactivation of the initial, now latent viral infection. Local symptoms of vaginal and cervical involvement include leukorrhea, abnormal bleeding, vaginal pain, dysuria (sometimes so painful as to lead to urinary retention), and dyspareunia.

DIAGNOSIS

Differential diagnosis will often include any of the other venereal diseases, other types of vaginitis and cervicitis, herpes zoster, condylomata lata, and erythema multiforme; the cervical lesions may even suggest carcinoma at times. A specific diagnosis can often be made on cytologic smear by recognition of the typical viral inclusion bodies. Furthermore, special cultures can be made from vulvar, vaginal, or cervical lesions, and the herpesvirus infection easily and quickly identified. Serologic tests for both type 1 and type 2 antibodies are also available.

TREATMENT

In the absence of a specific treatment for the disease, symptomatic management with drying and antipuritic agents and topical anesthetic agents has been used to relieve the local discomfort until the disease, usually short-lived, has run its course, and spontaneous healing of the lesions occurs. However, it has recently been discovered that the herpesvirus can be eradicated from the vulvar skin and mucous membranes by the local application of one of several tricyclic dyes (e.g., 1% aqueous solution of neutral red, or 0.1% proflavine), followed in a few minutes by exposure of the area so painted to incandescent (150-watt) or fluorescent (20 to 30 watt) light for 10 to 15 minutes at a distance of 6 to 8 inches. The same exposure to incandescent or fluorescent light is repeated by the patient 6 to 8 hours later and again 24 hours later. There is prompt relief of symptoms, often within 24 hours, and the lesions are usually completely healed within seven days. These photodynamic dyes are incorporated into the virus during replication, so that subsequent exposure to light results in inactivation of the virus. Symptomatic relief is universal, when such treatment is used in the primary phase of the infection, though the course of the disease is little altered. Where the recurrent form of the infection is concerned, the lesions disappear promptly along with the symptoms.

The possibility has been raised that inactivating the virus may potentiate its oncogenic properties, but this issue remains highly debatable and unsettled, though many authorities believe the risk to be slight or nonexistent. Obviously, all patients treated by photoinactivation must be followed very closely until this issue has been resolved, which may take years. But from the wealth of evidence already suggesting a possible link between herpesvirus type 2 infection and the subsequent development of cervical and even vulvar and vaginal neoplasms, all patients known to have had genital herpesvirus infections, regardless of the therapy they receive, should be followed closely with this possibility in mind. Nonetheless, recurrent herpesvirus infections may well pose more of an oncogenic risk than their treatment by photodynamic inactivation.

REFERENCES

1. Abrams, A. J. Lymphogranuloma venereum. *J.A.M.A.* 205:199, 1968.
2. Barnett, J. A., and Sanford, J. P. Bacterial shock. *J.A.M.A.* 209:1514, 1969.
3. Brown, T. K., and Munsick, R. A. Puerperal ovarian vein thrombophlebitis: A syndrome. *Am. J. Obstet. Gynecol.* 109:263, 1971.
4. Cavanagh, D., Dahm, C. H., and Rao, P. S. Shock as a complication of sepsis in the female genital tract. *Int. J. Gynecol. Obstet.* 11:61, 1973.
5. Collins, C. G. Suppurative pelvic thrombophlebitis. *Am. J. Obstet. Gynecol.* 108:681, 1970.
6. Davis, C. M. Granuloma inguinale. *J.A.M.A.* 211:632, 1970.
7. Decker, W. H., and Hall, W. Treatment of abortion infected with clostridium welchii. *Am. J. Obstet. Gynecol.* 95:394, 1966.
8. Eaton, C. J., and Peterson, E. P. Diagnosis and acute management of patients with advanced clostridial sepsis complicating abortion. *Am. J. Obstet. Gynecol.* 109:1162, 1971.
9. Friedrich, E. G. Relief for herpes vulvitis. *Obstet. Gynecol.* 41:74, 1973.
10. Hawkins, D. F., Sevitt, L. H., Fairbrother, P. F., and Tothill, A. U. Management of septic chemical abortion with renal failure: Use of a conservative regimen. *N. Engl. J. Med.* 292:722, 1975.
11. Henderson, D. N., Harkins, J. L., and Stitt, J. F. Pelvic tuberculosis. *Am. J. Obstet. Gynecol.* 94:630, 1966.
12. Josey, W. E. The sexually transmitted infections. *Obstet. Gynecol.* 43:465, 1974.
13. Knaus, H. H. Surgical treatment of genital and peritoneal tuberculosis in the female. *Am. J. Obstet. Gynecol.* 83:73, 1962.
14. Ledger, W. J., Sweet, R. W., and Headington, J. T. Bacteroides species as a cause of severe infections in obstetric and gynecologic patients. *Surg. Gynecol. Obstet.* 133:837, 1971.

15. McGruder, C. J., Jr. Surgical management of chronic pelvic inflammatory disease. *Obstet. Gynecol.* 13:591, 1959.
16. McKay, D. C., Jewett, J. E., and Reid, D. E. Endotoxin shock and the generalized Shwartzman reaction in pregnancy. *Am. J. Obstet. Gynecol.* 78:546, 1959.
17. Mickal, A., Sellman, A. H., and Beebe, J. L. Ruptured tuboovarian abscess. *Am. J. Obstet. Gynecol.* 100:432, 1968.
18. Nolan, G. H., and Osborne, N. Gonococcal infections in the female. *Obstet. Gynecol.* 42:156, 1973.
19. Robinson, D. W. Postpartum ovarian vein thrombophlebitis. *Am. J. Obstet. Gynecol.* 113:497, 1972.
20. Schaefer, G., and Sutherland, A. M. Tuberculosis of the genital organs. *Am. J. Obstet. Gynecol.* 91:714, 1965.
21. Schiffen, M. A., Elguezabal, A., Sultana, M., and Allen, A. C. Actinomycosis infections associated with intrauterine contraceptive devices. *Obstet. Gynecol.* 45:67, 1975.
22. Schwarz, R. H. *Septic Abortion.* Philadelphia: Lippincott, 1968.
23. Smith, R., Smith, L. F., and Tenney, B. Soap-induced abortion: Report of five cases. *Obstet. Gynecol.* 20:211, 1962.
24. Sparling, P. F. Diagnosis and treatment of syphilis. *N. Engl. J. Med.* 284:642, 1971.
25. Westrom, L. Effect of acute pelvic inflammatory disease on fertility. *Am. J. Obstet. Gynecol.* 121:707, 1975.

9
Disorders of Early Pregnancy

Any practicing physician, but particularly the gynecologist, is called on at least as often as the obstetrician to establish whether or not a patient is pregnant, and the gynecologist or general surgeon is perhaps the physician most frequently consulted regarding the various complications of early pregnancy. The most common and important of these complications will be discussed in this chapter. They include ectopic pregnancy, spontaneous abortion (threatened, incomplete, complete), therapeutic abortion, and the trophoblastic tumors, i.e., hydatidiform mole, chorioadenoma destruens, and choriocarcinoma. The subject of septic abortion has already received detailed consideration in Chapter 8, and certain aspects of habitual abortion are also taken up in Chapter 11.

DIAGNOSIS OF EARLY PREGNANCY

The various clinical tests and laboratory procedures that help to establish a definite diagnosis of early pregnancy and are sometimes useful in differentiating between disorders of early pregnancy and other gynecologic diseases with similar symptoms and findings have been reviewed in detail in Chapter 2. In addition to the history of the missed period in a woman whose cycles are invariably regular, and the subjective and hence only suggestive symptoms of breast fullness and tenderness, morning nausea, urinary frequency, and so on, which may appear within a few weeks after conception, there are certain physical findings that, being objective anatomic criteria, are fairly reliable guides to a correct diagnosis. These include the typical softening of the lower uterine segment, which is usually detectable at about six weeks after the last period (Hegar's sign), and the visible bluish hue taken on by the vagina and introitus, which usually appears near the end of the second month of pregnancy (Chadwick's sign). By this time the uterine fundus is usually one-and-a-half to two times enlarged and is soft and globular, and the breasts are visibly full and turgid, with heavily pigmented areolae and erect nipples from which colostrum can often be expressed, so that the diagnosis is now fairly definite on clinical grounds alone.

When the diagnosis of pregnancy is first established, the patient is usually most anxious to know the expected time of delivery. This can be estimated with some accuracy as being 280 days (± 2 to 3 days) following the first day of the last period. The expected time of arrival (ETA) can thus be rapidly calculated by counting ahead 1 year and subtracting 85 days, or by counting ahead 9 months and adding 5 days.

ECTOPIC PREGNANCY

Failure of the fertilized ovum to migrate or to be transported to the normal site of implantation within the endometrial cavity may result in implantation at an aberrant site in the tube, broad ligament, or on the ovarian surface, with the development of an ectopic gestation. (Although impossible to document or quantitate, it seems likely that many such misplaced fertilized ova never implant at all and simply undergo degeneration and absorption within the peritoneal cavity.) It is estimated that approximately 25,000 ectopic pregnancies occur each year in the United States, the ratio of ectopic to normal intrauterine pregnancies ranging from 1:300 to as high as 1:125 in various reported series. Although in recent years earlier recognition of this disorder with more prompt and effective treatment has brought about a reduction in deaths, ectopic pregnancy is still a significant cause of maternal mortality. Fatalities are nearly always the result of failure to make the diagnosis, delayed or inadequate surgery, or ineffective therapy for shock in patients with tubal rupture and massive intraperitoneal hemorrhage.

Etiology

A preexisting chronic salpingitis, whether of gonococcal, mixed bacterial (postabortal or puerperal), or tuberculous origin, is commonly found in association with ectopic pregnancy. The somewhat higher incidence of ectopic pregnancy in the Negro population of the United States is undoubtedly a reflection of the fact that black women also have a higher incidence of gonococcal salpingitis than do white women. It is currently estimated that approximately 25 percent of all ectopic pregnancies occur in association with preexisting chronic salpingitis, the majority of cases of which are of gonococcal origin. Obviously, the inflammatory disease in these cases has not resulted in complete occlusion, but the mucosal damage has been sufficient to produce luminal narrowing, distortion, and sometimes pseudodiverticula formation, with a resulting arrest and abnormal implantation of the migrating early embryo somewhere along the course of the tube, in a narrow, tortuous channel or postinflammatory sacculation. With the advent of more effective chemotherapy for both pyogenic and tuberculous salpingitis, control of the acute phase of the disease is now more often achieved before complete tubal closure has occurred. However, some degree of mucosal damage is usually sustained, and thus it is not surprising that within recent years there has been an apparent increase in the frequency of ectopic pregnancy.

Since any pathologic condition involving the tube or the uterotubal junction results in obstruction to the normal passage of the fertilized ovum, a number of other tubal, peritubal, or uterine disorders are similarly accompanied by a higher incidence of ectopic pregnancy. These disorders include the following: various of the congenital müllerian duct anomalies; benign tubal tumors and cysts (see Chap. 17); peritubal adhesions secondary to a prior appendicitis, endometriosis, or a previous pelvic or abdominal operation; uterine fibroids or adenomyosis in the cornual region near the uterotubal junction; and finally, a previous tubal plastic operation in which an attempt was made to restore patency and/or normal tubal pickup and transport function where these had been totally impaired by a prior chronic salpingitis or perisalpingitis. The subsequent rate of occurrence of ectopic tubal pregnancies following such tubal reparative procedures is notoriously high; although patency may be achieved, the effort to restore normal tubal transport function is often less successful.

Although the probable etiology of many ectopic gestations can thus often be traced to one of the specific preexisting disorders that impede the normal progress of the recently fertilized ovum to the endometrial cavity, the majority (50 percent or more) of ectopic pregnancies occur within fallopian tubes that are apparently anatomically and histologically normal. It can be assumed that premature arrest and ectopic implantation of the early embryo are therefore more commonly the result of a disturbance in tubal physiology, either on a hormonal or neurogenic basis. When one recalls the great dependence of normal tubal physiology, including both secretory and muscular activity, on adequate and properly timed ovarian hormonal stimulation of the secretory and ciliated cells of the mucosa and the smooth muscle layer of the tubal wall, it is obvious that even in ovulatory menstrual cycles, minor inadequacies in corpus luteum function and hormone output might well lead to an impairment of the tubal transport function. This in turn could result in prolonged retention of the ovum within the tube beyond the normal, approximately three-day interval required for fertilization and subsequent preliminary development of the zygote and early trophoblastic elements, as well as further conditioning of the ripening endometrium, both of which are essential if the early embryo is to be capable of implanting successfully once it has reached the endometrial cavity. In the face of such a delay, implantation within the tube might well result.

Another equally plausible mechanism for delay in tubal transport of the early zygote — and in support of which there is often empirical clinical evidence in many women presenting with an ectopic gestation — is neuromuscular rather than hormonal in nature. Although impossible to document objectively, it seems highly likely that in some cases emotional disorders and temporary psychological disturbances could well result in interference with the normal autonomic nervous system regulation of tubal muscular activity and lead to delay in passage of the fertilized ovum. (Such a neurogenic mechanism interfering in other aspects of reproductive physiology may also account for some instances of absolute infertility as well as certain cases of habitual abortion.) Some experienced observers think that ectopic pregnancies are more prone to develop in women who exhibit "spastic tubes" during attempts at tubal insufflation or hysterosalpingography. Certainly, in view of the known role and significance of psychosomatic mechanisms in the modification of other body functions and in the production of clinical disorders, it would be surprising if similar phenomena were not encountered in relation to female reproductive tract function.

One other probable way in which a delay in the migration of the fertilized ovum sufficient to result in ectopic implantation might occur is suggested by the observation that in a significant percentage (in some series as high as 50 percent) of tubal pregnancies, the corpus luteum of pregnancy is found in the contralateral ovary. This implies either that the ovum was fertilized within the free peritoneal cavity or that fertilization occurred in the ampullary portion of the tube on the same side as the corpus luteum and that the fertilized ovum subsequently transmigrated to the opposite tube. In either case, considerable delay would be inevitable, and the developing zygote could well enlarge sufficiently to be unable to pass through the narrow isthmic or cornual portion of the tube.

Finally, there has been recent interest in the possibility that delayed ovulation occurring around the twenty-first day of the cycle rather than at midcycle might be the cause of ectopic pregnancy in some cases. Such a delay in ovulation and fertilization could result in an initial failure of adequate uterine implantation due to a short and inadequate luteal phase, with subsequent uprooting of the poorly implanted conceptus and transfer to an ectopic site by tubal reflux during the menstrual flow. Retrospective histologic studies of the embryos in some series of ectopic pregnancies have verified that conception must have occurred around the twenty-first day of the cycle, and invariably the patient had experienced menstrual bleeding at the expected time, even though conception had taken place.

A dramatic example of the importance of functional disturbances of tubal physiology in the etiology of ectopic pregnancy is to be found in the reported observations on the relative rates of occurrence of ectopic pregnancy in the Jewish and Arab populations living side by side in Israel. Ectopic pregnancy is encountered many times more frequently in Jewish women than among Arab women even though chronic pelvic inflammatory disease, invariably the most common antecedent actual pathologic process found in tubes harboring ectopic gestations, is exceedingly rare among the Jewish population but extremely common in Arab women; the incidence of gonococcal salpingitis in the latter is five to six times higher than in Jewish women. Furthermore, these functional disturbances in tubal physiology are often of a fundamental sort and the resulting ectopic pregnancies are not simply isolated "accidents," since a large percentage of women experiencing an ectopic pregnancy have in the past and will in the future suffer from infertility and functional menstrual disorders. In addition, contrary to the often optimistic reassurance of their physicians, women who have had one ectopic pregnancy, even when the opposite tube appears grossly normal, have a seven to ten times greater chance of having another than do women who have never had such a pregnancy (roughly 10 percent will have another ectopic pregnancy at some future time). In fact, only about one-third will ever succeed in having a live baby, although a somewhat larger number will conceive, only to lose their pregnancies through abortion, miscarriage, or another ectopic gestation.

Closely related to these possible spontaneous types of tubal dysfunction leading to ectopic pregnancy may be the rare occurrence of ectopic pregnancy after postcoital prevention of an unwanted conception by the administration of large doses of diethylstilbestrol or other estrogenic compounds (the "morning-after pill" program), or the equally infrequent development of an ectopic gestation in the presence of an intrauterine contraceptive device. In both instances one assumes that interference with normal tubal transport by hormonal or mechanical inhibition respectively leads to arrest and implantation of the fertilized egg within the tubal lumen.

Sites of Ectopic Pregnancy

FALLOPIAN TUBE

The vast majority (95 percent) of ectopic gestations occur within the fallopian tube, most often in the ampullary or isthmic portion (Fig. 34). Interstitial or cornual pregnancies are considerably less frequent but of considerable significance when they do occur, since rupture of a cornual pregnancy usually takes place earlier and is often associated with the sudden onset of such massive hemorrhage that even the slightest delay in diagnosis and treatment can prove fatal.

Bilateral tubal pregnancies occurring simultaneously are extremely rare, but several such cases have been recorded. Similarly, the simultaneous occurrence of a tubal and a normal intrauterine pregnancy is only infrequently encountered, although a number of such instances have been reported in the recent literature.

OVARY

Primary ovarian pregnancies comprise approximately 1 percent of the total of all types of ectopic gestation (Fig. 34). Presumably, either the ovum fails to be properly extruded and is actually fertilized within the early corpus luteum, or, following fertilization within the tube or free peritoneal cavity, it fails to continue on its transtubal journey, implanting instead on the surface of the ovary, where it temporarily burrows into the ovarian cortex. Since the varying clinical manifestations are identical

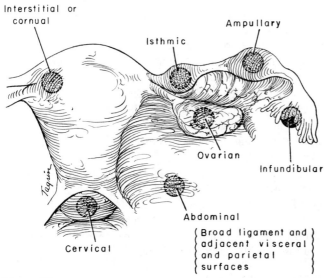

Figure 34
Sites of ectopic pregnancy.

with those of an ectopic tubal pregnancy, the diagnosis of an ovarian rather than a tubal gestation can only be made at laparotomy and only after the tube itself is clearly shown to be completely uninvolved in the implantation site. Not infrequently, an early ovarian pregnancy cannot be grossly distinguished from rupture or hemorrhage into a simple cyst, and it is often only when histologic examination of the resected specimen reveals chorionic villi that the true nature of the acute ovarian process becomes apparent. Of recent interest is the observation of a higher rate of ovarian pregnancies in women using intrauterine devices.

CERVIX

Cervical pregnancy (Fig. 34) appears to be the rarest of all types of ectopic gestation, probably because the chances are remote that a fertilized ovum that has passed completely through the uterus will nevertheless retain sufficient capacity to implant in the relatively unfavorable environment afforded by the cervical endothelium and glands.

ABDOMINAL SITES

Tubal, ovarian, or cervical pregnancies rarely survive more than two to three months and never reach the stage of fetal viability. The one type of ectopic gestation that occasionally does approach term with the development of a viable fetus is the so-called abdominal pregnancy. Actually, the weight of evidence suggests that nearly all abdominal pregnancies begin initially as tubal gestations. The latter are then "aborted" from the tube relatively early in their development and implant on the neighboring broad ligaments and adjacent uterus, bowel, and parietal peritoneum, the actual sites of placental development in abdominal pregnancy. The availability of an adequate blood supply in these areas makes the further growth possible. Thus prior pelvic inflammatory disease, known to be associated with an increased incidence of tubal pregnancy, is also considered to be the most important etiologic factor in the occurrence of abdominal pregnancy. Partial tubal obstruction leads to temporary tubal implantation, which later may be converted to an abdominal pregnancy if tubal abortion occurs while the early pregnancy is still capable of reimplantation. The incidence of abdominal pregnancy in a general population is roughly 1 per 15,000 live births, but it appears to be higher in blacks, possibly due to the greater frequency of chronic salpingitis in black women.

Migration of what was initially an intrauterine pregnancy via rupture of a previous cesarean section scar has been shown to be another mechanism by which an abdominal pregnancy can develop. (There is usually a demonstrable uteroplacental fistula in these cases.) Finally, initial implantation of a fertilized ovum on abdominal peritoneal surfaces with a resulting primary abdominal pregnancy has been fairly well documented in an occasional case, but this is exceedingly rare.

Diagnosis and Management of Abdominal Pregnancy

The patient frequently experiences mild abdominal pain and transient vaginal bleeding approximately six weeks following the last menstrual period (coincident with "tubal abortion"), and she then may be relatively asymptomatic for several weeks or months, presenting with what appears to both patient and physician to be a normal intrauterine pregnancy. Ultimately, as the pregnancy enlarges, abdominal pain and gastrointestinal or urinary tract disturbances develop, and on physical examination the physician alert to the possibility may detect obvious clues such as easily palpable superficial fetal parts or excessively loud fetal heart tones, or he may be able to demonstrate definitely that the fetal mass is separate from the uterus.

The finding of an abnormal fetal position (transverse lie or breech) with the presenting part high above the pelvic inlet should always raise the suspicion of abdominal pregnancy, since such fetal malpositions are inevitable in and characteristic of this condition. Pelvic roentgenograms utilizing soft-tissue techniques, occasionally hysterography, and aortography may be employed to confirm the diagnosis.

There are many recorded instances in which an abdominal pregnancy has been spontaneously and indefinitely retained without benefit of medical attention, with subsequent partial or complete resorption, skeletonization or lithopedion formation, or with the development of a pelvic abscess or a fistulous tract involving the vagina, abdominal wall, bladder, or rectum, through which fetal parts are extruded. Deliberate conservative medical management such as this is not to be recommended, however, and carries a high mortality. Once the diagnosis of abdominal pregnancy is definitely established, prompt laparotomy is indicated, regardless of the stage of gestation, in order to avoid dangerous complications, in particular, massive, spontaneous intraabdominal hemorrhage or serious pelvic sepsis. The fetus should be removed, ligating the umbilical cord close to the placenta, and if the stage of viability has been reached, a live baby that will survive and be relatively normal may be obtained in approximately 20 percent of cases.

The principal problem confronting the surgeon dealing with an abdominal pregnancy is the management of the placenta at laparotomy. If the blood supply of the placental attachments can be readily identified and completely and safely ligated (i.e., when essentially all of it is derived from the uterine and/or the ovarian vessels), then ligation and removal of the placenta should usually be done, since the risk of later hemorrhage is remote. Furthermore, the subsequent convalescence is greatly simplified by elimination of the need for spontaneous resorption of the placenta, which may in some instances be accompanied by sepsis, hemorrhage, and intestinal obstruction or fistula formation. On the other hand, if the placental attachment is broad and/or its blood supply diffuse and not readily identified or available for safe and complete ligation, the placenta should be left completely undisturbed after removal of the fetus, and the abdomen should be closed without drainage, accepting the possibility of a more prolonged and complicated convalescence and even the occasional need for reoperation. Any attempt to define the placental site and its vascular supply further in such cases — and particularly any ill-advised efforts at partial or total removal — are definitely contraindicated, since alarming and often fatal hemorrhage may result, either immediately or in the early postoperative period.

Tubal Pregnancy

PATHOLOGIC FEATURES

The tubal environment is not a favorable one, and even though implantation occurs, the embryo often fails to develop or is malformed. The wall of the tube becomes edematous, and there is vascular engorgement, but although chorionic villi usually undergo early development, there is little if any decidual response on the part of the tubal mucosa and no hypertrophy of the tubal musculature. Accordingly, the tubal wall remains thin as the tube becomes increasingly distended, and if tubal abortion does not occur first, as is frequently the case (such an event may go totally unrecognized or be accompanied by minimal symptoms and spontaneous resolution and recovery), rupture or actual penetration of the wall of the tube is inevitable, usually within six to eight weeks of onset.

If functional activity of the chorionic villi is sufficiently adequate in the early stages of a tubal pregnancy, the uterus will undergo enlargement, occasionally attaining the size of a three-months' pregnancy, and there will be a definite decidual change in the normal endometrium. With the onset of tubal abortion, or often well in advance of impending rupture of the ectopic gestation and as a result of a rapid decline in human chorionic gonadotropin (HCG) secretion, sloughing and hemorrhage from the uterine decidua now deprived of its hormonal support result in the onset of the abnormal vaginal bleeding so frequently seen in patients with tubal pregnancies. Occasionally, this sequence of events results in the passage of a decidual cast, which should further alert the physician to the possibility of ectopic pregnancy.

DIAGNOSIS

Signs and Symptoms

Only a minority of patients with tubal pregnancy, perhaps 15 percent, present the classic history: initial amenorrhea, with one or two missed periods accompanied by symptoms suggestive of early pregnancy, followed by the appearance of vaginal bleeding, signifying the impending termination of the pregnancy; then, after a variable interval of hours or days, the sudden development of abdominal pain, indicating rupture of the tubal pregnancy and the onset of intraperitoneal bleeding. At first, the pain is unilateral and pelvic in location, but shortly becomes generalized throughout the abdomen. It is often associated with shoulder pain as the hemoperitoneum increases and blood accumulates under the diaphragm. Thereafter, there is rapid progression to an obvious acute surgical abdominal emergency, with generalized abdominal tenderness and spasm, marked vaginal vault tenderness, and a characteristically exquisite pain on motion of the cervix. A tender adnexal mass is usually palpable, although this finding may be obscured if sufficient blood and clots are present in the pelvis. Cullen's sign, which is a bluish discoloration of the umbilicus, and a cul-de-sac that feels doughy and also may have a bluish color are sometimes present and further indicate massive hemiperitoneum. The classic textbook picture is completed by the obvious associated surgical shock, often with syncope, that promptly ensues as a result of the continuous, steady or abrupt massive hemorrhage.

On the other hand, the majority (85 percent) of patients exhibit subacute and atypical manifestations. Although some irregularity of the recent menstrual pattern has usually occurred, 25 to 40 percent of patients experience no interval of amenorrhea whatsoever; morning nausea, breast soreness and fullness, and other symptoms commonly associated with early pregnancy are also often absent or minimal. When it does appear, the abdominal or pelvic discomfort (present in 90 percent of cases) is frequently mild and sometimes poorly localized and intermittent at first, and the distress is often associated with similarly vague and inconstant symptoms of bowel or bladder irritability. Typically, the early pain is crampy or colicky in nature and generally is referred to one of the lower abdominal quadrants; only when bleeding or actual rupture occurs does it become severe and steady. Abnormal vaginal bleeding, a manifestation only slightly less frequent than abdominal pain and present in 80 percent of patients, is also often mild, intermittent, and frequently of considerable duration before the patient seeks medical advice. The patient is often more concerned about her pain, and the physician will frequently have to elicit specifically the information concerning the irregular flow. Finally, the findings on physical examination are frequently unremarkable or equivocal; there may or may not be significant pelvic or abdominal tenderness, and in 50 to 75 percent of the cases no definite adnexal mass will be palpable. Whether or not there is secondary uterine enlargement is also a highly variable feature. Occasionally, the temperature is slightly elevated, but the majority of patients are afebrile.

Thus it is the clinical picture in the vast majority of patients with subacute signs and symptoms that makes tubal pregnancy "the disease of diagnostic surprises" and the "great masquerader." Only by constantly maintaining a high index of suspicion toward the possibility of its presence in any woman of childbearing age who complains of abdominal pain and irregular bleeding can this disorder be consistently recognized, particularly in its early stages. Ectopic pregnancy represents a constant diagnostic challenge, not only because of its own frequently vague manifestations but also because a wide variety of other pelvic and abdominal disorders may be accompanied by similar signs and symptoms.

Differential Diagnosis

The differential diagnosis of tubal pregnancy should include the following:

1. Early normal intrauterine pregnancy, with some other cause of abdominal and/or pelvic pain and with or without a tender adnexal mass: e.g., a ruptured, bleeding corpus luteum of pregnancy; painful, tender, normal corpus luteum; painful stretching of the round ligaments; torsion of the ovary containing the corpus luteum or twisted ovarian cyst; spontaneous torsion of the fallopian tube in pregnancy; torsion or degeneration of a pedunculated fibroid; appendicitis; ureteral colic.
2. Intrauterine pregnancy with simple implantation bleeding or with "threatened," missed, or incomplete spontaneous abortion.
3. Pregnancy or hematometrium in a rudimentary uterine horn.

4. Anovulatory cycles with a painful, tender follicle cyst and irregular bleeding:
   a. Dysfunctional.
   b. In association with acute and chronic pelvic inflammatory disease.
   c. In association with the Stein-Leventhal syndrome.
5. Complications of endometriosis, pelvic inflammatory disease, ovarian tumors, pedunculated fibroids (torsion, rupture, hemorrhage into or from), or ovarian cysts (hemorrhage into and rupture or further bleeding from a corpus luteum cyst is a very common entity simulating ectopic pregnancy).

Diagnostic Plan

It should be emphasized again that prompt and accurate diagnosis is facilitated by constantly including ectopic pregnancy among the diagnostic possibilities in women of childbearing age who are suffering from abdominal pain and menstrual irregularities. In patients with a "textbook history" who are in shock with obvious internal bleeding, the diagnosis is nearly always apparent from the history and examination alone; confirmation by recovery of blood on cul-de-sac aspiration may also be sought but is often unnecessary. Operative treatment should proceed forthwith, following a brief period of preparation with transfusions to relieve shock and restore a satisfactory blood volume for safe anesthesia and surgery.

In patients with the more usual, atypical, subacute clinical picture, a period of observation in the hospital or even on an ambulatory basis has often been elected in the past, during which time the findings on repeated pelvic examinations, the results of pregnancy tests (positive in only 50 to 75 percent of cases), blood counts, vital signs, and the further clinical course of the illness are all utilized in attempting to arrive at a correct diagnosis. (A falling hemoglobin or hematocrit may be helpful; the white count may be normal or moderately elevated and is of no diagnostic value; the temperature usually remains normal or only slightly elevated.) Cul-de-sac aspiration has also frequently been employed as a guide to whether or not laparotomy is indicated. It is often helpful, but too great reliance on this maneuver can prove misleading, for in early, unruptured ectopic pregnancy, no blood will be obtained, whereas in many of the acute disorders simulating ectopic pregnancy but not necessarily requiring laparotomy, blood may well be obtained on culdocentesis.

A far more satisfactory and effective diagnostic approach is to carry out **laparoscopy** or **culdoscopy** almost immediately on all patients suspected of harboring an ectopic pregnancy (excluding the obvious cases, of course), because actual visualization of the tubes is the only way the diagnosis can really be established or excluded in the vast majority of patients. Prompt laparoscopy or culdoscopy completely eliminates the need for a prolonged, somewhat hazardous, and often expensive observation period and the various frequently inconclusive or even misleading laboratory studies and diagnostic maneuvers. It avoids an unnecessary laparotomy for diagnosis only, when conditions not requiring surgical treatment are responsible for the symptoms and findings.

When an ectopic pregnancy is not found, culdoscopy or laparoscopy has the added advantage in most cases of accurately identifying some other cause for the symptoms, which is information that may be important in itself in the further management of the patient. Some advocate actual culdotomy, or posterior colpotomy, in preference to culdoscopy or laparoscopy, but the former is a formal operative procedure, usually requiring general anesthesia and often presenting technical difficulties that prevent satisfactory visualization or palpation of the adnexa.

Finally, if a curettage has been done because a diagnosis of incomplete abortion was mistakenly entertained, a report by the pathologist of an atypical, decidual type of endometrium in the absence of any chorionic villi should immediately alert the physician to the possible existence of an ectopic pregnancy.

A specific histologic picture in the endometrium termed the *Arias-Stella phenomenon* is often seen in the presence of a bleeding tubal pregnancy, although it may be observed in aborting intrauterine pregnancies as well. It consists of marked secretory and proliferative activity (often within the same endometrial glands), piling up of cells within the gland lumens to form syncytial masses, and tall "bizarre" cells with foamy cytoplasm and hyperchromatic nuclei.

OPERATIVE TREATMENT

Obviously, the sooner the diagnosis is established, the more likely it is that a relatively conservative surgical procedure can be done. Depending on its size and the extent of local tubal damage produced by the ectopic gestation, several maneuvers may be considered.

1. Simple, manual extrusion by "milking" the ectopic pregnancy from the tube is often possible in the case of abortion with minimal bleeding of a very early tubal pregnancy located in the ampullary region.

2. Resection of the involved segment of tube and end-to-end anastomosis (over a splinting polyethylene catheter), or resection and tubal reimplantation if the ectopic pregnancy is in the isthmic or cornual region, can be done in the relatively small, early ectopic pregnancy with localized tubal damage when the remaining portion of the tube is normal. Obviously, conservation of even a portion of the affected tube is particularly desirable in patients who have already lost the opposite tube, although the considerable risk of a subsequent ectopic gestation will have to be accepted.

3. Salpingectomy is indicated in dealing with more advanced lesions where hemorrhage and rupture have produced extensive damage to the tube and mesosalpinx.

4. Salpingostomy. Favorable experiences have been reported by some when fairly large ectopic pregnancies were managed by incision of the distended tube with evacuation of the ectopic pregnancy, ligation of all bleeding points, and preservation of the tube if still viable. There is as yet insufficient follow-up information on the exact incidence of subsequent normal tubal patency and function, repeat ectopic pregnancies, permanent tubal occlusion, and so on, for proper evaluation of this procedure. However, its use should probably be seriously considered if the opposite tube has previously been removed.

5. Salpingo-oophorectomy will usually be necessary if tubal rupture and extensive vascular injury with dissection of the mesosalpinx, mesovarium, and infundibulopelvic ligament have occurred. Furthermore, if salpingectomy alone will be necessary in a patient in her middle or late thirties who has been infertile and remains hopeful of future pregnancies, concomitant removal of the ovary on the affected side may be wise, in order to guarantee that all her remaining ovulations will occur on the same side as the one remaining tube. In this way, at least theoretically, the chances of conception (the number of potentially fertile months per year) will thereby be greater than if she were left with two ovaries and a single tube.

Regardless of the particular operative approach employed, all gross blood and clots should be removed, for it is easier and quicker to give patients transfusions or iron therapy than to await resorption of peritoneal blood, and fewer intraperitoneal adhesions that might interfere with subsequent fertility will result. There is no evidence that there is any significant hazard per se to incidental appendectomy, so that it can and probably should be done routinely in most patients, assuming the patient's general condition is good and there are no other contraindications.

Postoperatively, if the patient is Rh-negative and does not already have an anti-D antibody, she should promptly receive RhoGAM, a purified human anti-Rh gamma globulin preparation. RhoGAM should be used to prevent sensitization whenever an Rh-negative woman may have received Rh-positive blood cells. Therefore it is indicated when such a patient has suffered an ectopic pregnancy, has undergone a spontaneous or therapeutic abortion, or has delivered an Rh-positive baby. RhoGAM appears to act by destroying Rh-positive blood cells before the recipient's immune system recognizes that an antigen is present (1 ml of RhoGAM will destroy approximately 10 ml of Rh-positive blood cells).

ABORTION

Any pregnancy that terminates before the fetus has attained the stage of viability can correctly be called a **miscarriage**, although this designation is customarily reserved for pregnancies ending between the twentieth and twenty-eighth weeks, and the term **abortion** is ordinarily applied when a pregnancy fails to survive 20 weeks. The problem of abortion in its various forms and with its associated diagnostic and therapeutic aspects is indeed a frequent and important one for the gynecologist, since approximately 10 to 15 percent of all known pregnancies end in abortions. Not only does this represent an immense fetal wastage, but the associated maternal mortality is not insignificant, ranging from 0.1 percent to as high as 1.0 percent in various reported series. Sepsis and hemorrhage are the chief causes of maternal deaths, with the higher mortality occurring in patient populations having a higher incidence of criminally induced abortions as well as a greater tendency to delay in seeking medical attention even for spontaneous abortions.

Abortions can obviously be classified in accordance with whether they are the result of termination of pregnancy through natural causes (**spontaneous abortion**)

or whether they have been induced by artificial means. The latter group can be
further subdivided into **criminal abortions**, if the induction has been attempted or
performed by the patient or another individual without medical indication or legal
sanction, and **therapeutic abortions**, if termination of the pregnancy has been for-
mally and openly carried out within a hospital or clinic, for proper and valid indications, and with full knowledge and medicolegal sanction of all parties concerned.

Etiology of Spontaneous Abortion

The majority of simple, nonrepetitive, spontaneous abortions occur in the second
or third month of gestation and are most commonly (in 50 to 75 percent) associated
with a blighted ovum and the inevitable subsequent abnormalities of both fetal and
placental development. In other words, these pregnancies were destined to fail at
the very outset, and the process of abortion simply represents the natural termination of an unproductive enterprise. It seems quite possible that the primary deficiency may be either maternal or paternal, or both, and, as noted in Chapter 3, may
often involve improper genetic transfers during the stage of fertilization and early
cell divisions within the zygote. The many recent studies indicating that major
chromosomal abnormalities are present in a high percentage of abortuses or stillborn
infants attest to the validity of this concept.

The maternal effects of serious acute or chronic systemic disorders (pulmonary,
renal, cardiovascular, and endocrine-metabolic), certain viral infections (e.g., rubella),
overwhelming bacterial infections, certain toxic drugs, and extensive local pelvic
trauma of the type sometimes encountered in automobile accident victims are occasionally followed by abortion of a previously normal pregnancy, though in most
such instances the resulting termination of pregnancy can hardly be considered
spontaneous. Some evidence has been advanced suggesting that fertilization late in
the cycle involving an "overripe" ovum may be a factor in causing chromosomal
aberrations, congenital malformations, and spontaneous abortions. Operations on
the ovary containing the corpus luteum during the first 30 to 90 days of pregnancy,
such as are sometimes necessary or prompted by torsion or a vascular accident in an
ovarian cyst, may also result in a "spontaneous" type of abortion of an otherwise
normally developing pregnancy due to premature withdrawal of ovarian hormonal
support before the immature placenta is capable of sustaining the gestation by an
adequate estrogen and progesterone production of its own.

As emphasized by Hertig and Livingstone [23], the potential role of a physical
trauma (e.g., a blow to the abdomen, a fall down stairs, an automobile accident) or
emotional trauma (e.g., a frightening experience, loss of a loved one) as etiologic
factors in the production of abortion is extremely dubious. Even in the presence
of a history suggesting such a train of events, careful histologic study of the fetal
and placental tissue obtained in instances of spontaneous abortion nearly always
reveals the typical features of a blighted ovum or maldeveloped fetus and placenta,
a situation that obviously antedates the apparent precipitating incident. Obviously,
this point has important medicolegal implications. It is usually only when direct

and severe accidental injury to the uterus, or to the fetus within, or to both has occurred that trauma per se can be incriminated as the actual cause of abortion of a previously normal pregnancy.

Clinical Types of Abortion

Depending on the apparent phase of abortion or impending abortion as indicated by the patient's history and findings when first seen, it is customary to classify abortions from a clinical standpoint as follows:

1. **Threatened abortion.** The patient gives the typical history of early pregnancy, with a missed period or two, and then notes the onset of vaginal bleeding, with or without uterine cramps. Pelvic examination reveals the cervix to be of normal length and the endocervical canal closed by an external os of normal diameter.

2. **Imminent abortion.** The same history, nearly always with cramps present. Examination reveals shortening and dilatation of the cervix.

3. **Inevitable abortion.** The same history, nearly always with cramps present. Examination discloses fetal or placental tissue or both within or protruding from the dilated, effaced cervical segment.

4. **Complete abortion.** The embryo, if present, and the entire placenta have been expelled. Obviously, diagnosis of this type of abortion depends on actual visualization by the physician of the tissue passed. Rapid cessation of bleeding and cramps and prompt early involution of the uterus subsequently are confirmatory.

5. **Incomplete abortion.** The fetus, with or without portions of the placenta, has been expelled, but some of the products of conception (usually fragments of placenta) remain within the uterus. Inspection of the tissue passed, together with persistence of cramps, bleeding, and cervical dilatation, usually is sufficient to indicate this type.

6. **Missed abortion.** Fetal death has occurred in utero before the twentieth week, but the pregnancy is retained for two months or longer. The presence of a missed abortion may be established before the onset of labor if amenorrhea persists but the uterus fails to enlarge further. More frequently, the patient is first seen because of the development of vaginal bleeding and cramps (the onset of the actual abortion) and is found to have a uterus "several months" smaller than would be expected from the duration of her amenorrhea.

7. **Septic abortion.** Any abortion complicated by intrauterine infection and fever (see Chap. 8). Although secondary infection of a spontaneous abortion is theoretically possible and may rarely occur, criminal induction can be assumed, or therapeutic interruption will be known, to have taken place in essentially all septic abortions.

8. **Habitual abortion.** By definition, the syndrome of habitual abortion is said to exist when a patient has had three or more successive pregnancies terminating in spontaneous abortion.

Clinical Features and Management of Abortions

THREATENED ABORTION

The category of threatened abortion includes the early phases of all pregnancies that ultimately terminate in abortion, as well as episodes of vaginal bleeding in many patients with fundamentally normal pregnancies but in whom bleeding occurs from marginal placental sinuses, polyps, cervical erosions, acute vaginitis, and so on. The latter situations are sometimes apparent on initial pelvic examinations, but in any event, the usual prompt cessation of bleeding and the subsequent continued normal progress of the pregnancy ultimately serve to distinguish those cases in which the initial clinical impression of threatened abortion was erroneous.

In those patients who ultimately proceed to termination of the pregnancy, the initial bleeding and signs and symptoms of uterine irritability are the first manifestations of failing corpus luteum and placental function, the deficient hormone production resulting in the beginning of placental circulatory failure and hemorrhage into the decidual basalis. Further progression of this process will lead to fetal death, placental separation, and eventually to active labor. In most instances, this sequence of events, once initiated, is probably completely irreversible by any therapeutic maneuvers now available. The actual number of patients who, initially, at least, experience a transient hormonal insufficiency that threatens continuation of normal placental function and the integrity of the pregnancy and whose pregnancies are capable of being "rescued" either by spontaneous return of normal hormonal support or by institution of the traditional regimen of bed rest, together with substitution therapy with progestational agents or estrogens, is probably very small. It is estimated that, when first seen, less than 30 percent of patients in whom abortion is actually threatened have viable fetuses and that 80 percent or more will proceed to abortion regardless of management. Currently, it is impossible to differentiate reliably either by the clinical picture or by any laboratory diagnostic aids the patients who may be fortunate enough to retain their pregnancies either as the result of or in spite of the therapy administered; hence all must be managed expectantly until either the abortion becomes obviously inevitable, or the signs and symptoms subside.

The possibility of the presymptomatic recognition of potential incipient threatened abortion by changes in the results of a number of laboratory tests suggestive of hormonal insufficiency has been discussed in Chapter 2. Quantitative gonadotropin assays, urinary pregnanediol excretion levels, and alterations in the cervical mucus arborization phenomenon or changes in the cellular pattern noted on vaginal smears all reflect progesterone or placental inadequacy and have been employed in attempting to identify patients most likely to abort. More recently, determinations of serum levels of human placental lactogen (HPL) (a rapid HPL radioimmunoassay method is now available) are being used as a guide to adequate placental function. Failure of the HPL level to rise with advancing pregnancy suggests inadequate function, and a sudden fall in the HPL level usually indicates acute placental failure and impending abortion or miscarriage. In such patients, various programs of supplemental hormone therapy employing a variety of the newer progestogens are under trial in the hope of reversing the presumed endocrine deficiency and decreasing the abortion rate in this group. However, the results in this field of clinical investigation continue to remain equivocal and extremely difficult to evaluate on a sound scientific basis.

IMMINENT AND INEVITABLE SPONTANEOUS ABORTIONS

In most instances of imminent and inevitable spontaneous abortion, provided that blood loss does not become excessive and the patient is reasonably comfortable, continued observation for a brief period of time seems justified in the hope that the abortion will be spontaneously concluded and the fetus and placenta completely expelled. If this expectant program does not yield the hoped-for results within a few hours, then intervention is indicated.

SPONTANEOUS COMPLETE ABORTION

In the majority of spontaneous complete abortions or early miscarriages the onset of labor is abrupt, and the fetus and placenta are expelled rapidly in an uncomplicated fashion with minimal cramps and bleeding, which cease promptly. Many such patients never visit the office or hospital; of those seen, examination even a few hours later usually reveals a firmly contracted fundus and a relatively tight cervix. If the subsequent course in such patients is uneventful, no further treatment is indicated. It should be noted, however, that in theory at least, no abortion or early miscarriage is actually complete, since, as the immature placenta separates from the uterine wall, the tips of the chorionic villi invariably remain attached. Thus many hold firmly to the belief that all abortions or early miscarriages, even though grossly "complete," should be managed by curettage to facilitate prompt convalescence and avoid postabortal complications that often ultimately require a D&C. Certainly, if any doubt exists as to whether or not the abortion is actually complete, or if cramps or bleeding persist in spite of the recovery of what appears to be a complete and intact placenta, curettage would seem to be the wisest policy.

SPONTANEOUS INCOMPLETE ABORTION

An incomplete abortion is the commonest disorder of early pregnancy that requires treatment, and surgical intervention is nearly always necessary. It is important to determine as promptly as possible whether an abortion is either in process (and therefore is inevitable) or has already been partially completed, so that definitive treatment can be instituted without undue delay rather than pointlessly pursuing a conservative waiting program as would be indicated in the earlier phase of threatened abortion. Ordinarily, the diagnosis of an incomplete abortion is rendered obvious by the typical history of persistent, severe uterine cramps, often accompanied by considerable bleeding and frequently by the passage of recognizable tissue. On examination, the cervical os is found to be dilated and patulous and the cervical segment effaced. The uterine fundus is still enlarged, soft, and boggy but is ordinarily not tender or painful on motion unless one is dealing with a septic, induced abortion.

Treatment

If no obvious tissue is present in the cervix, even though the latter is dilated, and if bleeding is not excessive and there is no evidence of sepsis, the following alternatives may be elected: (1) the physician may await possible spontaneous completion of abortion, or (2) attempt to hasten it with oxytocin (Pitocin), 0.5 ml subcutaneously every 30 minutes for four injections; this may be repeated in 4 to 6 hours. (3) If bleeding is excessive or persists, or if products of conception are visible in the cervical canal, the uterus should be promptly emptied surgically, carefully dilating the cervix further, if necessary, and then gently but thoroughly evacuating the uterine contents, by manual or finger curettage initially when possible, and then employing placental forceps and finally actual instrumental curettage to be absolutely certain that all placental and chorionic decidual tissue is removed. The preliminary intravenous administration of 10 units of oxytocin prior to curettage facilitates the latter by firmly contracting the fundus. At the conclusion of the procedure, intravenous or intramuscular injection of 0.2 mg of ergonovine also helps to maintain the uterus firmly contracted and is an aid to immediate hemostasis. A vacuum aspirator has been designed that can be introduced through a well-dilated cervical canal to carry out "suction curettage" of the intrauterine cavity. The suction technique has the advantages that little or no anesthesia is required, there is usually less bleeding, and in many cases the procedure can be completed in a few minutes. Occasionally, however, suction aspiration is not as effective as sharp curettage in completely removing all retained placental and decidual tissue. Once a diagnosis of incomplete abortion is definitely established, prompt curettage minimizes blood loss, reduces the chance of secondary infection, and shortens convalescence. Occasionally, a spontaneous abortion may be accompanied by a placenta accreta that resists persistent attempts at removal and is accompanied by continued hemorrhage of serious proportions. In such cases, which are fortunately rare, emergency hysterectomy may be the only alternative and is invariably lifesaving.

MISSED ABORTION

The existence of missed abortion, in which fetal death in utero precedes by two or more months the onset of symptoms of the actual mechanical aborting process, is most often not recognized until the development of cramps and bleeding indicates that the abortion is actively under way and causes the patient to seek medical attention. Actually, in the majority of these patients, spontaneous delivery will occur within two to three weeks after fetal death, and under these circumstances the problem is handled in the same fashion as any incomplete abortion. However, the diagnosis of intrauterine fetal death occasionally becomes apparent before the onset of labor, and a decision as to further management must be made. Fetal death is suggested if cessation of fetal movements is noted by patient and physician and if the fetal heartbeat is no longer audible to the physician. More definite evidence may be found in the disappearance of activity on the fetal electrocardiogram or in the demonstration on an abdominal x-ray film of elevation of the subcutaneous fat layer away from the fetal skull bones, the so-called *halo sign*. If fetal death is confirmed, it appears to be perfectly safe to treat the situation expectantly for three to four weeks and await the spontaneous onset of labor, which in 90 percent of cases will occur within one month and which will eventually take place in all cases.

In perhaps 25 to 35 percent of women who retain dead fetuses in utero for five weeks or longer, hypofibrinogenemia with secondary hemorrhagic phenomena will develop, and alarming hemorrhage may occur, both from the ·terus as well as at other body sites. Therefore, if labor does not occur within one month of the estimated time of fetal death, weekly determinations of the serum fibrinogen concentration (normal value roughly 350 mg per 100 ml) is a wise precautionary measure. In any case, the uterus should probably be emptied after one month, either by induction of labor (rupture of the membranes, with or without the additional use of oxytocins, or intrauterine injection of hypertonic saline solution) or by hysterotomy or curettage. Uterine evacuation is especially indicated if the fibrinogen level falls below 150 mg per 100 ml, or if bleeding occurs, regardless of the fibrinogen level. (The administration of fibrinogen alone, without emptying the uterus, is not effective in controlling the bleeding.) Not infrequently, the extreme apprehension of the patient and her family concerning the unfortunate situation is the most difficult aspect of all for the physician to manage. The ultimate labor itself is usually short and uncomplicated.

SEPTIC (CRIMINALLY INDUCED) ABORTION

The serious gynecologic emergency of septic abortion has already been discussed in detail in Chapter 8. It should be emphasized again that its management differs from that of a simple, spontaneous, incomplete abortion in that, unless massive hemorrhage dictates the need for earlier curettage, even in an early, uncomplicated septic abortion, control of or protection against invasive sepsis is achieved first by a short (6 to 12 hours), intensive preliminary antibiotic program, together with attention to restoration of normal fluid balance and blood volume prior to surgical emptying of the uterus. Prompt evacuation of the uterus shortly after institution of antibiotic therapy will frequently allow removal of the septic focus before extension beyond the confines of the uterine cavity can take place. Thus, spread of infection into the wall of the uterus and beyond, with the subsequent occurrence of septic and gram-negative endotoxemic shock, can be prevented. Should endotoxemic shock develop, the situation becomes critical, and the intensive therapeutic program presented in Chapter 8 will then be of vital importance.

HABITUAL ABORTION

By definition, a patient in whom three or more consecutive pregnancies have terminated in spontaneous abortion or miscarriage before the twenty-eighth week may be considered as potentially subject to habitual abortion. However, the chance that any pregnancy will end in abortion is roughly 15 percent, and a number of statistical analyses in large series of patients have shown that the probability of a second spontaneous abortion is only 20 percent, and that even after three consecutive miscarriages the risk is only 25 percent. Thus there are obvious shortcomings in such an empirical definition of habitual abortion, as well as many pitfalls for the unwary in the evaluation of programs of therapy designed for patients falling into this category. Nevertheless, there is little doubt that there is a group of women who exhibit a definite predisposition toward abortion and miscarriage, and patients in this category warrant careful study and management in the hope that obvious causes for their inability to maintain a pregnancy normally and carry it to term can be discovered and corrected in at least some of them.

Etiology and Management

Since the potential etiologic factors are many, and since multiple causes may operate simultaneously in the same patient, the diagnostic approach should include the following: (1) an evaluation of the nutritional and general health status of both husband and wife; (2) in the woman, a search for underlying chronic diseases that may foster placental insufficiency in early pregnancy (particularly, latent diabetes, thyroid disturbances, or primary ovarian dysfunction), a careful evaluation of potential, often subtle psychic factors, and finally, a thorough search for local anatomic defects that may mechanically predispose to premature termination of a pregnancy. There is also suggestive evidence that low-grade infections of the female and/or male genital tracts by T-strain *Mycoplasma* organisms may be a significant cause of repeated spontaneous abortions, and that elimination of these organisms by tetracycline or demeclocycline therapy will prevent subsequent fetal wastage (see Chap. 11). Obviously, it is preferable to carry out the diagnostic survey before the patient conceives again, correcting any deficiencies or abnormalities prior to the next pregnancy.

As far as general nutritional, endocrine-metabolic, or psychosomatic aspects of the problem are concerned, proper management of the so-called habitual aborter in early pregnancy includes assurance of adequate dietary and vitamin intake, and thyroid medication if indicated. Occasionally, it is desirable to give supplemental progesterone in the form of any of the newer progestational agents: e.g., Enovid, 20 mg orally, given daily beginning with the third or fourth week of pregnancy, with a gradual increase to 40 mg daily; or Delalutin, 500 mg intramuscularly, given weekly until the twenty-eighth week of gestation (no fetal masculinizing effects have been observed with either of these drugs in these dosages). However, the actual therapeutic value of supplemental progesterone is highly controversial, and it certainly should not be employed indiscriminately in these patients but only if there is valid evidence of progesterone deficiency (e.g., abnormal ferning on cervical mucous smears, low progesterone effects on vaginal smears, or low urinary pregnanediol excretion). Perhaps even more important is the development of a close, supportive relationship between physician and patient, the former constantly offering reassurance and encouragement at the regular prenatal visits and also remaining readily available in the intervals between. In this way it is often possible to relieve the stress and anxiety characteristically experienced by this group of patients by allowing them to relate their symptoms and verbalize their fears and apprehensions, which can then be sympathetically allayed and explained. Assuming that no local uterine abnormality or fundamental endocrinopathy exists, such a conscientious supportive program will allow 75 to 80 percent of these women who have habitually aborted in the past to carry to term. In nearly all reported series, no improvement in these results has been observed by adding routine progesterone medication to the regimen.

Another intriguing possibility is that in a certain percentage of women, habitual spontaneous abortion may be the result of immunologic rejection of the fetus due to excessive release of fetal antigens, especially in cases where tissue antigens from the husband and those from the wife are markedly dissimilar. Mitchell and his associates [2] have studied this problem extensively and have reported the accelerated rejection of skin grafts donated by the husband in a series of pregnant women who had been habitual aborters. Of considerable interest was their observation that 70 percent of the women who had received skin grafts from their husbands subsequently carried their pregnancies to term, suggesting the possibility that the grafting process might have induced immunologic tolerance to the fetal antigens of paternal origin. However, as Mitchell and co-workers were quick to point out, a 70 percent successful term pregnancy rate in a group of habitual aborters is no better than the success rate achieved by almost any of the regimens commonly employed in managing such patients. Nevertheless, the concept that some repetitive abortions might be the result of immunologic rejection merits consideration and remains the subject of continued investigation.

With regard to local, mechanical causes for repeated abortion or miscarriage, the principal conditions involved are (1) congenital anomalies of the uterus and vagina (see Chap. 3 for diagnosis and treatment), (2) submucous or intramural fibroids (see Chap. 12), and (3) incompetency of the cervix. Since this latter entity is of significance only in connection with habitual abortion or miscarriage, it seems appropriate to discuss it briefly here.

The Incompetent Cervix and Habitual Abortion

Although most abortions occur before the twelfth week and are associated with an abnormal embryo, a significant number of patients experience repeated premature terminations of otherwise normal pregnancies in the second, or occasionally early in the third, trimester of pregnancy (typically between the twelfth and thirty-fourth weeks). Such patients may be found to have an anatomic defect that involves the entire cervical segment and consists of an abnormal cervical dilatation, particularly at the level of the internal cervical os. This history of repeated second-trimester abortions occurring relatively rapidly and painlessly after spontaneous rupture of the membranes and usually unaccompanied by preliminary cramps or bleeding is characteristic and should be the clue that further studies are indicated to corroborate the diagnosis. If the patient first appears in the nonpregnant state, the diagnosis may be confirmed by the ease with which a No. 18 or larger cervical dilator may be introduced into the cervical canal and passed through the internal os, or by hysterosalpingography (either according to standard techniques or employing a special balloon catheter to retain the radiopaque dye within the cervical segment), which reveals the triangularly dilated internal os and upper endocervical canal. When, as is often the case, the patient is first seen while pregnant, the cervix will be observed to undergo painless dilatation over a period of several weeks, and ultimately the fetal membranes will be plainly visible as they bulge through a dilated, patulous cervix (Fig. 35A). Apparently, the incompetent cervix may occasionally be a primary congenital condition, some patients never having carried a pregnancy beyond the second trimester. However, the majority of patients give a history of one or more term pregnancies (often the last one was a difficult, traumatic labor and delivery) or have previously undergone what may have been a traumatic cervical dilatation and curettage, so that in most instances the defect appears to be an acquired one.

The management of the incompetent cervix during pregnancy involves surgical repair utilizing a vaginal approach and placing an encircling ligature strip of fascia, polyethylene, or Mersilene (Ethicon), a synthetic polyester fiber material; or, more recently, a dermal graft strip removed from the patient's lower abdominal skin, which is tied snugly about the cervix at the level of the internal os, closing the defect — the so-called Shirodkar operation, or cervical cerclage (Fig. 35B and C). To obtain best results in patients with the classic history, the procedure should preferably be done prophylactically, before actual dilatation and bulging of the membranes has occurred; but it is wiser to delay until after the sixteenth week to avoid performing the procedure prematurely, only to have a simple abortion due to a blighted ovum occur in the first trimester. Emergency cerclage in the face of an already dilated cervix and bulging membranes is also indicated if rupture of the membranes and actual initiation of early labor has not yet occurred. The membranes are gently reduced as the ligature is tied, and the procedure is often successful in halting the incipient premature labor. In either case, vaginal delivery can be accompanied by simply dividing the ligature at term and then either awaiting the spontaneous onset of labor or inducing labor in the usual manner; this will of course necessitate repeated cerclage with future pregnancies. If, on the other hand, an attempt at permanent repair is desired, cesarean section can be performed, but section will then be mandatory with all future pregnancies as well.

If the diagnosis of cervical incompetency is established in the nonpregnant state, the alternative procedure originally devised by Lash and Lash [31] can be utilized, and it has the advantage that it permits subsequent pregnancies to be delivered vaginally without seriously jeopardizing the cervical repair. The Lash operation is also carried out vaginally and involves removal of a longitudinal segment of the anterior cervical wall approximately one-half its circumference in width, thereby

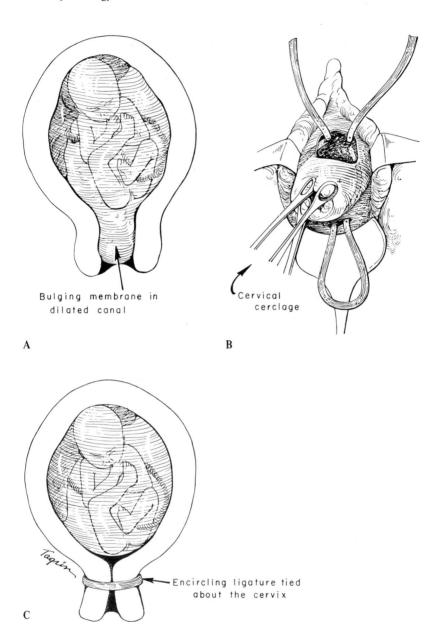

A

Bulging membrane in
dilated canal

B

Cervical
cerclage

C

Encircling ligature tied
about the cervix

Figure 35
A. Cervical dilatation in midtrimester pregnancy. B. Treatment by cervical cerclage,
showing placement of the encircling ligature. C. End result of cerclage, with restoration of adequate mechanical support of the pregnancy at the level of the internal
cervical os, forestalling progressive cervical dilatation and subsequent premature
initiation of labor.

reducing the previously dilated cervical canal and internal os to a normal diameter and state of competency.

THERAPEUTIC ABORTION

Medical Indications

Advances in general medicine in the past few decades have sharply reduced the number of valid, purely medical reasons for terminating a pregnancy. The mere presence of any degree of cardiac or renal disease, diabetes, tuberculosis, or other potentially chronic systemic disorder no longer warrants routine termination of pregnancy, for such diseases are now usually just as amenable to therapy in the pregnant as in the nonpregnant state. However, there remains a relatively small number of fairly generally accepted indications for seriously considering therapeutic abortion on medical grounds alone. Chief among these are the presence of maternal disorders that pose a real threat to the health or life of the mother and include the following:

1. Severe hypertensive cardiovascular disease.
2. Severe chronic renal disease.
3. Severe rheumatic valvular heart disease with uncontrollable cardiac decompensation.
4. Serious psychiatric disorders, especially when the threat of suicide is great.
5. Carcinoma of the breast or malignant melanoma coexisting with pregnancy. Although the primary therapy for either remains the same, regardless of the coexisting pregnancy, there is considerable evidence that the course of both neoplasms is adversely influenced by the high levels of placental steroids, particularly estrogen, present in association with the pregnancy, and that termination of the pregnancy may improve the chances for a favorable response to treatment.
6. Carcinoma of the cervix. In this situation, which is discussed more fully in Chapter 13, proper treatment is often facilitated by the preliminary performance of a therapeutic abortion; in any case, radiation or surgical treatment will, of course, terminate the pregnancy.
7. Miscellaneous medical disorders, under certain circumstances; e.g., lymphoma, ulcerative colitis, regional enteritis, multiple sclerosis, severe diabetes.

Another potential indication for therapeutic interruption of pregnancy involves situations in which it is suspected that there is a strong possibility that the fetus is abnormal. Obviously, therapeutic abortion on these grounds is a controversial, highly debatable subject, but nevertheless it is accepted as a legitimate and reasonable decision under certain special circumstances. The classic example of this type of indication is found in the case of the woman who contracts rubella (German measles) during the first trimester of pregnancy. On the basis of the high incidence of defective babies born to such mothers, the risks in the eyes of many women and their physicians are simply unacceptable. The accumulated figures from various reported series originally indicated that from one-third to one-half of all such patients would either lose the baby or give birth to a stillborn or seriously defective child with fetal abnormalities such as blindness in association with cataracts, deafness, congenital heart disease, microcephaly, or severe mental retardation. (As discussed in Chapter 4, other maternal viral diseases such as rubeola, mumps, chickenpox, and poliomyelitis may also be responsible for fetal anomalies, but the incidence of such abnormalities is considerably less.)

Although on the basis of subsequent careful prospective studies it appears that the overall risk may be more in the range of 10 to 15 percent, the problem is still a serious one, women contracting rubella during the first trimester having a six or seven times greater chance of giving birth to defective infants than a normal control group of pregnant women. (The risk is probably even greater if the disease occurs during the first two months of pregnancy, with a maximum risk of 50 to 60 percent the first four weeks, 25 to 35 percent in the next four weeks, 15 to 20 percent in the ninth to twelfth week, and only 5 to 10 percent in weeks 13 to 16.) Contraction of rubella during the early second trimester also increases the chance of an abnormal child or of premature delivery, but the risk is considerably less.

The safe, effective rubella vaccine now available promises virtually to eliminate this most common infectious cause of congenital abnormalities. Because 40 percent of adult women show definite symptoms and signs of the disease following inoculation, it is best administered during childhood, none of the vaccinated children or their contacts having exhibited any clinical evidence of disease despite the successful establishment of immunity in 97 percent of those vaccinated. Its use during pregnancy is definitely contraindicated, however, since even attenuated viruses are potentially teratogenic. In adult females of childbearing age, the safest time to give the vaccine is immediately postpartum, with strict avoidance of another pregnancy for three months following vaccination.

In general, the management of the unvaccinated woman who has been exposed to or contracts German measles during the first four months of pregnancy should be as follows:

1. An attempt should be made to determine whether or not the patient is already immune to the virus (80 percent of young adults in the United States have already been infected and are immune to rubella). This can be done by a standard serum hemagglutination inhibition test for antibodies against the rubella virus now performed by many state and hospital laboratories.

2. If the patient is shown not to be immune, serious consideration should be given to the early (within one week of exposure) administration of large doses (at least 20 ml intramuscularly) of gamma globulin, which, by virtue of the presence of neutralizing antibody for rubella, may prevent the development of the infection or modify its course sufficiently to reduce the incidence of subsequent abortion and fetal malformations significantly.

3. If the patient actually contracts the disease, consideration on the basis of all

the factors involved in each case should be given to whether therapeutic abortion is indicated or should be recommended. If there are religious or other contraindications to abortion, or if the situation affects a childless couple in the older age group whose future chances of conception are limited, then obviously the pregnancy should be allowed to proceed to term, accepting the risk of an abnormal child and the increased chance of other potential pregnancy complications. If, on the other hand, the patient is a young woman in her early childbearing years who is reluctant to accept the potential hazards of a deformed child, and if there are no religious or other contraindications to therapeutic abortion, then, barring any local legal obstacles, medical interruption of the pregnancy is probably indicated.

Other examples of similar types of situations in which the problem of whether or not therapeutic abortion is indicated may arise include a history of serious hereditary disorders, such as amaurotic idiocy and hemophilia, particularly if previous offspring have exhibited these disorders, as well as exposure to drugs known to produce serious fetal damage, such as the sedative thalidomide, which produced phocomelia in a high percentage of infants born to mothers to whom it had been administered early in pregnancy. Since it is now possible to establish definitely the presence of many inherited fetal disorders by amniocentesis (e.g., virtually all chromosomal abnormalities, including Down's syndrome; certain biochemical disorders such as Tay-Sachs disease and Hurler's disease; and sex-linked diseases carried by females but affecting only males, such as hemophilia), it is likely that there will be an increasing use of therapeutic abortion for this type of indication.

Elective (Voluntary) Therapeutic Abortion for
Unwanted and Unplanned Pregnancy

During the past few years, a much more liberal viewpoint toward therapeutic interruption of pregnancy has come into existence among both the lay population and the medical profession. This has resulted not only in the adoption of more permissive legislation in most states but also in a steady increase in the number of voluntary therapeutic abortions done each year. This has served to reduce the number of criminal abortions performed in the United States but has by no means eliminated them, and morbidity and mortality from the illegal procedures still remain a major problem.

Nowadays, the vast majority of legal interruptions are performed because the patients do not desire to continue the pregnancy. The decision is thus a voluntary one on the part of the patient, with the advice and consent of the physician who is counseling and treating her. Most of these women are single, many of them are in their early twenties, and a significant percentage are teenagers. Certainly, the facts of these situations usually favor the concept that the individual should not have to carry the undesired pregnancy to term, with the risk of further emotional and socioeconomic damage, just because of an unplanned, unwanted, accidental conception, the result of irresponsibility, emotional disorders, ignorance, or the unavailability of contraceptives.

However, to concentrate entirely on this approach to the problem of unwanted pregnancy seems questionable on both moral and practical grounds. Rather, there must be greater emphasis placed on improving both the quality and the availability of contraceptive methods for those who need them most. There should be no restrictions on the provision of birth control services or the availability of contraceptives for any sexually active person, regardless of age, sex, or marital status. Stating it another way, it would seem more rational to approach the general solution of what is now primarily a sociocultural and economic problem by better education in combination with public health or preventive medicine measures rather than by a surgical operation. There is no question, however, but that liberalization of abortion laws and their broader application in specific, individual circumstances has been long overdue, and each case must be considered on its own merits.

By the late 1960s, the majority opinion of the medical profession (including the American Medical Association and the American College of Obstetricians and Gynecologists, both of which issued official policy statements) was in favor of uniform state laws providing that a licensed physician can terminate a pregnancy in an accredited hospital if he can reasonably establish in consultation with two other licensed physicians that:

1. There is substantial risk that continuance of the pregnancy would threaten the life or gravely impair the physical or mental health of the mother; or
2. There is substantial risk that the child would be born with grave physical or mental defects; or
3. The pregnancy is the result of legally established statutory or forcible rape or incest.

By mid-1970, both these organizations had adopted even more liberal resolutions supporting the concept, and several state legislatures had already passed laws to the effect that therapeutic abortion should only require the consent of the woman and her licensed physician. New York was one of the first states to pass such legislation, and New York physicians, hospitals, and special abortion clinics carried out elective abortions on a large scale in the early 1970s.

In 1973, the United States Supreme Court ruled that the decision for or against abortion was and is the prerogative of the pregnant woman in consultation with her physician, paving the way for elective abortions during the first two trimesters to be done legally in all states; since then, more than a million legal abortions have been performed annually in this country.

First-trimester abortions are relatively simple, inexpensive, and free of significant risk of serious complications. Second-trimester abortions are much more complicated, and the potential for serious complications and an unpredictable outcome is much greater. Therefore, certain state and federal regulations aimed at protecting the health of the pregnant woman undergoing the abortion are valid, but there is no legal barrier to the performance of elective, or voluntary, abortion in the second trimester.

After the second trimester, and at the time when the fetus first becomes viable (potentially capable of leading an independent life outside the mother), the safety and rights of the potential new life now also become a proper subject for legal protection by state or federal laws. Most state laws, as well as the 1973 Supreme Court ruling, therefore continue to restrict therapeutic abortions after the second trimester to those necessary to preserve the life or health of the mother, and public opinion has strongly supported the obvious wisdom of this concept. When necessary and indicated, third-trimester abortions are even riskier and more complicated and almost invariably require hysterotomy if they are to be safely and expeditiously done; therefore they should be avoided as much as possible. Ideally, elective (voluntary) abortions should be done early in the first trimester.

Management of Therapeutic Abortion

It is generally accepted that for abortions on medical grounds it is advisable to have on the patient's record the written opinions of two or more physicians, or of a hospital committee organized for the purpose, all recommending therapeutic abortion and the reasons therefor. For voluntary abortions, the patient (and, though not legally required, if she is married, her husband also) should sign a statement that she (or they) is (or are) requesting and concur in the decision to proceed with the therapeutic abortion. If the patient is a minor and unmarried, it is wise to obtain parental consent, if possible, although even if one or both parents refuse consent, the abortion can still legally be done. The decision to abort should be made early, preferably before the end of the first trimester, so that the pregnancy can be interrupted safely and in the simplest way, by suction curettage, or, when necessary, formal dilatation and curettage. A variation involving vacuum aspiration of the uterine contents (an office procedure) within 14 days of a missed menstrual period is also widely practiced and has been euphemistically termed *menstrual regulation* or *menstrual extraction.* There are even fewer complications than with the preceding methods, and only 3 to 4 percent of women so managed in early pregnancy require further treatment because of method failure. Most therapeutic abortions carried out by suction curettage can be done in the transient operating room section of the hospital or clinic and require only paracervical block or a very short period of general anesthesia. Although uterine perforation is rare during suction curettage, should it occur, there is the possible danger that the powerful suction may draw parametrial tissues and other adjacent structures, including the uterine artery, ureter, bladder, and ileum, through the perforation in the uterine wall and into contact with the suction cannula, with resulting hematomas and traumatic lacerations. Hence suction curettage requires just as much care as regular curettage if complications are to be prevented or recognized and treated promptly if they occur.

In addition to accidental perforation and related trauma during D&C or suction curettage, the other common potential complication is retention of fetal or placental fragments, with subsequent bleeding, or intrauterine and pelvic sepsis, or both. Patients should be alerted to these possibilities and warned to report the development of cramps, abdominal pain, vaginal bleeding, or fever immediately. Such symptoms will require hospitalization for a formal D&C, as well as vigorous management of pelvic infection as discussed in Chapter 8.

Curettage is not a safe or feasible technique for interruption of pregnancy after the third month, especially in primigravidas. Instead, the intraamniotic injection of hypertonic saline solution has proved to be an effective method of inducing labor after the third or fourth month, although it is not without hazard. The technique is as follows:

1. The patient's bladder is emptied, and the lower abdomen is surgically prepared and draped.
2. Under local anesthesia, a No. 16 or No. 18 needle trocar is introduced into the amniotic cavity, inserting it in the midline and well below the top of the fundus to avoid loops of bowel.
3. A total of 100 to 200 ml of amniotic fluid is removed, and then 200 to 300 ml of a 20% saline solution is instilled and the needle withdrawn.

Although a certain percentage of failures is encountered, labor usually occurs within 8 to 20 hours, and delivery is ordinarily accomplished within a few hours. Subsequent curettage is not infrequently necessary to complete the removal of all placental and decidual tissue.

Aside from the dangers of introducing infection or accidental injury to adjacent viscera, the most serious complications, including several deaths, have occurred as a result of the accidental intravenous injection of the hypertonic saline solution. Cerebral convulsions and acute renal failure, the latter presumably due to hemolysis, and acute tubular necrosis have occurred, with fatal outcomes reported in several cases. Furthermore, a number of instances of disseminated intravascular coagulation and secondary maternal hemorrhage have been observed, presumably secondary to the release of tissue thromboplastin from the edematous, fragmenting placenta.

An alternative approach now being utilized is the intraamniotic instillation of the natural or synthetic prostaglandins F_2 and $F_{2\alpha}$. These compounds induce strong uterine contractions that usually result in cervical dilatation and expulsion of fetus and placenta within 24 hours. In some clinics, in addition to the prostaglandins, "laminaria tents" are used. These are insertable plugs made from dried seaweed (available commercially from Milex Products, Inc.), with an action similar to that of the old-fashioned "slippery elm" (i.e., gradual swelling occurs when the substance absorbs moisture), so that dilatation of the cervix is further promoted and speeded up by this mechanical means. (Laminaria tents have also been employed by some as a preliminary step prior to suction curettage, inserting one 12 hours before, especially in young nulligravidas with tight cervical canals that are otherwise difficult to dilate.) The use of prostaglandins appears to be a safer method than hypertonic saline, because their use avoids the dangers of disseminated intravascular coagulopathy and hypernatremia.

The physician should be on the lookout for psychological problems secondary to guilt feelings over the abortion, for they are encountered occasionally, especially in women who were emotionally unstable beforehand, and may require psychiatric consultation. However, emotional disturbances following abortions have not been as frequent or as serious as had been anticipated, and proper preabortion counseling, together with reassurance and sympathetic support during and after the procedure, will tend to minimize the emotional trauma suffered by women undergoing elective abortions.

Finally, postabortion counseling regarding an effective contraceptive program is of vital importance. Without a conscientious and sympathetic follow-up program, a significant number of patients who have undergone their first abortion may become "repeaters."

If the therapeutic termination of pregnancy is indicated for chronic medical or psychiatric conditions that will be in existence at the time of any subsequent pregnancy, sterilization at the time of abortion should be seriously considered. This would be particularly true in the case of a woman who already has children. Sterilization can be done by bilateral laparoscopic tubal ligations after evacuation of the uterus.

TROPHOBLASTIC TUMORS: HYDATIDIFORM MOLE, CHORIOADENOMA DESTRUENS, AND CHORIOCARCINOMA

Hydatidiform Mole

Although minor degrees of hydatidiform swelling of placental villi are observed in at least two-thirds of all spontaneously aborted pathologic ova, the generalized and more advanced degree of this process present in older pathologic ova results in the development of a true hydatidiform mole. Although apparently somewhat more common in Asian countries than in the United States, hydatidiform mole occurs roughly once in every 2000 pregnancies and is a more common complication of pregnancies in older women in their late forties or early fifties than in younger women. It is in essence a "missed abortion" of a blighted ovum whose chorionic villi persist and continue to undergo increasing hydatid swelling. This hydropic degeneration occurs because the immature villi, in spite of the absence of a fetal circulation (the embryo either does not form or dies during the third to fifth week of development), possess a functioning trophoblast and stroma, and hence continue to take up fluid from the maternal circulation, making progressive accumulation of fluid within their connective tissue spaces inevitable. In addition to gross swelling of villi, there is frequently histologic evidence of hyperplasia of trophoblastic elements as well as of myometrial invasion, even in so-called benign moles, and these observations, together with the fact that 50 percent of all choriocarcinomas follow molar pregnancies, tend to support the concept that hydatidiform moles should probably be considered true neoplasms of trophoblastic origin, usually benign but always potentially malignant. Occasionally, clinically and histologically benign moles may give rise to demonstrable "metastases" (usually pulmonary, but occasionally vaginal or vulvar). In this connection it must be remembered that even normal trophoblast frequently undergoes so-called physiologic deportation by virtue of its normal "invasion" of maternal blood vessels, with subsequent dispersion of groups of trophoblastic cells via the bloodstream, perhaps occasioned by the milking effect of uterine contractions or "placental commotion." However, such trophoblastic deportation does not of itself imply malignancy, although malignant trophoblast is probably disseminated by this same mechanism. The difference lies in the limited survival of normal trophoblast or benign mole when deported and its ultimate auto-lysis; malignant trophoblast persists as metastatic choriocarcinoma. It is still far from clear whether the underlying cause of trophoblastic tumors involves an ovarian insuf-ficiency with inadequate estrogen levels or an immunologic deficiency (lack of syn-cytiolysins), whether they may be produced by an intracellular infectious agent, or whether they represent a true neoplastic change.

CLINICAL FEATURES AND DIAGNOSIS

Clinical manifestations of hydatidiform mole commonly first appear in the fourth or fifth month of pregnancy, with abnormal vaginal bleeding the most frequent and cardinal symptom, usually unaccompanied by cramps or other pelvic discomfort. Occasionally, the patient will report having passed "grapelike bodies," the typical fragments of swollen, hydatid villi. On examination, the uterus will be found to be soft and of a rather characteristic doughy consistency, and the degree of enlarge-ment is usually out of proportion to the calculated duration of the pregnancy. (For example, although by dates the pregnancy may be known to be of only four to five months' duration, the uterine size may be more consistent with a pregnancy of five to six months.) Absence of the embryo is readily established by the lack of fetal heart sounds or palpable fetal structures, as well as by failure to visualize a fetal skeleton on a plain x-ray film of the abdomen. Transabdominal injection of radi-opaque dye into the uterine cavity (amniography) and subsequent visualization of a typical moth-eaten or honeycombed appearance on the abdominal x-ray film is another method by which an early differentiation between normal pregnancy and hydatidiform mole can often be made. Ultrasonography, if available, also permits a definite diagnosis of molar pregnancy in most cases. Definite laboratory confir-mation of the diagnosis may be obtained by virtue of the fact that hydatidiform mole or any of the other trophoblastic tumors are invariably associated with a high level of HCG, one that often continues to rise and be maintained at high levels far beyond the 90- to 100-day peak followed by a significant fall in titer observed in normal pregnancy; this may be quantitated by any of the bioassay techniques described in Chapter 2. Other frequently associated clinical features include some form of toxemia of pregnancy in roughly 40 percent of patients, and palpable bilat-eral ovarian enlargement due to the frequent presence of multiple theca-lutein cysts that develop in response to the persistently high titer of HCG.

INITIAL TREATMENT

If abortion is in process in a case of suspected or definitely established early molar pregnancy (on the basis of the gross and/or histologic features of tissue already passed), immediate and thorough evacuation of the uterus by careful suction curettage and forceps exploration is indicated. Special care should be taken to avoid perforating the cervix or fundus of the typically soft molar uterus. In the case of larger moles, particularly if the patient is not in labor and the cervix is not dilated, either an attempt to induce labor by intravenous oxytocin drip or evacuation of the uterus by abdominal hysterotomy may sometimes be preferable to primary curettage. However, in general, hysterotomy should be avoided if possible, and suction curettage is usually successful even in the face of considerable uterine enlargement, unless massive bleeding ensues, which may necessitate emergency hysterotomy. In any event, following evacuation of the mole itself, gentle, sharp curettage of the endometrial cavity should be done and these scrapings submitted separately to the pathologist. Their careful histologic examination, together with study of the microscopic features of the actual molar tissue, will be of considerable help in determining the likelihood of further complications and the need for further therapy. Finally, in the case of patients age 35 to 40 or older, especially those not desirous of retaining childbearing function, primary hysterectomy rather than evacuation of the mole is probably the treatment of choice, since it minimizes the chance of further complications and greatly simplifies subsequent management.

Although prophylactic postevacuation chemotherapy, usually with actinomycin D, has been advocated and used successfully by some, the majority opinion favors withholding chemotherapy until there is evidence of persistent trophoblastic disease. On the one hand, only 10 to 20 percent of molar pregnancies are followed by the development of malignant trophoblastic tumors, and these should be detected promptly in their early, curable phase if a proper follow-up program is instituted. On the other hand, there is a significant toxicity and morbidity associated with even a prophylactic chemotherapy regimen, and it seems unwise to subject all patients with benign molar pregnancies to these uncomfortable side effects and risks unless it is really essential to do so in order to increase the curability of the 10 to 20 percent who are at risk, and as yet there is no evidence that this is the case. There is some suggestion that in the presence of uterine enlargement greater than expected for the menstrual history dates and bilateral ovarian enlargement, the patient has a greater-than-usual chance (55 to 60 percent as compared with 10 to 20 percent for the overall group) of malignant sequelae after a molar pregnancy. Perhaps it is in this type of patient that the use of prophylactic chemotherapy might be worth considering. However, the cure rate with delayed chemotherapy given only to those 10 to 20 percent of patients who subsequently manifest persistent trophoblastic disease is essentially 100 percent, so it is hard to make a strong case for prophylactic chemotherapy.

FURTHER MANAGEMENT

Careful follow-up of all patients is mandatory for these reasons: (1) the possibility of retention of fragments of molar tissue exists even following thorough curettage; (2) the potential for malignant transformation may reside in any mole; and (3) it is impossible to predict this potential with complete accuracy even by histologic examination (although the more anaplastic the histologic appearance, the greater the chance for malignant sequelae). The principal features of the follow-up program and the indications for and types of subsequent therapy may be outlined as follows:

1. In addition to an initial or baseline quantitative HCG assay (the highly sensitive serum or 24-hour urine HCG radioimmunoassays are the recommended ones; simple pregnancy tests, either biologic or immunologic, are of no value whatsoever in follow-up programs), a chest film should also be obtained, since the first manifestation of the malignant nature of the abnormal trophoblast may be a silent pulmonary metastasis. If a pulmonary lesion is seen on the initial chest x-ray, a diagnosis of choriocarcinoma should probably be assumed and the patient given intensive chemotherapy, since the earlier chemotherapy is begun, the greater the chance for successfully controlling the disease. The potentially lifesaving benefits of prompt institution of therapy far outweigh the slight chance that the pulmonary shadow might represent a focus of "physiologically" deported benign mole that would probably regress spontaneously. Even if the chest film is negative, it will nevertheless serve as another useful baseline for further evaluation and should be repeated periodically every one to two months during the next 12 months.

2. The patient should avoid conception for at least 12 to 18 months, since a new pregnancy would confuse the follow-up picture by producing a sudden recurrence of uterine enlargement and a rising HCG titer. Thereafter, pregnancy is perfectly safe, and a normal gestation is the usual result.

3. Initially, the patient should be carefully checked every one to two weeks for evidence of subnormal uterine involution or the return of abnormal bleeding, and HCG assays should be done at each visit to detect a persistent or rising titer. (In the absence of retained molar tissue, HCG titers ordinarily fall below the level of 500 m.u. per 24 hours, above which a positive pregnancy test is obtained [5 m.u. per ml if serum assay is employed] , and reach the normal range of 200 to 500 m.u. per 24 hours or less within a few weeks [six weeks at most] after evacuation of a mole.) If follow-up studies remain consistently negative for two to three months, they should then be continued every one to two months for at least one year.

4. On the other hand, persistent or recurrent bleeding, persistent uterine enlargement, and/or a persistent or rising HCG strongly suggests either retention of benign molar tissue or some more serious manifestation of trophoblastic disease. Any of the preceding symptoms or findings is sufficient indication for a repeat chest film and another curettage. The latter will usually suffice to reveal and remove any residual trophoblastic tissue within the uterus, with the exception of the occasional invasive mole (chorioadenoma destruens) or, even more rarely, a choriocarcinoma that is situated either deep within the myometrium or high in the cornual region or has extended to the adnexal or parametrial regions and hence is inaccessible to the curette. If histologic examination of all tissues removed at the time of repeat curettage shows only apparently benign trophoblast, if the chest film remains negative, and if the patient is otherwise asymptomatic, the program of careful, frequent

follow-up observations should be repeated. However, should bleeding, subinvolution, or persistent elevation of the HCG titer continue following the second curettage, then prompt, aggressive chemotherapy and probably hysterectomy thereafter are indicated as discussed under Chemotherapy of Trophoblastic Tumors, because persistence of these abnormal symptoms and findings after the second curettage is invariably due to retained but inaccessible trophoblastic tissue, usually chorioadenoma destruens.

5. However, if secondary curettings show definite malignant trophoblast (either chorioadenoma destruens or choriocarcinoma), but there is no evidence of distant metastasis, two possible forms of management may be employed:

a. Prompt institution of chemotherapy, as later described, is probably preferable and offers a good chance for cure. Also, preservation of childbearing function is thus achieved. A number of instances of complete eradication of chorioadenoma destruens or local uterine choriocarcinoma with subsequent normal pregnancies are now on record.
b. When preservation of the uterus is no longer essential, hysterectomy may also be advisable, although only in a minority of patients will it add significantly to the cure rate achieved by chemotherapy alone.

(If uninvolved, the ovaries may safely be preserved if this seems desirable, for although often grossly enlarged and distorted by the presence of multiple thecalutein cysts, they will resume normal appearance and function once the abnormal trophoblastic tissue is removed.) If a definite diagnosis of choriocarcinoma is established on examination of the final hysterectomy specimen, in view of its uniformly fatal course in the past, regardless of whether and when hysterectomy was performed, additional chemotherapy and continued close follow-up supervision are indicated. If the lesion proves to be a locally invasive mole or chorioadenoma destruens, postoperative chemotherapy is certainly optional and is probably unnecessary in most cases, since this lesion rarely metastasizes.

6. Regardless of the presence or absence of uterine disease, if local (e.g., vaginal, vulvar) or distant (e.g., pulmonary, abdominal) metastases are demonstrated, immediate institution of chemotherapy is indicated. The commonest site of metastasis is the lung, and the most frequent initial manifestation of the malignant nature of the trophoblastic tumor is a small, silent, often single focus of metastatic disease noted on the routine chest film; as often as not, there may be no local disease in the uterus. In any case, when metastatic disease is unequivocally present, hysterectomy appears to have no influence on the chances of a successful outcome following chemotherapy, and it is therefore probably not indicated, even when local uterine disease is present. Furthermore, when cure of choriocarcinoma with metastases is achieved by chemotherapy, resumption of normal menses and even subsequent normal pregnancies have been reported, so that in the younger woman still desirous of future childbearing, avoidance of hysterectomy has an additional advantage.

The rationale for the overall plan just outlined for the management of patients with apparently benign hydatidiform moles rests in the original clinically oriented pathologic classification proposed by Hertig and Sheldon [24] in 1947 and summarized in the next section. Although the subsequent discovery of an effective chemotherapeutic approach to the problem of malignant trophoblastic tumors has altered some of the details of the program in important ways and has vastly improved the outlook for cure of choriocarcinoma, the fundamental principles of management remain essentially the same.

PATHOLOGIC CLASSIFICATION OF APPARENT HYDATIDIFORM MOLES

The following classification, based on the histologic appearance of the mole and of associated scrapings from the uterus, is modified from Hertig and Sheldon [24]:

1. Histologically benign moles, 70 to 75 percent. (One-half or more of these patients subsequently have normal pregnancies.)
2. Histologically apparently malignant moles, 25 to 30 percent.
   a. Chorionepithelioma in situ, 3.5 percent. (Clinically benign; cured by curettage alone.)
   b. Syncytial endometritis, 4.5 percent. (Clinically benign; cured by curettage alone.)
   c. Chorioadenoma destruens (invasive mole), 16 percent. (Usually highly curable by hysterectomy; also responsive to chemotherapy.) Rarely accompanied by distant metastases. Usually manifested by subinvolution, bleeding, and rising HCG level within five to six weeks after original mole passed.
   d. True chorionepithelioma (choriocarcinoma), 2.5 percent. Invariably metastasizing, often with extensive local spread. Before specific chemotherapy became available, it was uniformly fatal and incurable, regardless of the treatment given, but the current chemotherapeutic approach appears to effect cure in 75 percent or more of cases.

Chorioadenoma Destruens

So-called invasive mole or chorioadenoma destruens can only develop in association with a molar pregnancy (cf. Choriocarcinoma), for by definition it is a lesion in which one or more molar villi have invaded the myometrium. This same potentially more invasive quality of some molar tissue may also give rise to the relatively uncommon but related lesion, metastatic mole, in which one or more molar villi have been transported to a distant site (vaginal or pulmonary foci of metastatic mole are the ones most commonly seen) but retain their villous morphology. The trophoblastic elements of either chorioadenoma destruens or metastatic mole are nearly always histologically benign, though in rare instances they may be sufficiently hyperplastic or even anaplastic to resemble choriocarcinoma in microscopic appearance.

CLINICAL MANIFESTATIONS

Although undoubtedly many such lesions undergo spontaneous regression, the invasive nature of those that persist ultimately leads to the development of an excavated, hemorrhagic lesion of the uterine wall and, in more advanced cases, even to perforation of the uterus. The usual clinical manifestations appear within five to eight weeks of the time when the original mole was passed or surgically evacuated and include subinvolution of the uterus, persistent bleeding (due to invasion of blood vessels within the uterine wall in the depths of the lesion, which usually retains its original communication with the endometrial cavity), and a rising HCG level. Distant metastases are extremely rare. The clinical approach to this sequence of events has already been described and involves repeat curettage, but because invasive mole tends to develop deep within the myometrium, it is often impossible to document its existence by curettage. Hence the absence or paucity of chorionic villi on secondary curettage in the presence of this clinical picture is highly suggestive of invasive mole, particularly when symptoms persist after the second curettage. Pelvic angiography has also proved helpful in demonstrating the presence and extent of local pelvic spread in the case of any of the malignant trophoblastic tumors.

TREATMENT

Although the lesion is invariably benign, ultimately it will become extensive enough to penetrate the uterus completely and lead to serious complications and even death from hemorrhage and sepsis. It is thus a potentially very serious disorder if not recognized and treated early. As already noted, hysterectomy, usually with conservation of the ovaries, is the standard treatment of choice. However, the evidence is now quite clear that even benign trophoblastic tissue is highly responsive to chemotherapy, and this approach is usually preferable in young women desiring more children. Chemotherapy is probably also indicated as an adjunct to the surgical management of the occasional locally metastatic benign molar lesion (e.g., vaginal or parametrial) that either cannot be completely excised by hysterectomy or recurs following attempted complete excision.

Choriocarcinoma (Chorionepithelioma)

The one unquestionably true malignant neoplasm of trophoblastic origin, but fortunately relatively rare, is the choriocarcinoma. From the standpoint of pathologic classification, it is a pure epithelial tumor that on histologic examination is seen to be composed of interlacing strands of syncytiotrophoblast and cytotrophoblast, both elements usually presenting a highly anaplastic appearance. Although the development of choriocarcinoma may accompany or follow any form of pregnancy, it, too, most commonly appears in association with an abnormal type of gestation. In Hertig and Sheldon's original report [24], the relative frequency of occurrence of choriocarcinoma with respect to the various types of pregnancy was estimated as follows: Of all choriocarcinomas, 50 percent occur in association with a molar pregnancy, the actual incidence being roughly 1 choriocarcinoma for every 40 molar pregnancies; 25 percent occur after abortion (actual incidence, 1:15,400); 22 percent occur after normal pregnancy (actual incidence, 1:160,000); and 3 percent occur after ectopic pregnancy (actual incidence, 1:5300). A later survey by Brewer et al. [7] yielded somewhat similar results in a large collected series of cases, 32 percent having been preceded by hydatidiform mole, 35 percent by abortion, and only 33 percent by a pregnancy that had progressed beyond 20 weeks. Occasionally, choriocarcinoma may not manifest itself for many years after the last pregnancy, and, although uncommon, intervals of 5 to 10 years between the pregnancy and the clinical appearance of the malignant tumor have been reported.

CLINICAL FEATURES

The existence of choriocarcinoma is nearly always completely unsuspected when it follows normal pregnancy, spontaneous abortion, or ectopic gestation. Furthermore, its presence locally in either the uterus or placenta following term pregnancy is rare, and even when it follows hydatidiform mole, there will be no evidence of a primary uterine focus in 50 percent of cases. Thus it is frequently impossible to establish a definite diagnosis by histologic examination of molar tissue or of scrapings obtained at the time of the initial evacuation of a mole or an abortus, and it is extremely rare that a diagnosis can be made by examination of a resected ectopic pregnancy or from study of the placenta after delivery of a normal pregnancy.

Most often, the initial clinical manifestations arise in connection with metastatic foci, the commonest sites of metastases being the lung, vagina, cervix, and vulva; spread to the liver and brain is also frequent, and even involvement of the gastrointestinal tract and bones is occasionally seen. In advanced cases, local extension to involve the ovaries and broad ligaments may also occur if a primary uterine tumor is present. Grossly, the lesions are purplish-red, granular, and usually markedly hemorrhagic, and hence those presenting externally (e.g., vulva, vagina, or cervix) or involving a viscus communicating externally (e.g., uterus, lungs, or gastrointestinal tract) characteristically have bleeding as their most prominent symptom.

Excision biopsy of an accessible cervical, vaginal, or vulvar metastasis will of course establish a definite diagnosis. In the case of suspected remote metastases in which biopsy is not feasible (e.g., suspicious pulmonary lesion on routine follow-up chest film), a quantitative HCG assay should be done, a markedly elevated level confirming the diagnosis. Occasionally, the diagnosis of choriocarcinoma is first established on the basis of examination of the complete uterus after hysterectomy has been performed for presumed chorioadenoma destruens or retained mole. As already noted, the pathologist's initial impression of the presence or absence of significant anaplastic features in the histologic appearance of the original hydatidiform mole is of some prognostic value, and patients in whom the molar tissue appears "malignant" should be followed particularly closely. However, only approximately 50 percent of this small group of patients with histologically malignant-appearing moles will ultimately have a malignant trophoblastic tumor: 40 percent will have chorioadenoma destruens and 10 percent, choriocarcinoma. Therefore, careful follow-up observations as previously described, rather than precipitant hysterectomy, are indicated, particularly in young women, since 50 percent will never have a choriocarcinoma. Furthermore, in the 40 percent who subsequently have an invasive mole, the condition in essentially all is completely curable by hysterectomy later on, when the diagnosis is definitely proved. On the other hand, the condition in 10 percent of this small group of patients in whom choriocarcinomas develop later can be considered as essentially incurable by hysterectomy alone from the very outset because of the early occurrence of blood vessel invasion and almost universal presence of metastatic disease outside the uterus.

TREATMENT

Prior to the advent of chemotherapy, the clinical course of most patients with choriocarcinoma was characterized by rapid and progressive dissemination of metastatic disease, often complicated by massive hemorrhage and secondary infection in the pelvis if a local uterine focus was also present and extensive enough to perforate the wall of the uterus. Therefore, even in the presence of known metastases, total hysterectomy was formerly felt to be indicated in most cases and was often effective in preventing further extension of the local growth, thus avoiding the secondary local complications. Excision of solitary or well-localized multiple metastases (e.g., vaginal, vulvar, pulmonary) has also been effectively carried out in the past in selected patients, with a number of recorded cases of apparent cure. Furthermore, occasionally, remote metastases were observed to regress, with subsequent long-term remissions, after removal of the primary tumor. Although in the past the disease has always been highly lethal in most instances, with a fatal termination within two years or less in all but a few patients, evidence has now been accumulated that such has not uniformly been true. The report of Brewer et al. [7] on 21 patients with well-documented choriocarcinoma (these cases were also histologically verified by Hertig) who had survived free of disease for periods of from 5 to 34 years following hysterectomy, 6 of them with metastases that were either excised, radiated, or underwent spontaneous regression, contradicts the old belief that bona fide choriocarcinoma was universally fatal. (These 21 patients represent 14.4 percent of the total group of 147 cases on file at the Albert Mathieu Chorionepithelioma Registry.)

Chemotherapy of Trophoblastic Tumors

The formerly hopeless outlook confronting the vast majority of patients with choriocarcinoma has been dramatically altered by the introduction of effective chemotherapy. In fact, the malignant trophoblastic tumors represent the only group of neoplasms in which actual cure has been accomplished through the use of anticancer drugs alone, although thousands of patients suffering from all types of malignant tumors have received a wide variety of chemotherapeutic agents during the past 20 years. Of the various compounds employed in the treatment of choriocarcinoma, the antimetabolite methotrexate, a folic acid antagonist, was the first to be successfully utilized and even at the present time probably remains the drug of choice for an initial trial of chemotherapy. Other drugs now employed that appear to be yielding good results include actinomycin D, an agent falling into the general class of antibiotics, and vinblastine (available as Velban), an oncolytic plant alkaloid. Patients who fail to respond or become resistant to methotrexate frequently obtain favorable remissions following treatment with one of the other two drugs. In those who fail to respond to single-drug therapy, remissions can sometimes be induced by means of multiple drug therapy with methotrexate, actinomycin D, and chlorambucil. Finally, although the chemotherapy is usually given systemically, in the case of some patients with local pelvic disease that fails to respond, arterial infusional chemotherapy has also been utilized and appears to have been highly successful in selected cases. Preliminary arteriography has also proved very helpful in defining the precise site and extent of the local pelvic disease.

Treatment with any of these compounds, which are highly toxic, is accompanied by a number of potentially hazardous systemic side effects, including severe bone-marrow depression, dermatitis, stomatitis, alopecia, and various manifestations of central nervous system, hepatic, and renal toxicity. This type of chemotherapy must therefore be carried out with the patient hospitalized and under the closest supervision by personnel highly experienced in the choice and regulation of drug and dosage as well as in the prevention and management of any of the numerous manifestations of drug toxicity. Response to treatment during and after each course of drug therapy is carefully evaluated, utilizing both clinical and roentgenographic observations and, most important, the subsequent changes in the quantitative HCG excretion levels, the latter being the most sensitive and reliable indicator of whether or not the disease has been arrested or is progressing. A highly sensitive radioimmunoassay test that is specific for HCG is now available for this purpose.

For details of treatment regimens, the interested reader is referred to any of several comprehensive reports included in the references at the end of this chapter.

Hertz and his colleagues published an early report in 1961 [25] indicating that approximately 50 percent of the patients they had treated during the preceding five years had achieved complete remissions of from six months' to five years' duration. All 63 patients had received methotrexate, and 13 who had failed to respond had also received vinblastine, 2 of the latter group also attaining the status of apparent cures. In addition, many of the patients who ultimately succumbed to the disease experienced temporary regressions and worthwhile palliation, in some instances of three to four years' duration. Analysis of their initial results emphasized that probably the most important single factor affecting the chances for cure by chemotherapy was the duration of the disease prior to the institution of treatment. With this key factor in mind, and as a result of a subsequent larger experience with both methotrexate and actinomycin D, the latter drug appearing to be at least as effective as methotrexate and far more effective than vinblastine, it is apparent that with early treatment, survival rates of between 75 and 90 percent can be achieved by chemotherapy in patients with choriocarcinoma. This prediction has indeed been an accurate one, as shown by subsequent reports from a number of institutions.

The possible role of drug therapy in the management of patients with benign hydatidiform moles or in the treatment of chorioadenoma destruens has also been explored. There are now sufficient data to show definitely that methotrexate and actinomycin D are equally successful in controlling benign trophoblastic disorders. On the basis of numerous clinical trials, it is apparent that chemotherapy is a safe, effective, and simpler alternative to surgery in dealing with these potentially pre-malignant lesions. The ability to achieve complete cure without the need for hyster-ectomy and loss of childbearing function represents a great advance for the many younger women encountered with persistent or invasive moles. In this regard, a number of reports of successful normal pregnancies following treatment by chemo-therapy of patients with choriocarcinoma, chorioadenoma destruens, and benign moles have already appeared in the literature.

REFERENCES

1. Asherman, J. G. Etiology of ectopic pregnancy: A new concept. *Obstet. Gynecol.* 6:619, 1955.
2. Bardawil, W. A., Mitchell, G. W., Jr., McKeogh, R. P., and Marchant, D. J. Behavior of skin homografts in human pregnancy: I. Habitual abortion. *Am. J. Obstet. Gynecol.* 84:1283, 1962.
3. Barter, R. H., Dusbabek, J. A., and Riva, H. L. Surgical closure of the incompe-tent cervix during pregnancy. *Am. J. Obstet. Gynecol.* 75:511, 1958.
4. Berlind, M. The contralateral corpus luteum: An important factor in ectopic pregnancies. *Obstet. Gynecol.* 16:51, 1960.
5. Breen, J. L. A 21 year survey of 654 ectopic pregnancies. *Am. J. Obstet. Gynecol.* 106:1004, 1970.
6. Brenner, W. E., Edelman, D. A., and Kessel, E. Menstrual regulation in the United States. *Fertil. Steril.* 26:289, 1975.
7. Brewer, J. I., Rinehart, J. J., and Dunbar, R. W. Choriocarcinoma. *Am. J. Obstet. Gynecol.* 81:574, 1961.
8. Brewer, J. I., Torok, E. E., Webster, A., and Dolkart, R. E. Hydatidiform mole. *Am. J. Obstet. Gynecol.* 101:556, 1968.
9. Carr, D. H. Chromosome anomalies as a cause of spontaneous abortion. *Am. J. Obstet. Gynecol.* 97:283, 1967.
10. Clark, J. F. J., and Guy, R. S. Abdominal pregnancy. *Am. J. Obstet. Gynecol.* 96:511, 1966.
11. Connell, E. B. Abortion: Patterns, technics, and results. *Fertil. Steril.* 24:78, 1973.

12. Curry, S. L., Hammond, C. B., Tyrey, L., Creasman, W. T., and Parker, R. T. Hydatidiform mole: Diagnosis, management, and long-term follow-up of 347 patients. *Obstet. Gynecol.* 45:1, 1975.

13. Goldstein, D. P. The chemotherapy of gestational trophoblastic disease. *J.A.M.A.* 220:209, 1972.

14. Goldstein, D. P. Prevention of gestational trophoblastic disease by use of actinomycin-D in molar pregnancies. *Obstet. Gynecol.* 42:475, 1974.

15. Graff, G., Lancet, M., and Czernobilsky, B. Ovarian pregnancy with intrauterine devices in situ. *Obstet. Gynecol.* 40:535, 1972.

16. Grant, A. The effect of ectopic pregnancy on fertility. *Clin. Obstet. Gynecol.* 5:861, 1962.

17. Green, T. H., Jr. The role of culdoscopy in the diagnosis of tubal disorders. *Clin. Obstet. Gynecol.* 5:799, 1962.

18. Hall, R. E. The Supreme Court decision on abortion. *Am. J. Obstet. Gynecol.* 116:1, 1973.

19. Hallatt, J. G. Repeat ectopic pregnancy: A study of 123 consecutive cases. *Am. J. Obstet. Gynecol.* 122:520, 1975.

20. Halpin, T. F. Ectopic pregnancy: The problem of diagnosis. *Am. J. Obstet. Gynecol.* 106:227, 1970.

21. Hammond, C. B., Borchert, L. G., Tyrey, L., Creasman, W. T., and Parker, R. T. Treatment of metastatic trophoblastic disease. *Am. J. Obstet. Gynecol.* 115:451, 1973.

22. Hammond, C. B., Hertz, R., Ross, G. T., Lipsett, M. B., and Odell, W. D. Primary chemotherapy for nonmetastatic gestational trophoblastic neoplasms. *Am. J. Obstet. Gynecol.* 98:71, 1967.

23. Hertig, A. T., and Livingstone, R. G. Spontaneous, threatened and habitual abortion: Its pathogenesis and treatment. *N. Engl. J. Med.* 230:797, 1944.

24. Hertig, A. T., and Sheldon, W. H. Hydatidiform mole: A pathologico-clinical correlation of 200 cases. *Am. J. Obstet. Gynecol.* 53:1, 1947.

25. Hertz, R., Lewis, J., Jr., and Lipsett, M. B. Five years' experience with the chemotherapy of metastatic choriocarcinoma and related trophoblastic tumors in women. *Am. J. Obstet. Gynecol.* 82:631, 1961.

26. Ingersoll, F. M. Operations for tubal pregnancy. *Clin. Obstet. Gynecol.* 5:853, 1962.

27. Javert, C. T. Repeated abortion: Results of treatment in 100 patients. *Obstet. Gynecol.* 3:420, 1954.

28. Jones, G. S. Abortion and corpus luteum deficiency. *Obstet. Gynecol. Surv.* 14:243, 1959.

29. Jones, W. B., and Lewis, J. L., Jr. Treatment of gestational trophoblastic disease. *Am. J. Obstet. Gynecol.* 120:14, 1974.

30. Keyser, H. H., Iffy, L., and Cohen, J. Basal body temperature recording in ectopic pregnancy. *J. Reprod. Med.* 14:37, 1975.

31. Lash, A. F., and Lash, S. R. Habitual abortion: Incompetent internal os of cervix. *Am. J. Obstet. Gynecol.* 59:68, 1950.

32. Lauerson, N. H., and Wilson, K. H. Midtrimester abortion induced by serial intramuscular injections of 15(s)-15-Methyl-Prostaglandin $F_{2\alpha}$. *Am. J. Obstet. Gynecol.* 121:273, 1975.

33. Mann, E. C. Habitual abortion, a report in two parts on 160 patients. *Am. J. Obstet. Gynecol.* 77:706, 1959.

34. Pasnau, R. O. Psychiatric complications of therapeutic abortion. *Obstet. Gynecol.* 40:252, 1972.

35. Persaud, V. Etiology of tubal ectopic pregnancy. *Obstet. Gynecol.* 36:257, 1970.
36. Smythe, A. R., II, and Underwood, D. B., Jr. Ectopic pregnancy after post-coital diethylstilbestrol. *Am. J. Obstet. Gynecol.* 121:284, 1975.
37. Stim, E. M. Saline abortion. *Obstet. Gynecol.* 40:247, 1972.

look up Hall, R.E. & Todd, W.D.

Am J. Obst. & Gynec 81:1229;

1961

10
Endometriosis

Historically speaking, endometriosis is a twentieth-century disease. Its very existence as a pathologic entity, as well as that of its near relative, adenomyosis, was first recognized around the turn of the century. Furthermore, social changes peculiar to the civilization of this century and influencing profoundly the pattern of reproductive function of the modern female in many areas of the world may in part, at least, be responsible for the steadily increasing incidence and significance of endometriosis since 1900. Because it is such a common, important, and fascinating disease, and since the sum total of our knowledge about it is literally a product of our times and has occurred simultaneously with the development of gynecology as a specialty, a brief historical résumé of the initial phases of its discovery and understanding may be of some interest.

Although the earliest description of the lesion now called endometriosis was probably given by von Recklinghausen in 1895, he applied the term **adenomyoma** to the general pathologic process, perhaps because in retrospect most, if not all, of his small group of cases were in fact instances of what is now termed *adenomyosis,* rather than *endometriosis.* This distinction, which is subsequently clarified in detail, is a significant one, but another 30 years passed before the differences in the nature and probable etiology of the two histologically similar lesions came to be understood and generally accepted. Cullen of Baltimore in 1897 was the first American to describe and discuss the occurrence of aberrant endometrial tissue within the uterine wall (adenomyosis), and his further researches and published work during the next 25 years ultimately defined the disorder we now recognize as adenomyosis and accurately demonstrated its true pathogenesis. Meanwhile, isolated reports of aberrant endometrium having been found in sites other than the uterus began to appear in the literature: Pfannenstiel (1897) reported a case involving the rectovaginal septum; Russell, in Baltimore (1899), reported the first case documented in the ovary; and Meyer, in Berlin (1909), reported the first recognized case of bowel endometriosis, the patient ultimately having a bowel resection performed by Mackenrodt.

The real beginnings of the sort of comprehensive studies and investigations that have led to our current knowledge of the disease, its origins, and its significance came in 1921 with the first report of the observations of John A. Sampson of Albany, New York, concerning "perforating hemorrhage (chocolate) cysts of the ovary." Thereafter, Sampson maintained a lifelong interest in the disease and for the next 20 years wrote numerous papers recording his enlightened observations and continual weighing of the accumulating evidence for and against his seven proposed theories of origin, the most famous of which is his tubal reflux and implantation theory. In 1922, a year after Sampson's first paper appeared, Blair-Bell of Liverpool, in reporting a series of cases with aberrant endometrium in the ovary, first used the terms **endometriosis** and **endometrioma**, the former for the disease, the latter for the individual cystic lesion.

327

In the past four decades, an increasingly intense interest in the disease, its natural history, clinical implications, and management is reflected in the many careful investigations and clinical surveys reported in the now massive literature on the subject. Among the valuable contributions by many over the past 20 to 30 years, the work of Meigs and the studies of Te Linde and Scott should be noted as particularly outstanding, the former because of his broad and long-term interest in all aspects of the disease and its clinical management, as well as for his concept of the importance of early marriage and childbearing in its prevention; the latter because of the excellence of their experimental investigations of the probable pathogenesis of the disease and, in particular, their critical evaluation of the tubal reflux and implantation theory.

DEFINITION

Endometriosis may be defined as a disorder resulting from the presence of actively growing and functioning endometrial tissue (both glandular and supporting stromal elements are usually found) in aberrant sites outside the uterus. The precise mechanism by which the ectopic endometrium appears in its abnormal site is still not conclusively proved. Theories of origin will be discussed, but in view of the widespread anatomic locations in which endometriosis may be encountered, several etiologic mechanisms undoubtedly exist, since no single theory can satisfactorily explain its appearance at all sites where it is known to occur.

Adenomyosis, on the other hand, though similar in histologic appearance, is a condition wherein islands of endometrial glands and stroma are found within the myometrium, interspersed between and surrounded by the smooth-muscle fibers. Cullen clearly showed nearly 40 years ago, however, that a direct connection between these aberrant islands and the surface endometrium lining the uterine cavity can invariably be demonstrated. Thus the etiologic mechanism involved in the development of adenomyosis would seem to be an entirely different one. The validity of the concept of adenomyosis and endometriosis as two separate disease entities, each with a different pathogenesis, is further supported by the fact that the former characteristically is found in older, multiparous patients, whereas the latter typically appears in the young, nulliparous female. Formerly, it was customary to refer to adenomyosis as **internal endometriosis**, and "true" endometriosis occurring outside the uterus was classified as **external endometriosis**; a few continue this usage even today. However, this terminology ignores completely the previously noted obvious differences between the two lesions and should be discarded, since it serves only to perpetuate confusion. Further discussion of adenomyosis will be found in Chapter 12, where it is deliberately treated separately to emphasize this distinction.

Occasionally, lesions clinically resembling endometriosis in their behavior are encountered in which the ectopic epithelium bears a histologic resemblance to tubal epithelium or to endocervical epithelium. The terms **endosalpingosis** and **endocervicosis** have been applied to these pathologic curiosities, which, because of their rarity, will not be discussed further here.

One other entity, frequently termed **stromal endometriosis** (a variety of other terms have also been used to designate this lesion, most of them more accurate and appropriate), should be mentioned for clarification. As suggested by the term, the aberrant tissue consists of endometrial stromal cells without glandular elements, but the primary lesion has never been found outside the uterus. Clinically, it behaves as a uterine neoplasm, and since it often pursues a highly malignant course, extrauterine and extrapelvic metastases and local extension do occur. Obviously, "stromal" endometriosis bears no clinical resemblance to the "true" endometriosis under discussion here. Occasionally, in true endometriomas of long standing, repeated hemorrhage with necrosis or pressure atrophy may cause degenerative changes in the endometrial glands and produce a histologic picture in which glandular elements are absent and only stromal cells are found; this situation also bears no relation to so-called stromal endometriosis. Although some believe the latter may be a variant of the commoner form of endometriosis, the majority opinion favors a different pathogenesis. (Stromal endometriosis will therefore be considered as a uterine malignancy and is discussed more fully in Chapter 14.)

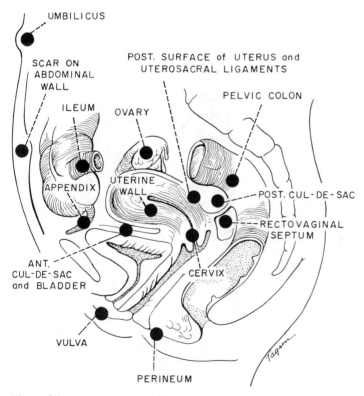

Figure 36
Sites of occurrence of endometriosis.

SITES OF OCCURRENCE

The areas involved by endometriosis are widespread, and usually multiple (Fig. 36). Within the pelvis, it is found most frequently in the ovaries and on the peritoneal coverings of the uterosacral ligaments, posterior cul-de-sac, and posterior wall of the lower uterine segment. Figure 37 depicts the characteristic findings at laparotomy in a typical patient with pelvic endometriosis. It is also commonly encountered in the tubal serosa, the anterior cul-de-sac peritoneum and other pelvic peritoneal surfaces, the rectovaginal septum, the broad ligaments, the round ligaments, including the portions within the inguinal canals, and the sigmoid colon. Less often, it involves the cervix, vagina, vulva, perineum, bladder (the actual vesical wall itself), and ureters or periureteral tissues. Elsewhere in the abdomen, it occasionally involves the appendix, small bowel, umbilicus, and scars of previous anterior abdominal incisions, and there have even been isolated reports of endometriosis of the gallbladder, liver, and kidneys, though its presence within the peritoneal cavity above the level of the umbilicus is rare. It has been found in pelvic and inguinal lymph nodes, and, more rarely, it has been encountered in the pleura, lung, and skeletal muscle and bone of the extremities.

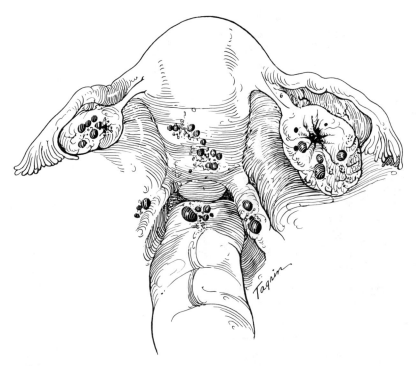

Figure 37
Characteristic findings at laparotomy in pelvic endometriosis.

INCIDENCE

There is no question but that an increasingly widespread interest in the disease during the past 40 years has resulted in its being recognized with greater accuracy and frequency than formerly. But it is equally certain that endometriosis has actually undergone an absolute increase in frequency during the same period of time, particularly in whites of the Western world. At the present time, reports from various hospital centers indicate that it is found in from 10 percent to as high as 30 percent of all patients undergoing pelvic laparotomies for whatever cause, with a strikingly higher incidence in private patients as compared with ward patients. Meigs was the first to note and appreciate the significance of this disparity, dramatically illustrated in Table 3, which summarizes his data. The only significant differences between the two patient groups over the 15-year observation period were the marked delays in marriage and in childbearing in the private-patient series. Although less striking, the private-patient group also showed decreased fertility (66 percent versus 90 percent fertility in ward patients) and decreased parity (78 percent with two children or less versus only 66 percent with fewer than three children in the ward series). The percentage of married patients was almost identical in the two groups (75 percent versus 80 percent), emphasizing again that it is the late marriage, late childbearing, and diminished fertility that are undoubtedly of importance in the increased incidence of endometriosis.

Meigs repeatedly emphasized that regardless of the fundamental mechanisms of origin of the disease, the lesion is more apt to occur and attain clinical significance in women who have postponed fulfillment of their normal reproductive function of childbearing, since prolonged cyclic ovarian function, uninterrupted by the multiple pregnancies nature undoubtedly intended, results in a continuous stimulus to proliferation and extension of the disease; thus its significance in developed Western societies, which favor postponement of marriage and childbearing among its youth. It is noteworthy that in areas such as China, India, Africa, and many of the South

Table 3
Incidence of Endometriosis in Routine Consecutive Pelvic Laparotomies[*]

	Percentage of Cases			
Patient Group	Number of Consecutive Cases	Endometriosis Confirmed Microscopically	Age at Marriage 25 or Over	Age at First Child 25 or Over
Private patients				
Series I (1936-1941)	400	28.0	54	60
Series II (1945-1947)	400	30.5	57	70
Series III (1949-1952)	400	23.8	64	63
Ward patients				
Series I (1936-1941)	400	5.0	16	23
Series II (1944-1947)	400	5.8	11	14
Series III (1949-1952)	400	4.3	24	27

[*]Modified from Meigs [15].

American countries, where cultural tradition and socioeconomic factors still favor early marriage and early, frequent childbearing, endometriosis is a rarity even today. This very same factor may well account for the known rarity with which endometriosis has thus far been encountered among blacks.

ETIOLOGY

Of the many theories of the histogenesis of endometriosis to be advanced over the years, perhaps only four or five still merit any serious consideration and are outlined briefly here.

Theory of Tubal Reflux and Direct Implantation

Although Sampson at one time considered that there were seven possible mechanisms for the development of endometriosis (including most of the others mentioned here), he ultimately favored the theory of tubal reflux and direct implantation of normal, desquamated endometrium, which is forever linked with his name. He believed that fragments of endometrium regurgitated with menstrual blood during each period might often traverse the oviducts in retrograde fashion, retain their viability, and implant on the peritoneal surfaces of any pelvic or abdominal structures on which they came to rest, thereafter eroding and burrowing into the subserosal tissues. He further believed that with succeeding menstrual cycles these ectopic areas would grow and function as normal endometrial tissue and that they might ultimately be responsible for additional implantation. Sampson's theory is generally accepted as the most plausible one, and Te Linde and Scott, among others, have shown in animal investigations that this phenomenon can indeed be reproduced under experimental conditions in monkeys.

Furthermore, there is no question but that under some circumstances, implantation by endometrium does take place; e.g., in surgical incisions of the abdominal wall, cervix, vagina, vulva, and perineum, numerous instances have been reported in which this was the only possible explanation for the occurrence of endometriosis at these sites. Similarly, although endometriosis involving the tubal mucosa and presenting as an intraluminal mass is uncommon, it has recently been observed in the proximal stumps of one or both fallopian tubes following bilateral tubal ligations in a number of women. It is postulated that the intraluminal lesions in these proximal stumps must develop as a result of endometrial reflux, with subsequent implantation of the endometrial cells trapped in the ligated tubal stumps. Moreover, this type of tubal endometriosis may account for some instances of the syndrome of posttubal ligation pain and dysmenorrhea that is experienced by a sizable number of women following the rapidly increasing number of tubal sterilization operations currently being performed.

However, Sampson's theory is not a completely satisfactory explanation for all the known facts about the disease as it is normally encountered. It does not even entirely explain the precise details of the anatomic distribution and most frequent sites of pelvic endometriosis and obviously cannot explain at all the appearance of endometriosis in remote, extraperitoneal areas. Furthermore, although it cannot be detailed here, some investigative work fails to corroborate the belief that desquamated menstrual endometrium retains its viability and capacity for implantation often enough to be the etiologic agent of such a common disease.

Coelomic-Epithelium Metaplasia Theory

The coelomic-epithelium metaplasia theory was advanced independently by Meyer of Berlin and Iwanoff of Russia, who by their different concepts complemented and supported each other. Since dormant, immature cellular elements whose origins may be traced embryologically to the müllerian epithelial system are known to persist into adult life over a widespread area, but particularly throughout the central region of the pelvis, Meyer and Iwanoff postulated that metaplasia of these cells could account for the appearance of endometriosis in many areas. Presumably, following the menarche, repeated cyclic ovarian stimulation of these coelomic epithelial cell elements, with their totipotential capacities for histologic differentiation, could result in the metaplastic formation of functioning endometrial tissue in ectopic sites. Actually, this hypothesis can better explain many cases of endometriosis of the rectovaginal septum, for example, than the implantation theory, and, since coelomic epithelium is known occasionally to become pinched off in the embryologic development of the thorax and limb buds, can even account for the rare instances of endometriosis in the lung, pleura, arm, thigh, and buttocks. Thus this theory is a most attractive one and has been championed by many, including Meigs, Novak, Gruenwald, and Ranney; conceivably, it could be the explanation for almost all instances of endometriosis.

Theory of Lymphatic Dissemination

Halban, and later Javert, suggested that normal endometrium might "metastasize" via lymphatic channels and thus spread to extrauterine sites where implantation and growth would produce the characteristic lesions of endometriosis. The belief that this phenomenon does occur has been strongly supported by the finding of benign endometriosis in pelvic lymph nodes, though conceivably the coelomic metaplasia theory could also account for this.

The Vascular Theory

In attempting to explain a case of endometriosis of the arm, Navratil suggested the possibility of the deportation of normal endometrium via venous channels, with vascular dissemination to remote areas of the body. Although either of the mechanisms suggested by Halban and Navratil could explain certain of the cases of endometriosis in distant sites, and may in fact be operative occasionally, it seems very unlikely that they are involved in the development of endometriosis in its commonest forms and locations.

Müllerian Cell Rest Theory

Originally advanced by Russell, the first to report endometriosis in the ovary, the müllerian cell rest theory assumes that isolated cell rests of embryonic müllerian epithelium are stimulated by cyclic ovarian function in the postmenarchal female, with resulting maturation into functioning endometrium in ectopic areas. Although a few isolated cystic endometriomas of the retroperitoneal area may well have arisen on this basis, it is again extremely doubtful that this is the basis for the origin of endometriosis in general.

A number of other etiologic theories have been proposed and discarded long ago for lack of any supportive evidence. It would seem that the most valid and universally applicable hypotheses remain the tubal reflux and implantation theory of Sampson and the coelomic metaplasia theory of Iwanoff and Meyer. Perhaps elements of both must be invoked in any complete explanation of the origins of this interesting disease.

PATHOLOGIC FEATURES

Although the microscopic picture will vary somewhat with the anatomic location and duration of the lesion, the three diagnostic histologic features of endometriosis are: (1) endometrial glands, (2) endometrial stroma, and (3) evidence of hemorrhage, either fresh (red cells and hemosiderin pigment) or old (hemosiderin-laden macrophages). The typical lesion also shows an abundance of inflammatory cells and fibrous connective tissue indicative of the intense reaction of the surrounding normal cellular elements to the presence of the functioning ectopic endometrial tissue.

Because of its precise microscopic resemblance to normal endometrium and its known responsiveness to ovarian hormonal stimulation, the functioning epithelium of an endometrioma sometimes duplicates closely the phases of the normal intrauterine endometrium, showing proliferative change in the preovulatory portion of the menstrual cycle and secretory changes in the postovulatory or progestational phase. However, more often, the ectopic endometrial tissues of the areas of endometriosis, particularly the more advanced lesions, are out of phase with the normal endometrium within the uterus and are found in the proliferative stage even during the secretory phase of the normal menstrual cycle. Presumably, this is due to the difference in blood supply and to the effects of the increasing tissue fibrosis surrounding the endometriosis. This altered responsiveness to the normal ovarian hormonal cycle occasionally results in a microscopic picture of cystic hyperplasia or even a pseudodecidual reaction in the ectopic endometrium of endometriosis. As previously mentioned, destruction of the glands by hemorrhage and pressure atrophy in lesions of long standing may occur, with only the endometrial stromal cells and evidence of old hemorrhage remaining as histologic guideposts to the true nature of the process.

In pregnancy, a marked decidual reaction will be noted microscopically, with softening and some gross shrinkage of the areas of endometriosis. At the conclusion of the pregnancy, with subsidence of the decidual reaction, microscopic atrophy and a pronounced tendency to regression of the visible and palpable gross lesions of endometriosis are usually seen. On this long-known, beneficial effect of pregnancy on endometriosis is based the current medical treatment of the disease by "pseudo-pregnancy," as discussed later.

From the standpoint of gross pathologic anatomy, the characteristic appearance of endometriosis again differs somewhat with the location and duration of activity of the lesions. In the ovary the process is almost always bilateral and the tendency is for the formation of cystic structures varying from tiny, bluish or dark-brown blisters to large chocolate cysts, some of the latter attaining a size of 20 cm or more in diameter. There is usually considerable fibrosis and puckering of the ovarian surface in the region of the cyst, as well as adherence to neighboring structures (sigmoid, uterus, broad ligament, or pelvic wall). This occurs because of the intermittent rupture (usually during or just after a period) and partial spillage of the contents of the endometrioma, with resulting local peritonitis and fibrosis, which seals off the leak and produces scar-tissue fixation. It is this scar tissue's puckering and dense adherence to its surroundings that is so indicative of endometriosis, not simply the chocolate contents of the cyst, for the latter may be encountered in hemorrhagic corpus luteum cysts or any cystic lesion of the ovary in which hemorrhage has occurred and old blood is present.

In the other most frequently involved areas, namely, the uterosacral ligaments, cul-de-sac, posterior uterine surface — in fact, throughout the pelvic peritoneum — the lesions are smaller and often more numerous, consisting of multiple "blueberry spots" or "powder-burn" lesions surrounded by a stellate pattern of dense, fibrous scar tissue, the latter making up most of the bulk of the visible and palpable puckered nodules. The intense fibrotic response to the presence of active ("menstruating") ectopic endometrium in these areas is undoubtedly the limiting factor in the growth in size of the lesions. This same scar-tissue contraction tends to draw up or down and create fixation of any and all of the neighboring structures (e.g., the uterus, which characteristically becomes fixed in a retroverted position, the rectosigmoid, adnexa, and small bowel) with ultimate obliteration of the cul-de-sac and marked anatomic displacement and functional impairment of the pelvic viscera.

In some areas and organs the process may spread or "invade" in cancerlike fashion (e.g., the rectovaginal septum and posterior vaginal fornix, rectum, sigmoid, bladder, ureter, and small bowel). The endometriosis burrows in from the serosal surface, penetrating deeply into the muscular and submucosal layers of the walls of these structures, where it may spread further in a longitudinal direction but rarely involves the mucosa.

Intermittent bleeding into the gastrointestinal or urinary tract may result, usually coinciding with the menses, but this is due to periodic congestion of the overlying mucosa and not to actual mucosal ulceration. Eventually, the accompanying extensive fibrosis may produce a tumor mass indistinguishable grossly from carcinoma, particularly in the colon, and the resulting constriction of and encroachment on the bowel lumen may produce variable degrees of obstruction. Ureteral obstruction may occur in a similar way. Small-bowel obstruction may also result, but it is usually due to fixation and kinking rather than to actual narrowing of the lumen.

CLINICAL MANIFESTATIONS

It is apparent from the discussions of its pathologic features and probable etiology that endometriosis is a disease of the active reproductive life of women. It is never seen before the menarche and is most frequent in women in their twenties and thirties. It is rare for endometriosis to become clinically significant before the age of 20, although there have been occasional reports of the disease in adolescence; during the past 20 years the author has personally treated two such cases in girls who were 16 and 17 years of age and who had both experienced the rupture of an ovarian endometrioma requiring laparotomy. It is possible that the minimal symptoms and findings that would ordinarily be present in the early phases of the evolution of the disease during adolescence are simply insufficient to render its recognition possible in all but a minority of those in whom it is actually present at this time of life. Thus pelvic endometriosis in teenagers may actually be somewhat more common than has generally been appreciated. In any case, the diagnosis should be considered, even in this age group, if there are any suggestive physical findings, or if the menstrual discomfort differs from that usually accompanying essential adolescent dysmenorrhea in its nature, location, and response to standard therapy.

As would be predicted, it ceases almost entirely to be a problem after the menopause, for with cessation of cyclic ovarian function the lesions ordinarily atrophy and regress, leading to softening and almost complete disappearance of the secondary surrounding fibrotic nodules and scar-tissue deformities. Occasional exceptions to the postmenopausal inactivity of the disease have been encountered and reported, but these are rare. In some cases, reactivation may have been induced by hormonal therapy. Occasionally, at the time of laparotomy for other cause in postmenopausal women, persistent scarring in the form of cul-de-sac obliteration, old adnexal adhesions, or pelvic tissue plane distortions may point to the probable prior presence of pelvic endometriosis, but microscopic proof is invariably absent due to the total atrophy of the endometrial glands and stroma.

Thus the typical patient is in her late twenties or early thirties, is either single or has married late and voluntarily delayed childbearing, or is suffering from involuntary sterility. Many are nulliparous, and, of the rest, the majority have had only one pregnancy or at most two. When a pregnancy has occurred, it has usually been after the age of 25, and, if more than one, the interval between them will usually have been more than five years. Early childbearing is not sufficient in itself to protect the susceptible woman from the potential development of clinically significant endometriosis unless multiple pregnancies follow at intervals of no more than five years until she is well along in her thirties. Under these circumstances, it is rare for the disease to appear or produce any symptoms.

SYMPTOMS

The classic history is one of so-called acquired (or secondary) dysmenorrhea, a poor descriptive phrase, perhaps, since the pain of endometriosis rarely resembles the typical uterine cramps of primary or "essential" dysmenorrhea, either in character, severity, duration, or timing with respect to the onset of menstrual flow. However, use of the phrase does imply the onset of a new and different pelvic discomfort after a variable number of years of relatively normal, painless menses, the new pain related to, but not necessarily occurring simultaneously with, each period. In actual fact, the pelvic pain of endometriosis is more likely to begin a day or two before the onset of flow, though its intensity may increase during the early days of menstruation. It tends to be a deep-seated aching or bearing-down pain in the lower abdomen, posterior pelvis, vagina, and back. There is often radiation into the rectal and perineal areas with rectal tenesmus and symptoms of bowel irritation, this distribution being secondary to the characteristic involvement of the uterosacral ligaments, cul-de-sac, and adjacent surfaces of the uterus and rectum, with or without rectovaginal septal disease. If, as is often the case, endometriomas of one or both ovaries are present, dull unilateral or bilateral lower abdominal pain, often with radiation to the thighs, may be noted.

Usually, the discomfort tends to abate after two or three days, subsiding completely toward the end of or just after the period, and the patient will then be completely comfortable once more until a day or two before the onset of the next flow. However, as the disease progresses, the pain in these typical areas tends to increase in severity and may also come to occupy more and more of the latter half of each cycle. Two additional points deserve emphasis. First, not all patients with endometriosis have pain. In spite of extensive disease palpable on pelvic examination or found at laparotomy, 15 to 20 percent of patients will report no discomfort whatsoever, though they may suffer from other manifestations of the pathologic process, notably infertility, or may simply present with a "pelvic mass." Second, the small "peritoneal implant" type of lesion may produce intense pain due to the extreme sensitivity to stretching of the overlying peritoneum that is tightly constricted about it by the marked fibrosis it incites. On the other hand, the presence of a large chocolate cyst of the ovary, which is accompanied by little if any fibrosis and is relatively free to expand, may produce little discomfort until the cyst becomes distended or ruptures.

Other chronic symptoms, varying with the anatomic areas involved and the extent of the disease, include dyspareunia, cyclic bowel disturbances with painful defecation and rectal bleeding, and even subacute intestinal obstruction, as well as the rarer manifestations, such as cyclic painful inguinal swellings (endometriosis of the round ligament, inguinal glands, or inguinal canal peritoneum) and bladder irritability and hematuria (bladder wall involvement). Occasionally, if ovarian involvement is bilateral and sufficiently extensive to impair ovarian function, premenstrual or postmenstrual staining, menorrhagia, and irregular cycles may result. Ordinarily, however, even women with extensive endometriosis continue to have regular, normal,

ovulatory menstrual flow "to the bitter end." In fact, endometriosis is rarely encountered in women prone to anovulatory cycles and dysfunctional bleeding.

Not infrequently, leakage or frank rupture of an enlarging ovarian endometrioma
may produce generalized peritonitis and an acute abdominal emergency. Spillage of
old blood (the chocolatelike contents of the endometrial cyst) produces an intense
local irritation and inflammatory response, which results in a chemical peritonitis.
As might be expected, the acute episode usually commences at or shortly after a
menstrual period, rupture having been prompted by fresh bleeding into the cyst
cavity, with resulting sudden increase in intracystic pressure. Although small leaks
may have occurred previously, with rapid sealing-over and prompt subsidence of the
local peritoneal reaction, the majority of the acute episodes will require immediate
laparotomy, the mortality of nonsurgically treated cases in the past having approached
50 percent.

Finally, infertility is an extremely common initial complaint, either absolute or
relative ("one-child sterility") and often exists in the absence of any other symptoms
or significant abnormalities on pelvic examination. Impairment of fertility is usually
secondary to interference with the tuboovarian mechanism for ovum pickup and
transfer by periadnexal adhesions and fixation, and the latter can be created by
relatively minimal pelvic endometriosis.

PHYSICAL FINDINGS

Although the findings on pelvic examination are somewhat variable and may occasionally be minimal or even absent in the early stages, the characteristic, almost
diagnostic, finding is the hard, fixed, fibrotic nodule, usually noted as a beaded or
shotty thickening in the uterosacral ligaments, cul-de-sac, or posterior surface of
the lower uterine wall or cervix. Actually, this nodularity in these specific locations
is almost universally present in patients with endometriosis and is pathognomonic of
the disease. Although these thickenings may be palpable vaginally, they are best
appreciated on rectal examination, particularly in patients with minimal involvement,
where the palpating finger can more readily reach and explore these posterior structures (Fig. 38). If the disease is sufficiently extensive, the cul-de-sac may have been
completely obliterated and the uterus drawn back and adherent to the rectum in
fixed retroversion. If ovarian endometriomas are present, they will be palpable as
cystic ovarian enlargements, typically bilateral but often of different size and characteristically fixed to the pelvic walls, cul-de-sac, or adjacent structures. In the case
of endometriosis of the rectovaginal septum, bidigital rectovaginal examination will
be helpful in defining the nature of the pathologic condition, and occasionally the
bluish nodule or nodules may be visible behind the cervix on speculum examination.
Tenderness and pain on motion of any of the involved structures is characteristic,
although not diagnostic, and typically is maximal just before and during each period.

DIAGNOSIS

In typical cases the correct diagnosis is often strongly suggested by the history alone,
and even in patients with minimal involvement and mild symptomatology, a careful,

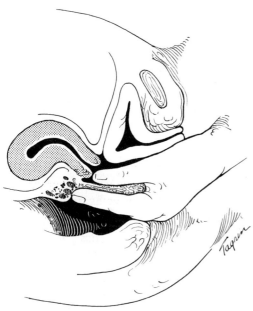

Figure 38
Rectal examination in the typical patient with pelvic endometriosis. The tender
nodularity of the uterosacral ligaments and cul-de-sac and the fixed retroversion
of the uterus are almost diagnostic of the disease.

detailed history may raise the suspicion that endometriosis is present. Usually, a
presumptive diagnosis based on the characteristic symptoms and their chronological
relationship to the menstrual cycle can be verified with almost absolute certainty if
on vaginal and rectal examination the tender uterosacral ligament or cul-de-sac
nodules are palpable, and if the often-associated fixed retroversion of the uterus is
present.

If the history is typical, but the physical findings minimal and equivocal, laparoscopy or culdoscopy may prove extremely valuable in establishing a definite diagnosis.
When the disease is of limited extent and has not produced a fixed retroversion with
obliteration of the pouch of Douglas, cul-de-sac puncture with excellent visualization
of the usual areas of involvement is ordinarily carried out readily under local anesthesia with the culdoscope. However, laparoscopy will be necessary and preferable
if the disease has produced an obliteration of the cul-de-sac, or fixation of the uterus
in retroversion, or both. When a trial of medical therapy rather than surgery is being
considered as the initial step in management, it is obviously important to establish
a precise diagnosis before treatment, and pelvic endoscopy using the laparoscope or
culdoscope has proved to be the answer in such cases. As discussed in more detail
in Chapter 11, "unexplained infertility" is sometimes due to minimal endometriosis
producing tuboovarian adhesions in the absence of symptoms or of palpable disease
on physical examination. Here again, laparoscopy or culdoscopy in such patients
has proved extremely helpful in the discovery of their otherwise silent endometriosis.

Not infrequently, endometriosis is first discovered at the time of laparotomy performed for some other lesion or with another diagnosis in mind, and recognition of the lesions, the characteristic gross appearance of which has already been described, presents no special problem. Microscopic confirmation will of course be forthcoming when resected lesions (ovarian endometriomas) or peritoneal excisions ("blueberry spots" or "powder burns") are examined in the pathology laboratory. In the case of endometriosis in the less common superficial sites such as abdominal scars, the umbilicus, groins, posterior vaginal fornix, vulva, or perineum, simple direct biopsy confirmation will be possible.

Other diagnostic aids include the following: (1) pelvic examination under anesthesia, which is occasionally of help where office examination is unsatisfactory or equivocal; (2) a barium cnema, to reveal the typical roentgenologic pattern of sigmoid endometriosis (see Fig. 39); (3) an intravenous pyelogram (when involvement of the ureter or periureteral tissues is suspected, the location and degree of obstruction, if present, can be determined); (4) cystoscopy (when endometriosis of the bladder is suspected, cystoscopy performed at the time of the period will usually reveal the typical bluish-black submucosal cystic lesions).

DIFFERENTIAL DIAGNOSIS

From the standpoint of symptomatology, patients with adenomyosis (not surprisingly), pelvic inflammatory disease, and the so-called pelvic congestion syndrome (see Chap. 5) may present with cyclic pelvic discomfort superficially resembling that of endometriosis. Occasionally, the complaints of women in their twenties and early thirties in whom lifelong essential dysmenorrhea has persisted and grown more severe may also raise the suspicion of endometriosis. However, in each of these other situations, details of the past history, the age and circumstances at the onset of symptoms, the location of the pain, and so on, are helpful clues as to the more likely nature of the underlying disorder. Furthermore, the absence of the characteristic physical findings of endometriosis will argue strongly against its probable presence in patients with any of the preceding disorders. Although bilateral adnexal masses and a fixed uterus may result, only rarely are the gross anatomic changes of chronic pelvic inflammation such as to simulate the typical nodular changes of endometriosis, and except for the frequent uterine enlargement associated with adenomyosis, the findings of pelvic examination in the other three disorders will usually be unremarkable. It should be noted, however, that endometriosis not infrequently coexists with adenomyosis and also with fibroids, and that the latter alone may occasionally cause cyclic menstrual discomfort. Thus there will be some patients in whom multiple disorders are present and palpable, all contributing to the symptomatology, and in whom differential diagnosis may be difficult.

Ovarian endometriomas must of course be distinguished from other cystic lesions of the ovary. Their tendency to fixation, in contrast to the usual mobility of most benign ovarian cysts, the usual presence of other areas of palpable endometriosis in the cul-de-sac and uterosacral ligament regions, and the typical history will nearly always render the diagnosis obvious. Rarely, cystic ovarian cancers with peritoneal

ovarian endometriomas

seeding may produce cul-de-sac nodularity, but again, the patient's age and history usually suggest the correct diagnosis. The acute picture produced by rupture of a chocolate cyst may simulate a ruptured ectopic pregnancy, hemorrhage into, or rupture or torsion of, an ovarian cyst, acute salpingitis, appendicitis, or, for that matter, any acute intraabdominal emergency. Although a correct preoperative diagnosis may not be made in over 50 percent of the cases, attention to details of the prior history, particularly the pattern of menstrual discomfort, and a careful search for and recognition of the diagnostic significance of the classical nodularities in the cul-de-sac and uterosacral ligaments, if present in association with the cystic lesion, should permit a much higher percentage of accurate preoperative diagnoses than otherwise.

PREVENTION

Since the potential for the development of endometriosis would seem to be an intrinsic feature of the embryology and physiology of the human female, the vast majority of women perhaps having an inherent susceptibility to the disease, prevention in an absolute sense is probably not possible. However, prophylaxis against the occurrence of clinically significant endometriosis (extensive, progressively increasing involvement, with disabling symptoms and disorders of pelvic function, including infertility) may be achieved by women who choose to avoid undue delay in childbearing and have several pregnancies at intervals no longer than five years. That such a pattern of reproductive function effectively decreases the incidence of detectable endometriosis, even at laparotomy, has already been mentioned. This is not to suggest a program that would further complicate the growing world population problem. It is only necessary that unduly late childbearing be avoided and that whatever number of children a couple deems desirable and reasonable be borne without prolonged delay during the early part of the woman's childbearing years. Such a program in itself might reduce considerably the incidence of significant pelvic endometriosis, and should endometriosis nevertheless develop later on, the tragedy of involuntary sterility would already have been obviated. Nor is such a program incompatible with effective, voluntary participation in any world population-control scheme that might ultimately be advocated, for it simply suggests when to have the children, not the optimal number to have. Although encouragement of young couples to marry and have their families early, to say nothing of fostering conditions to make this feasible and desirable, is more a problem for society in general than for the medical profession, the physician may find this concept useful in the management of individual patients, as noted in the next section.

TREATMENT

Nonoperative Treatment

Nonsurgical therapy is often called conservative treatment, but this is not necessarily a valid designation, because the plan and goal of many of the operations performed for endometriosis are also directed toward conserving and restoring the normal anatomy and function of the female reproductive organs.

SIMPLE OBSERVATION

In many young unmarried women, although typical physical findings may be present, symptoms are either absent or inconsequential, the actual extent of involvement is often only minimal, and no immediate treatment of any kind is indicated. The situation and facts of the disease should usually be explained in a reassuring way, with the favorable effects of childbearing on the future course of the disease pointed out to the patient, so that she may take this factor into account in her future planning. The importance of regular follow-up examinations at least once or twice yearly to check on further progression of the disease in such patients is obvious, for with continued supervision, any necessary change in the plan of management can be made before the potentially destructive effects of the disease become too far advanced for effective treatment that will also preserve reproductive function.

A similar approach is indicated in the woman in her late thirties or early forties, whether married or unmarried, in whom symptoms are mild and easily managed with simple analgesics, and in whom, in spite of the sometimes more extensive disease palpable, possible infertility is no longer a matter of concern. If the disease remains relatively quiescent under observation, these women can be carried along to the menopause, when atrophy ensues and the problem is solved. The only difficulty occasionally posed by such a patient will be the need to differentiate between moderately extensive endometriosis and some other pelvic lesion, particularly an ovarian neoplasm. In such cases, exploratory pelvic laparotomy frequently becomes essential, and if endometriosis is found, surgical extirpation should be done.

In the young married woman with moderate symptoms and only a moderate amount of disease palpable, the ideal treatment is pregnancy, if it can be achieved and if it is desired. Again, the facts should be presented to the couple and an adequate time allowed for them to attempt to conceive before instituting active therapy, since a significant number of women with known minimal endometriosis will successfully conceive without treatment of any kind. However, if pregnancy does not occur after approximately a year of trial, a complete fertility investigation should be done to discover other possible factors. Following this, some form of active therapy for the endometriosis should be instituted.

MEDICAL (HORMONE) THERAPY

As already suggested, patients who seem most suitable for hormone therapy are those in whom the diagnosis is certain, symptoms are mild, infertility is not the primary problem, and large masses are not present.

Pseudopregnancy

On the basis of the known salutary effect of pregnancy on the disease, attempts to produce a similar physiologic amenorrhea by pituitary inhibition and suppression of ovulation have been utilized in the treatment of endometriosis since the mid-1930s. Originally, massive doses of estrogen were tried, but management was difficult, with patients often unable to tolerate the medication at the required high-dose levels and with frequent secondary complications of uterine bleeding, ovarian cyst formation, and rupture of ovarian endometriomas. Furthermore, the results of treatment were erratic and in general not satisfactory. In the early 1960s, with the development of newer, more potent progestational compounds, reliable production of a more effective, prolonged pseudodecidual change in the areas of endometriosis was rendered easier and somewhat more tolerable to the patient. The resulting decidual change is then followed by necrosis and atrophy, and it is this subsequent atrophy that is responsible for the beneficial effect on the disease and the temporary inhibition of its further progression.

The exact biochemical mechanisms by which either normal pregnancy or hormone therapy with estrogens or progesterone exerts this beneficial effect are not precisely known, but the endometrial atrophy probably results from both pituitary blockage of follicle-stimulating hormone (FSH) production as well as from interference with the metabolism of the endometrial tissue locally. A number of these agents have been employed, Enovid having been the one most widely used, and considerable success was initially reported. Once treatment is instituted, it is customary to continue it for 6 to 12 months in accordance with several typical programs outlined by Kistner [12], who has done extensive work in this field. Objective regressions of the disease were initially reported to occur in as high as 80 percent of patients so treated, and the subsequent pregnancy rate has ranged from 35 to 50 percent in some series. Assessment of reported results has been difficult because of the all-too-frequent uncertainty of the pretreatment diagnosis (this uncertainty should always be dispelled prior to hormone therapy, by pelvic endoscopy if possible) and the problems posed by the frequent need to judge the success or failure of treatment on the basis of subjective response alone.

The following dosage regimens are based on those suggested by Kistner cited above:

Enovid:
    2.5 mg daily for one week (orally)
    5.0 mg daily for one week
    10.0 mg daily for two weeks
    15.0 mg daily for two weeks
    20.0 mg daily for rest of treatment program

(If breakthrough uterine bleeding occurs, the daily dose is increased by 10 mg and maintained at that level until termination of therapy.)

Norlutate: 5 mg orally daily for two weeks. Increase by 5 mg every two weeks until a maintenance dose of 15 to 20 mg is reached. (Add an oral estrogen if breakthrough bleeding is encountered.)

Deluteval 2X: 1 ml (250 mg Delalutin with 5 mg estradiol valerate) intramuscularly at weekly intervals. Increase by 0.5 ml every six weeks, or whenever breakthrough bleeding occurs.

Depo-Provera: 2 ml (100 mg) intramuscularly every two weeks for four doses; then 2 ml every four weeks. (Add an oral estrogen for breakthrough bleeding.)

The nausea that may occur in the early weeks of therapy with any of these medications is minimized by slowly increasing the dose. However, it is still a problem for 35 percent of patients. If encountered, it will sometimes subside with temporary reduction in dosage. In addition to complete amenorrhea and absence of ovulation, most patients will experience many of the other symptoms and signs of early pregnancy, including moderate uterine enlargement, breast swelling and discomfort, and weight gain. In addition to the breakthrough uterine bleeding previously noted, heavy bleeding with the passage of decidual tissue (pseudoabortion) may occur, either during drug therapy or shortly after its termination, and be sufficient to require curettage for control.

Initial swelling of an ovarian endometrioma following institution of a program of hormone therapy may occasionally simulate the signs and symptoms of an ectopic pregnancy or, more important, may actually cause rupture and leakage of the endometrioma, requiring an emergency operation. For this reason — and also because possible ovarian cancer must be excluded — large ovarian cysts presumed to be endometriomas are a contraindication to this type of therapy and are instead an indication for conservative surgical treatment.

It would seem advisable to carry out laparoscopy or culdoscopy in all patients prior to instituting treatment by pseudopregnancy, particularly in women suffering from infertility, both to confirm the diagnosis and to ascertain that the extent and location of endometriosis in the individual patient are potentially responsive to hormone treatment with restoration of fertility. Patients with extensive adhesions surrounding the adnexa and producing gross mechanical interference with ovum pickup and transport, regardless of tubal patency or the extent of disease elsewhere in the pelvis, can obviously be offered a better chance for restoration of function as well as relief of discomfort by conservative surgery, and time should not be wasted attempting hormone therapy, particularly in the woman already in her early thirties.

Initially, there was evidence to suggest that a planned course of preoperative hormone therapy for six to eight weeks prior to surgery might greatly facilitate the dissection and conservative resection of areas of the disease. Presumably, the operation would be rendered easier by virtue of the softening effect on the lesions and the fibrosis surrounding them and as a result of the delineation of tissue planes by the slight edema accompanying the decidual change that would be induced. However, not all surgeons are convinced that such preoperative medical therapy is helpful, and many report that the increased vascularity actually makes the dissection more difficult. Furthermore, the use of medical therapy subsequent to a conservative operation in which it was not technically feasible to excise all the disease has been employed as an adjunct to operative therapy in the belief that it might improve the chances of such a patient achieving pregnancy, or gaining relief from symptoms, or both. However, the end results in most reported series have not substantiated this belief.

Use of Androgens

Through mechanisms that again are not entirely clear, but perhaps acting either indirectly through an antiestrogen effect or more directly on the endometrial cell metabolism locally, the administration of androgens will also frequently cause softening and regression of endometriosis, with marked alleviation of symptoms. Although originally tried in large doses with a view to obtaining pituitary suppression and anovulation, the use of low-dosage schedules that do not inhibit ovulation has proved far superior and has many practical advantages over therapy by pseudopregnancy with progestogens: it is less expensive; there are fewer side effects; and since ovulation is not suppressed, pregnancy is possible during the course of treatment. In fact, there have been a number of reports of patients with proved pelvic endometriosis and infertility of long duration who have conceived while on, or immediately subsequent to, a course of androgen therapy. The plan of treatment is simple, and the usual drug employed is methyltestosterone (e.g., Metandren Linguets, 5 mg); a course of medication consists of the sublingual or buccal administration of 5 mg of the drug once daily for three to six months. This dosage rarely produces significant side effects, though a temporary mild acne or slight increase in hair may occasionally be noted, usually in certain brunettes who already exhibit a mild tendency to hirsutism. All the temporary side effects disappear at the conclusion of therapy, and voice changes or clitoral hypertrophy are unheard of with this dosage. In addition to reported pregnancies after androgen therapy, the majority of women so treated will experience gratifying relief of symptoms and objective regressions of palpable disease, often with remissions lasting several years.

Summary

The conservative therapy of endometriosis with either progestogens or androgens can be useful in young women desiring to postpone either conservative or definitive surgery temporarily, or in older women who wish to obtain temporary relief from troublesome symptoms (e.g., pelvic pain, bowel and urinary tract disturbances). This applies not only to patients who have had no previous treatment but also to patients who have had previous conservative surgery or who have undergone hysterectomy with preservation of ovarian tissue and then experience symptomatic recurrences. Often, such patients complain primarily of rectal symptoms, with alternating diarrhea and constipation, rectal pain, and bleeding; occasionally, cyclic pelvic pain or, more rarely, painful pseudomenstruation from vaginal vault endometriosis occurs after hysterectomy. Some of these women can be kept relatively asymptomatic with intermittent courses of hormone medication until the problem ceases with the onset of the menopause, cessation of ovarian stimulation, and atrophy of any residual endometriosis.

This approach received widespread trial during the 1960s, but as experience with its results was accumulated and carefully evaluated, the initial enthusiasm waned. Although a significant but variable and unpredictable percentage of patients were afforded temporary relief by pseudopregnancy programs, symptoms promptly recurred, and the disease continued to progress when the medication was discontinued. Ultimately, the majority of medically treated patients required surgical intervention of some type. Furthermore, the program of medication was extremely expensive, and the unpleasant side effects of the pseudopregnancy regimens often proved as troublesome to the patient as the symptoms produced by the endometriosis. Finally, medical therapy is considerably less successful than conservative surgery in correcting infertility due to endometriosis, rarely relieves the symptoms of patients with extensive disease, and is contraindicated in patients with adnexal masses, a situation always warranting surgical exploration.

Thus, a certain disenchantment with medical therapy has come to replace the overly optimistic expectations accompanying its initial widespread use. Nevertheless, it remains a useful therapeutic approach in some patients if its very definite limitations, contraindications, and the often temporary nature of the end results are borne in mind. It is also possible that new drugs will be forthcoming that will have greater, more predictable effects on endometriosis and that will be better tolerated by the patient. A case in point may be the new steroid compound isoxazole ethisterone (Danazol), a substance with antigonadotropic action now undergoing careful clinical trials [4]. The drug can be taken orally, is well tolerated, and has minimal side effects. Early results have been promising in terms of objective regression of the lesions, subjective relief of symptoms, and subsequent pregnancies in 40 percent of patients whose chief complaint had been infertility.

RADIATION THERAPY

The use of x-ray castration is briefly mentioned, because there have in the past been patients who ordinarily would have been selected for total extirpative surgery, in whom clinical judgment of the facts of the individual situation dictated irradiation as the most suitable means of ovarian ablation to produce regression of endometriosis. Although the results have often been satisfactory, both the nature of the gross pathology produced by endometriosis, with its tendency to adhesions and fixation of adjacent pelvic and lower abdominal viscera, as well as the potential danger of future malignant change in pelvic organs exposed to sterilizing doses of radiation, make its use for this purpose unduly hazardous. It should therefore probably be restricted to the occasional exceptional case.

Surgical Treatment

There are many who feel that when active therapy is indicated, the treatment of endometriosis remains primarily surgical because of the potentially destructive nature of the pathologic process, its erratic pattern of progression, and its unpredictable response to medical therapy. Obviously, acute complications of the disease, notably ruptured endometriomas of the ovary, are emergency situations that must be dealt with surgically. Such acute episodes account for 5 to 10 percent of all patients requiring treatment for endometriosis. Since the symptoms and signs of the resulting chemical peritonitis usually become progressively worse within 24 to 48 hours, the majority of these patients should have prompt laparotomy. In the younger patient, conservative surgery is the treatment of choice; in the older patient in whom preservation of childbearing function is no longer a consideration, total hysterectomy and bilateral salpingo-oophorectomy are preferable. This definitive surgical procedure can usually be done perfectly safely, provided the patient's general condition has not deteriorated as a result of undue preoperative delay.

Where the chronic manifestations of the disease are concerned, surgical treatment will be selected when medical therapy fails or is inappropriate to the total goal of treatment. Management in each case must be individualized, and the type and extent of surgery performed will depend largely on the age and childbearing requirements of the patient and, to a lesser extent, on the amount and distribution of the disease present. In general, so-called conservative surgery is indicated in young women and more radical extirpative surgery, in older patients.

CONSERVATIVE SURGERY

Although it may be selected as the primary method of management in any young woman with symptomatic endometriosis, conservative surgery is particularly called for in patients known to have large endometriomas or such extensive adnexal adhesions that even a symptomatically successful program of hormone therapy is unlikely to render them fertile. This type of surgical approach is not, strictly speaking, conservative, implying minimal dissection or resection, since it in fact strives to excise as much of the endometriosis as possible, conserving all tissue necessary for reproductive function and attempting to restore functional capacity to this conserved tissue. It should again be emphasized that a complete fertility investigation should be done on both husband and wife to uncover all potential factors in their sterility prior to contemplating or undertaking a conservative operation for endometriosis when infertility is the major problem.

In a typical case the operative maneuvers will consist of the following: resection of ovarian endometriomas, when present, shelling the chocolate cyst out of the surrounding normal ovarian tissue, which can then be reconstituted and preserved; mobilization of the uterus and adnexa with excision of all gross areas of endometriosis on the surface of the uterus, tubes, uterosacral ligaments, cul-de-sac, bladder flap, and other areas of the pelvic peritoneal cavity; reperitonealization of all raw areas, with or without the help of omental grafts in the denuded cul-de-sac, as necessary, together with anterior suspension of the uterus (preferably by the Coffey or Baldy-Webster technique), both steps aimed at preventing adherence of the uterus, tubes, and ovaries posteriorly again, with immobilization and interference with the proper function of the adnexa. If pelvic pain has been a prominent symptom, concomitant presacral neurectomy is usually advisable as a further means of preventing recurrence of dysmenorrhea and central pelvic pain, both of which are possible additional factors in disturbed uterotubal function. Some also advocate division and partial resection of the uterosacral ligaments for the same purpose, since the additional autonomic nerve supply of Frankenhäuser's plexus, which travels in these structures, is thereby also interrupted.

The results of this type of extensive but "conservationistic" surgery have been eminently satisfactory, and the ideal end result, subsequent pregnancy, should be achieved in 50 to 65 percent of women so treated, if the operation is properly and meticulously done. Even if pregnancy does not occur, the majority will have little or no future trouble, and only rarely will they require another operative procedure at a later date.

RADICAL EXTIRPATIVE SURGERY

More radical surgery for endometriosis should be carried out in women in their late thirties or forties who desire no further pregnancies, since this is even more certain to relieve their symptoms and effect a permanent cure of the disease than is a conservative procedure. Total abdominal hysterectomy is performed, removing all gross endometriosis, including any ovarian endometriomas. Often, however, particularly if the patient is 10 to 15 years premenopausal, some normal ovarian tissue can and should be preserved. If, on the other hand, the patient is within 5 to 10 years of the menopause, or has extensive rectosigmoidal endometriosis likely to result in future symptoms or bowel obstruction, bilateral salpingo-oophorectomy should also be done. (If this proves necessary in a younger patient, symptoms of the premature artificial menopause so produced can be managed by the cautious administration of small doses of estrogens without risking reactivation of any areas of disease remaining behind.)

Further difficulties after this type of procedure, even with preservation of one or both ovaries, are unusual. When they do occur, conservative medical therapy with androgens or progestogens may be all that is required to keep the patient free of symptoms and the disease in abeyance until, with the onset of the menopause, the process undergoes atrophy and complete resolution. Only rarely (most often for rectosigmoidal endometriosis manifesting itself several years after hysterectomy with ovarian preservation and producing increasingly severe rectal bleeding, pelvic pain, and progressive bowel obstruction) will reoperation and castration or, less preferably, x-ray sterilization be necessary.

CLINICAL MANIFESTATIONS AND MANAGEMENT OF ENDOMETRIOSIS IN LESS FREQUENT SITES

Rectosigmoid and Sigmoid

The pathology and symptomatology of involvement of the colon by endometriosis have already been mentioned, and in the presence of typical endometriosis elsewhere in the pelvis, the diagnosis is often obvious. There are times, however, when the clinical symptoms, the size and characteristics of the actual mass within the bowel wall, and the degree of obstruction it produces are such as to render the differentiation from carcinoma extremely difficult, even at laparotomy. Sigmoidoscopy, when the lesion is within reach of the instrument, as is frequently the case, does not usually permit a definite diagnosis of endometriosis, since the actual lesion rarely, if ever, involves the mucosa and is not accessible for biopsy. However, it will reveal the narrowed lumen, and this fact in the absence of any ulceration or mucosal lesion at the constricted point tends to favor the diagnosis of endometriosis. On the other hand, the roentgenologic findings on barium enema are usually so characteristic as to be almost diagnostic (Fig. 39). In typical cases, a filling defect of considerable

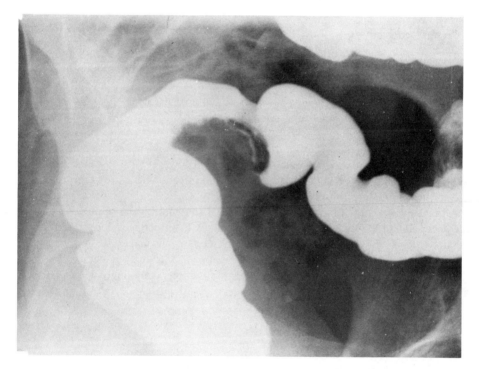

Figure 39
Barium enema examination revealing characteristic roentgenologic appearance of endometriosis of the rectosigmoid colon. Note filling defect with sharply defined borders and a normal mucosal pattern throughout. During fluoroscopy the lesion was tender to palpation and relatively fixed. The patient was a 41-year-old nullipara, infertile during 10 years of marriage, with a 9-year history of increasingly frequent and troublesome bouts of lower abdominal cramps, diarrhea, and rectal bleeding, most of the episodes occurring premenstrually. The diagnosis of endometriosis was confirmed at laparotomy, at which time total hysterectomy and bilateral salpingo-oophorectomy were performed, with subsequent complete relief of all symptoms.

length (4 to 7 inches) with sharply defined borders will be seen, but the mucosal pattern will be intact and normal throughout; a cardinal associated feature will be the fixation and tenderness to palpation in the area of the lesion during fluoroscopic examination.

In the older woman, management presents no problem, since castration will cause complete regression, with relief of all symptoms as well as the element of obstruction. In this situation it is the treatment of choice, and bowel resection should not and need not be attempted. In the rare instance of extensive rectosigmoidal involvement in a young woman in whom it is imperative to preserve childbearing potential, local resection of the involved segment of colon may occasionally be indicated, with an attempt at medical management by inducing pseudopregnancy as a possible alternative, but one much less likely to be successful.

Bladder and Ureters

Cyclic hematuria and the other symptomatology accompanying vesical involvement as well as its cystoscopic recognition have already been described. Usually, the vesical lesions are situated anteriorly in the vertex of the bladder, well away from the trigone, and are best treated by resection of the involved area, which is simply and safely accomplished by a transabdominal approach. If castration is contemplated, bladder resection is unnecessary.

Intermittent ureteral obstruction with cyclic renal colic related to the menses and a more chronic, slowly progressive constriction of the lower ureter with increasing hydronephrosis above it and recurrent urinary tract infection have been reported, though such cases are relatively infrequent. Usually, the obstruction is produced by constrictive scar tissue in the vicinity of peritoneal endometriosis at some point in the pelvis along the course of the ureter. Only rarely is the actual wall or lumen of the ureter invaded by the endometriosis; in such cases, cyclic hematuria may occur. In the older patient, surgical castration is the treatment of choice and almost always results in return of normal ureteral anatomy and function. Only rarely will a direct attack on the ureter itself be indicated or necessary, either in the form of lysis of adhesions or resection and reanastomosis.

Miscellaneous

Symptomatic endometriosis of the umbilicus, abdominal scars, groin, vulva, perineum, cervix, or vagina is uncommon. Endometriosis of the various cutaneous sites often seems to have occurred as a result of direct implantation, but in some instances, lymphatic spread or possibly even metaplasia of adjacent coelomic epithelial derivatives may better account for its appearance in these distant sites. The nature of the pathologic condition is often apparent from the obvious relation to the menstrual cycle of symptoms and changes in size and appearance of the visible and palpable lesions. Treatment is simple excision, both for relief of symptoms and for histologic confirmation of the diagnosis.

Endometriosis of the appendix is not infrequently found during laparotomy for more widespread pelvic disease, and incidental appendectomy should, of course, be done. Instances of intussusception of an appendix involved by endometriosis have been reported. In some patients, the result may be recurring attacks of right lower quadrant pain, mimicking appendicitis, often with a palpable abdominal mass or actual acute or subacute intestinal obstruction. In others, the lesion manifests itself as an asymptomatic pseudotumor of the cecum or right colon, accidentally discovered during routine abdominal exploration or in the course of a barium-enema examination. In other patients, endometriosis of the appendix may give rise to a clinical picture of recurring bouts of premenstrual abdominal pain referred to the right lower quadrant but without other signs or symptoms suggestive of appendicitis. Finally, in a great many patients, the lesion may be a completed asymptomatic one, discovered as an incidental finding during exploratory laparotomy.

The serosal surfaces of the small bowel are frequently involved in older patients with extensive pelvic and lower abdominal disease of long duration. In such patients, even though they may be 10 to 15 years premenopausal, bilateral oophorectomy should probably always accompany hysterectomy to forestall potential future difficulty with small-bowel obstruction. Depending on the size and location of the small-bowel lesions, local excision or even limited small-bowel resection represents an alternative approach in younger women in whom a conservative operation to restore or maintain fertility is both desirable as well as technically feasible. Furthermore, even in patients undergoing bilateral oophorectomy, small-bowel resection may have to be done if the fibrotic scarring accompanying the lesion has already narrowed the bowel lumen to such an extent that obstructive symptoms are likely to develop or have already appeared.

Endometriosis of the kidney is extremely rare, fewer than a dozen cases having been reported. Back and flank pain with associated gross or microscopic hematuria are the usual clinical features, but only occasionally are the symptoms cyclic and related to the premenstrual phase. Intravenous pyelograms will reveal a definite but nonspecific abnormality that often suggests renal cell carcinoma. Thus the correct diagnosis of endometriosis is invariably made only following pathologic study of the nephrectomy specimen.

Rarely, involvement of the sciatic nerve sheath by areas of endometriosis lying deep beneath the broad ligament has been reported, with cyclic sciatica occurring in relation to the menses. Here again, in view of the serious nature of the potential disability, castration would seem the wisest and most effective therapy, though an attempt at local excision or hormone therapy might be made under exceptional circumstances.

Finally, there have been scattered case reports of thoracic endometriosis involving either the lung or the pleura. Thoracic lesions may produce either cyclic, recurring hemoptysis or recurring spontaneous pneumothorax, with symptoms coincident with menstruation.

Although cyclic external bleeding from areas of endometriosis located in extragenital sites such as the bladder, gastrointestinal tract, or thorax produces a type of "vicarious menstruation," this form of aberrant cyclic bleeding should be distinguished from a somewhat more common, truly functional type of vicarious menstruation. An example of the latter is vicarious nasal menstruation, which accounts for 30 percent of extragenital cyclic bleeding and is secondary to cyclic vascular congestion and hyperemia of the nasal mucosa induced by cyclic elevation of serum estrogen levels. Less often, these same estrogen-induced vascular disturbances may occur in the oral cavity, bladder, stomach, retina, conjunctiva, or skin, especially of the hands, and result in so-called vicarious menstruation from these sites.

MALIGNANT CHANGE IN ENDOMETRIOSIS

Although it rarely occurs, carcinoma may arise in the aberrant endometrium of endometriosis, just as it does in the endometrium lining the uterine cavity. The known frequency of endometriosis and the rarity of malignant change within it suggest that for various, as yet unknown reasons, malignant epithelial tumcrs are less likely to develop in areas of ectopic endometrium than in nonaberrant endometrium. When malignant change does take place, it invariably occurs in the ovary.

Sampson considered the possibility of the development of carcinoma in endometriosis, and in 1925 he set forth the pathologic criteria for its recognition as follows: (1) Benign and malignant tissues must coexist in the same ovary and have the same histologic relationship as in carcinoma of the body of the uterus; (2) the carcinoma must actually be seen arising in the benign tissue and not invading it from some other source.

The majority of the reported instances of cancers arising in ovarian endometriosis in which the evidence for this transformation was incontrovertible and Sampson's pathologic criteria had been satisfactorily fulfilled have been adenoacanthomas. These are neoplasms of low-grade malignancy that characteristically arise only in connection with endometrial or endocervical tissue; this same histologic type also accounts for 10 to 15 percent of the adenocarcinomas arising in the endometrial cavity. (Adenoacanthomas of the ovary are discussed more fully in Chapter 15.) Adenoacanthomas are simply specific histologic variants belonging within the broader category of primary endometrioid carcinomas of the ovary, so termed because of their striking resemblance to primary carcinomas of the endometrium. The apparent origin of pure endometrioid tumors of the ovary (endometriallike adenocarcinomas without the malignant or metaplastic squamous cell elements that characterize adenoacanthomas) in areas of ovarian endometriosis has also been documented in a number of instances. Finally, the transition from ovarian endometriosis to malignancy has also been established in some cases of the so-called clear cell adenocarcinomas of the ovary (formerly called mesonephromas); these tumors are probably of müllerian rather than mesonephric origin, however, and hence may well be simply another variant or near-relative of the endometrioid tumor category. Since Long and Taylor [13], Scully et al. [22], and others have emphasized both the existence and relative frequency of primary endometrioid tumors of the ovary, recognition and increased accuracy of classification of these lesions have led to the realization that this histologic type of tumor actually accounts for 10 to 15 percent or more of all primary ovarian malignant tumors. However, the vast majority of these endometrioid tumors appear to arise de novo from the ovarian germinal epithelium, which, like the endometrium itself, is of müllerian origin; only a small number develop as a result of malignant transformation of ovarian endometriosis.

There have also been isolated case reports of malignant tumors apparently arising in endometriosis of the broad ligament, cul-de-sac, rectovaginal septum, and vagina, but these are extremely rare occurrences.

It is apparent from the foregoing remarks that the possibility of malignant change in endometriosis is not a factor to be considered in the management of the overall problem in a given patient, and it is certainly no indication for prophylactic surgery. Far more significant from the clinical standpoint is the frequent need to distinguish an endometrioma from an ovarian tumor, or to exclude the possibility of an ovarian tumor's coexisting with pelvic endometriosis. In either circumstance it often becomes mandatory to carry out surgical exploration, even when the patient is asymptomatic.

REFERENCES

1. Andrews, W. C., and Larsen, G. D. Endometriosis: Treatment with hormonal pseudopregnancy and/or operation. *Am. J. Obstet. Gynecol.* 118:643, 1974.
2. Bullock, J. L., Massey, F. M., and Gambrell, R. D. Symptomatic endometriosis in teen-agers. A reappraisal. *Obstet. Gynecol.* 43:896, 1974.
3. Fathalla, M. F. Malignant transformation in ovarian endometriosis. *J. Obstet. Gynecol. Br. Commonw.* 74:85, 1967.
4. Friedlander, R. L. The treatment of endometriosis with Danazol. *J. Reprod. Med.* 10:197, 1973.
5. Golditch, I. M. Endometriosis presenting as an acute abdominal emergency. *Obstet. Gynecol.* 26:780, 1965.
6. Gray, L. A. The management of endometriosis involving the bowel. *Clin. Obstet. Gynecol.* 9:309, 1966.
7. Green, T. H., Jr., and Meigs, J. V. Pseudomenstruation from posthysterectomy vaginal vault endometriosis. *Obstet. Gynecol.* 4:622, 1954.
8. Green, T. H., Jr. Conservative surgical treatment of endometriosis. *Clin. Obstet. Gynecol.* 9:293, 1966.
9. Gruenwald, P. Origin of endometriosis from mesenchyme of celomic walls. *Am. J. Obstet. Gynecol.* 44:470, 1942.
10. Hajdu, S. I., and Koss, L. G. Endometriosis of the kidney. *Am. J. Obstet. Gynecol.* 106:314, 1970.
11. Kerr, W. S., Jr. Endometriosis involving the urinary tract. *Clin. Obstet. Gynecol.* 9:331, 1966.
12. Kistner, R. W. Current status of the hormonal treatment of endometriosis. *Clin. Obstet. Gynecol.* 9:271, 1966.
13. Long, M. E., and Taylor, H. C., Jr. Endometrioid carcinoma of the ovary. *Am. J. Obstet. Gynecol.* 90:936, 1964.
14. Meigs, J. V. Endometriosis. *Ann. Surg.* 127:795, 1948.
15. Meigs, J. V. Endometriosis: Etiologic role of marriage age and parity; conservative treatment. *Obstet. Gynecol.* 2:46, 1953.

16. Ranney, B. Etiology of endometriosis (collective review). *Surg. Gynecol. Obstet. (Int. Abst. Surg.)* 86:313, 1948.
17. Ranney, B. Endometriosis. I. Conservative operations. *Am. J. Obstet. Gynecol.* 107:743, 1970.
18. Ranney, B. Endometriosis. II. Emergency operations due to hemoperitoneum. *Obstet. Gynecol.* 36:437, 1970.
19. Ranney, B. Endometriosis. III. Complete operations. *Am. J. Obstet. Gynecol.* 109:1137, 1971.
20. Rio, F. W., Edwards, D. L., Regan, J. F., and Schmutzer, K. J. Endometriosis of the small bowel. *Arch. Surg.* 101:403, 1970.
21. Sampson, J. A. Perforating hemorrhagic (chocolate) cysts of the ovary. *Arch. Surg.* 3:245, 1921.
22. Sampson, J. A. The development of the implantation theory for the origin of peritoneal endometriosis. *Am. J. Obstet. Gynecol.* 40:549, 1940.
23. Schmidt, F. R., and McCarthy, J. D. Intussusception of the appendix with endometriosis presenting as a cecal tumor. *Arch. Surg.* 103:515, 1971.
24. Scully, R. E., Richardson, G. S., and Barlow, J. F. The development of malignancy in endometriosis. *Clin. Obstet. Gynecol.* 9:384, 1966.
25. Spangler, D. B., Jones, G. S., and Jones, H. W., Jr. Infertility due to endometriosis: Conservative surgical therapy. *Am. J. Obstet. Gynecol.* 109:850, 1971.
26. Steck, W. D., and Helwig, E. B. Cutaneous endometriosis. *J.A.M.A.* 191:167, 1965.
27. Te Linde, R. W., and Scott, R. B. Experimental endometriosis. *Am. J. Obstet. Gynecol.* 60:1147, 1950.
28. Uohara, J. K., and Kobara, T. Y. Endometriosis of the appendix. *Am. J. Obstet. Gynecol.* 121:423, 1975.

11
Infertility

Many of the fundamental advances toward a more precise understanding of both the normal and abnormal physiology underlying reproductive tract function made during the past 30 years have been stimulated by and have contributed to the steadily increasing interest in the broad problem of human infertility. This increased knowledge of reproductive tract physiology, together with the continuing development and refinement of special diagnostic techniques and programs of therapy, both medical and surgical, has led to the growth of what is now a subspecialty within the field of gynecology and obstetrics. This subspecialty has its own major national and regional scientific societies, with a burgeoning literature and its own medical journals, and with a significant number of physicians and scientists concentrating their major clinical and research efforts on the study, diagnosis, and treatment of disorders accompanied by sterility. The intense interest and activity along these lines may at first glance seem paradoxical in the light of the equally serious concern over the potential impact of the world population explosion, of which currently there has been a noticeably increased awareness. It is perhaps unnecessary to point out, however, that the worldwide population explosion has little meaning for the unfortunate couple desperately anxious for children, whose marriage has thus far been barren. Furthermore — and quite rightly and logically so — the same individuals and groups engrossed in the study of sterility have also long been conscious of the seriousness of the problem of potential overpopulation in the world and have pioneered in the study, development, and testing of methods of conception control. Thus, the two problems, far from being mutually antagonistic, are actually separate facets of the broad subject of reproductive physiology and biosociology.

It is immediately obvious that disorders accompanied by impaired fertility include a wide range of anatomic and structural abnormalities such as congenital anomalies, tumors, pelvic inflammation, and endometriosis, as well as the various physiologic or endocrinologic disturbances of reproductive tract function, almost all of which are discussed in other chapters. (The physiology underlying normal conception in the female has been presented in Chapter 5.) In fact, the potential subject matter of the field of infertility tends to run the entire gamut of gynecologic physiology and pathology. Therefore, to avoid needless repetition, the major emphasis in this chapter will be on the approach to diagnosis and management of the couple who present themselves to the physician primarily because of infertility. The general diagnostic plan will be outlined, and certain diagnostic techniques employed almost exclusively in a sterility investigation will be presented in some detail here, having been purposely omitted from Chapter 2. A general survey of methods of therapy for the various conditions associated with infertility will follow, merely outlining those that have been considered more fully in other chapters but presenting in somewhat more detail those used in dealing with certain specific abnormalities whose chief or only manifestation is impaired fertility.

DEFINITION AND SCOPE OF THE PROBLEM

By definition, and from a practical clinical standpoint as well, the problem of infertility does not arise until a couple fails to conceive after a year or more of normal marital endeavor. An occasional couple will become apprehensive about their ability to conceive within less than a year, but in general it is wiser to adopt a reassuring attitude and postpone a complete sterility investigation for at least one year, provided that a careful history and thorough physical examination reveal no obvious barrier to conception. Among normal and ultimately fertile couples, approximately 65 percent will conceive within six months of trial and roughly 80 percent, after a year of trial; of the remaining 20 percent, half will achieve pregnancy by the end of two years, the other half requiring more than two years. It seems reasonable to consider the 20 percent as relatively infertile rather than absolutely infertile, but they, too, will of necessity often be accepted for a sterility investigation. They may in fact be aided in achieving a pregnancy sooner than might otherwise have occurred by virtue of the element of mental and emotional reassurance (and possibly even through occasional actual, local therapeutic benefits, e.g., possible beneficial effect of a diagnostic tubal insufflation) obtained during the course of a careful investigation by an understanding physician, one equally cognizant of and sympathetic toward the many subtle psychosocial as well as basic anatomic and endocrinologic factors at work in this vital, emotionally charged aspect of marital life.

When the total population of married couples is considered, as has been done in a number of studies of sizable populations, the reported proportion of couples with absolute infertility ranges from 10 to 20 percent. With the figure of 15 percent involuntarily sterile couples representing the approximate average for the total population of married couples in the United States, the magnitude of the problem that infertility potentially poses for the physician can readily be appreciated, involving as it does 3.5 million childless couples in this country alone.

DIAGNOSTIC APPROACH TO INFERTILITY

At the outset of a sterility investigation it should be carefully explained to the couple that it is their reproductive capacity as a biologic unit that is under scrutiny and that therefore both husband and wife must be completely evaluated. The responsibility for initiating and supervising the study customarily falls to the gynecologist for several reasons: e.g., the naturally predominant interest and concern of the female partner in the problem; the higher incidence of disturbances in female reproductive tract anatomy and function adversely affecting fertility as compared with reproductive system disorders in the male; and the greater number of female factors to be analyzed and the more complicated techniques of study required. The gynecologist may also carry out the investigation of the husband, although more often the male partner will be referred to a urologist with a special interest and competence in the evaluation of male fertility, the urologist cooperating in the total study program and carrying out the diagnostic studies and any indicated therapy in the male. The gynecologist should, however, be completely familiar with the diagnostic aspects and general therapeutic principles of male infertility, since the status of the husband obviously influences the course of study and therapy of the wife, and since information concerning both partners is essential to him in his role as principal counselor and chief administrator of the total diagnostic and treatment program. Hence for complete orientation the studies to be carried out in the male will also be briefly outlined.

The specific factors that must be studied and the various tests by which this is accomplished should be enumerated and described to the couple in advance to ensure their subsequent understanding and cooperation. It should be emphasized that multiple factors are often responsible for a couple's failure to conceive, and the physician himself must always bear this in mind, for the entire investigation must for this reason be carried through to completion before undertaking therapy for any obvious abnormality discovered early in the course of the evaluation. It should be pointed out initially that a proper study and any subsequently indicated therapeutic measures will require time (often a year or more) and patience on the part of all concerned if success is to be achieved.

OUTLINE OF BASIC DIAGNOSTIC STUDIES IN THE INFERTILE COUPLE

Both husband and wife must initially be carefully assessed from the standpoint of the possible existence of any generalized disorders or conditions that might be major or contributing causes of their failure to achieve pregnancy. Thereafter, the major portion of the investigation is carried forward by more specific inquiry, examination, and special diagnostic studies focused on the inherent anatomic and functional status of both their reproductive tracts in order to assess the four principal factors involved in the process of conception. These factors are: in the male (1) the seminal factor; in the female (2) the ovarian factor, (3) the tubal factor, and (4) the cervical factor. Other less readily categorized aspects of the reproductive process, disturbances of which may result in impaired fertility, are evaluated simultaneously and may be considered as frequently significant miscellaneous factors. A general idea of the relative frequency with which disturbances of the various factors are the major cause of infertility may be gained from the following composite estimates based on the reported experience of various individuals and clinics engaged in the diagnosis and treatment of sterility patients: male factor, 25 to 35 percent; ovarian factor, 15 to 25 percent (failure of ovulation in 10 to 20 percent; inadequate progesterone production alone, with ovulation occurring, or the so-called luteal phase defect, in 5 to 10 percent); tubal factor, 25 to 35 percent (the percentage may be higher in areas where there is an increased incidence of venereal disease or tuberculosis); cervical factor, 15 to 20 percent. In roughly 35 percent of infertile couples, multiple factors are probably responsible for the problem; in 20 percent, the infertility is the result of a combination of male and female factors.

General Evaluation

HISTORY AND EXAMINATION

A complete general history is taken of both partners, and each has a physical examination, as well as basic laboratory tests (blood counts, urinalyses, serology, thyroid
function studies) to discover or rule out the following: obvious systemic disease;
gross anatomic disturbances; generalized endocrine disorders (e.g., thyroid, adrenal,
or pituitary); nutritional deficiencies; toxic exposures (e.g., male occupational
exposures to heavy metals or radioactive substances) and so on; and a particular
effort should be made to determine whether or not prior illnesses, injuries, or
surgical procedures in or near the genital tract might conceivably have resulted in
impaired function. Examples of the latter include:

Male: Previous mumps orchitis with testicular atrophy; a history of medications
(a number of drugs, including some antibacterial agents such as the nitrofurantoins
and a variety of psychotropic drugs, can cause oligospermia, or sexual dysfunction,
or both); previous venereal disease; varicocele; undescended testes; hypospadias or
other congenital anomalies; chronic prostatitis; previous groin injuries or hernior-
rhaphies, in which possible damage to the vas deferens may have been sustained;
a history of tuberculosis.

Female: Previous venereal disease, especially a history of symptoms suggesting
prior pelvic inflammatory disease; history of appendicitis or appendectomy; prior
abortions or miscarriages; obvious congenital anomalies of the uterovaginal tract;
history of tuberculosis.

SEXUAL AND PSYCHOLOGICAL FACTORS

A detailed inquiry is made concerning marital adjustment, coital technique, frequency, and timing, and various psychosocial factors that may inhibit normal reproductive function. The importance of obtaining complete information along these
lines by thoughtful and tactful questioning cannot be overemphasized, for coital
infrequency, unsatisfactory and ineffective coital performance due to ignorance or
psychic inhibitions, or tensions associated with inability to achieve a satisfactory
overall marital adjustment will often prove to be the sole or an important contributing factor in the failure to achieve pregnancy. Although this information should be
sought reasonably early in the course of the sterility investigation, it is often wiser
to postpone detailed discussion of these matters for a few visits until the physician-
patient relationship is sufficiently well established to permit the patient or the
couple to speak of them more freely and openly. Less often, serious personality
disturbances or even major psychiatric disorders may be discovered and prove to be
the primary cause of sterility in one or the other of the marital partners.

Evaluation of the Male (Seminal Factor)

SEMEN ANALYSIS

At least two or three semen specimens should be examined, especially if the initial
one is substandard. The specimen should be collected in a clean, dry jar (preferably

after four to six days' abstinence), kept at or below room temperature, and examined within 2 to 4 hours with reference to the following:

1. **Volume:** Normally 2.5 to 5.0 ml, with an alkaline pH, and initially rather viscid.
2. **Liquefaction:** Normally complete within 10 to 30 minutes.
3. **Motility:** Normally at least 50 percent active, motile sperm at 4 hours, or 60 to 80 percent at 2 hours. Examine a drop of semen on a slide with coverslip edges sealed with petrolatum.
4. **Cell count:** Use a white blood cell pipette, filling it with semen to the 0.5 mark and diluting to the 1:20 mark with tap water; using a red cell counting chamber, count the sperm in five small blocks (as for a red cell count). The total figure obtained yields count in millions per milliliter. The average of several counts should be used for the final estimate. Normal range: 40 to 150 million per milliliter, with average normal count of 60 to 100 million per milliliter. (However, occasional pregnancies have occurred in the presence of sperm counts of 10 to 20 million per milliliter or, rarely, even lower counts.)
5. **Cell morphology:** The semen smear is prepared in the same way as a routine blood smear. Stain with Wright's stain and evaluate and count several hundred sperm heads. **Normal:** 60 to 80 percent or more of the sperm heads should exhibit normal morphology.

In evaluating the significance of semen analysis in the individual patient, it should be kept in mind that, given a reasonable sperm count, the factors of motility and morphology are probably the most decisive ones with respect to fertility.

TESTICULAR BIOPSY

If complete absence of sperm is discovered on semen analysis, or in the face of marked oligospermia, testicular biopsy may be indicated to differentiate between primary testicular failure and a mechanical block in the vas deferens or epididymis, or as a diagnostic and prognostic guide in the case of oligospermia.

Special Diagnostic Tests in the Female

The gynecologic history, particularly with regard to menstrual function, together with the findings of the pelvic examination, may or may not be immediately suggestive of abnormal ovarian function or palpable disease of the uterus, or adnexa, or both. In any case, detailed investigation of the three major female reproductive factors is carried out by the special tests described in the sections that follow.

OVARIAN FACTOR AND ENDOMETRIAL RESPONSE

The procedures that follow are to establish whether or not there is regular ovulation and production of a progestational endometrium satisfactory for implantation.

Basal Body Temperature Chart

The basal body temperature chart should be kept for four or more cycles, including
a record of coital frequency and timing. Typical biphasic temperature curves will
be indicative of regular ovulation, whereas irregular, monophasic curves will indicate
failure of ovulation and absent or inadequate progesterone production (Fig. 40).

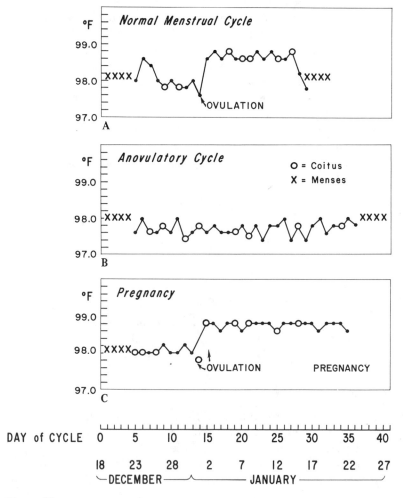

Figure 40

Basal body temperature chart. A. Typical biphasic temperature curve indicative of
ovulation and normal progesterone effect. B. Irregular monophasic curve characteristic of anovulatory cycles. C. Ovulatory curve with sustained temperature elevation
following conception and the first missed period.

Endometrial Biopsy

Endometrial biopsy confirms the presence or absence of ovulation and also evaluates whether or not the development of a mature secretory endometrium suitable for implantation and maintenance of a fertilized ovum is occurring regularly. For maximal information, endometrial biopsy should be done within 12 hours of the expected appearance of menstrual flow, or at the most within a few days of the calculated onset of the period. (When performed at this time, it may also prove valuable in the discovery of unsuspected pelvic tuberculosis.) A biopsy may also be done immediately following the onset of flow, but this is usually difficult for both patient and physician to arrange. Ovulation is indicated if microscopic study reveals a definite secretory endometrium. Furthermore, the degree of secretory maturation can usually be accurately estimated by histologic study and will serve as an index of whether or not progesterone production is adequate.

Other Tests for Ovulation and Progesterone Production

Other tests for ovulation and progesterone production as described in Chapter 2 may also be employed, but these are rarely necessary for clinical purposes.

Not infrequently, determination of the actual time of ovulation as precisely as possible may also be important, especially if study reveals either that the husband is subfertile, with a depressed sperm count or poor sperm motility, or that the quality of the wife's cervical mucus is poor and unresponsive to the usual methods of treatment. In such situations, more accurate estimates of the most fruitful time for coitus may help to improve the couple's chances for conception. (Precise timing of ovulation is also of obvious importance in determining the optimal period for therapeutic insemination.) The most useful methods for determining the time of ovulation with reasonable accuracy include observations of the thermal shift on the basal body temperature chart (ovulation is believed to occur 24 to 48 hours before the rise) and detection of the specific preovulatory and ovulatory changes in the vaginal cytologic smear, in the cervical mucus fern test, in the characteristics of the cervical mucus itself, especially the spinnbarkeit (see Cervical Factor), and in the glucose content of the cervical mucus. The latter is the basis for the Tes-Tape test, now commercially available for use by the patient herself, although the reliability of such a "do-it-yourself" test is questioned by many.

Parsons and his associates [10] have developed a technique for measuring the electrovaginal potential (EVG). On the basis of daily measurements they believe that the time of ovulation can be even more precisely detected by a definite, sharply defined change in the EVG pattern. They are the first to admit, however, that these electropotential changes have as yet to be absolutely correlated with the day of ovulation. Nevertheless, it is of some interest that as a result of such studies in over 600 patients, their data have suggested that ovulation may be occurring considerably earlier in the usual 28-day cycle (day 8 to 10 instead of day 12 to 14) than has been assumed on the basis of most other methods for ovulation timing. Their conclusions are therefore still tentative and controversial and the method itself remains as yet a research tool, but one that may prove extremely valuable in studying other aspects of female reproductive tract physiology, whether or not their concept of "earlier ovulation" is ultimately substantiated.

TUBAL FACTOR

The tests to be described are to determine whether or not the tubes are normal and patent and the ovarian-tubal transfer mechanism is normal. It should be emphasized again that not only must the tubes (or at least one tube) have a patent lumen, but the tubal anatomy and physiology must also be sufficiently normal to ensure that proper peristaltic and secretory activity is present to maintain viability and aid in the movements and function of the sperm and ovum, as well as to provide a suitable milieu for the early days in the life of the zygote. Equally important, the fimbriated ends and distal portions of the tubes must be sufficiently free within the pelvic cavity to come into normal apposition with the ovaries at ovulation time, and the surfaces of the latter and the intervening peritoneal space must not be separated from the tubes by adhesions that impede or completely block the passage of the ovum to the fimbriated tubal opening. This latter aspect of tubal function — or, more correctly, of the ovarian-tubal transfer mechanism — is sometimes referred to as the *peritoneal factor,* since, strictly speaking, it relates to the peritoneal space surrounding both the tubes and the ovaries that must be traversed by the ovum. Interference with the normal operation of this factor is encountered in the presence of local intraperitoneal adhesions secondary to disorders such as endometriosis, previous pelvic inflammation, or prior appendicitis. Thus, complete assessment of tubal function involves not only determination of patency but also whether or not the ovum transfer and pickup mechanism is unimpeded (peritoneal factor). Precise clinical assessment of the physiological and biochemical performance of the fallopian tubes is as yet not possible, although normal tubal anatomy and histology is usually an indication of normal function, provided that ovarian hormonal control of tubal activity is normal.

Rubin Test (Uterotubal Insufflation with Carbon Dioxide)

For greatest reliability the Rubin test should be done during the 7 to 10 days immediately following a period. If an initial test is negative, insufflation should be repeated once or twice in subsequent cycles before proceeding with further studies. Because of the danger of gas embolism, it should never be done in the presence of uterine bleeding.

Technique. With the patient in lithotomy position, the cervix is exposed by speculum, the anterior lip is grasped with a tenaculum, and the cervical os is swabbed clean and painted with Schiller's solution (used here as an antiseptic). A uterine sound is passed to determine the direction and depth of the uterine canal and to dilate gently the endocervix and internal os. A special insufflation cannula (metal, with a rubber acorn for an airtight seal and a detachable, terminal plastic tip beyond; or a completely plastic, disposable, combined one-piece acorn and tip) is introduced, the airtight seal adjusted and the outer end of the cannula connected by rubber tubing to

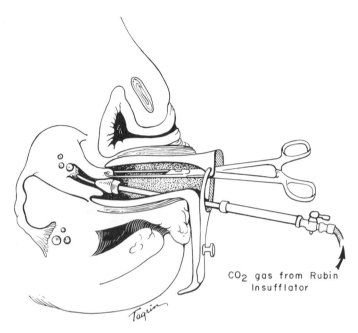

CO₂ gas from Rubin
Insufflator

Figure 41
Tubal insufflation (Rubin test). Cannula secured in place and insufflation with
carbon dioxide administration in progress.

the Rubin insufflator, which delivers the carbon dioxide (Fig. 41). Either the kymo-
graphic type, which yields a permanent record of pressure fluctuation, or the simpler
model, with mechanical flowmeter and attached pressure gauge, may be used; 100 ml
of carbon dioxide is allowed to flow slowly and steadily, the pressure changes in the
system being constantly observed; occasional slight manipulations of the cervix to
alter the position of the uterus may aid in establishing free flow. Occasionally,
inhalation of an ampule of amyl nitrite may result in flow when none occurs initially
because of functional obstruction due to spasm in the cornual region. Tubal patency
is suggested if an abrupt drop in pressure of 20 to 40 mm occurs after an initial rise
to levels of 80 to 120 mm Hg or more. When the insufflation is completed and the
apparatus removed, further confirmation is obtained by having the patient sit upright,
whereupon any carbon dioxide free in the peritoneal cavity rises beneath the diaphragm, producing the typical shoulder pain characteristic of a positive test. The
development of this characteristic shoulder pain is the only valid end point signifying
a positive test. The pain is usually abrupt in onset, occurs within 15 to 60 seconds,
and is sharp but transient. If the onset of pain is delayed (several minutes or even
hours), patency of one or both tubes, but with peritubal and pelvic or abdominal
adhesions trapping the gas and slowing its ascent, is suggested. Tubal spasm is a frequent cause of negative test results and should be differentiated by the previously
mentioned maneuver with amyl nitrite as well as by repeating the test on one or

more separate occasions. If several negative Rubin tests are obtained, hysterosalpingography, or culdoscopy, or both is indicated for further evaluation.

Hysterosalpingography

Hysterosalpingography for the study of tubal anatomy and patency is usually best employed as an adjunct to carbon dioxide insufflation when the latter indicates apparent tubal occlusion. Since the cervical canal and the endometrial cavity are also outlined, this test may also detect uterine abnormalities of significance with regard to the infertility, e.g., submucous fibroids or congenital anomalies, such as bicornuate or septate uterus.

Technique. The procedure is entirely similar to that of the Rubin test and is most conveniently done in the x-ray department on a special table such as is commonly employed for cystoscopy and retrograde pyelography. A wooden (nonradiopaque) speculum is helpful though not essential. An insufflation cannula is introduced in the same manner as for tubal insufflation; a special adapter attached to the cannula permits the cervical tenaculum to be locked in place anterior to the cannula, mechanically applying countertraction and maintaining an airtight seal at the cervix, and has a Luer-Lok outer end for attaching the syringe of radiopaque dye. The entire system should be filled with dye before insertion of the cannula to avoid introducing air bubbles that might cause artifacts suggestive of intrauterine or tubal disease; either Ethiodol, an oil-based medium, or one of the aqueous iodide media (e.g., Salpix) is employed. Only 1 or 2 ml is injected initially, and a film is taken for optimal study of the uterine cavity (an excessive amount of dye at this point may mask intracavitary abnormalities such as polyps or submucous fibroids). Following the first film (developed and examined immediately before proceeding) and depending on the apparent size of the uterine cavity and the extent to which tubal filling has already been achieved, 2 to 4 ml more of dye is instilled and a second (and usually last) film obtained. (**Note:** Fluoroscopy should *not* be used, since the danger of excessive radiation for both patient and physician is much too great.) Patency of the tubes may already be suggested on the first or second x-ray film (Fig. 42). If apparent cornual block is present, amyl nitrite inhalation may be tried to eliminate the possibility that the failure of tubal filling is due to temporary cornual spasm. Fimbrial occlusion may also already be suspected because of the demonstration of obvious dilatation of the tubal lumen and droplet formation of the dye (due to contact with the watery fluid contained in a hydrosalpinx or pyosalpinx in the fimbriated end). In any event, if Ethiodol or a similar oily medium has been employed, a third x-ray film taken 24 hours later is usually advisable. This will definitely settle the question of whether or not dye has reached the free peritoneal cavity or has been trapped in diseased and occluded tubes.

Culdoscopy or Laparoscopy

Culdoscopy or laparoscopy affords direct observation of the tubes during uterotubal instillation of an aqueous solution of methylene blue, indigo carmine, or a similar

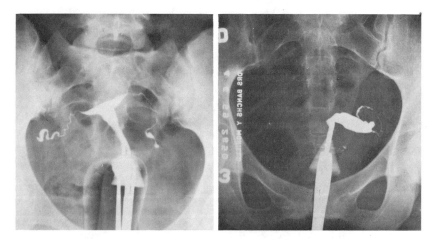

Figure 42
Hysterosalpingography. A normal uterine configuration and normal, patent tubes
are seen in the film on the left. On the right is the hysterosalpingogram of a 26-
year-old woman complaining of infertility of 4 years' duration, the x-ray revealing
a bicornuate uterus with a rudimentary right uterine horn and nonpatent tube,
findings that were confirmed at a subsequent laparotomy.

dye. This approach has frequently proved more accurate and is certainly often more
informative than tubal insufflation, or hysterosalpingography, or the two techniques
combined, because it not only demonstrates tubal occlusion, if present, but also
permits visualization of the nature and exact anatomy of the pathologic process producing the block. It is especially useful when the results of the latter two studies,
together with the history and findings on pelvic examination, are equivocal with
respect to the presence or absence of tubal obstruction. In the presence of old
appendicitis, endometriosis, or minimal chronic pelvic inflammatory disease, the
tubes are frequently still patent, and hence the results of Rubin's test and the hysterosalpingogram will often be normal in spite of the peritubal pathologic condition
present.

Perhaps most important, laparoscopy or culdoscopy permits direct visual inspection of the adnexal regions, and often it is only by this means that can one detect
interference with the normal transfer of ovum to tubes by periadnexal adhesions,
with resulting restriction of normal tuboovarian mobility.

Parenthetically, it is worth pointing out that almost the entire basic female fertility study can be accomplished at a single culdoscopy or laparoscopy performed at
the proper time in the menstrual cycle. Not only can the tubal (and peritoneal)
factor be thoroughly investigated, but the status of ovarian function is also readily
apparent, even to the point of demonstrating recent ovulation or the absence thereof.
Certainly, if the other routine diagnostic maneuvers are not revealing and infertility
persists after another year of study and attempted treatment, and assuming the

husband is found normal, most patients deserve to have laparoscopic or culdoscopic examination, and, in many instances, an unexpected pathologic condition will be discovered in this way.

CERVICAL FACTOR

Examination of the cervical mucus reveals whether or not it undergoes favorable changes at ovulation time, enabling penetration, survival, and normal progression of sperm.

Postcoital Cervical Mucus Test (Sims-Huhner Test, "PK" Test)

For a postcoital cervical mucus test the patient reports to the office within 6 to 12 hours after coitus, on or within 24 to 48 hours of the day of the cycle that the basal body temperature chart or other tests indicate to be the probable time of ovulation. Without use of a lubricant, the cervix is exposed by speculum, and a sample of endo-cervical mucus is aspirated by medicine dropper or special cannula from the level of the internal os and examined immediately, using a clean glass slide with a coverslip. A sample of vaginal secretion is also examined for sperm to exclude the possibility of faulty coital technique, in case the cervical mucus should be found to contain no sperm whatsoever.

Normal findings: 5 to 20 sperm per high-power field, 50 percent active at 4 hours and 25 percent active at 12 hours.

In addition to the actual cervical-mucus sperm count, simple observations of the volume and physical characteristics of the ovulatory cervical mucus usually yield valuable clues as to whether or not the normal, temporary changes favorable to sperm penetration and progression have occurred. The cervical secretion should at this time (for a period of perhaps 48 to 72 hours) be abundant in amount and crystal-clear, thin, and watery, yet with a characteristic consistency that permits it to be drawn in long threads (spinnbarkeit); and it should be relatively free of leuko-cytes and epithelial cells on microscopic examination. On the other hand, if the cervical secretion is scanty, cloudy, viscid, and cellular, an abnormal postcoital test is invariably obtained. Under these conditions the abnormal test can usually be assumed to be the result of poor ovulatory cervical mucus, unless studies in the husband suggest that a low sperm count or poor sperm motility is also a potential factor.

An abnormal test should be verified two or three times before it is considered conclusive. Excluding faulty coital technique or performance of the test on the wrong day of the cycle, an unsatisfactory test usually indicates one of the following abnormalities: (1) poor sperm quality, (2) poor seminal fluid (chronic prostatitis, and so on), (3) poor cervical mucus quality due to chronic endocervicitis, or (4) poor cervical mucus quality due to inadequate estrogen effect or other hormonal imbalance.

Further confirmation that an abnormal postcoital cervical mucus test is the result of poor quality of the cervical mucus itself may often be obtained by performing a preovulatory cervical mucus fern test. If the fern phenomenon does not occur, the presence of either chronic cervicitis or a lack of adequate estrogen stimulation is probably the basis for the deficiency in the normal secretory activity of the endocervical glands and the resulting quantitative and qualitative abnormalities of the ovulatory cervical secretions that render them unsuitable for sperm penetration and survival.

MISCELLANEOUS IMPLANTATION AND MAINTENANCE FACTORS

In considering female infertility, a fourth category must be added to the usual three (or a fifth, if one treats the peritoneal factor as independent of the tubal factor) to include certain disorders affecting female fertility that are less directly related to the basic physiology of reproduction and do not fall under any of the preceding three (or four) headings. Since all these disorders concern abnormalities of uterine anatomy, this category might quite properly be termed the *uterine factor.* Some of these conditions may result in apparent primary infertility due to immediate failure of implantation (no delay in the onset of the next normal period is experienced), but many of them result in repeated abortions, a form of sterility in the broad sense of the word (see Chap. 9). Most frequent among such conditions are submucous or intramural fibroids; endometrial or endocervical polyps; traumatic intrauterine adhesions (Asherman's syndrome); congenital uterine anomalies (primarily the various duplications, including bicornuate and septate uterus); and incompetent internal cervical os, an acquired defect (following obstetric or surgical trauma to the cervix) that is often the cause of repeated second-trimester abortions (see Chap. 9). The diagnosis of these conditions rests primarily on the findings on pelvic examination supplemented by study of the anatomy of the uterus by hysterosalpingography.

IMMUNOLOGIC FACTORS IN INFERTILITY

One other explanation for unexplained infertility in certain couples has been brought to light by the studies of Behrman and associates [1], Franklin and Dukes [3], and others who investigated the possibility that immunologic phenomena might be the cause of some barren marriages. At first, it appeared that cervical secretions might contain immune antibodies of the ABO(H) blood-group system that could selectively neutralize, inhibit, or agglutinate sperm cells in some immunologically incompatible matings by virtue of the fact that the male possessed an antigen for which the female had the corresponding antibody. Thus a wife with group 0 blood would have ABO(H) antibodies not only in her serum but also in her uterine, cervical, vaginal, ovarian, follicular, and other body secretions, while the husband, if his blood group were A, B, or AB, would have an ABO(H) antigen not only in his erythrocytes but also in many body secretions, including semen. If the husband were heterozygous (OB or OA), pregnancy might occur and result in group 0 children, since his group 0 spermatozoa would not be agglutinated. However, if he were homozygous (A, B, or

AB) the marriage might be irrevocably sterile, since either or both of group A and group B spermatozoa would be agglutinated and rendered incapable of fertilization.

Whether or not these blood-group incompatibilities were important factors in a given couple would be determined by whether or not any antibodies appeared in the secretions of the female reproductive tract (they are most common in group O women, rare in group A or B, and nonexistent in group AB), and, if so, whether or not they were present in sufficient titer to have a significant effect, as well as whether or not the spermatozoa contained any or sufficient amounts of antigen. In view of the millions of fertile ABO(H) incompatible marriages, it has become apparent that the percentage of unfavorable effects on conception is small. However, though they ultimately showed that ABO(H) incompatibility plays little role in infertility, these initial investigations did bring to light the existence in some infertile women of acquired, even more specific antisperm antibodies of both sperm-agglutinating and sperm-immobilizing types. Furthermore, some men have been shown to possess sperm antibodies of autoimmune origin that cause spontaneous agglutination following ejaculation, rendering it impossible for the clumped sperm to penetrate the cervical mucus. Hence, in couples in whom there is no apparent cause for infertility, it is important to keep these possibilities in mind. Autoimmune agglutinating antibodies are considered to be present in the husband if a sample of sperm mixed with semen clumps after 1 to 2 hours of incubation.

Similarly, a simple serologic test can be used to demonstrate sperm agglutination in the female by mixing a suspension of fresh sperm from the husband with the wife's serum; the presence of circulating sperm-agglutinating antibodies in the female is indicated when, after incubation of the mixture for a few hours, agglutination of sperm is noted on microscopic examination. (Tests with a number of other sperm samples from donors are run simultaneously as controls.) A more sensitive and precise laboratory method employing radioactive-iodine—labeled serum gamma globulin from the woman detects and quantitates sperm agglutination phenomena. By measuring how much of the tagged immune globulin coats the male sperm sample when the two are mixed, the degree to which the wife's antibodies oppose and inactivate the husband's sperm can be assessed and compared with the results in the control series run with donor sperm samples.

The presence of circulating sperm-agglutinating or sperm-immobilizing antibodies has been detected in less than 10 percent of normally fertile women but has been reported in over two-thirds of several large groups of women with unexplained infertility and is thought to be the major factor in the infertility in 15 to 20 percent of these couples. In some women the antibody reaction is specific for the husband's sperm; in others, immunologic incompatibility has been found for the majority of sperm cells tested. It is also clear that circulating sperm-agglutinating antibodies may be only an indicator of and not actually involved in the immunologic mechanism responsible for the infertility. Furthermore, evidence is accumulating that failure of implantation rather than in vivo sperm agglutination and failure of fertilization, may be the fundamental problem resulting from the immunologic incompatibility between husband and wife.

OUTLINE OF THERAPY FOR THE VARIOUS DISORDERS ASSOCIATED WITH INFERTILITY

In the general management of the infertile couple, the therapeutic benefits that often appear to be achieved simply by carefully carrying out the total study program should not be overlooked. It is well known that roughly 20 percent of couples undergoing a sterility investigation conceive while under study and before any specific treatment has been given. This phenomenon may be due to inadvertent local therapeutic effects of tubal insufflation and endometrial biopsy on tubal or cervical anatomy and physiology, or even to indirect effects on ovarian function, or the beneficial effects may be of a more general neuroendocrine nature. Thus, favorable changes in reproductive tract physiology may be promoted by reassurance and by the couple's more relaxed attitude as they proceed with the study under the sympathetic guidance of an interested physician.

A word should also be said concerning the couple in whom thorough investigation using all the standard studies fails to reveal a cause for failure to conceive. In the past, such "normal infertile" couples with "unexplained infertility" have all too often suffered from a policy of watchful neglect and cautious optimism inspired by the normal findings encountered during the routine diagnostic tests of a complete fertility evaluation. In actuality, the female in the situation will be found in roughly 50 percent of cases to have an unsuspected pelvic pathologic condition, usually, minimal endometriosis or pelvic adhesions secondary to prior pelvic inflammation or appendicitis, which, though not palpable and not affecting tubal patency tests, has seriously interfered with normal ovum pickup and tubal transport functions. Therefore such women should often be offered laparoscopy or culdoscopy (or exploratory laparotomy, if gynecologic endoscopy is unavailable) without undue delay, since actual visualization of the pelvic viscera is the only way in which this situation can be recognized or the possibility of its existence definitely excluded.

If evidence of an underlying organic disease still cannot be demonstrated, the possibility that an immunologic incompatibility is responsible for an unaccountably barren marriage should be considered, as already emphasized. When the woman is found to have a high circulating sperm-agglutinating or sperm-immobilizing antibody titer with respect to her husband's sperm, a marked reduction in or even complete disappearance of the antibody titer can sometimes be achieved by use of a condom during intercourse for periods of several months to as long as a year, thereby preventing repeated exposure to sperm antigens. In a significant number of couples so managed, pregnancy has occurred when use of the condom was discontinued and normal intercourse resumed at the time of expected ovulation.

Obviously, any general health or psychosocial factors that have been demonstrated and may be adversely affecting reproductive tract function and impeding conception should receive careful attention and treatment at the outset. The importance of recognizing and adequately dealing with psychological or emotional factors that by virtue of inhibiting normal reproductive tract function may be the fundamental reason for the inability of the couple to conceive cannot be overemphasized. If the underlying psychological disturbance is relatively mild, the gynecologist himself may be able to cope with the problem, but deep-rooted anxieties or more profound psychic disturbances may require the combined efforts of the psychiatrist and marriage counselor or psychiatric social service worker. It should also be remembered that for most couples a variable amount of anxiety inevitably accompanies the continuing failure to achieve a much-desired pregnancy and that awareness of this and sympathetic reassurance by the physician during the course of study and treatment may prevent a "vicious circle": anxiety → interference with neuroendocrine aspects of reproductive tract physiology → persistent sterility → increased anxiety.

Moreover, the couple should thoroughly understand the basic facts of reproductive anatomy and physiology. Faulty coital technique and timing, which at times may be the principal or only problem, should of course be corrected. In most women, ovulation probably occurs about two days before the average middle day of the menstrual cycle (or 24 to 48 hours before the rise in basal body temperature). Because of month-to-month variation in the precise timing of ovulation, the fertile period in the human female may be considered as extending from two days before to five days after this day. Since the human ovum remains fertilizable for from 4 to 20 hours, and human spermatozoa retain their fertilizing capacity for 12 to 48 hours, there is a significant latitude of from 12 to possibly as long as 48 hours in any one cycle when a single coitus may prove fruitful; intercourse more often than once in every 24 to 48 hours rarely increases the chances of conception. If, however, the intervals between intercourse during the fertile period become much longer than two to three days, a definite increase in the number of cycles of trial before pregnancy ensues can in general be predicted, and if intercourse is even less frequent, prolonged delay (apparent infertility) may result. Most couples should therefore be advised of the likely fertile period based on the woman's careful record of her cycle lengths, employing temperature chart data as a cross-check, and she should be informed that intercourse approximately every other night represents a reasonably optimal frequency as far as ensuring maximal chance for conception is concerned. They should be cautioned against the tendency to conduct their marital life by the calendar, however (such a program can well be self-defeating), and should approach this aspect with as much spontaneity and normal individual variation as possible.

Although in the past, periods of sexual abstinence have been recommended immediately prior to the woman's fertile period in the hope of improving the husband's fertility, the evidence of the value of this maneuver is dubious. In some cases it may increase the total sperm count (daily or more frequent intercourse may decrease it), but usually the quality and motility of the aged sperm present after an interval of four to six days' abstinence is considerably reduced, and the chances of conception may thereby be impaired rather than improved. Again, optimal sperm vitality, motility, and fertilizing capacity seem to be favored when ejaculation occurs approximately every 48 hours.

In addition to these general aspects of the overall plan of management, specific forms of therapy will be indicated for any definite reproductive tract abnormalities discovered during the course of the survey of the key factors involved in conception and are discussed in the following sections.

Therapy for Disturbances of the Male Factor

Although detailed discussion of therapy for male infertility is beyond the scope of this book, a brief summary seems indicated.

1. If the sperm count is in the low normal range, and/or sperm morphology, sperm motility, or semen volume or quality is poor, in the absence of infection or local anatomic or pathologic disorders, general measures that may improve male fertility include the following: insistence on an adequate diet, rest, exercise, and relaxation from a too-strenuous living pace; avoidance of excessive alcohol and tobacco consumption; and occasionally the judicious use of thyroid medication if a hypometabolic state is suspected. In some couples, too frequent intercourse may result in sufficient reduction in the husband's semen quality and sperm count to prevent conception; if this is suggested by the results of repeated semen analyses following varying intervals of abstinence, a reduction in the frequency of intercourse and a period of abstinence just before ovulation may improve the chance of conception. Although it enjoyed a passing vogue a few years ago, the use of testosterone or other steroid hormone preparations in an attempt to improve sperm counts and motility in otherwise normal males has proved essentially worthless as far as either spermatogenesis or male fertility is concerned. Although a relatively uncommon cause of male infertility, impotence on the part of the husband may be discovered to be the source of the infertility. This may respond to thorough examination, explanation that no physical abnormality exists, and simple reassurance, although at times intensive psychotherapy will prove necessary.

2. Chronic prostatitis and cytourethritis often result in poor-quality semen and sperm, and vigorous treatment of the chronic infection may improve this situation and restore fertility.

3. Because of the importance of the heat-regulatory mechanism of the scrotum in maintaining an optimal testicular temperature for normal spermatogenesis, marked obesity, confining sedentary occupations, the wearing of excessively tight clothing (e.g., skintight jockey shorts or athletic supporters), frequent steam or sauna baths, or chronic occupational exposure to high temperature (bakers, certain industrial workers) may significantly affect sperm count and quality, and correction of these factors may improve fertility in the male. There is evidence that the presence of a significant degree of varicocele may also impair male fertility by interfering with scrotal thermal control (or possibly causing retrograde venous blood flow from the renal vein into the spermatic vein, with a resulting abnormal adrenal hormone or metabolic effect), and surgical repair of a large varicocele is often successful (in 60 to 70 percent of cases) in elevating the sperm count in infertile oligospermic males, with return of normal fertility (a 50 to 60 percent pregnancy rate in one series). These results are particularly significant, since it is estimated that varicocele may be

responsible for at least 20 to 25 percent of the cases of male infertility (39 percent in one reported series).

4. Although orchiopexy for bilateral undescended testis rarely results in normal spermatogenesis if carried out after puberty, it deserves mention as an important measure for the prevention of potential male infertility if performed in time.

5. Congenital or acquired anomalies of the penis and urethra such as hypospadias, epispadias, phimosis, or urethral stricture, any of which may interfere with normal ejaculation and semen placement, may sometimes be corrected by surgical measures.

6. If semen analysis reveals a complete absence of sperm, but testicular biopsy shows normal testicular histology and spermatogenesis, obstruction in the epididymis or vas deferens is nearly always present. At times, this can be successfully relieved or bypassed by surgical procedures, e.g., epididymovasostomy or resection of the area of block and reanastomosis in the case of an occluded vas deferens.

7. Rarely, a hypogonadal state in the azospermic male with absent spermatogenesis on testicular biopsy and with low or absent follicle-stimulating hormone (FSH) excretion may be due to a primary pituitary deficiency, and this may sometimes respond favorably to chorionic gonadotropin therapy.

8. In the face of complete azospermia and absence of testicular function as established by testicular biopsy, the possibility of employing artificial insemination using semen from carefully selected donors should be considered and discussed with the couple. Although the legal implications for the resulting offspring are as yet not completely clarified, no real problems in this regard have been encountered or are anticipated, and therapeutic insemination is now a well-established procedure and has successfully brought the joys and satisfactions of parenthood to thousands of couples. The other alternative is, of course, adoption.

Therapy for Disturbances of the Ovarian Factor

The various disturbances in ovarian physiology that may result in female infertility include all the essentially functional disorders as well as the basic endocrine diseases discussed in Chapter 5 and Chapter 6 respectively, and there is no need to repeat the details of their diagnostic recognition and treatment here. In the majority, simple ovarian dysfunction will be present, and proper management will involve primarily a medical approach employing supplemental hormone therapy to restore and maintain normal ovulation and adequate progesterone production. The importance of not overlooking the possible existence of the so-called luteal-phase defect should be emphasized again, for it may not be suspected if the occurrence of ovulation is used as the sole criterion of normal ovarian function. However, careful inspection and interpretation of the basal body temperature curve in the luteal phase, or a properly timed premenstrual endometrial biopsy, or both will reveal any "progesterone inadequacy," and subsequent supplemental therapy with progesterone (e.g., Provera, 5 mg daily from day 18 to day 28, and, if pregnancy occurs, continuing thereafter at a 10-mg daily dose for two to three months) may render conception and normal implantation possible. On the other hand, a surgical approach may be indicated in the treatment of patients with certain types of pathologic ovarian endocrine conditions; bilateral ovarian wedge resections for the Stein-Leventhal syndrome and resection of the various functioning ovarian tumors are the chief examples. Medical therapy with clomiphene may be an alternative in selected cases of the Stein-Leventhal syndrome. (The management of this and other anovulatory disorders with clomiphene, menotropins [Pergonal], or purified human pituitary gonadotropins is discussed in Chapter 6.)

Therapy for Disturbances of the Tubal Factor and the Tuboovarian Ovum Transfer Mechanisms (Peritoneal Factor)

Occasionally, repeated tubal insufflations or hysterosalpingograms will be followed by pregnancy in previously infertile women in whom impaired tubal patency had been suggested by initial abnormal results in tests of tubal function. It is nearly always impossible to determine whether the successful outcomes might be due to disruption of filmy tubal or peritubal adhesions, to dispersal of mucus plugs within the tubal lumina, or simply to overcoming chronic tubal spasm by the insufflation; perhaps they are most often merely coincidental events. Nevertheless, on the basis of such favorable experiences, which occur sporadically in the practice of any gynecologist, there are firm advocates of this nonoperative technique as the initial approach in women with apparent impaired tubal function. However, a critical appraisal of reported results makes it seem unlikely that such an approach will be successful in the presence of unequivocal bilateral tubal occlusion. Minimal pelvic tuberculosis with impaired tubal function, so often first discovered during the course of a sterility investigation, perhaps represents an exception. The conservative treatment of this disease, with preservation of childbearing potential and an occasional subsequent successful pregnancy, has been discussed in Chapter 8.

Where actual anatomic distortion by a pelvic disease that produces a mechanical tubal block or interferes with the tubal ovum pickup and transfer mechanism exists, a reparative surgical procedure usually offers the only hope of restoring normal tubal function. As indicated by the following, the nature and extent of the pathologic process will determine the best procedure:

1. Pelvic endometriosis with adherent uterus and adnexa and extensive peritubal adhesions, with or without fimbrial occlusion. **Treatment:** A conservative operation with excision of all gross areas of endometriosis; mobilization and suspension of the adherent uterus; mobilization of the adnexa with lysis of peritubal adhesions and fimbrioplasty, if necessary; and usually a concomitant presacral neurectomy. (See Chapter 10 for a more detailed consideration of the indications and techniques of conservative surgical procedures and a discussion of medical therapy with progestational agents in certain selected patients with endometriosis accompanied by infertility.)

2. Uterine fibroids so situated as to cause tubal obstruction in the cornual regions.

Treatment: Myomectomies, with care to avoid injury to the adjacent cornual portions of the tube.

3. Tubal occlusion secondary to previous pelvic inflammatory disease or salpingitis isthmica nodosa. The occlusion may involve either or both of the fimbrial and cornual ends of the tubes and is often associated with extensive pelvic adhesions. **Treatment:** One type of tuboplasty or a combination of the various types, which, depending on the site of block, may involve cornual resection and tubal reimplantation, midtube resection and end-to-end anastomosis, or fimbrioplasty (Fig. 43). The development and refinement of meticulous, atraumatic surgical techniques, the use of polyethylene splinting catheters in performing tubal anastomosis and reimplantations, and the use of special polyethylene hoods devised to protect the area of fimbrioplasty temporarily during the healing phase (the hoods are later removed at a second laparotomy or through the laparoscope), together with the employment of antibiotics, corticosteroid and antihistamine antiinflammatory agents, and solutions of heparin and related fibrinolytic substances in an effort to promote healing and inhibit adhesion formation, have all tended to improve the ultimate results of these procedures in recent years. However, the success rate is still relatively low, the most favorable results in terms of restoration of tubal patency being achieved when cornual resection and reimplantation suffices (roughly 30 to 40 percent are successful); patency is reestablished by fimbrioplasty in only 10 to 20 percent of patients with complete fimbrial occlusion. However, Grant [4] has succeeded in improving these results by early and frequently repeated postoperative tubal irrigations (hydrotubation), and he has observed subsequent pregnancy in 40 percent or more of his patients.

Because of the underlying damage to the tubal endothelium and muscular wall and the resulting impairment of normal secretory and peristaltic activity present in the majority of these cases, the percentage of patent tubes resulting from operative repair will far exceed the percentage of subsequent pregnancies. However, ectopic gestation is frequently encountered among the latter because of persistence of abnormal function despite restoration of patency. Thus, in terms of the ultimate index of success, that is, the occurrence of a normal intrauterine term pregnancy, favorable results following tuboplasty occur in only 20 to 30 percent of cases at best. It is therefore important that the couple be made aware of the limited chances for success before proceeding with tuboplasty. Nevertheless, the procedure is invariably worth attempting, since it usually represents the sole chance for restoration of fertility, and the risk and morbidity of the operation are essentially nonexistent. On the other hand, if only lysis of peritubal adhesions is required to restore normal tubal function, the tubes themselves being basically normal, a 60 to 70 percent subsequent pregnancy rate can be anticipated.

Therapy for Disturbances of the Cervical Factor

When thorough investigation of the husband has eliminated him as a factor in repeatedly poor results in postcoital cervical mucus tests, examination of the cervix itself,

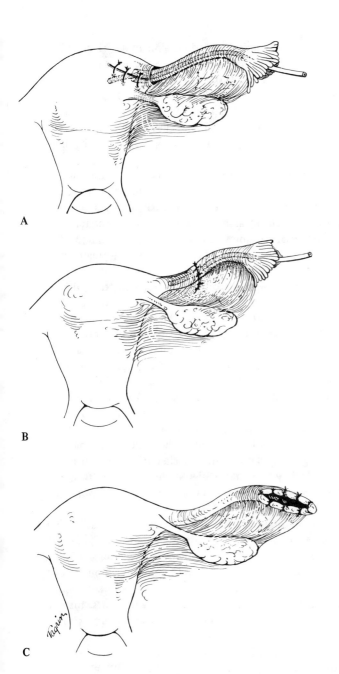

Figure 43
Various types of tuboplasty. A. Cornual resection and tubal reimplantation.
B. Partial tubal resection and end-to-end anastomosis over a splinting polyethylene
catheter. C. Salpingostomy (or fimbrioplasty).

together with the additional studies of cervical secretions already described, will usually confirm that the difficulty stems from primary cervical disease (chronic infection) or inadequate secretory activity. Chronic vaginitis with its invariably associated cervicitis should be vigorously treated. If an extensive congenital cervical erosion or chronic endocervicitis is found and appears to be the most likely cause of poor cervical mucus, careful cauterization of the cervix is indicated in an effort to eradicate the infection while preserving the normal secretory capacity in the uninvolved cervical glands.

In the absence of chronic cervicitis, poor cervical mucus (thick, opaque, and cellular instead of thin, clear, and watery) may be the result of inadequate estrogenic stimulation of the cervical glands during the critical preovulatory and ovulatory phases of the cycle. At times, the resulting abnormal cervical factor is simply one of many manifestations of the abnormal physiology of anovulatory reproductive tract function, all of which are contributing to the resulting infertility, and treatment must be directed at the overall problem of ovarian dysfunction.

However, it is not uncommon to encounter women in whom ovulation with adequate progesterone production is occurring regularly but in whom preovulatory estrogen levels are apparently inadequate to bring about the normal quantitative and qualitative changes in cervical secretory activity necessary for the production of a favorable cervical mucus at ovulation time. In this situation, a useful program of medication consists of the administration of diethylstilbestrol in a dosage of 0.1 to 0.2 mg daily from day 5 through day 12 of the cycle for three or four cycles, a dose level that will not interfere with ovulation but frequently improves both the quality and the quantity of cervical mucus. A somewhat different approach employs larger, "flood" doses of estrogen, prescribing 1.0 to 2.0 mg of diethylstilbestrol (or 1.25 to 2.5 mg of Premarin) daily from day 1 through day 24 of the cycle, in alternate months. Although ovulation is prevented every other cycle during the course of treatment, there are some who believe that the massive stimulation and "flushing out" of the cervical glands achieve better results as far as the eventual improvement in the quality of the cervical mucus is concerned.

At times, persistently poor postcoital test results may be due to premature semen loss from the vagina or inadequate cervical contact with the seminal pool, in turn secondary to faulty coital technique or minor vaginal anatomic variations. If this is suggested on the basis of the history, pelvic findings, and failure to demonstrate any abnormality of the semen or of the cervix and its secretions, the use of special plastic vaginal tampons that the patient inserts immediately following intercourse may be tried in an attempt to facilitate retention of the semen in close apposition to the external cervical os.

Finally, if in spite of the various therapeutic efforts that have been described, satisfactory sperm penetration of the cervical canal cannot be achieved in the usual way, artificial insemination using the husband's semen should be considered. The semen can be introduced by placing it in a snug-fitting plastic cap that is then applied to the cervix, or by careful, direct injection into the cervical canal or intrauterine cavity. In any case, the optimal time for insemination is of course selected as accurately as possible on the basis of the basal body temperature chart, or other indexes of ovulation, or both.

Therapy for Miscellaneous Factors Responsible for Implantation and Maintenance Failures (Uterine Factor)

The treatment of abnormal uterine factors implicated in infertility is as follows:

1. Intramural and submuccous fibroids: Myomectomy.
2. Endometrial or endocervical polyps: Dilatation and curettage with excision of polyps.
3. Asherman's syndrome (traumatic intrauterine adhesions): Surgical removal of intrauterine adhesions by curettage or hysterotomy.
4. Congenital anomalies and their treatment:
   a. Complete duplications: Unification operation of Strassman (see Fig. 21).
   b. Uterine septa: Resection of septa.
   c. Rudimentary uterine horn: Resection of rudimentary horn.
   d. Bicornuate uterus: Unification operation of Strassman.
5. Incompetent internal cervical os with repeated second-trimester abortions (see also Chap. 9):
   a. If discovered during pregnancy but before abortion: surgical closure of internal os (method of Shirodkar; see Fig. 35).
   b. If discovered between pregnancies: plastic surgical repair of incompetent cervix (Lash procedure) by resection of a segment of appropriate size from the circumference of the endocervical canal.
6. T-strain *Mycoplasma* infection of the cervix, vagina, and/or endometrium. There is some evidence that the presence of mycoplasmas within the lower genital tract may be responsible for some cases of infertility and perhaps an even larger number of repeated spontaneous abortions. Administration of tetracycline or demeclocycline (Declomycin) to affected infertile women has seemed to increase fertility in some, though not all, reported series, and in a number of clinical trials has definitely appeared to reduce the number of spontaneous abortions in women who had previously shown a high rate of spontaneous abortion.

RESULTS OF THE STUDY AND TREATMENT OF INFERTILITY

It is estimated that by careful study and treatment between 25 and 50 percent of all infertile couples can be cured of their involuntary sterility and helped to achieve one or more successful pregnancies. An adequate therapeutic program may require several years of continuing investigation and may involve prolonged or repeated treatment of various factors with all the potentially helpful measures before a successful outcome is obtained. The great variation in the percentage of favorable results and the length of time required to achieve them is of course markedly influenced by the age of the couple, the nature of the disease or functional disorder present, and whether or not there are multiple factors responsible for the infertility. For example, the results in terms of subsequent fertility and normal pregnancy following the surgical treatment of the infertile woman with the Stein-Leventhal syndrome are favorable in 85 to 90 percent of patients (the normal fertility range), whereas successful pregnancy following tuboplasty occurs in only 10 to 20 percent of patients. Occupying an intermediate position, conservative surgery for infertility due to pelvic endometriosis restores fertility in approximately 50 to 60 percent of patients. The majority of patients suffering from infertility do not require operative therapy, and although it is difficult to assess the percentage of favorable results following the various forms of medical therapy, or even to be certain that the treatment was responsible for the successful outcome, persistent and patient efforts are probably rewarded by successful pregnancy in 40 to 50 percent of this larger group.

Although there is no absolute upper age limit above which couples should be advised that the study and attempted treatment of their infertility are unlikely to be worth the effort, the older wife and husband in their late thirties or early forties should understand that the chances of achieving a successful pregnancy are considerably less than in the case of couples under the age of 35. This is in part a reflection of the decline in fertility experienced after the age of 30 even by couples with no fertility problems. Furthermore, there tends to be a higher incidence of serious organic disease in the group of women over 35 who suffer from infertility — extensive endometriosis, multiple fibroids, chronic pelvic inflammatory disease, or previous pelvic surgery that has resulted in the loss of an ovary or both one tube and ovary. Nevertheless, many couples with sterility of long standing can be helped to have children by careful treatment of the often multiple factors that a thorough investigation has shown to be contributing to their impaired fertility, and they therefore should not be unduly discouraged from embarking on a standard program of study and therapy.

MANAGEMENT FOLLOWING UNSUCCESSFUL THERAPY

If it is soon obvious that an incurable barrier to conception exists, or if after a period of years the program of therapy has failed to achieve pregnancy, the possibility of adopting children should be considered seriously. It should be part of the physician's responsibility to aid the couple in reaching this decision, to refer them to adoption agencies known to him to be reliable and ethical, and to cooperate fully in helping them secure a child. The other alternative, that of artificial donor insemination, may also be considered if, as previously discussed, the sterility is solely on the basis of an abnormal male factor.

Even if an irremedial impairment of fertility is ultimately demonstrated, a thorough sterility investigation will have accomplished an extremely worthwhile purpose. For only by a complete study of the problem and an adequate trial of all known therapeutic measures will a couple be assured that everything possible has been done, be willing to abandon further anxiety-ridden and fruitless efforts, and be able to achieve the peace of mind necessary to accept and live with the final reality of the situation.

They are then in a position to proceed with adoption or with a mature readjustment of their marital goals.

REFERENCES

1. Ansbacher, R., Keung-Yeung, K., and Behrman, S. J. Clinical significance of sperm antibodies in infertile couples. *Fertil. Steril.* 24:305, 1973.
2. Dubin, L., and Amelar, R. D. Varicocelectomy as therapy in male infertility: A study of 504 cases. *Fertil. Steril.* 26:217, 1975.
3. Franklin, R. R., and Dukes, C. D. Further studies on sperm-agglutinating antibody and unexplained infertility. *J.A.M.A.* 190:682, 1964.
4. Grant, A. Reconstruction of the Fallopian Tube in the Infertile Patient. In M. L. Taymor and T. H. Green, Jr. (Eds.), *Progress in Gynecology*, Vol. VI. New York: Grune & Stratton, 1975. Pp. 705–727.
5. Horne, H. W., Jr., Kundsin, R. B., and Kosasa, T. S. The role of mycoplasma infection in human reproductive failure. *Fertil. Steril.* 25:380, 1974.
6. Jette, N. T., and Glass, R. H. Prognostic value of the postcoital test. *Fertil. Steril.* 23:29, 1972.
7. Jones, G. S., and Pourmand, K. An evaluation of etiologic factors and therapy in 555 private patients with primary infertility. *Fertil. Steril.* 13:398, 1962.
8. Li, T. S. Sperm immunology, infertility, and fertility control. *Obstet. Gynecol.* 44:607, 1974.
9. Moghissi, K. The function of the cervix in fertility. *Fertil. Steril.* 23:295, 1972.
10. Parsons, L., MacMillan, H. J., and Whittaker, J. O. Abdominovaginal electric potential differences, with special reference to the ovulatory phase of the menstrual cycle. *Am. J. Obstet. Gynecol.* 75:121, 1958.
11. Peterson, E. P., and Behrman, S. J. Laparoscopy of the infertile patient. *Obstet. Gynecol.* 36:363, 1970.
12. Robboy, M. S. The management of cervical incompetence: UCLA experience with cerclage procedures. *Obstet. Gynecol.* 41:108, 1973.
13. Schulman, S. Immunologic barriers to infertility. *Obstet. Gynecol. Surv.* 27:553, 1972.
14. Umezaki, C., Katayama, K. P., and Jones, H. W., Jr. Pregnancy rates after reconstructive surgery on the fallopian tubes. *Obstet. Gynecol.* 43:418, 1974.
15. Wallach, E. E. The uterine factor in infertility. *Fertil. Steril.* 23:138, 1972.
16. Young, P. E., Egan, J. E., Barlow, J. J., and Mulligan, W. J. Reconstructive surgery for infertility at the Boston Hospital for Women. *Am. J. Obstet. Gynecol.* 108:1092, 1970.

12
Leiomyomas, Adenomyosis, and Other Benign Diseases of the Uterus

LEIOMYOMAS

Popularly known as fibroids, leiomyomas are sometimes also called **myomas** or **fibromyomas**. In actuality, they are true benign tumors of smooth muscle cell origin, and it is only after atrophic and degenerative changes have occurred that the grossly and histologically obvious element of fibrosis is introduced. Leiomyomas may develop in any structure or viscus that contains smooth muscle cells. For example, they occur occasionally throughout various portions of the gastrointestinal tract, arising in the muscular layer of the esophageal, gastric, or intestinal wall and usually projecting within the lumen as an intramural, extramucosal tumor with a characteristic, almost diagnostic, roentgenologic appearance.

Leiomyomas are far more frequent in the reproductive tract, however, represent the most common pelvic tumor, and indeed may be encountered in any of the pelvic structures where smooth muscle elements are to be found. Thus various sites for their occurrence include not only the uterus itself but also the fallopian tubes, vagina, vulva, and round and uterosacral ligaments. Although brief reference in the appropriate chapters is made to their appearance and varying manifestations at extra-uterine sites, the vast majority of leiomyomas develop within the uterus, a fact that is undoubtedly related to the various as yet relatively poorly understood etiologic and developmental factors that influence both their initial formation as well as their subsequent rate and pattern of growth. It is estimated that uterine leiomyomas develop in at least 20 to 30 percent of all women sooner or later; many of these remain completely asymptomatic and relatively insignificant in size and represent mere incidental findings.

Etiology

Histologically, a leiomyoma in its initial stages is a localized proliferation of smooth-muscle cells. The precise nature of the stimulus to the original proliferative process is unknown, but there is reason to believe that it may be mechanical or physical in nature and operate at points of maximal local stress and strain within the constantly contracting muscular bundles of the myometrial layer of the uterine wall. The process may thus be analogous to the physical reorientation and increased activity of osteoblasts that occur in the callus at a fracture site in the lower extremity once weight bearing is resumed. The contours and the nature of the contractions of the uterine muscular wall are such that multiple points of stress along the myometrial layer are inevitable, and this is reflected in the invariable multiplicity of uterine fibroids. Only rarely is a solitary fibroid encountered, usually in a young, white female, in whom others nearly always develop ultimately. Furthermore, the genesis of uterine fibroids is continuous in point of time, and new ones may appear throughout the active reproductive life of susceptible women. It is thus extremely common to find "crops" or generations of fibroids of different sizes in any multinodular fibroid uterus, the latter probably corresponding roughly with their respective times of onset.

It is not at all clear why leiomyomas develop in some women and not in others. It is apparent, however, that black women are far more likely to have leiomyomas than are white women (the incidence is perhaps 50 percent or more in black women but only about 20 percent in white women). Moreover, clinically significant fibroids develop in black women at a considerably younger age, and the growth rate of their leiomyomas appears to be more rapid. Whether or not there is any relationship between these facts and the greater tendency to keloid formation in blacks is problematical but intriguing.

Finally, the growth-promoting effects of estrogen with respect to leiomyomas are well known. This is clinically apparent in the sudden increase in the growth rate of uterine fibroids frequently noted in association with pregnancy (although much of the enlargement noted during pregnancy may be due to edema superimposed on the actual increase in proliferation of smooth-muscle cells), the invariable cessation of growth following the menopause, and also in the resumption of growth and occasionally dramatic increase in size of known fibroids in postmenopausal women to whom estrogens are given. There is little evidence that the actual origin of leiomyomas is dependent on an endocrine imbalance wherein estrogen in relative excess (unopposed by adequate amounts of progesterone) serves as the inciting stimulus for the local benign neoplastic proliferation of smooth-muscle cells. The frequent association of fibroids with an anovulatory or progesterone-deficient type of menstrual pattern, with its often accompanying endometrial hyperplasia and simple ovarian follicle cysts, is frequently cited in support of this concept. Since fibroids are extremely common, however, this association could well be simply coincidental; certainly, there is no actual evidence that an endocrine imbalance is present prior to the genesis of a leiomyoma, and fibroids develop in vast numbers of women who by all clinical and laboratory criteria have perfectly normal ovarian function.

Pathologic Anatomy

The original areas of smooth-muscle cell proliferation appear within the myometrial layer; if the leiomyoma maintains this same relative position within the wall of the uterus as it enlarges, it is termed an **interstitial,** or **intramural**, fibroid (Fig. 44A). This is probably most likely to occur if the area of smooth-muscle proliferation arose initially in the central portion of the myometrium. Since intramural fibroids are thus surrounded on all sides by approximately equal thicknesses of myometrium, they also tend to remain spherical in shape.

Because the surrounding muscular wall of the uterus is in a perpetual state of intermittent contraction about these initially small interstitial tumors, there is also

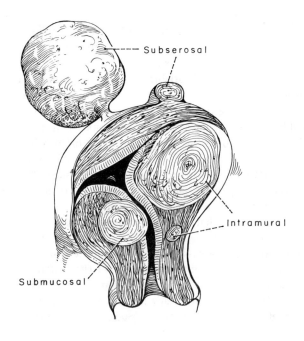

A

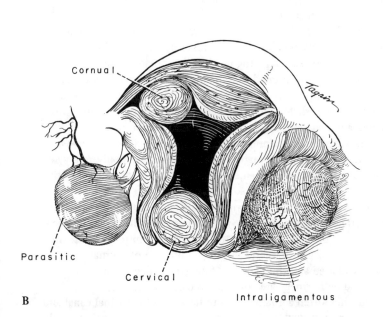

B

Figure 44
Uterine fibroids. A. Types. B. Various locations.

a considerable tendency for them to be pushed either inward toward the endometrial cavity or outward toward the peritoneal surface of the uterus, particularly
if they originally arose in the inner or outer portions respectively of the myometrium.
When this occurs, leiomyomas tend to lose their original spherical shape and develop
varying degrees of asymmetry. Furthermore, as they become more or less extruded
from the muscle layer, the thin connective-tissue attachment, with its contained
relatively sparse vascular and lymphatic channels, invariably becomes increasingly
attenuated, and the fibroid may assume the form of a pedunculated tumor with a
narrow pedicle. When the leiomyoma protrudes into the cavity of the uterus, it is
termed a **submucosal**, or **intracavitary**, fibroid; when it bulges through the outer
surface of the uterine wall it is termed a **subserosal** fibroid (Fig. 44A). In either case,
such fibroid tumors often ultimately become markedly pedunculated.

If the original leiomyoma is so situated that on its subsequent outward extrusion
it appears and continues its growth between the leaves of the broad ligament, it is
termed an **intraligamentous**, or **broad-ligament**, fibroid (Fig. 44B). Leiomyomas in
this location are of considerable significance for two reasons: (1) Their lateral location sometimes makes it difficult or impossible to be certain that they are uterine
fibroids and not ovarian tumors (this is true also of any laterally placed pedunculated
subserosal fibroid), and (2) the distortion of the uterine blood supply and the displacement of the ureter from its normal course through the broad ligament produced
by the intraligamentous fibroid often makes hysterectomy technically more difficult
than usual and exposes the ureter to a greater risk of accidental injury if the operation
is carelessly or improperly carried out.

Occasionally, in pedunculated fibroids of considerable age, the pedicle and the
accompanying vascular channels may become progressively smaller, while at the same
time adherence to adjacent tissues — e.g., the neighboring broad ligament or, less
often, the omentum — may result in the development of an accessory blood supply
that grows in from such a secondary, external source. If under these circumstances
the blood supply of the true pedicle eventually becomes totally inadequate, thrombosis and infarction of the pedicle alone may occur, with the fibroid completely
separating from the uterus and maintaining its viability through its now well-established accessory vascular channels. Although they are encountered only rarely, such
"wandering" leiomyomas of the broad ligament or omentum are termed **parasitic**
fibroids.

Finally, although the vast majority of uterine fibroids develop in the wall of the
fundus, perhaps 5 to 10 percent appear in the muscular wall of the cervix (**cervical
fibroids**) (Fig. 44B). Here, there is a universal tendency for them to protrude into
the endocervical canal as they grow larger, the surrounding rim of normal cervix
becoming progressively dilated and thinned out. Superficial ulceration, necrosis,
secondary infection, and hemorrhage are common in cervical fibroids, and as they
become pedunculated, they often actually come to lie within the vaginal canal and
can be surgically removed by a local, transvaginal resection. A considerable number
retain their endocervical location, however, and large cervical fibroids in this position
pose the same potential technical problems during hysterectomy as do broad-ligament

fibroids, since by their size they often make adequate exposure of the uterine vessels and adjacent ureter difficult.

Degenerative Changes

From a histologic standpoint, the original pure collection of proliferating smooth-muscle cells soon begins to undergo atrophy and hyaline degeneration, particularly within the central portion of the growing tumor, for the blood supply of a leiomyoma is relatively sparse at best, and with continued growth it becomes increasingly limited with respect to those areas farthest removed from the capsular vascular channels. Areas in which atrophy and degeneration have occurred are most often replaced by fibrous tissue, which gives the usual fibroid its typical firm consistency, particularly noticeable in the hard central core.

At the periphery, a pseudocapsule is permanently maintained, and there is always a distinct line of cleavage between the leiomyoma and the surrounding normal myometrium. As a result, local removal of the fibroid (myomectomy) is readily accomplished by incising the overlying muscular wall down to the surface of the pseudocapsule of the fibroid itself, which is then invariably easily shelled out.

As the smooth-muscle atrophy, fibroblast replacement, and progressive impairment of blood supply proceed, further chronic degenerative changes, particularly prone to occur in large tumors, may result in a myxomatous type of degeneration with diffuse edema and a soft, gelatinous consistency. In some instances this process may progress to actual cystic change within the softer areas of the fibroid. More often, fatty necrosis and, ultimately, calcification take place. In fact, calcification of fibroids (Fig. 45) is commonly seen in older, postmenopausal women in whom the fibroids have obviously been present and undergoing degenerative change over a period of many years; involution of the uterus and its normal blood supply and superimposed arteriosclerotic vascular disease have both led to further impairment of the vascular supply to the tumor.

CARNEOUS DEGENERATION

On much the same basis, acute degenerative change amounting to a sudden infarction of all or a large portion of a leiomyoma may also take place. This is particularly prone to occur in pedunculated fibroids, when, as a result of torsion or spontaneous thrombosis of the narrow pedicle, the blood supply is suddenly cut off completely. A specific form of acute degenerative change of this type, termed **red degeneration,** or **carneous degeneration,** is most commonly seen during pregnancy. In this situation the increased growth of the fibroid, abruptly stimulated by the extremely high and rising estrogen levels, leads to an equally rapid outstripping of the precarious blood supply, a situation that is further aggravated by the often marked edema of the fibroid as well as by the pressure of the enlarging uterus. At some point, whether due primarily to arterial or venous insufficiency or to a combination of both, sudden vascular impairment develops, often in the nature of acute venous thrombosis, and

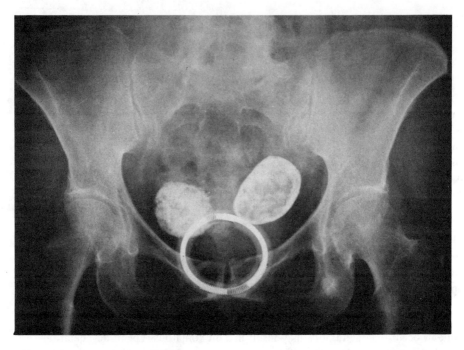

Figure 45
Typical x-ray appearance of calcified fibroids. The patient was a 70-year-old woman with asymptomatic pedunculated fibroids. The ring pessary she wore for an associated uterine prolapse is also visible on the film.

may or may not proceed to total infarction. On cut section, a leiomyoma that has undergone acute carneous degeneration looks like raw, red meat, and on microscopic examination, marked edema, pronounced vascular engorgement with evidence of extravasation of blood into tissue spaces, and varying degrees of hyaline degeneration are seen. From a clinical standpoint, this acute vascular accident poses obvious problems in differential diagnosis as well as in management in both the pregnant and nonpregnant patient. In the former, the resulting increased uterine irritability predisposes to abortion, miscarriage, or premature delivery; however, myomectomy is at least as hazardous in this respect. In general, since the acute process will often subside without the development of actual infarct necrosis, a conservative program of observation and supportive therapy is usually indicated initially in the pregnant patient. Increasing evidence of ischemic necrosis and deterioration of the patient's general condition may ultimately make exploration necessary, however, and the risk that myomectomy may further increase the likelihood of loss of the pregnancy will have to be accepted. In the nonpregnant patient, the process is usually less acute and dramatic, but persistence of symptoms for more than a day or two, or a steady increase in their severity, is usually sufficient indication for exploration and myomectomy or hysterectomy, depending on the individual circumstances.

A rare complication is the development of a gas abscess within a degenerated leiomyoma. Organisms such as the coliforms, streptococci, or staphylococci enter the degenerated fibroid directly from the uterine cavity or via hematogenous or lymphatic spread, producing suppuration and gas formation; the latter is readily demonstrated on a plain abdominal x-ray. If this gas abscess is unrecognized and untreated, rupture into the peritoneal cavity, with resulting generalized peritonitis, or perforation into the bowel or bladder may occur. Occasionally, spontaneous drainage into the uterine cavity will take place. Although the roentgenographic picture is fairly characteristic, the possibility of gas formation accompanying either a tuboovarian abscess or a pelvic abscess developing on some other basis (e.g., diverticulitis) must also be considered.

SARCOMATOUS DEGENERATION

Whether or not a true sarcomatous change can take place in what was originally a completely benign leiomyoma is a somewhat controversial issue. Obviously, the occurrence of such a malignant transformation is exceedingly difficult to prove in most instances, although suggestive evidence is at hand in some cases in which a leiomyosarcoma is found growing in a local area within the capsule of what appears grossly to be a simple fibroid, all other areas of which are histologically benign. Circumstantial clinical evidence of the possibility of sudden change in the character of a leiomyoma is also present in some patients who, having been followed for many years with clinically benign "fibroids" that have not increased in size, abruptly show evidence of rapid growth of their tumors, which are found to be leiomyosarcomas following excision.

Granting that malignant change may sometimes occur in a benign leiomyoma, there is nevertheless a considerable difference of opinion in the literature as to its frequency; some authors place the incidence of such sarcomatous degeneration in uterine fibroids as high as 1 to 4 percent, although the majority of reports on the subject have estimated it to be in the neighborhood of 0.5 percent. Since benign leiomyomas are extremely common, and uterine sarcoma is encountered only rarely, either figure would seem to be excessively high in comparison with the experience in most institutions. A possible explanation for this discrepancy may lie in the fact that some leiomyomas are actually highly cellular (the so-called **cellular myoma**), and on microscopic examination show frequent mitoses, hyperchromatic nuclei, and even giant cell types with multinucleated patterns. Such a cellular myoma is not a sarcoma at all but may occasionally be mistaken for one; thus, in hospitals where this distinction is not always carefully made, the incidence of uterine sarcoma arising in fibroids might be unduly high. It seems likely, however, that if sarcomatous degeneration does take place, it would tend to occur in this type of benign but highly cellular leiomyoma.

In any case, leiomyosarcomas of the uterus that appear to have arisen in leiomyomas are not as highly malignant and uniformly fatal as are true endometrial sarcomas. Grossly, they give the appearance on cut section of soft, meaty tissue resembling raw pork, and often they contain areas of hemorrhage and necrosis. Histologically the tumor is usually of the spindle rather than the round cell type; occasionally, sufficient numbers of giant cell types are present to warrant classification as a giant cell sarcoma.

Intravenous Leiomyomatosis and Benign Metastasizing Leiomyoma

Intravenous leiomyomatosis and benign metastasizing leiomyoma are two benign forms of leiomyomatous tissue spread that may simulate malignancy and thus be erroneously considered manifestations of leiomyosarcoma. Both are rare and usually occur in patients who also have ordinary uterine fibroids as well. In intravenous leiomyomatosis, smooth muscle cells enter and grow within vascular spaces and venous channels, sometimes implanting in the vena cava, heart, and lungs. However, the clinical course in these patients is relatively benign and usually prolonged. The microscopic appearance of the leiomyomatous tissue remains benign, with no cellular atypia and few mitotic figures.

Similarly, in benign metastasizing leiomyoma, a patient who appears to have simple uterine fibroids is found at the time of planned hysterectomy or myomectomy to have numerous intraperitoneal nodules of varying size, superficially resembling implants of metastatic carcinoma and involving omentum as well as visceral and parietal peritoneal surfaces. On close inspection of these nodules, however, even their gross appearance is seen to be that of small, benign leiomyomas, and this is confirmed by detailed microscopic examination of both the uterine leiomyomas and the "metastatic implants." All the "metastatic" leiomyomas that are technically easy to remove should be resected, and hysterectomy or myomectomy should be carried out as planned. The patient is very unlikely to have any further manifestations of this unusual form of benign metastatic spread of a benign leiomyoma.

Secondary Pathologic Changes in the Fibroid Uterus

The wall of the uterus surrounding a leiomyoma may thin out as a result of the pressure atrophy produced by the enlarging fibroid; or, on the other hand, the myometrium surrounding multiple fibroids may hypertrophy as a result of the stimulus to increased contractility produced by their presence, the result being a large, thickwalled uterus. Endometrial polyps are also commonly found in association with uterine fibroids, and their development may be the result of interference with the blood supply to the endometrium overlying the fibroids, with a consequent disturbance in the endometrial growth pattern, leading to local hyperplastic change and eventual polyp formation. Since there is good evidence that both endometrial polyp formation and an increased rate of growth of fibroids are often secondary to a relative preponderance of estrogen, ovarian hormone imbalance may also be a factor in their frequent coexistence.

Symptoms and Clinical Manifestations

Although probably the majority of uterine fibroids remain small and clinically insignificant, symptoms sufficiently severe to require treatment develop in a large number of women with these tumors. Subserosal fibroids, even those attaining considerable size, are most likely to remain asymptomatic, whereas submucosal (intracavitary) or intramural fibroids are more likely to cause difficulty and may do so even when relatively small. The symptomatic manifestations produced by fibroids vary considerably and depend primarily on their size, number, and location. The chief symptoms are described in the sections that follow.

PAIN

If experienced, pain is usually crampy in nature and secondary to the presence of submucous and intramural fibroids. Most typically it occurs at the time of menstruation; less often, it occurs intermenstrually. Acute pain may be caused by infarction due to sudden degeneration or torsion of a pedunculated subserosal or intracavity fibroid.

PRESSURE SYMPTOMS

Pressure symptoms occur due to the enlarging mass and include the following: pressure effects on the bladder (frequency, urgency, incontinence), colon (constipation, rectal pain, difficult defecation), and small bowel (abdominal cramps); pelvic and lower abdominal discomfort.

ABNORMAL BLEEDING

Usually abnormal bleeding takes the form of menorrhagia, with increased amount and duration of flow, and it ordinarily occurs only in association with submucous or multiple intramural fibroids, which may:

1. Produce a large increase in the endometrial surface area from which bleeding can occur, the increased surface area being the result of the secondary dilatation of the uterine cavity caused by the enlarging fibroids.
2. Interfere with the normal myometrial contraction about the spiral uterine arterioles, normally an important auxiliary hemostatic mechanism.
3. Impair normal endometrial vascular reactions and homonal responses by interference with the normal blood supply, particularly in the endometrium directly overlying the fibroids (in spite of normal ovarian hormonal production and balance).
4. Actually undergo necrosis and ulceration, often with extremely heavy bleeding, an event particularly likely to occur in the presence of submucous fibroids.

The increasingly excessive chronic blood loss occurring over the course of months or years often occasioned by the presence of uterine fibroids may not be obvious to the patient, who gradually becomes accustomed to the heavier flow. However, a severe simple iron deficiency anemia frequently develops in this way, and it is not uncommon to find the hemoglobin levels in the range of 4 to 5 gm in women whose menorrhagia is due to fibroids.

Irregular menstrual cycles or intermenstrual bleeding are rarely due to the presence of fibroids alone, and some other cause for this type of abnormal menstrual function should be sought, even though fibroids may be present. In fact, it is important to point out that in many patients with abnormal uterine bleeding, coexisting fibroids will be completely unrelated to the actual source of the abnormal flow, which is most often due to hormonal imbalance (dysfunctional bleeding) or occasionally to endometrial hyperplasia or polyps or to carcinoma of the cervix or fundus. Hence, before deciding that the bleeding is related to the presence of fibroids, one must take into account their number, size, and location and exclude dysfunctional bleeding and other organic causes for uterine hemorrhage.

INFERTILITY

Less often, infertility may result from interference with the normal tuboovarian pickup and transport mechanisms by intramural or multiple large subserosal fibroids, particularly if they are located in the cornual regions; or infertility may be secondary to abnormal early implantation and habitual abortion in the presence of submucous or multiple intramural fibroids. Obviously, before concluding that a known uterine fibroid may be playing a significant role in a couple's failure to conceive, both the wife and husband should first undergo a complete sterility investigation to be certain that other, often far more important factors are not overlooked. Only when all other possible causes have been excluded or corrected and pregnancy still fails to occur should myomectomy be considered. When such a thorough preliminary investigation has been done, however, the results following myomectomy in the management of the otherwise normal infertile woman with uterine fibroids are often highly successful and gratifying with respect to subsequent fertility and pregnancies carried to term.

POLYCYTHEMIA

Although relatively rare, secondary polycythemia is occasionally encountered in patients with large uterine leiomyomas. A number of such cases have been recorded in the literature, and in none could any other cause for erythrocytosis be demonstrated. The hemoglobin, hematocrit, and red cell counts, which were usually markedly elevated preoperatively, rapidly fell to normal following hysterectomy in these patients, with no subsequent recurrence of polycythemia. The mechanism for the secondary erythrocytosis is obscure. Various explanations postulated include the possibility that a large fibroid acts as a peripheral arteriovenous shunt, or, even more likely, that it may produce sufficient quantities of a humoral factor, erythropoietin, which either stimulates erythropoiesis or inhibits the normal red cell storage and reservoir function of the spleen.

MISCELLANEOUS SYMPTOMS

Miscellaneous situations warranting surgical intervention include rapid growth of apparent fibroids (particularly at or after the menopause), which may suggest the possibility that a sarcoma rather than a fibroid is present, and inability to differentiate between a lateral fibroid and an ovarian tumor. In this latter instance, laparoscopy or culdoscopy may provide the needed information and avoid a laparotomy merely for diagnosis in patients in whom the fibroids are asymptomatic and who otherwise will require no treatment once the possibility of an ovarian tumor is excluded. One other unusual complication requiring surgical intervention is the occasional occurrence of sudden and often massive intraperitoneal bleeding from dilated veins on the surface of a pedunculated subserosal fibroid. The resulting acute hemoperitoneum produces generalized abdominal symptoms and signs with associated hemorrhagic shock, so that the need for prompt laparotomy is invariably obvious, although the precise nature of the intraabdominal catastrophe often remains obscure until the abdomen is opened.

Diagnosis

The findings on careful abdominal, vaginal, and rectal examinations, occasionally supplemented by examination under anesthesia, usually suffice to establish that a uterine enlargement or "pelvic tumor" indicates the presence of a leiomyoma. It is obviously of great importance to be certain that the lesion in question is indeed simply a fibroid and not an adnexal mass — in particular, not an ovarian tumor — even if it is asymptomatic. And when symptoms are present, as already emphasized, one must not be too quick to assume that they are due to fibroids, if present, since the latter frequently coexist with other more significant pelvic disease.

Culdoscopy or laparoscopy may be of value, as previously mentioned, in differentiating a laterally situated uterine fibroid from an ovarian mass in questionable cases. Occasionally, the presence of a submucous fibroid may be demonstrated or confirmed by hysterosalpingography or by curettage. Frequently, the typical pattern of calcification in older, degenerated fibroids will be noted on abdominal x-ray films, and the roentgenographic appearance is usually sufficiently characteristic to be diagnostic of a leiomyoma (Fig. 45).

Treatment

In the majority of women, conservative management is possible, but it is wise to check the pelvic findings every six months for a year or two, both to avoid any possibility of a mistake in diagnosis and to obtain a general impression of the rate

of growth of the fibroids and whether or not symptoms are likely to develop. Thereafter, a regular annual checkup program is all that is required, unless symptoms arise.
Because the growth rate of leiomyomas is usually very slow, most patients can be
carried through to the menopause, if when originally seen they are asymptomatic or
having only minimal symptoms. It is important to avoid the postmenopausal use of
estrogens in such patients, lest growth of the fibroids be stimulated and symptoms
result.

If symptoms are sufficient to warrant treatment (removal), whether myomectomy
or hysterectomy is done will be determined largely by whether or not the individual
circumstances make preservation of childbearing function desirable and important.

MYOMECTOMY

Myomectomy, the local removal of leiomyomas with preservation of the uterus, is
invariably possible, regardless of the size, location, or number of fibroids. Large
submucous fibroids may require that the uterus actually be opened (hysterotomy),
but the leiomyomas can then be dealt with and removed in the usual manner. A
helpful technical maneuver of aid in minimizing blood loss during myomectomy
involves the local intrauterine injection of vasopressin solution and seems superior
to the technique of applying clamps or rubber-band tourniquets to the uterine or
ovarian vessels (see Chap. 21). It is important to resuture the wall of the uterus
carefully in layers to obliterate all dead space and create a strong, solid scar.
Properly closed myomectomy incisions in the nonpregnant uterus heal extremely
well, and cesarean section will thus not necessarily be mandatory if the patient
subsequently becomes pregnant.

Undoubtedly depending largely on the patient's age and the care and completeness with which the fibroids are removed, the recurrence rate after myomectomy
(the subsequent development of new leiomyomas) has been in the vicinity of 30
percent in most large reported series, with 10 to 20 percent of these women eventually requiring hysterectomy. However, the subsequent uncomplicated term
pregnancy rate following myomectomy has been most satisfactory, approaching
closely that for normal women of comparable age. The results in women undergoing myomectomy because of infertility (after a thorough infertility investigation
has excluded other significant factors) have been particularly gratifying in many
instances, with 40 to 50 percent conceiving successfully. In view of these results,
the risk of recurrence, which should be known and accepted by both patient and
physician, seems well worth taking in younger women who have been infertile or
who desire additional children.

HYSTERECTOMY

In the older woman who has completed her family and who has multiple, symptomatic leiomyomas, it is usually wiser to carry out hysterectomy, preserving the ovaries
when this is possible and indicated. Ordinarily, the presence of fibroids poses no

special problems during hysterectomy. However, as previously noted, in the case of broad-ligament or cervical fibroids it is particularly important to bear in mind at all times the course and location of the ureters and bladder and to mobilize the fibroid and dissect and display carefully the displaced ureters and uterine vessels before beginning the actual removal of the uterus.

ADENOMYOSIS OF THE UTERUS

Adenomyosis is a condition resulting from the ingrowth and pinching off within the muscular wall of the uterus of islands of normal endometrial glands and stroma derived from the endometrial cavity proper. It has been termed **internal endometriosis**, but as emphasized in Chapter 10, this term should probably be discarded, since the lesion appears to be unrelated both in nature and etiology to true or "external" endometriosis, although the two are essentially identical in histologic appearance. Although these endometrial islands are situated within the myometrium and interspersed between the smooth muscle bundles, they frequently retain a direct anatomic connection, however tortuous and hidden, with the surface endometrium lining the uterine cavity. Cullen in his classic studies of this disorder [14] was able to demonstrate clearly the persistence of these connections by careful serial sections and reconstructions of the uterine wall and underlying endometrial lining in areas involved by adenomyosis, thus laying the foundations for a correct understanding of the entirely different pathogenesis of adenomyosis as contrasted with that of endometriosis. This difference in etiology is also reflected in the fact that adenomyosis is essentially a disease of multiparous women in their late thirties and forties, whereas endometriosis is characteristically seen in the young, relatively infertile woman. It therefore seems likely that the myometrial dispersion of islands of normal endometrium found in adenomyosis may often be secondary to the traumatic and disruptive effects on the uterine wall produced by repeated pregnancy, delivery, and postpartum involution. A less common causative factor in some cases may be an unduly deep and vigorous curettage. Finally, since adenomyosis is frequently (in 35 to 50 percent of cases) accompanied by varying degrees of cystic and adenomatous hyperplasia of the surface endometrium, it seems possible that a hormone imbalance with a preponderance of estrogen may favor the persistence, growth, and activity of the aberrant endometrial islands within the myometrium. Such an ancillary causative mechanism could perhaps also account for the somewhat increased incidence of fibroids, endometrial polyps, and even endometrial carcinoma (invasive or intraepithelial) that has been noted in adenomyomatous uteri. (Pelvic endometriosis is also found in approximately 10 percent of cases, an incidence considerably less than is ordinarily encountered in women undergoing pelvic laparotomy for all causes.)

Pathologic Features

Grossly, the disease exhibits two forms (Fig. 46). On the one hand, it may consist of a diffuse and uniform involvement of the entire uterine wall, the myometrium

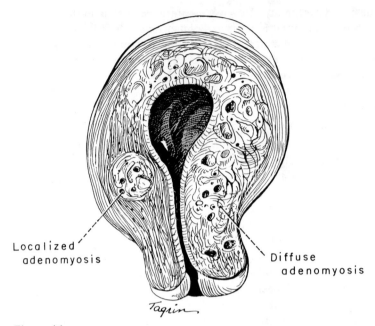

Localized
adenomyosis

Diffuse
adenomyosis

Taquin

Figure 46
Adenomyosis of the uterus. Diffuse involvement of the uterine wall (right) and the
localized form, the so-called adenomyoma (left).

presenting a characteristic trabeculated appearance on cut section, with occasional
blood-filled cystic spaces also visible. The myometrium itself invariably undergoes
hypertrophy, so that the uterus becomes symmetrically enlarged in most cases,
although the lesion may exist occasionally in a normal-sized or even atrophic uterus.
Less often, on the other hand, the process may be more focal and produce an adenomyoma, a localized tumor that is clinically indistinguishable from a leiomyoma.
However, in either case, the process is in the nature of an infiltration of the surrounding myometrium, and there is no tendency to encapsulation. Thus, although
a local adenomyoma can be resected, it cannot be "shelled out" like a leiomyoma,
since no capsule is present. Adenomyosis is most often found in the posterior wall
of the fundus, less commonly on the anterior wall, and only infrequently in the
cornual or cervical segments. Rarely, a focal adenomyoma may become pedunculated and behave like a submucous fibroid.

From a histologic standpoint, the endometrial tissue in areas of adenomyosis
consists of both glands and stroma and is often immature or atrophic; it presents
evidence of normal cyclic changes (occasionally, decidual transformation in the
presence of pregnancy) in only 25 to 50 percent of cases. This "progesterone unresponsiveness" probably results primarily from the involvement of the basal layer of
the surface endometrium in the invasion of the myometrium. The myometrial cells
exhibit hypertrophy and hyperplasia surrounding the islands of endometrium.

Hemosiderin deposits within phagocytes are often observed in the myometrium adjacent to areas of adenomyosis. Not infrequently, the aberrant endometrial glands show cystic hyperplasia, and occasionally even glandular atypicalities are seen, but true malignant change rarely, if ever, occurs. This is in sharp contrast to the situation encountered in the entity known as stromal endometriosis of the uterus, which, in spite of the fact that it, too, involves an infiltration of the myometrium by endometrial elements (in this case, stromal cells unaccompanied by glands), cannot properly be considered a variant of adenomyosis. For although this stromatosis of the uterine wall may in some instances exhibit a benign microscopic appearance and benign clinical behavior, the evidence suggests that it is in reality a true neoplastic process and one that is more frequently encountered in its highly malignant form of endometrial stromal sarcoma. (For a discussion of stromal endometriosis, see Chapter 14.)

Clinical Manifestations

Although the not infrequent coexistence of other uterine and pelvic disease, as well as the often nonspecific nature of its symptomatology, frequently tends to obscure the manifestations of adenomyosis and render a definite preoperative diagnosis difficult, there is a tendency to certain characteristic and progressive symptoms and signs that should enable it to be correctly recognized in many instances. It is a more common disorder than has generally been appreciated, with an estimated incidence in the range of 15 to 25 percent of all women. (In some reports based on study of multiple sections from autopsy or hysterectomy specimens, the incidence has been as high as 50 to 60 percent.) As already noted, it is encountered more frequently in older women, with a peak incidence in the fifth decade, and patients in whom it is found are invariably multiparas. In many women it remains minimal and asymptomatic and is either never discovered or is detected simply by chance as an incidental finding in a hysterectomy specimen removed for other reasons.

The classic symptom complex accompanying adenomyosis, and the one most often encountered, is the following triad: increasing menorrhagia, the menstrual flow becoming both heavier and of longer duration; an acquired type of dysmenorrhea that becomes progressively more severe; and a steadily enlarging uterus that is usually symmetrical, extremely firm and globular, and typically tender to palpation, especially around the time of the menses. Occasionally, the uterus is somewhat irregularly nodular to palpation ("nutmeg uterus"), and, not infrequently, pelvic findings mistakenly suggests the presence of uterine fibroids; in the case of a localized adenomyoma, differentiation from a leiomyoma may be impossible. Other symptoms often present include metrorrhagia, dyspareunia, a sense of pelvic pressure or diffuse pelvic and lower abdominal pain, secondary bladder or bowel irritability, and a "pelvic congestion" type of premenstrual syndrome produced by the appreciably increased vascular supply to the uterus that uniformly develops if the adenomyosis is extensive.

Although the presence of associated disease may well be responsible for part or all the symptoms in many cases, adenomyosis per se can and does produce this characteristic complex of symptoms and signs in the absence of other lesions. Its presence alone can seriously interfere with the usual endometrial and myometrial hemostatic mechanisms and produce menorrhagia, and the marked distention of the uterine wall honeycombed with the highly vascular, swollen areas of adenomyosis readily accounts for the severe dysmenorrhea, dyspareunia, and painful, tender uterine enlargement.

Treatment

Resection of localized areas of adenomyosis with preservation of the uterus, especially in cases of true adenomyoma formation, is often feasible and is occasionally indicated in younger women in their late twenties or thirties, particularly if they have yet to have all the children they desire. Hormone therapy with oral contraceptives or cyclic estrogen or progesterone does not alleviate the symptoms; in fact, estrogens alone given in the second half of the menstrual cycle will definitely increase the menorrhagia (Halban's test). For the older woman with symptoms severe enough to warrant definitive treatment, total hysterectomy will usually be the treatment of choice, preservation of the ovaries frequently being possible and desirable in premenopausal patients.

MISCELLANEOUS BENIGN UTERINE DISORDERS

Fibromas and Cysts

Fibromas, or true benign connective-tissue tumors, occasionally arise in the wall of the fundus or cervix, but they are relatively rare in comparison with the ubiquitous leiomyoma. Cystic lesions of the uterus are also uncommon; the majority are actually pseudocysts that result from areas of degeneration and cystic change within what were originally leiomyomas or adenomyomas. However, in rare instances, a true cyst, congenital in origin and derived from mesonephric duct remnants or cell rests, may be encountered. (These are thus related both in nature and etiology to parovarian cysts and to Gartner's duct cysts of the vagina.)

Polyps

The frequently encountered **endometrial polyp**, together with the common **cervical and endocervical polyps** discussed in Chapter 7, make up another large group of benign uterine tumors. Whereas cervical polyps usually arise on an inflammatory basis in connection with chronic cervicitis, endometrial polyps most often develop in association with endometrial hyperplasia, both in turn being due to a hormonal imbalance. Prolonged stimulation by estrogen in relative excess leads to diffuse cystic or adenomatous endometrial hyperplasia as well as to focal areas of gross mucosal hypertrophy that ultimately become polypoid in structure. Although they may occur at any age, endometrial polyps are most commonly seen in premenopausal or postmenopausal women, at a time when ovarian endocrine dysfunction is also almost universal. When symptomatic, their principal manifestation is intermenstrual or postmenopausal bleeding. Diagnostic curettage is indicated in either case to rule out the possibility of cancer of the fundus or endocervix, and when polyps are found, they are readily removed by a combination of curettage and careful exploration of the uterine cavity with curved polyp forceps. Malignant change in an initially benign endometrial polyp is extremely rare; when it does occur, it is usually superficial and of low histologic grade. Although hysterectomy is undoubtedly indicated in such cases, there is usually no tumor elsewhere in the uterus, the lesion having been confined to the polyp, and the cure rate is therefore essentially 100 percent.

One additional type of benign polypoid lesion is the so-called **placental polyp**. Here again, a localized area of mucosal proliferation and heaping-up of a somewhat hyperplastic endometrial lining takes place about a fragment of retained decidual tissue, the constant uterine contractions about the area gradually leading to polypoid transformation. Except that it follows pregnancy and hence occurs in a relatively younger age group, the symptoms are essentially identical with those produced by a simple endometrial polyp; it should be noted, however, that the interval between the antecedent pregnancy and the appearance of a symptomatic placental polyp may be a lengthy one, sometimes amounting to several years.

Uterine Adhesions

Uterine adhesions (**Asherman's syndrome**, or **traumatic intrauterine synechiae**) may develop, most often following too vigorous postpartum or postabortal curettage (the vast majority of cases thus follow mechanical trauma to the endometrium during pregnancy or during the critical interval from the seventh to the twenty-eighth postpartum day), but occasionally after endometritis or operative procedures on the uterine wall such as myomectomy or cesarean section. Although many patients probably remain asymptomatic, and some may undergo spontaneous cure, in the typical case, following the traumatic curettage, the patient has a secondary amenorrhea or hypomenorrhea, an acquired dysmenorrhea, and either infertility or a tendency to abortion. Such a history is highly suggestive of the cause of the patient's symptoms, but the diagnosis can and should be readily confirmed by hysterography, which usually reveals a distorted or even linear-shaped uterine cavity, partially or almost totally obliterated by extensive adhesions and adherence of the uterine walls. Thereafter, a metal uterine sound is used to verify the presence of the intrauterine adhesions and locate them precisely. Endocrine causes of postpartum amenorrhea are usually readily excluded by the history and findings and by simple endocrine studies, if indicated. If the adhesions primarily involve the cervix, dysmenorrhea, infertility, and amenorrhea are the most prominent symptoms. If the cervical stenosis is complete, hematometria and hematosalpinx sometimes develop. If the adhesions are largely limited to the fundus, hypomenorrhea and repeated abortions are the more typical clinical features. Treatment involves surgical removal of the adhesions, most often by dilatation and curettage, following which the uterine cavity is kept expanded and the walls separated by an inlying balloon catheter or a plastic intrauterine device until complete healing has occurred. In some cases an abdominal approach with hysterotomy will be required, particularly if there are extensive thick and rigid adhesions in the uterine fundus. Antibiotics are administered prophylactically both preoperatively and postoperatively to prevent intrauterine infection; cortisone and antihistamines are also employed by some as an aid to the prevention of new adhesions; and cyclic estrogen-progesterone is administered for two to three months to promote good endometrial proliferation during the healing phase. It is possible that Asherman's syndrome is largely a preventable disorder if uterine curettage is strictly avoided whenever possible during the critical three weeks' interval from the seventh through the twenty-eighth postpartum day by anticipating the possibility, detecting the presence of retained secundines promptly, and doing the indicated curettage in the early postpartum period.

Pyometra

A pyometra is defined as the development of a collection of "pus" (sterile in 40 to 50 percent of cases) within the cavity of the uterine fundus as a result of interference with the normal dependent drainage of the uterus. Invariably, the obstruction occurs within the cervical canal (usually within the endocervix), but it occasionally is secondary to an obliteration of the external cervical os. Although carcinoma of the cervix or endometrium is sometimes the cause of the condition (in 15 to 20 percent of cases), benign cervical stenosis due to atrophic changes similar to those affecting the vagina postmenopausally or to old inflammatory changes or old obstetric trauma with secondary scarring and fibrosis is actually a more common cause, accounting for roughly 40 percent of cases. Prior radiation for cervical cancer and previous cervical surgical procedures (including D&C, cauterization, cone biopsy, and trachelorrhaphy) are other frequent causes and account for the remaining 40 percent of cases.

Pyometra usually occurs in postmenopausal women, with a peak incidence in the age range 55 to 70. The most common presenting symptom is an abnormal vaginal discharge, usually yellowish-brown, or vaginal bleeding; less often, the patient complains of lower abdominal pain due to the uncomfortable uterine distention from backed-up secretions and old blood. Roughly one-fourth of patients will be asymptomatic, an enlarged, soft, "cystic-feeling" uterus being noted on routine pelvic examination. It is rare for the condition to be associated with fever, leukocytosis, or other signs or symptoms of a true infection.

A pyometra should be managed by careful cervical dilatation and then meticulous fractional curettage of the endometrial cavity and endocervix to confirm or rule out the possibility of cervical or endometrial carcinoma. (Occasionally, the actual curettage will have to be delayed until the cavity has been allowed to drain for a week or two, permitting the uterine wall to involute and regain its normal thickness.) If either cervical or endometrial cancer is detected, drainage of the uterine fundus for several weeks with a rubber T-tube (such as is employed for drainage of the common bile duct) anchored by a suture to the cervix is indicated before either radiotherapy is begun or radical surgery contemplated. If only a benign stricture is present, simple T-tube drainage for one month after completion of the D&C should suffice to correct the condition, with follow-up cervical dilatations in the office as indicated. Postoperative antibiotics are usually not necessary unless there is some suspicion that uterine perforation has occurred during the procedure.

Idiopathic Uterine Hypertrophy

Finally, an entity termed **idiopathic uterine,** or **myometrial, hypertrophy,** or **diffuse myometrial sclerosis** (also sometimes called **fibrosis uteri,** or **chronic subinvolution**) is occasionally encountered. The uterus is symmetrically enlarged, and the patient is prone to excessive bleeding for which there is often no other explanation, since the process is frequently unaccompanied by any other pathologic process in the uterus or ovaries. The patient is invariably a multipara and frequently complains of dysmenorrhea, low backache, and a constant sense of pelvic pressure. Thus, both symptomatically as well as on pelvic examination, myometrial hypertrophy may simulate either adenomyosis or a solitary, large, centrally located submucous or intramural fibroid. The uterine enlargement and considerably thickened uterine wall are due in part to an actual hypertrophy of smooth muscle fibers, which in turn may be secondary to progressively increasing subinvolution of the uterus after multiple pregnancies. There is also a marked increase in the amount of fibrous tissue between the smooth muscle fibers, and this is the factor most responsible for the sometimes dramatic increase in the volume of the uterine fundus. The reason for the tendency to excessive bleeding is not entirely clear, but it may well be that it is the result of impaired myometrial contractility at the time of the menstrual flow. However, in many patients, there may be associated uterine disease (leiomyomas or adenomyosis) that could equally well be the cause of the pain and excessive flow.

Although the majority of hypertrophied uteri are probably either asymptomatic or cause minimal difficulty, when symptoms are severe and menorrhagia is marked, hysterectomy may be required for relief.

REFERENCES

1. Asherman, J. G. Traumatic intra-uterine adhesions. *J. Obstet. Gynecol. Br. Emp.* 57:892, 1950.
2. Bird, C. C., McElin, T. W., and Manalo-Estrella, P. The elusive adenomyosis of the uterus — revisited. *Am. J. Obstet. Gynecol.* 112:583, 1972.
3. Carmichael, D. E. Asherman's syndrome. *Obstet. Gynecol.* 36:922, 1970.
4. Cullen, T. S. The distribution of adenomyoma containing uterine mucosa. *Arch. Surg.* 1:215, 1920.
5. Emge, L. A. The elusive adenomyosis of the uterus. *Am. J. Obstet. Gynecol.* 83:1541, 1962.

6. Ingersoll, F. M. Fertility following myomectomy. *Fertil. Steril.* 14:596, 1963.
7. Ingersoll, F. M., and Malone, L. J. Myomectomy: An alternative to hysterectomy. *Arch. Surg.* 100:557, 1970.
8. Jensen, P. A., and Stromme, W. B. Amenorrhea secondary to puerperal curettage: Asherman's syndrome. *Am. J. Obstet. Gynecol.* 113:150, 1972.
9. Lewis, P. L., Lee, A. B. H., and Easler, R. E. Myometrial hypertrophy. *Am. J. Obstet. Gynecol.* 84:1032, 1962.
10. Molitor, J. J. Adenomyosis: A clinical and pathologic appraisal. *Am. J. Obstet. Gynecol.* 110:275, 1971.
11. Murphy, E. S. Diffuse myometrial sclerosis. *Am. J. Obstet. Gynecol.* 103:403, 1969.
12. Oelsner, G., Ammon, D., Insler, V., and Serr, D. M. Outcome of pregnancy after treatment of intrauterine adhesions. *Obstet. Gynecol.* 44:341, 1974.
13. Rothman, D., and Rennard, M. Myoma-erythrocytosis syndrome. *Obstet. Gynecol.* 21:102, 1963.
14. Spurlin, G. W., Van Nagell, J. R., Jr., Parker, J. C., Jr., and Roddick, J. W., Jr. Uterine myomas and erythrocytosis. *Obstet. Gynecol.* 40:646, 1972.
15. Whiteley, P. F., and Hamlett, J. D. Pyometra — a reappraisal. *Am. J. Obstet. Gynecol.* 109:108, 1971.

13
Carcinoma of the Cervix

GENERAL REMARKS ON PELVIC NEOPLASMS

One-fourth of all malignant diseases in women arise in the genital tract, and the vast majority are carcinomas, the order of frequency as to site of origin being the cervix, endometrium (uterine fundus), ovary, vulva, vagina, and fallopian tube. An idea of the relative incidence of the various cancers of the female genital tract can be obtained from the experience of the Pondville (Massachusetts Department of Public Health) State Cancer Hospital (Table 4). As also suggested in Table 4, a change in the relative incidence of the various female genital tract cancers may have taken place in recent years for a variety of reasons, some of which will be noted in this and the following four chapters.

Because of the accessibility of most of these tumors, female genital cancer is particularly susceptible to simple methods of early detection, and, relatively speaking, cure rates are potentially the highest of any area of the body if the lesions are recognized in their early phases and are treated promptly and properly. An appreciation of when to suspect the possible existence of a pelvic malignancy and how to approach the problem of diagnosis and evaluation in the individual patient is therefore even more important than a precise knowledge of the details of current therapy. The principles and techniques of a sound cancer detection program for gynecologic cancers are presented in Chapter 1.

Proper treatment must be based on a complete understanding of the differing natural histories of each type of gynecologic cancer as well as on a thorough knowledge of the possibilities and limitations of all the applicable forms of therapy: surgery, radiation, and, more recently, chemotherapy. Although complete and permanent cure is the natural and ideal goal of all therapy, in many instances even the "incurable" patient may be given untold benefit in the way of long-term palliation by the intelligent use of these various therapeutic tools.

Carcinoma of the cervix accounts for 11 percent of all cancer and for 50 to 65 percent of all malignant tumors of the female reproductive tract and is a close second to carcinoma of the breast in frequency among all cancers in women. Approximately 30,000 new cases of invasive cervical cancer are discovered each year in the United States alone, and nearly 10,000 women die annually from this disease in this country. A number of statistical studies have indicated that cervical carcinoma will ultimately develop in roughly 2 percent of all women.

However, the incidence and death rate of invasive squamous cell carcinoma of the cervix is steadily declining because of the increasingly widespread early detection and treatment of its antecedent lesions, carcinoma in situ and severe, persistent cervical dysplasia. The number of deaths from cervical cancer in the United States has been reduced by roughly 50 percent in the last decade alone. In 1930, it was the number one cause of death from cancer in women; now it is fourth on the list.

Table 4
Relative Incidence of Carcinomas of the Female Genital Tract Encountered at the Pondville State Cancer Hospital (Massachusetts Department of Public Health)

Site	1927–1961		1962–1974	
	Number of Patients	Percentage of Total	Number of Patients	Percentage of Total
Cervix	2052	64.0	407	45.3
Endometrium	596	18.7	218	24.2
Ovary	310	9.7	176	19.6
Vulva	170	5.3	68	7.6
Vagina	70	2.2	25	2.8
Fallopian tube	2	0.1	4	0.5
Totals	3200	100.0	898	100.0

Nevertheless, the overall incidence of cervical cancer, if one includes the preinvasive stage, carcinoma in situ (40,000 new cases of carcinoma in situ are discovered annually in the United States), has remained the same and may now even be increasing as the result of increasing and more promiscuous sexual activity among the teenage and young adult population, with a corresponding increase in the exposure of a much younger group of women to some of the potential etiologic factors discussed in the next section.

ETIOLOGY

The development of carcinoma of the cervix in women who have never had sexual intercourse is so extremely rare as to be a medical curiosity, and only 10 to 12 percent of cases are encountered in women who have never been pregnant. These facts have long suggested that sexual activity and childbearing are important predisposing factors. Actually, the most striking epidemiologic correlations are to be found in the effects of early marriage and early childbearing, roughly 50 percent of all cervical cancers appearing in women who were married and/or had their first child before the age of 20. This would tend to indicate either the significance of the duration of exposure to whatever causal factors may be linked to sexual activity and childbearing, or possibly that there is a constitutional predisposition to the disease, perhaps endocrinologic in nature, that is also manifested by an irrepressible urge and drive toward early sexual activity. This phenomenon is perhaps even more apparent in the even greater incidence of cervical cancer in women who are sexually precocious and promiscuous. Thus, the most significant epidemiologic features of cervical cancer are such as to suggest that it can almost be characterized as a venereal disease.

That there may in addition be hereditary, ethnic, socioeconomic, and cultural factors in the background is indicated by a variety of epidemiologic observations. For example, cervical cancer is only one-fifth as common in Jewish women as compared with non-Jewish white women living in the United States, whereas it is twice as common in the American black population as in non-Jewish white women. In both instances the explanation might also lie in the differing specific local vaginal and cervical factors, as follows:

1. The etiologic role of sexual intercourse has been postulated as secondary to potential carcinogenic effects of human smegma. Cervical carcinoma has been produced in laboratory animals (rats and mice) following prolonged and repeated exposure to human smegma, and what appears to be a carcinogenic virus has been isolated from horse smegma. The relative infrequency of cervical carcinoma in Jewish women might thus be explained by the fact that Jewish males are universally circumcised, since circumcision is known to reduce the accumulation of smegma markedly. A similar relationship between the status of the marital partner with respect to circumcision and the incidence of cervical carcinoma has been observed in certain non-Jewish female populations, a notable example being the women of the Fiji Islands, among whom cervical cancer is eight times more common in wives of noncircumcised men as compared with those whose husbands have been circumcised. The higher incidence of cervical cancer in American black women might be at least partially explained on this same basis. The extreme rarity of cervical carcinoma in virgins (e.g., a careful study of 13,000 Canadian nuns reported by Gagnon [12] uncovered not a single bona fide case during a 20-year period), and the increased incidence associated with early and/or promiscuous sexual activity lends additional support to the hypothesis that the uncircumcised male with poor penile hygiene (who also has a higher incidence of carcinoma of the penis) may be an important etiologic factor in the genesis of female cervical cancer.

2. From time to time over the years, evidence has been presented linking the development of cervical cancer with repeated childbirth lacerations in the multiparous cervix and the resulting prolonged state of chronic cervicitis; with congenital erosions of the nulliparous cervix and the consequent constant exposure of the externally displaced squamocolumnar junction to the bacterial flora and acid environment of the vagina; and even with the chronic presence of trichomonal vaginitis and accompanying secondary inflammation of the cervical epithelium and glands.

In each instance a carcinogenic influence might be attributed to the constant state of epithelial proliferation in the cervix engendered by chronic inflammation and/or the repeated sequence of cervical trauma followed by healing or attempted regeneration of the cervical epithelium, or to the effects on cellular growth and metabolism in the critical area of the squamocolumnar junction of a cervical epithelium abnormally exposed to vaginal acidity and a bacterial or protozoal environment. With respect to the latter point, it is perhaps of some interest that cervical carcinoma develops with considerably less frequency in the prolapsed uterus, a situation wherein the cervix, although frequently lacerated and often actually eroded, lies completely outside the vagina.

The possible status of the traumatized, chronically infected cervix as a frequent site of epithelial dysplasia and ultimately an increased incidence of frank malignant change has already been discussed in Chapter 7. Although much of the statistical evidence in support of these concepts is inconclusive, the clinical impressions of several generations of gynecologists to the effect that cervical cancer more commonly appears in the lacerated, chronically infected cervix and is exceedingly rare in the well-epithelialized, relatively normal-appearing cervix cannot be denied a considerable degree of validity. The implications of these concepts with respect to prophylaxis against the development of cervical cancer by the proper postpartum care of the cervix and the treatment of "benign" cervical abnormalities such as erosions, severe lacerations, and significant chronic cervicitis by cauterization, repair, or amputation are equally obvious. It is perhaps unnecessary to reemphasize that it is also incumbent on the physician before treatment of the "abnormal cervix" to determine positively (by means of cytologic study, the Schiller test, and cervical biopsy) that an early malignant change does not in fact already exist.

Possible Etiologic Role of Type 2 Herpesvirus Hominis Infection of the Female Genital Tract

An even more promising alternative explanation for the apparent significance of precocious and promiscuous sexual intercourse in the genesis of cervical carcinoma is currently under intensive study, namely, the possible role of type 2 herpesvirus genital tract infection (see also Chap. 8). It is postulated that this strain of herpes simplex, which is genitotropic and is transmitted venereally, might be the carcinogenic agent responsible for the development of cervical neoplasia. Such a theory is attractive because it also accounts for the fact that cervical cancer does possess many of the epidemiologic characteristics of a venereal disease. Although the vulvar and vaginal lesions accompanying herpes progenitalis infection are often the most obvious and the most symptomatic, it is now known that the cervix is actually the more frequent site of herpesvirus infection (75 percent or more of cases).

Infection with type 2 herpesvirus can be detected by cytologic examination of cervical smears or vaginal aspirates or by actual recovery of the virus from these secretions, as well as by the presence of serum antibodies in infected patients. In several ways, the use of one or more of these screening tests shows that the incidence of type 2 herpesvirus infection in the general population is 0.10 to 0.15 percent. However, there is now well-documented evidence of an increased incidence of cervical dysplasia and carcinoma in patients with type 2 herpesvirus infections, as well as an increased incidence of type 2 herpesvirus infections among women with cervical carcinoma and dysplasia. In one such study, 23 percent of 245 women with proved type 2 herpesvirus infection had either cervical dysplasia, carcinoma in situ, or invasive carcinoma, as compared with a 2.6 percent incidence of these lesions in a group of 245 women of similar age, race, and background without clinical or laboratory evidence of herpetic infection. In another investigation, 83 percent of a group of women with invasive cervical cancer had type 2 herpesvirus antibodies as contrasted with a 0 to 20 percent incidence of herpesvirus antibodies in several groups of matched controls without cervical cancer. In another such study, an antibody to AG-4, an early antigen associated with herpesvirus type 2, was found in the blood of 35 percent of women with dysplasia, 68 percent of patients with carcinoma in situ, and 91 percent of patients with invasive cervical cancer. The antibody was essentially absent in matched controls and in groups of women with cancer in other sites such as the breast, ovary, or lung. The antibody was also absent in a series of women who had been successfully treated for cervical cancer. Another investigating team studying this same correlation found that 95 percent of patients with dysplasia and 100 percent of patients with either carcinoma in situ or invasive carcinoma of the cervix had strongly positive herpesvirus type 2 antibody titers, as opposed to only one-third to one-half of matched controls.

Because the only tumor occurring in primates known to be caused by a virus is the herpesvirus-induced reticulum cell sarcoma in monkeys, a potential oncogenic role for type 2 herpesvirus hominis is definitely within the realm of possibility. It is equally possible that type 2 herpesvirus might not be the sole agent responsible but could be acting as a mandatory cocarcinogen to potentiate the effect of some other agent (e.g., a carcinogenic substance in smegma). There is, in fact, an experimental animal model in which skin cancer develops with methylcholanthrene only when a herpesvirus infection is introduced to potentiate its carcinogenic effect.

Thus, although far from proved, a causal relationship is definitely suggested by all these observations, with the possibility that herpesvirus acting over a latent period of several years eventually provokes the development of cervical anaplasia and neoplasia. It is also apparent that the more precocious and promiscuous the woman's sexual exposure, the more likely she is to be infected by the genital herpesvirus. It has also been shown that the male genital tract frequently (in 10 to 15 percent of men) serves as a reservoir for herpesvirus type 2, so that women who begin sexual activity early in their teens and have multiple partners are much more likely to become infected, and at an earlier age.

Certainly, women known to have had genital herpes infections should be followed closely in order to detect as soon as possible any evidence of the development of cervical dysplasia or carcinoma. Finally, since herpetic genital infections do not normally appear until adolescence (and assuming that a mandatory etiologic role for type 2 herpesvirus infection were to be firmly established), the possibility that immunization procedures could be carried out during childhood that would completely prevent the development of cervical cancer looms as a potential dramatic breakthrough in the field of cancer prevention.

Of course, it is also possible that some other agent transmitted during coitus may be the principal oncogenic factor, or possibly a cofactor. The nuclear protein of the sperm head has its proponents for nomination to this role, as do the vaginal *Mycoplasma* organisms, which also occur frequently in sexually active women and promiscuous women. The theory then assumes that one or more of these agents is active at a time when the cervical epithelial cells (more specifically those of the so-called transformation zone, the area just above the squamocolumnar junction where a process of squamous metaplasia of the adjoining columnar epithelium normally takes place) are vulnerable to such agents, prior to completion of the usual benign process of squamous metaplasia.

PATHOGENESIS

Epidermoid or squamous cell carcinomas constitute 90 to 95 percent of all cervical carcinomas, and, with few exceptions, they are either derived from the squamous epithelium bordering on the squamocolumnar junction or arise in areas of squamous metaplasia or from the so-called reserve cell components in the columnar epithelium of the endocervical canal (the so-called transformation zone). The remaining 5 to 10 percent represent either pure adenocarcinomas, adenoacanthomas (adenocarcinomas with benign squamous metaplasia), or adenosquamous carcinomas in which there is a mixture of both adenocarcinoma and squamous cell carcinoma, all three of these glandular types of carcinoma originating in the columnar epithelium lining the surface or glandular structures of the endocervical canal. As noted later, there has been some evidence lately of a recent trend toward an increasing incidence of primary adenocarcinomas of the cervix, including the adenosquamous variety. However, it is too soon to verify the existence and significance of this trend or to venture a possible explanation for it.

Microscopically, the epidermoid carcinomas can be classified into three principal cellular types:

1. Keratinizing squamous cell carcinomas (usually well differentiated).
2. Large cell, nonkeratinizing carcinomas (usually of moderate degrees of cellular differentiation).
3. Small cell, nonkeratinizing carcinomas (most often undifferentiated tumors).

Large cell nonkeratinizing carcinomas have the most favorable prognosis; they appear to be the most radiosensitive, but in addition the cure rates are the highest of all, whether therapy is by radiation or radical surgery. Keratinizing tumors, on the other hand, have the least favorable prognosis and the greatest frequency of lymph node metastases; they appear to respond less favorably to radiation therapy and to be more curable by radical surgery in most, but not all, reported series. The small cell nonkeratinizing tumors also have a slightly less favorable prognosis, but when selection of treatment is on a random basis, appear to do equally well whether treated by radiation or by radical surgery.

Adenocarcinomas are usually readily identifiable microscopically on the basis of their typical glandular pattern. Occasionally, a highly undifferentiated adenocarcinoma may be difficult to distinguish from a large cell nonkeratinizing cervical carcinoma, but the periodic acid-Schiff (PAS) stain can be done, and if PAS-positive material is demonstrated, the tumor can be assumed to be of glandular origin. The five-year survival rate for cervical adenocarcinomas, especially of the mixed adenosquamous variety, has been less favorable than that for squamous cell cancers in most reported series. These tumors are thought by many to be less radiosensitive, and treatment by radical surgery, when feasible, is probably to be recommended, with or without adjunctive radiotherapy, as circumstances may indicate.

It has already been noted in Chapter 7 that intraepithelial carcinoma and invasive carcinoma of the cervix frequently, although probably not invariably, are preceded by and represent progressively advancing stages of the cervical epithelium's fairly generalized tendency to dysplasia and anaplasia. Although it is clear that some of the simple, benign, mild to moderate cervical dysplasias never undergo neoplastic transformation and may even regress in a significant percentage of cases (25 to 30 percent or more), there is a considerable body of evidence suggesting that the histologic lesion designated as severe cervical dysplasia is often the forerunner of carcinoma in situ (and in fact is often difficult to distinguish from it microscopically), and that the latter lesion in turn is even more intimately related to invasive carcinoma, being in fact the preinvasive stage of invasive carcinoma in the vast majority of instances. In one follow-up study of 520 women with dysplasia, 25 percent had progressed to carcinoma in situ within six years of the initial diagnosis of dysplasia. In another prospective study involving 127 women with cervical dysplasia followed for periods of up to 20 years, invasive cancer developed in 35 percent of the group. A review of the best available data suggests that at least 35 to 50 percent of cases of carcinoma in situ eventually progress to invasive cervical cancer; with adequate long-term follow-up, the percentage may prove to be even higher.

Detailed microscopic study of cervical biopsy specimens or of complete surgical specimens obtained from women with cervical cancer frequently reveals all three histologic lesions (invasive cancer, carcinoma in situ, and squamous cell anaplasia) coexisting in various areas of the same cervix. In fact, in small cervical cancers one often finds a definite margin of intraepithelial carcinoma surrounding the borders of the gross malignant lesion, an observation that suggests the latter's origin from what was originally a larger area of carcinoma in situ. As might be expected, areas of squamous cell anaplasia can be identified even more frequently in cervices harboring only carcinoma in situ. The phenomenon of carcinoma in situ with early microscopic invasion of the cervical stroma (the so-called microcarcinoma, a lesion that is nevertheless by definition a true invasive carcinoma) represents another link in the chain of evidence supporting the concept that intraepithelial carcinoma ultimately progresses to invasive cervical cancer in many, if not all, instances. Even in patients in whom a final clinical diagnosis of carcinoma in situ has been carefully established by curettage and conization or multiple cervical biopsies, serial microscopic sections have been reported to reveal early stromal invasion in from 3 percent to as many as 25 percent of cases. Furthermore, by more retrospective and a small number of prospective types of studies, a number of well-documented instances have been recorded wherein patients whose initial lesions were shown by biopsy to be carcinoma in situ ultimately exhibited invasive cervical cancer after intervals of from 2 to 10 years.

Finally, certain statistical data concerning the similar rates of occurrence, ethnic incidence, and parallel age-distribution curves of squamous cell anaplasia, carcinoma in situ, and invasive carcinoma furnish additional circumstantial evidence for their fundamental relationship and indicate roughly the time factor involved in the spectrum of progressively increasing epithelial abnormalities. With regard to rate of occurrence, the only meaningful data concern carcinoma in situ and invasive carcinoma, the figures available revealing an entirely comparable attack rate for both lesions of roughly 30 to 50 cases per 100,000 female population per year in the United States. With respect to ethnic incidence, both carcinoma in situ and cervical cancer are one-fifth to one-sixth as common among Jewish as compared with non-Jewish white women, and both are twice as common in the black female population as compared with the white female population of the United States.

The age-distribution curves for the three lesions are parallel and similar in configuration, with an upward trend in average age proceeding from anaplasia through carcinoma in situ to early and advanced invasive carcinoma. Most revealing in this regard are the data reported by Younge and Hertig and associates [35] at the Free Hospital for Women in Boston, who maintained an active interest for over 30 years in this and other facets of the problem of the genesis of cervical cancer. In their series of cases, the average age of 243 patients with cervical anaplasia was 34.9 years; of 201 patients with carcinoma in situ, it was 38.0 years; of 38 patients with probably early stromal invasion, it was 42.2 years; of 131 patients with clinically unsuspected invasive cancer (very early, or microcarcinoma), it was 48.5 years; and for a much larger group of patients with grossly obvious invasive cancer of the cervix (Stages I to IV) the average age was 51 years. The conclusion that the three histologic lesions represent progressive stages of the same basic neoplastic process seems inescapable.

One other observation by Younge and his colleagues is pertinent and concerns the increasing accuracy with which the three lesions were detected by vaginal smears. In their series, anaplasia yielded positive or suspicious smears in 67 percent of cases, whereas smears were positive in 82 percent of patients with carcinoma in situ and in 98 percent of women with invasive cancer. Happily, this increasing diagnostic accuracy of exfoliative cytology parallels the progression of the neoplastic process itself.

PATHOLOGIC FEATURES

Histologic Appearance

CERVICAL DYSPLASIA

In cervical dysplasia, a variable degree of disturbance of the normal, orderly arrangement of the epithelial cells is noted, with mitoses in the layers above the basalis and with the nuclei of many cells enlarged, irregular, and hyperchromatic; giant or multinucleated cells are frequently present. The microscopic appearance thus closely resembles that of intraepithelial carcinoma, with the exception that good surface stratification is frequently maintained.

EPIDERMOID CARCINOMA IN SITU

A complete or nearly complete loss of the normal stratification involving all layers, as well as a loss of the polarity so characteristic of the normal squamous epithelial pattern, is seen in epidermoid carcinoma in situ. Marked cellular pleomorphism and the presence of numerous mitoses, many of them abnormal, are observed throughout the entire thickness of the squamous epithelium. (In normal squamous epithelium, mitotic activity is minimal, orderly, and limited to the lower third of the epithelial layers.) Typically, the edges of the intraepithelial neoplasm are discrete microscopically, and there is an abrupt, sharply defined margin between it and the adjacent normal squamous epithelium. At no point does abnormal cellular proliferation penetrate beneath the basement membrane. Although this morphologically malignant change is frequently limited to the surface epithelium of the cervix, in more extensive lesions it also tends to involve the epithelium of the cervical and endocervical mucous glands, appearing to spread into the glandular lumina and even to replace the entire thickness of the columnar epithelium normally present there. Such a lesion is designated carcinoma in situ with glandular involvement, but because the basement membrane of the glands remains intact and uninvaded, it is nevertheless still an intraepithelial carcinoma, although it should probably be considered a somewhat more advanced phase of preinvasive carcinoma.

INVASIVE EPIDERMOID CARCINOMA

Microcarcinoma

Microcarcinoma by definition is an early invasive lesion in which the diagnosis can be established only by histologic study, since there will be no grossly visible or obvious malignant tumor in the cervix. Unfortunately, there has been a tendency to group all such early invasive cancers of the cervix into the single category, microcarcinoma, erroneously implying that all exhibit a similar histologic picture, represent the same degree of progression of the invasive process, and pose an identical threat to the patient that is considerably less than that posed by clinically recognizable early Stage I cancers. This oversimplified abuse of the term **microcarcinoma** has led to the even more unfortunate impression in the minds of some physicians that the treatment in nearly all such cases can be identical to that of carcinoma in situ (simple hysterectomy) with equally favorable results. Such is emphatically not the case; in fact, the majority of true microcarcinomas should be treated like any Stage I carcinoma of the cervix, whether by radiation or by radical surgery.

Histologically, the term **microcarcinoma** really covers a wide spectrum of invasive change. In some cases the lesion is largely carcinoma in situ, but foci are seen where the basement membrane has been disrupted and stromal invasion has occurred. If these foci are infrequent and actual stromal penetration dubious, it may be reasonable to consider such a lesion as carcinoma in situ with questionable invasion and treat it as intraepithelial cancer. (Beecham [1] has wisely suggested that these be termed Stage 0-Ia lesions.) However, when there are many such foci of basement membrane breakthrough, and when the unquestioned stromal invasion is more diffuse and deeply penetrating, sometimes even with foci of cells within lymphatic channels, a true microcarcinoma (Stage Ia) is present, with all the malignant potential of any invasive cancer. Pelvic lymph node metastases from such a lesion, although theoretically possible and occasionally reported, are uncommon; however, microscopic permeation to the immediate paracervical areas does occur in a significant number. Therefore this type of microcarcinoma should receive the same therapy as any Stage I carcinoma of the cervix, and if proper treatment is given, the prognosis is excellent, with cure rates approaching 100 percent.

Two other types of microcarcinoma fall in the "twilight zone." The first type is in actuality a small, early invasive cancer discovered prior to ulceration of the superficial layers of the cervical epithelium and hence presenting no lesion of the cervix visible to the naked eye. Although on microscopic examination it may be seen to contain areas of carcinoma in situ, histologically it is readily seen to be basically almost entirely an invasive cancer. The second type is better termed an **occult carcinoma**, since it is really a small invasive carcinoma that would have been clinically visible were it not hidden out of sight in the endocervical canal above the external os. The former should probably still be classified as Stage Ia; the latter might be more accurately considered Stage Ib, the subgroup under Stage I to which all clinically recognizable carcinomas confined to the cervix should be assigned. In any case, there should be no dispute that both types are true invasive cancers and that both should be treated as such by adequate radiation therapy or radical surgery.

Clinically Obvious Invasive Squamous Cell Carcinoma of the Cervix

Grossly visible invasive carcinomas of the cervix exhibit the typical microscopic features of epidermoid carcinoma arising at any site. The well-differentiated (microscopic grade I) so-called spinal cell carcinomas showing abundant keratinization and frequent pearl formation are relatively uncommon (15 percent), the vast majority of cervical carcinomas (70 percent) being of the transitional cell variety, with an intermediate degree of differentiation (microscopic grades II and III). The highly malignant and undifferentiated carcinomas (microscopic grade IV) are usually composed principally of spindle cells and at times are so anaplastic in appearance as to resemble sarcomas; fortunately, they are only occasionally encountered (in 10 percent of cases).

ADENOCARCINOMA OF THE CERVIX

The common variety of adenocarcinoma originates from the columnar epithelium of the surface lining and glands of the endocervical canal and constitutes approximately 5 percent of all cervical cancers. Possibly as a result of the steady decline in the incidence of invasive squamous cell cervical cancer that has resulted from the early detection and treatment of its precursors, severe dysplasia and carcinoma in situ, there has been a relative increase in the number of primary cervical adenocarcinomas. In fact, several institutions have reported a marked increase in the incidence of adenocarcinoma of the cervix recently, with this lesion now accounting for 30 to 35 percent of their cervical cancer cases, suggesting that there may actually be a trend toward an absolute, not just a relative, increase in the number of glandular carcinomas. Histologically, cervical adenocarcinomas tend to exhibit a glandular pattern and to retain their mucus-secreting characteristics, but papillary adenocarcinoma is also common. In the more undifferentiated varieties the histologic appearance may be highly anaplastic and the glandular origin barely recognizable. It is usually impossible on histologic grounds alone to distinguish adenocarcinoma of the cervix from adenocarcinoma of the endometrium, although special staining techniques may be used in preparing the sections for histologic study (e.g., PAS or alcian blue) and help in making the distinction, since endocervical epithelial cells differ from endometrial cells in their staining properties. It is of course extremely important to differentiate a primary adenocarcinoma of the cervix from an adenocarcinoma of the endometrium that has extended downward to involve the cervix (carcinoma corporis et cervicis), since the plan of management will be somewhat different in the latter. As in the case of endometrial carcinoma, squamous metaplasia may occur in association with adenocarcinoma of the cervix, giving rise to the lesion designated as adenoacanthoma. Occasionally, carcinomas with both malignant epidermoid and glandular elements are encountered, i.e., adenosquamous carcinoma. Rare forms of primary glandular carcinoma of the cervix include mesonephric carcinoma, medullary carcinoma, and adenoid cystic carcinoma.

Mention should be made of a specific group of mixed adenosquamous carcinomas of the cervix that are highly anaplastic and may be subdivided into two subtypes in accordance with whether the predominant neoplastic element is composed of signet-ring cells or of the so-called glassy cells. The chief significance of this special group lies in the fact that unlike the vast majority of adenocarcinomas of the cervix, which show a response to radiation therapy comparable to that of epidermoid carcinoma, these highly anaplastic mixed tumors, particularly the glassy cell type, appear to be radioresistant and hence should definitely be treated by radical surgery or a combination of preliminary radiation therapy and radical surgery [13]. Unfortunately, survival rates following treatment are not quite as favorable in patients with adenocarcinomas arising in the cervix because within this histologic category are found some of the very anaplastic, highly invasive, widely metastasizing types, including the mixed adenosquamous carcinomas, of which the so-called glassy cell tumor is the most common and lethal type.

Regardless of the therapy utilized, glassy cell carcinomas, as well as the other varieties of mixed adenosquamous cancers, carry a very poor prognosis. Cure rates are extremely low even in the early clinical stages, and these tumors are prone to rapid local extension and widespread vascular and lymphatic involvement with early distant metastatic spread.

Finally, mention should also be made of the clear cell carcinomas of the cervix (probably often termed **mesonephric adenocarcinomas** in the past), histologically entirely similar to the much more common clear cell carcinomas of the vagina seen in adolescent and young adult females whose mothers were exposed to diethylstilbestrol (DES) or similar synthetic, nonsteroidal estrogens during their pregnancies (see Chap. 4). As was true for its vaginal counterpart, clear cell carcinoma of the cervix was seen, though rarely, even prior to the era of DES therapy for threatened or habitual abortion. However, both tumors, though still relatively uncommon, are now seen more frequently than in the past, and the occurrence of clear cell carcinoma of the cervix is also almost invariably linked with prenatal exposure to DES.

These lesions are also somewhat more aggressive than ordinary adenocarcinomas or the far more common squamous cell cancers, but the prognosis is not nearly so bad as is the case for the glassy cell tumors.

Gross Pathologic Features

Carcinoma in situ and microcarcinoma do not produce any visible alterations of the cervix, but their presence can often be detected by Schiller's test, neither of these epithelial lesions staining with iodine. Clinically obvious epidermoid carcinoma may present as a proliferative or exophytic tumor, growing out from the cervix as a bulky, cauliflowerlike mass of friable, easily bleeding tissue. Or it may instead present as an invasive or endophytic type of lesion, the deeper substance of the cervix being taken up and expanded by a firm mass of tumor, often with a palpable, hard nodular extension of the disease into the paracervical areas or submucosally along the vaginal walls. Finally, it may take the form of an ulcerating type of tumor, the cervix simply being destroyed to a varying degree, leaving a central excavation surrounded by the hard, irregular advancing margins of the lesion itself and its deeper extensions. In the case of carcinomas arising higher in the endocervical canal, whether epidermoid or glandular in type, the lesion itself may not be visible, but as a result of growth into the canal, or into the deeper substance of the cervical wall, or both, the cervical segment becomes abnormally hard and irregularly broadened and expanded. This is the so-called barrel-shaped cervix characteristic of endocervical carcinoma.

Routes of Spread

Direct local extension to involve the vagina, either on the mucosal surface or submucosally in the stromal tissue or along vaginal lymphatic, perivascular, or perineural channels, tends to occur frequently. Similarly, lateral spread into the paracervical and parametrial areas is common, the tumor following the same type of tissue pathways and ultimately reaching the walls of the pelvis in advanced cases. The ureters, by virtue of their close proximity to the cervix at the level of the main uterine vascular and lymphatic pedicles, lie directly in the path of the laterally spreading tumor and thus are frequently encroached on once the disease has undergone significant extension beyond the cervix. As a result, ureteral obstruction with secondary renal impairment on one or both sides is extremely common in the late stages, and urinary tract complications are the most frequent cause of death in both untreated and unsuccessfully treated patients. Direct spread anteriorly or posteriorly may eventually lead to invasion of the wall of the bladder or rectum respectively, since both organs lie in close approximation to the cervix and upper vagina. Large-bowel obstruction and ureteral or urethral obstruction may be produced in this manner, and when complete penetration of the walls of these viscera occurs, vesicovaginal or rectovaginal fistulas or both result.

Spread of cervical cancer via lymphatic channels with involvement of the pelvic lymph nodes is also frequent (Fig. 47). The intermediate paracervical (ureteral) and

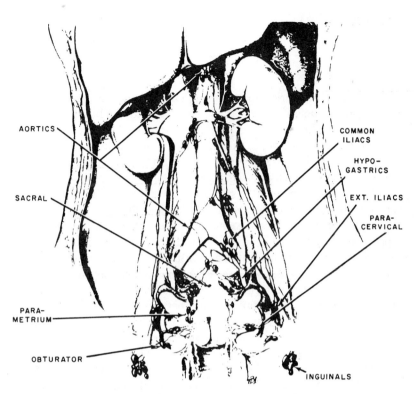

Figure 47
Routes of lymphatic spread in cervical cancer. (From E. Henriksen. The Lymph
Nodes and Lymph Channels of the Pelvis. In J. V. Meigs [Ed.], *The Surgical Treat-
ment of Cancer of the Cervix.* New York: Grune & Stratton, 1954.)

parametrial nodes are sometimes the first to be affected, but direct metastatic extension to the pelvic wall nodes is much more common (external iliac, obturator, and
hypogastric node groups); in more advanced cases, the common iliac, sacral, aortic,
and even inguinal nodes may be involved. The more extensive the local lesion, the
more frequently will lymph node metastases be observed. The approximate incidence
of lymph node metastases with respect to each of the progressively more advanced
clinical stages of the disease (see the next section) as determined by studies of surgical specimens reported by various clinics is as follows: Stage I, 15 percent; Stage II,
25 to 35 percent; Stage III, 35 to 60 percent; Stage IV, 50 to 65 percent.

Metastatic spread of cervical cancer via the bloodstream is decidedly uncommon,
although pulmonary, skeletal, and even cerebral metastases are occasionally encountered, usually in the presence of hopelessly advanced disease or in the presence of
rapidly growing, highly anaplastic tumors. It is thus apparent that although cervical
cancer may undergo extensive local spread and has a marked proclivity for lymphatic
involvement, it tends, even in its advanced stages, to remain confined to the pelvis

and pelvic lymph nodes. This feature of its natural history has an important bearing
on the management of cervical cancer in its more advanced phases.

Clinical Stages

Originally established as a basis for comparing the results of therapy by various
methods and in various treatment centers throughout the world, the International
Classification (formerly the League of Nations Classification) of the Stages of Carcinoma of the Uterine Cervix also serves as an extremely useful guide to prognosis.
Furthermore, it provides a helpful framework within which to plan and discuss
general principles of therapy as well as specific details of treatment applicable to
individual patients with approximately the same extent of disease. Clinical staging
is in essence an estimate of the extent of the disease based on the local, palpable
findings on abdominal, pelvic, and rectal examinations, preferably done under
anesthesia, supplemented by any information obtained by cystoscopy, proctoscopy,
and chest and skeletal roentgenograms that might further define the local extent or
possible distant spread of the disease. With the exception of large, palpable pelvic
lymph node metastases, the clinical staging depends primarily on the extent of the
local disease and, for example, is not influenced by whether or not the lymph nodes
in a patient with Stage I carcinoma treated by radical Wertheim hysterectomy and
pelvic lymphadenectomies prove on microscopic examination to be involved by
tumor. (Such a case is still classified as Stage I, with positive lymph nodes.) It
should also be remembered that clinical staging completely disregards the histology
of the tumor, and furthermore that the clinical **Stages I, II, III,** and **IV** are completely
unrelated to, and should not be confused with, the histologic estimate of the degree
of malignancy, the microscopic **grades 1, 2, 3,** and **4.**

The International Classification of the Clinical Stages of Cervical Cancer (Fig. 48)
may be briefly outlined as follows:

Stage 0: Intraepithelial carcinoma (carcinoma in situ).

Stage I: The lesion is entirely confined to the cervix, regardless of the size of
the tumor. The very early, subclinical microcarcinomas also fall in this category
and are now classified as Ia (1), a lesion that is predominately carcinoma in situ
but with penetration of the basement membrane and invasion of the adjacent
stroma to a depth of less than 1 mm; and Ia (2), which is occult invasive cancer —
either an extensive microinvasive cancer with deeper penetration of the stroma
but without a gross clinical lesion, or a clinically recognizable invasive lesion that
is hidden from view in the endocervical canal. If tumor emboli are present in
blood vessels or lymphatics on microscopic examination, a microinvasive lesion
should probably always be assigned to Stage Ia (2), and the patient should probably also always receive the same therapy as patients with Stage Ib lesions, i.e.,
radical surgery or adequate radiation therapy. All other frankly invasive, clinically
recognizable Stage I carcinomas are placed in Stage Ib. Lesions accompanied only
by extension upward to involve the body of the uterus are also included in Stage I,

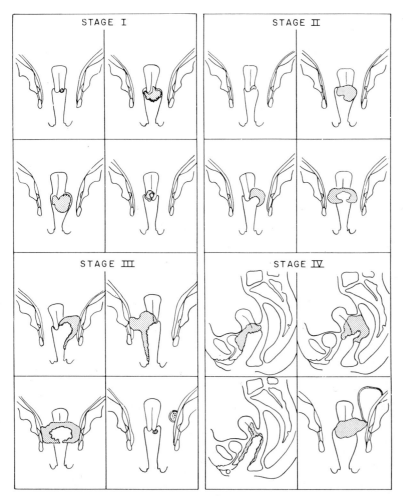

Figure 48
Clinical stages of cervical cancer (International Classification). (From T. H. Green, Jr. Gynecology. In G. L. Nardi and G. D. Zuidema [Eds.], *Surgery: A Concise Guide to Clinical Practice* [3rd ed.]. Boston: Little, Brown, 1972, Chap. 39.)

even though they are no longer strictly confined to the cervix, since spread to the corpus is usually along the surface of the endocervical canal and appears to have no unfavorable prognostic significance.

Stage II: The lesion has spread beyond the cervix to involve the vagina (but not the lower one-third) and/or the paracervical region on one or both sides but does not extend to the pelvic walls. Further subdivision into Stage IIa (vaginal extension only) and Stage IIb (with paracervical extension) is also employed and is meaningful, because the IIa lesions are potentially more curable than the IIb lesions.

Stage III: The lesion involves the lower one-third of the vagina (IIIa, no extension to the pelvic walls), or has infiltrated the paracervical tissues all the way to the pelvic wall on one or both sides (IIIb), or is associated with palpable, unequivocally involved lymph nodes on the pelvic wall. Ureteral obstruction on one or both sides, as demonstrated by intravenous pyelography, has recently been included among the criteria for classifying the lesion as Stage IIIb.

Stage IV: The lesion has invaded the bladder or rectum (IVa), or has extended outside the true pelvis (IVb), (e.g., vulvar metastases; huge pelvic-wall metastases palpable as abdominal masses; distant metastases in the upper abdomen, lungs, skeleton, inguinal, or supraclavicular nodes).

SYMPTOMATOLOGY

As already noted, the typical patient with clinically obvious epidermoid cervical cancer is a multipara between 45 and 55 years of age (primary adenocarcinoma of the cervix has tended to reach its peak incidence in a slightly older age group) who married and delivered her first child at an early age (often before the age of 20).

It should be noted at this point, that with the recent trend toward earlier and more promiscuous sexual activity, dysplasia, carcinoma in situ, and even early invasive cervical cancer are beginning to be encountered in a much younger age group nowadays, with all three of these lesions occurring even in teenagers. Thus, even the teenaged female, if she is "on the pill" or is engaging in sexual activity, regardless of her contraceptive program or lack of one, should be offered the benefits of regular examinations and annual cytologic screening. Several studies have shown that the rate of "significant cervical epithelial atypias" in this group of sexually active, often promiscuous teenagers was two or three times that of the general population of women of all ages.

Probably the first symptom of early carcinoma of the cervix is a thin, watery, sometimes blood-tinged vaginal discharge that is frequently ignored by the patient. The cardinal and universal symptom is intermittent, painless, abnormal intermenstrual bleeding, often initially only spotting occurring postcoitally or after douching. As the tumor enlarges, the bleeding episodes become heavier, more frequent, and of longer duration, and the patient may also describe what seems to her to be an increase in the amount and duration of her regular periods; ultimately, the bleeding becomes essentially continuous. In the older women, the occurrence of obviously abnormal postmenopausal bleeding often results in the patient's seeking medical attention somewhat more promptly. There tends to be a delay in the appearance of symptoms in primary adenocarcinomas of the cervix, since the majority arise higher up in the endocervical canal. For the same reason, they often remain undetected by either clinical or cytologic examinations until they are considerably larger and more extensive. Further, some varieties of adenocarcinoma are not very responsive to radiation and some are highly anaplastic lesions that metastasize early and widely. All these facts help to account for the much poorer prognosis with adenocarcinomas.

Late symptoms of the more advanced stages of the disease include: the development of pain referred to the back, flank, or leg, usually secondary to involvement of the ureters, pelvic walls, or sciatic nerve roots or resulting from pressure from involved and enlarging paraaortic lymph nodes on lumbar nerve roots; the occurrence of dysuria, hematuria, rectal bleeding, or constipation due to bladder or rectal invasion; or the appearance of edema of one or both lower extremities as the result of lymphatic and venous blockage by extensive pelvic-wall infiltration and nodal metastases. Massive hemorrhage and the development of uremia and profound cachexia may occur as preterminal events.

DIAGNOSIS, DETERMINATION OF THE EXTENT OF DISEASE, AND GENERAL EVALUATION OF THE PATIENT

Carcinoma In Situ and Early Invasive Carcinoma

Carcinoma in situ as well as early invasive carcinoma (microcarcinoma) are invariably asymptomatic, and either may exist even though the cervix appears to be normal on speculum examination. However, both may be detected in the asymptomatic phase by (1) routine cytologic study (vaginal smears, endocervical smears) and/or (2) Schiller's test with biopsy of "Schiller-negative" areas of the cervical epithelium (abnormal areas of nonglycogen-containing epithelium that do not stain with Schiller's iodine solution); (3) colposcopy and colpomicroscopy (see Chap. 2) have also been shown in the hands of those skilled and experienced in their use to be valuable in the detection of early lesions and to be particularly useful in selecting specific sites for biopsy in asymptomatic patients with abnormal cytologic findings but negative or equivocal findings on clinical examination.

In the case of asymptomatic patients in whom pelvic examination seems normal, but routine cytologic smear is reported positive for squamous carcinoma cells, the following diagnostic routine is suggested:

1. Multiple punch biopsies of the squamocolumnar junction of the cervix at 6, 9, 12, and 3 o'clock sites, and/or from abnormal areas of cervical epithelium as indicated by Schiller's test. (These procedures can be done in the office or clinic.)

2. If any of these biopsies reveal invasive carcinoma, further studies and treatment should be carried out as subsequently outlined. (Diagnostic conization is obviously unnecessary in this situation.)

3. If the biopsy findings are positive but are reported as showing only carcinoma in situ or only dysplasia of varying degrees of severity, then hospitalization for cold-knife cone biopsy of the cervix (removing the entire squamocolumnar junction) and fractional curettage (separate specimens from the endocervix and endometrial cavity) may be necessary to be absolutely certain that the preliminary biopsy specimens were not taken from the periphery of an early invasive carcinoma. In other words, the presence of carcinoma in situ in a simple cervical biopsy specimen does not yet rule out the presence of invasive cancer elsewhere in the cervix; rather, it in fact

implies that invasive cancer may already exist elsewhere in the cervix (or that invasive cancer may appear later on if the cervix is allowed to remain). It is estimated that 5 to 10 percent of patients in whom simple, cervical biopsies reveal only carcinoma in situ will be found to have invasive cancer if an adequate cone biopsy is performed. (In patients in whom a simple biopsy reveals severe dysplasia, 25 to 50 percent will be found to have intraepithelial cancer, and 1 to 2 percent will have early invasive cancer.) The cone biopsy should be carefully cut into small blocks by the pathologist and multiple sections from each block examined microscopically. If a diagnosis of carcinoma in situ is confirmed, and no invasive cancer is demonstrated, therapy is as outlined under Treatment.

If colposcopy is available — and it is currently becoming widely used — a much better alternative to routine cone biopsy in this situation will be careful colposcopic study and colposcopically guided, multiple biopsies of the most suspicious areas of the cervix, plus endocervical curettage with a small, sharp endocervical biopsy curet suitable for office use. If a colposcope and a trained and experienced colposcopist are at hand, this program for the systematic study of the cervical epithelium will render cone biopsy unnecessary in roughly 90 percent of this group of asymptomatic patients without clinical evidence of cancer but with abnormal cytologic findings. In about 10 percent of such patients, cold-knife conization will still be essential for one or more of the following reasons:

a. Colposcopy has revealed the abnormal epithelial lesion to be large and/or to extend out of sight within the endocervical canal, or the so-called cervical transformation zone in which most cervical neoplasms originate extends out of sight within the endocervical canal.
b. Colposcopically directed or random biopsies have revealed lesions that are histologically less serious than would have been predicted on the basis of the degree of cytologic abnormality.
c. Any of the biopsies have revealed early or questionable stromal invasion in what otherwise would be considered only carcinoma in situ.

In (a) and (b), cone biopsy is essential to confirm or rule out invasive cancer; in (c), cone biopsy is mandatory to determine the degree of microinvasion in order to plan proper therapy.

Obviously, if an experienced colposcopist is not available, cone biopsy remains the only safe diagnostic alternative.

4. If the punch biopsy findings are negative, the patient should also be hospitalized for total cone biopsy of the cervix and fractional curettage, studies that will usually reveal the source of the malignant cells and suggest the proper treatment.

If these further studies are also negative, however, and if carcinoma of the vagina, vulva, urethra, and bladder have also been ruled out, it may be elected to:

1. Follow the patient carefully, and if subsequent smears are negative, continue regular follow-up observations indefinitely. (The positive smear may have been a

rare false-positive, perhaps the result of atypical cervical epithelial changes; or the lesion may have been a tiny carcinoma in situ, excised by the cone biopsy but missed histologically in the multiple section technique.) If subsequent smears are positive, however, hysterectomy is warranted and advisable. An exception might occasionally be made in the case of a young woman desirous of further pregnancies, provided that she could be kept under surveillance, would agree to indefinite follow-up, and was aware that further treatment could not be postponed for long in the face of continuous abnormal smears.

2. Carry out simple total hysterectomy immediately, an approach that is probably justified in many cases, particularly in women no longer of childbearing age or in whom prolonged cooperation in a regular follow-up program cannot be guaranteed.

In the case of asymptomatic patients in whom routine cytologic smear is reported positive for adenocarcinoma cells, prompt hospitalization for fractional curettage and examination under anesthesia is indicated. The lesion will usually prove to be a carcinoma of the endometrium or endocervix, but occasionally the malignant cells will be found to have been shed by an early primary ovarian or tubal carcinoma or, more rarely, by a distant abdominal neoplasm (e.g., stomach, pancreas). Thus, in spite of negative findings on a D&C, if repeated cytologic smears positive for adenocarcinoma cells are obtained, exploration and removal of the uterus with both adnexa must seriously be considered.

Invasive Carcinoma of the Cervix

Vaginal smears are invariably positive in invasive carcinoma of the cervix, although cytologic recognition of malignant cells is occasionally difficult or impossible because of associated heavy bleeding.

INSPECTION AND BIOPSY

Lesions arising at the squamocolumnar junction are usually obvious on speculum examination, and biopsy confirmation is readily obtained. Lesions arising within the endocervical canal may not be visible. However, the cervical segment frequently takes on a typical barrel shape due to the expanding growth within. Histologic confirmation is obtained by fractional curettage, which will also distinguish between primary carcinoma of the endocervix and a primary carcinoma of the endometrium with secondary involvement of the cervix (carcinoma corporis et cervicis).

ESTIMATION OF EXTENT OF PRIMARY TUMOR

Clinical staging is done in accordance with the International Classification. When doubt exists as to the correct stage, final decision should be postponed until the patient is examined under anesthesia.

OTHER STUDIES

Other studies to complete the evaluation of the local lesion and all potential avenues of direct and metastatic spread include an intravenous pyelogram, chest and skeletal roentgenograms and bone scan, cystoscopy, proctoscopy (occasionally a barium enema also), liver scan, and lymphangiography, or lymph node scan.

EVALUATION OF THE PATIENT

Hemoglobin, hematocrit, blood volume studies, total protein, nonprotein nitrogen (NPN), serum electrolytes, and general medical status are especially valuable and necessary if bleeding has been excessive or prolonged, urinary tract function has been impaired by extension of the tumor, or weight loss and poor nutrition in the more advanced stages of the disease have complicated the picture. It is extremely important to restore a normal blood volume and normal protein and electrolyte balance prior to treatment, whether radiation therapy or radical surgery is contemplated. Whether or not urinary tract impairment will also have to be dealt with before beginning treatment of the cancer will depend on the nature and extent of the impairment.

TREATMENT

Carcinoma In Situ

In young women, when preservation of childbearing function is desirable, an approach involving attempted total excision of the lesion by cold-knife conization of the cervix or treatment by cryosurgery or electrocautery, and prolonged, regular follow-up observation is permissible. The facts of the situation should of course be carefully explained to the patient and her husband, emphasizing the need for careful and prolonged follow-up. Reassurance can be given that there is little, if any, risk involved in conservative management, since not only is the lesion frequently totally excised and permanently controlled by the cone biopsy, cryosurgery, or electrocautery, but there is also a wide safety margin implicit in the interval of 5 to 10 years usually required for progression to invasive cancer and during which persistence or recurrence of the intraepithelial neoplastic process will surely be detected by a program of regular follow-up examinations. One should constantly bear in mind, however, that even when conization, cryosurgery, or electrocautery has been properly performed, the cervix may harbor residual carcinoma in situ in as many as 25 to 30 percent of cases, and that even microinvasive carcinoma may be missed occasionally (in 1 to 2 percent) by what seems to have been an adequate cone biopsy. Therefore, if positive smears persist or recur, immediate repeat biopsy study is imperative. Occasionally, further management by conization is warranted, but a definitive hysterectomy will usually then be required if the development of frank invasive carcinoma has again been excluded.

In essentially all others, simple total hysterectomy is indicated, with removal of a wide vaginal cuff (see Fig. 51B) (at least 2 cm all around — or more if a preoperative Schiller's test performed on the vaginal mucosa delineates areas that do not take the stain normally and suggests more extensive involvement of vaginal vault epithelium by carcinoma in situ). Whether or not the ovaries are preserved will depend primarily on the age of the patient. Total hysterectomy with removal of a generous vaginal cuff should cure essentially 100 percent of patients with carcinoma in situ of the cervix. The recurrence rate is less than 0.5 percent in most series when an adequate operation is properly done, while the recurrence rate when carcinoma in situ is treated by conization is roughly 4 to 5 percent. When there is a recurrence, it is usually because (1) a preliminary colposcopy with guided biopsies plus endocervical curettage (or a diagnostic cone biopsy, as indicated, plus endocervical curettage) were omitted, improperly performed, or the specimens subjected to inadequate microscopic study, and the cervical lesion in retrospect was a microcarcinoma (early stromal invasion), not carcinoma in situ; or (2) the upper vagina was inadequately evaluated prior to hysterectomy by Schiller's test and/or biopsies of suspicious areas, and, as a result, the vaginal cuff removed with the uterus failed to include areas of vaginal carcinoma in situ. Patients treated by total hysterectomy and excision of a generous vaginal cuff should be followed at regular intervals by examination and cytologic study to detect the occasional recurrence of intraepithelial carcinoma or development of invasive cancer in either the remaining vaginal epithelium or the vulva. For it must be remembered that the entire squamous epithelial lining of the lower female genital tract tends to show a regional predisposition to both intraepithelial and invasive carcinoma. Although the cervix is by far the most frequent site of malignant change, simultaneous or sequential development of carcinoma in situ or invasive cancer in the vagina or vulva occurs in perhaps 10 percent of women who have had carcinoma in situ of the cervix. The removal of the upper 2 to 3 cm of vagina eliminates the second most common site of malignant change, and the chances of subsequent development of carcinoma in the lower vagina and vulva are relatively slight.

It should be emphasized again that cases in which microscopic study of specimens from colposcopically directed or cervical cone biopsies reveals **carcinoma in situ with definite early stromal invasion** (microcarcinoma) must be classified as Stage Ia (2) invasive cancer of the cervix, and their proper management requires that they be treated as such. As previously noted, simple "glandular involvement" does not imply invasion, nor does the presence of "questionable stromal invasion" by an occasional cell in an area or two along the basement membrane justify altering the diagnosis of carcinoma in situ or modifying the standard treatment. However, if the stromal invasion is definite and significant in amount, the lesion should definitely be considered as Stage Ia. If the stromal invasion is less than 1 mm (2 mm at most) (only a very few consider 4 to 5 mm to be a "safe depth" for conservative management) and is not accompanied by the appearance of tumor cells within vascular or lymphatic channels, i.e., Stage Ia (1), standard total abdominal hysterectomy (or vaginal hysterectomy) with removal of a wide vaginal cuff is probably adequate treatment.

At the other extreme are patients in whom the final histologic diagnosis is cervical anaplasia, "not sufficiently advanced to be classified as frank carcinoma in situ"; such patients can often safely and properly be treated by conization alone with continued observation, particularly if preservation of childbearing function is desirable. The follow-up program must be a regular and indefinite one, however, even in the case of dysplasia. In the older woman, a strong case can be made for hysterectomy if the lesion is extensive and severe, especially if abnormal smears persist after conization.

Microcarcinoma

As has already been made abundantly clear, many patients with microinvasive carcinoma of the cervix should be treated by adequate radiation therapy or radical surgery, not by simple hysterectomy. If the stromal invasion extends to a depth of more than 1 to 2 mm (only a minority continue to feel that stromal invasion should extend at least 4 to 5 mm deep before being considered "potentially serious"), and/or if there is lymphatic or vascular permeation visible in the biopsy specimen, i.e., Stage 1a (2), the lesion must be treated as an early small but definitely invasive Stage I cervical carcinoma. That these are truly invasive cancers is also attested to by the 3 to 4 percent incidence of lymph node metastases in this group as compared with a 15 percent incidence in Stage Ib cases. A strong case can be made for radical surgery rather than radiotherapy in the management of microcarcinoma, because it permits preservation of the ovaries and avoids radiation changes in the remaining vagina in this group of women, who are usually younger than those with clinically obvious cervical cancer. The importance of employing a radical Wertheim hysterectomy rather than a simple hysterectomy with a generous vaginal cuff lies in the need for wide paracervical, paravaginal, and parametrial resection even for this type of microinvasive lesion if maximal potential cure rates (95 percent or more) are to be obtained.

Although simple total hysterectomy will cure a considerable number of true microcarcinomas, i.e., Stage Ia (2), numerous reports indicate that the cure rates achieved will be significantly less, in the range of only 40 to 75 percent at best, depending on where in the histologic spectrum of microcarcinoma the particular microinvasive lesion happens to fall. The difficulties and poor results achieved in the treatment of recurrences where inadvertent simple hysterectomy has been performed in the presence of unsuspected early cervical carcinoma (the ultimate cure rate in this unfortunate group of patients has ranged from 22 to 57 percent in a number of reported series) also attest to the inadequacy of simple hysterectomy in the management of early invasive cervical cancer. Therefore, to employ simple hysterectomy routinely for microcarcinoma does not really seem to be in the best interests of the patient who, as a result of modern methods and programs of cancer detection, is fortunate enough to have her cervical cancer discovered at an early stage when cure rates approach 100 percent if adequate treatment is given. The added argument, still sometimes heard, that radical surgery (or adequate radiotherapy) carries too high a risk or morbidity to warrant use in the management of these early invasive cancers is fallacious, since the mortality of radical surgery is essentially zero, and the "10 to 15 percent incidence of fistulas and other serious postoperative complications" still sometimes cited is now a relic of the past, modern methods of operative technique and postoperative management having reduced this incidence to 1 percent or less. The same can be said with regard to the morbidity of modern radiotherapy.

One cannot, however, fault the attempts to "tailor" the radical surgical procedure somewhat to these early cervical cancers. But it should be pointed out that the "modified Wertheim procedure" used by some pelvic surgeons in dealing with microinvasive carcinoma of the cervix actually involves essentially the same dissection performed in the radical Wertheim operation, perhaps not quite so extensive, and often omitting lymphadenectomy. However, it is a far cry from simple total hysterectomy, and therein lies the secret of its success in achieving highly satisfactory cure rates for microcarcinoma. Pelvic lymphadenectomy is perhaps less important, since lymph node metastases are much less frequent with microinvasive cancers. However, since nodal metastases do occur occasionally, and since node dissections add nothing to the morbidity of the procedure when done by properly trained and experienced pelvic surgeons, omitting lymphadenectomy makes little, if any, sense.

Invasive Cervical Carcinoma

METHODS OF TREATMENT

Radiation Treatment

Ever since the discovery of radium and x-rays, radiation has been the most frequently applied form of treatment for cervical cancer and is still considered to be the primary treatment of choice in the majority of clinics. Even in the early years of its use, its results were far superior to those then being obtained by the relatively newly conceived and at the time hazardous attempts at radical surgical excision. The basic plan currently employed in most centers consists of the use of intrauterine and intravaginal radium sources to deliver approximately 5000 to 6000 R to the primary tumor and the immediately adjacent paracervical and paravaginal tissues. The general principles of therapy are the same whether the Stockholm, Manchester, or some other technique is followed in the application of the radium, and regardless of the design and configuration of the radium applicators themselves. They may be Stockholm "vaginal boxes" plus intrauterine "stems," Manchester "vaginal ovoids" plus intrauterine "stems," or one of the combined types of uterovaginal radium holders such as the Ernst applicator (Fig. 49), all of which are available in different sizes to conform to the varied anatomy in each individual case, but the basic plan of therapy follows that shown in Figure 50. Usually one half of the total radium dosage is given in each of two courses approximately three weeks apart, the radium usually remaining in place roughly 36 to 40 hours on each occasion. Each application requires a short period of general anesthesia, at which time the clinical staging can be even more accurately confirmed. Anteroposterior and lateral roentgenograms of

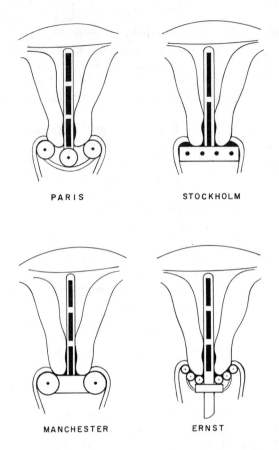

PARIS   STOCKHOLM

MANCHESTER   ERNST

Figure 49
Various types of radium applicators employed in radiation therapy of cervical cancer.

the pelvis are obtained as soon as feasible after placement of the radium sources as a final check on their correct position and to provide a basis for a more precise calculation of the amount of radiation delivered to various areas of the pelvic cavity. Two or three weeks after the final radium application, external x-ray therapy is instituted to each lateral pelvic region to bring the roentgen dosage delivered there and at the pelvic walls up to levels comparable with those attained in the tumor and central pelvic area.

Following the introduction in 1970 of the "afterloading" technique and specially designed afterloading applicators, as well as more flexible, smaller sources of radium-266 or cesium-127 (less often, iridium-192, cobalt-60, or gold-198), it is now possible virtually to eliminate radiation exposure to physicians and other personnel involved in the implantations. These modifications in technique have also improved the accuracy of placement, simplified the procedure, and in some cases have shortened the time period or entirely eliminated the need for anesthesia.

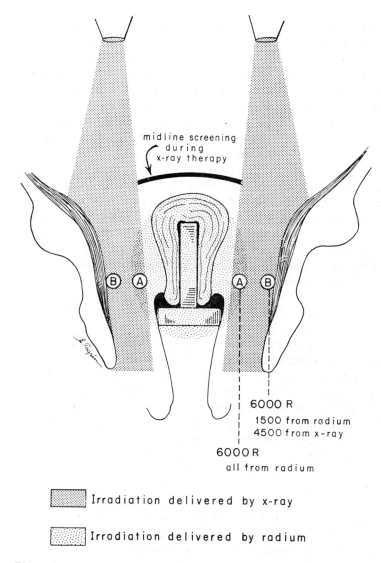

midline screening
during
x-ray therapy

(B)(A)   (A)(B)

6000 R
1500 from radium
4500 from x-ray

6000 R
all from radium

Irradiation delivered by x-ray

Irradiation delivered by radium

Figure 50
Basic plan of radiotherapy of cervical cancer. (From T. H. Green, Jr. Gynecology.
In G. L. Nardi and G. D. Zuidema [Eds.], *Surgery: A Concise Guide to Clinical
Practice* [3rd ed.]. Boston: Little, Brown, 1972, Chap. 39.)

In most institutions, supravoltage therapy has replaced conventional orthovoltage,
with the 22-Mev betatron currently representing the most sophisticated equipment
in terms of greater effectiveness with less morbidity. In some clinics the cobalt-60
beam is still used as the source of external irradiation, and in a few institutions
external irradiation delivered through a vaginal field or port (vaginal cone therapy)

has for years been utilized in place of radium. Maximal success with any method of radiation therapy depends on the skill and experience of the therapist, especially on his ability to tailor the details of therapy (dosage, type of application, and the order in which radium and external irradiation are given) to the requirements of each individual case. Great care must be exercised in the proper placement of the radium applicators and judicious selection of the proper dosages to be administered by means of radium and external irradiation. Only in this way will maximal curability be achieved while minimizing the severity and morbidity of the radiation reaction in the normal tissues and structures adjacent to the tumor. Despite all precautions, serious complications (e.g., proctitis, vaginal vault necrosis, hemorrhagic cystitis, parametritis, rectovaginal fistula, ureteral obstruction due to periureteral radiation fibrosis, bowel necrosis, obstruction, and perforation, vesicovaginal fistula, massive hemorrhage from radiation necrosis, to list the most common in descending order of frequency) will occur in 25 to 30 percent of patients, and a 2 to 3 percent mortality from radiation complications has been reported in many series. (See also Chapter 22 for a discussion of the complications of radiation therapy and their management.)

There are some advocates of pretreatment exploratory laparotomy prior to beginning radiotherapy, especially in patients with advanced Stage II or Stage III lesions, in order to "stage the extent of disease" more accurately and particularly to determine whether or not paraaortic lymph node involvement is present. If such proves to be the case, the x-ray treatment program can be planned in advance to include the paraaortic areas within the field of therapy. A more feasible plan is to perform pretreatment lymphangiography, since 75 to 80 percent of patients with paraaortic lymph node metastases will be detected in this way without the need for major surgery in the form of exploratory laparotomy. Only a small percentage of patients, most of whom have Stage II disease, will benefit from paraaortic radiation therapy. Because of significant complications in 20 to 25 percent of cases, it should not be given prophylactically to all patients, but only to those with known paraaortic metastases proved by lymphangiogram or lymph node biopsy.

Radical Surgery

The origins of the radical surgical attack on cervical cancer are to be found in the pioneer efforts of Wertheim, Amreich, Schauta, and others among their colleagues in the Austrian-German school of surgery that flourished at the turn of the century. Although enthusiasm waned when radiation therapy first appeared on the scene, interest in the surgical approach was kept alive by its continued use in a few centers during the twenties and thirties (notably throughout Austria and Germany and also by Bonney in England) and was rekindled, particularly in the United States, by the outstanding work of Meigs [24, 25]. Largely through his efforts in perfecting and extending the radical operation of Wertheim, to which he also added bilateral pelvic lymph node dissections, and as a result of his demonstration in a large series of patients that such an extended radical abdominal hysterectomy with bilateral pelvic lymphadenectomy could be carried out with essentially no mortality and that it was highly effective in the cure of the early stages of cervical cancer, radical surgery has now become an equally important and accepted method of treatment. Similarly, the radical vaginal hysterectomy originally popularized by Schauta has been further perfected and extensively utilized in some centers, notably by Navratil in Austria, Bastiaanse in Holland, Mitra in India (who added simultaneous extraperitoneal lymphadenectomies with the hope of increasing the curability of patients with lymphatic spread), and by McCall [23] in this country. Finally, during the past 20 years, the surgical approach has been further extended to encompass the advanced stages of cervical cancer through the development and clinical trial by Brunschwig [3, 4] and others of the so-called superradical procedures termed **pelvic exenterations**, the rationale for and the results of which are further described in the discussion of the management of Stage III and Stage IV lesions.

The modifying adjective **radical** applied to either the Wertheim abdominal hysterectomy or the Schauta vaginal hysterectomy refers to the wide removal of the paravaginal, paracervical, parametrial, and uterosacral tissues, along with a portion of the cul-de-sac and a generous length of vaginal canal, all in direct continuity with the uterus. Thus essentially all the tissue between the pelvic walls laterally, the bladder and pubic rami anteriorly, and the floor of the pelvis and rectum posteriorly is resected with the uterus, leaving only the cleanly dissected ureters traversing the essentially skeletonized pelvis. Furthermore, the lymphatic channels and pelvic lymph nodes that accompany and surround the common iliac, external iliac, and hypogastric artery and vein and that lie in the obturator fossa are also completely resected, cleanly dissecting these major vessels and the subjacent pelvic walls on both sides. The extent of the dissection is perhaps best illustrated by the typical final specimen obtained by either the Wertheim or Schauta radical hysterectomy, as contrasted with a simple hysterectomy specimen (Fig. 51A and C), and by the final appearance of the pelvis at the completion of a radical Wertheim hysterectomy and pelvic lymphadenectomy (Fig. 51D).

The chief arguments favoring a more widespread use of radical surgery in the primary management of the early stages of cervical cancer are (1) the admitted existence of the phenomenon of radioresistant tumors (in 15 to 20 percent of clinically favorable Stage I carcinomas, for example, tumor persists in the cervix despite adequate radiation therapy, and whether the "resistance" is a property of the tumor, the host, or the host-tumor relationship, is beside the point); and (2) the probability that radiation therapy alone does not offer the best hope of curing the patient with pelvic lymph node metastases in association with Stage I or Stage II cervical cancer. In numerous reported series, the expected incidence of pelvic node metastases is roughly 15 percent in Stage I and 30 percent in Stage II. In patients undergoing pelvic lymphadenectomies after radiation therapy, the incidence of positive lymph nodes falls to only 10 percent in Stage I and 20 percent in Stage II, indicating that radiation therapy has apparently eradicated lymph node disease in only one third of the patients. Radical hysterectomy and bilateral pelvic lymphadenectomy achieve somewhat better results, since of Stage I and early Stage II patients with positive nodes, nearly 50 percent are alive and well at 5- and 10-year follow-up examinations. In the hands of experienced pelvic surgeons, the results of radical surgery in the

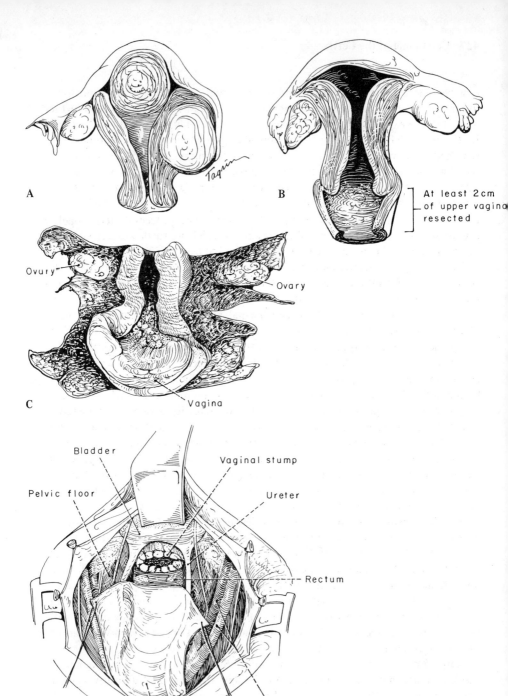

A

B

At least 2 cm
of upper vagina
resected

Ovary

Ovary

C

Vagina

Bladder

Vaginal stump

Pelvic floor

Ureter

Rectum

Iliac vessels

D

Peritoneum

treatment of Stage I and early Stage II cancer of the cervix are slightly better than the results of radiotherapy. However, because of the limited number of such skilled and highly trained surgeons, radiation therapy continues to be the primary treatment modality in the majority of institutions, with a surgical approach reserved for radiation failures.

Obviously, the Wertheim and Schauta procedures are primarily designed to deal with Stage I and Stage II lesions. When the tumor has invaded the bladder or rectum — a situation formerly considered hopelessly incurable surgically and even today only rarely cured by radiation therapy — the more recently evolved superradical surgical procedures now offer a chance for cure to a significantly greater number of patients. The pelvic exenteration operations involve the same wide dissection previously described for the radical Wertheim hysterectomy, often with actual ligation and removal of the hypogastric vessels, together with en-bloc removal of the bladder, lower ureters, entire vagina, often with the vulva and perineum, and the rectum (total pelvic exenteration). In selected cases, where the tumor has not extended posteriorly, the rectum may be spared (anterior exenteration); less often, when the direction and extent of the tumor spread affects the rectum alone and has left the region of the bladder and lower ureters uninvolved, only the rectum need be sacrificed (posterior exenteration). If the rectum is removed, sigmoid colostomy is of course required.

When the bladder and lower ureters have been resected, urinary diversion is accomplished either by transplanting the ureters into the colon a few inches proximal to the colostomy (this technique has now largely been abandoned) or, preferably, into an isolated short segment of distal ileum brought out through the right lower quadrant of the abdominal wall (the procedure devised by Bricker and known as the Bricker pouch, ileal loop, or bilateral ureteroileostomy) (Fig. 52). A modification of Bricker's technique of urinary diversion applicable when total pelvic exenteration is done involves use of an isolated segment of sigmoid rather than an ileal loop for the urinary conduit. The sigmoid conduit provides equally satisfactory function without complications and avoids the need for a small-bowel operation; the ileal loop remains the best choice in patients undergoing only anterior exenteration. Whatever procedure is performed, suitable colostomy or ileostomy bags are available for the constant collection of urine, and the situation is not as troublesome for the patients as might be supposed, most of them being able to lead normal, active lives, with the exception of permanent loss of normal sexual function. Obviously, patients undergoing pelvic exenteration must be in good general physical condition and mentally and emotionally capable of adjusting to and coping with their postoperative situation; only rarely do they fail to meet these requirements, however. From a philosophical

---

Figure 51
Operative approach to the early stages of carcinoma of the cervix. A. Simple total hysterectomy specimen (for comparison with B and C). B. Total hysterectomy with resection of a wide vaginal cuff for carcinoma in situ of the cervix. C. Radical Wertheim hysterectomy specimen. D. Skeletonized pelvis following radical Wertheim hysterectomy and bilateral pelvic lymphadenectomy.

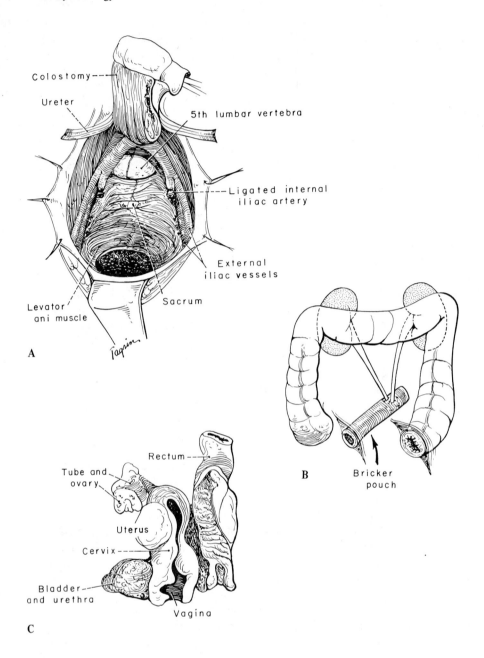

Figure 52
Total pelvic exenteration. A. The completely dissected pelvis. B. The bilateral ureteroileostomy, employing an isolated ileal segment (Bricker pouch). C. The resulting surgical specimen.

viewpoint, the operation of pelvic exenteration, although anatomically mutilating, usually seems justifiable in the eyes of the patient, her family, and her physicians, since it offers a potential chance for cure in what is otherwise a hopeless situation. (See also Chapter 22 for a discussion of the complications of radical surgery and their management.)

GENERAL PLAN OF PRIMARY TREATMENT ACCORDING TO CLINICAL STAGE

Stage I

Either radiation therapy or radical surgery (the Wertheim-Meigs radical abdominal hysterectomy with pelvic lymphadenectomy or the Schauta radical vaginal hysterectomy) may be elected with the expectation of approximately equal cure rates. Radical surgery is probably to be favored over radiation therapy in younger women with Stage I and even early Stage II lesions, since it avoids exposing them to the long-term hazards of pelvic irradiation (i.e., late complications involving the gastrointestinal and urinary tracts and an increased risk later on of malignancy in other pelvic organs) and also leaves them a shortened but normal vaginal epithelial canal, with more normal function. There is reason to suspect that many patients in whom radiation treatment proves unsuccessful have radioresistant tumors (or an unsuitable host-tumor relationship with respect to radiation response) and might have been cured by radical surgery, and that, on the other hand, certain apparently favorable early lesions that rapidly recur following radical surgery might have proved highly responsive to radiation therapy with resulting cure of the disease had radium and x-ray been employed instead. Ultimately, a method may evolve for the selection of one or the other as the optimal mode of therapy for each individual patient, giving radiation to those with known radiosensitive tumors and performing radical surgery on those with demonstrably radioresistant lesions.

A variety of attempts have been made over the years to solve the early, preferably pretreatment recognition of the radioresistant tumor, the initial efforts involving study of histologic changes induced in the tumor during the early phases of radiation therapy. These observations proved little more valuable than a simple clinical appraisal of gross tumor response; nor have efforts to correlate the specific histologic features of the tumor with its ultimate response to radiation been consistently fruitful. The most promising approach to date, introduced by Graham and Graham [14], has been the use of cytologic criteria based on study of specific alterations in the nuclear and cytoplasmic details in some of the benign vaginal cells both before treatment (sensitivity response [SR] cells) and, in the case of patients receiving radiation therapy, after the first radium application (radiation response [RR] cells). The percentage frequency with which SR or RR cells appear in the smear is employed in the attempt to judge whether in a given patient a favorable response to radiation is to be expected or whether a greater expectation of cure will be realized by a surgical approach. A long-term study of the end results of this cytologic method of selection, together with a review of other related approaches, has been reported by the author [16] and would be of interest to readers desiring more details.

Although the value and validity of any of the various techniques for the prediction of radiation response has yet to be established firmly, it is certainly to be hoped that a reliable method will ultimately be found for selecting the optimal treatment for the individual patient — radiation or radical surgery — for only then will both forms of therapy realize their true potential as co-partners in the overall management of the disease. Parenthetically, it should be noted that, in an effort to obtain the benefits of both, trials of combined therapy are in progress in some clinics, using either (1) radiation therapy first, using radium alone, sometimes supplemented by a reduced course of x-ray therapy, followed by radical hysterectomy, or (2) radical hysterectomy with postoperative full-pelvis external irradiation. Reported results have in some, but not all, instances suggested somewhat improved cure rates over those obtained by either treatment modality alone, but the incidence of serious complications has been significantly higher. There is also some evidence that patients with primary pure adenocarcinoma of the cervix are more effectively treated by radical surgery or a combination of irradiation and surgery than by radiotherapy alone (either a preliminary, reduced dosage of preoperative irradiation followed by radical hysterectomy, or a full course of radiotherapy followed by simply hysterectomy).

Stage II

Early Stage II lesions (only vaginal involvement, or with minimal paracervical involvement) are also suitable for either primary radiation therapy or a primary surgical attack by the Wertheim-Meigs radical abdominal or the Schauta radical vaginal procedure, the latter more recently often supplemented by extraperitoneal lymphadenectomy, with the expectation of comparable results. More advanced Stage II lesions, however, are probably best treated by primary radiation therapy. If the tumor fails to respond to radiation, a surgical approach can then be considered; either radical hysterectomy (abdominal or vaginal) or more extensive pelvic exenteration procedures may be necessary.

Posttreatment Early Follow-Up Program for Stage I and Stage II

Frequent, careful follow-up examinations are vital in the early weeks and months after treatment for Stage I and Stage II lesions. Particular attention should be paid to continued bleeding and discharge or to persistence of a suspicious visible cervical or palpable endocervical lesion, and endocervical curettage or cervical or vaginal biopsy would be indicated in either case. Regular follow-up cytologic smears should be taken; smears should be negative following radical surgery, and persistence of abnormal cells in the smear for more than two to three months after radiation therapy strongly suggests persistent disease. In this situation, if biopsy findings are positive, radical surgery should be immediately considered, since 10 to 20 percent of all postradiation recurrences in Stage I patients are still confined to the cervix, and an additional 30 to 40 percent are still within the field of, and potentially curable by, either radical hysterectomy or some type of pelvic exenteration.

Stage III

Primary treatment in Stage III should be by radiation, since approximately 25 percent will respond favorably and a cure will be achieved, whereas a primary surgical approach in this stage, assuming the lesion would prove at laparotomy to be resectable, would nearly always involve some form of pelvic exenteration. Because of the extent of the disease in Stage III it is sometimes impossible to apply radium initially. Under these circumstances, external x-ray therapy to the entire pelvis (approximately 5000 R) should be given first, and if regression occurs, the radium therapy can usually then be administered without difficulty. These patients should be followed extremely closely during and immediately after radiation therapy. If and as soon as it is apparent that radiation therapy has not controlled the disease, an attempt at radical surgery (pelvic exenteration) should be considered if the patient's general condition permits.

This plan of therapy assumes at least one normally functioning kidney and ureter and normal NPN and electrolyte balance. If the ureters are involved bilaterally, but hydronephrosis and hydroureter are not too severe, renal function adequate, and uremia absent or mild, radiation therapy can be cautiously begun in the hope that favorable response will relieve the obstruction. However, the situation should be watched closely, constantly checking the NPN and serum electrolytes and repeating the pyelograms at intervals as indicated. If one encounters bilateral complete or nearly complete ureteral obstruction with marked impairment of renal function and impending uremia, either when the patient is first seen or during the course of radiation therapy, the procedures to accomplish urinary diversion must be carried out. The choice of the type of urinary diversion and when it is to be performed will depend on the overall therapeutic plan, provided that the treatment still offers some hope of control of the disease and the effort is not merely a palliative one. (If there is no hope, progressive uremia may well prove a far more comfortable and kinder alternative to the prolongation of a hopeless situation, and urinary diversion would therefore be pointless and contraindicated.)

MAINTENANCE OF URINARY FUNCTION

If **radiation therapy** is selected as the primary mode of treatment and there is a reasonable expectation of cure, unilateral or bilateral temporary nephrostomy may be elected. Should it become apparent that radiation therapy is not causing regression, and an attempt at radical surgery is then contemplated, more definitive and permanent urinary diversion (e.g., bilateral ureteral anastomosis to an ileal pouch) can be accomplished at the time of laparotomy if the lesion proves resectable.

When **radical surgery** is selected as the primary form of treatment:

1. If the general condition of the patient is satisfactory, and if impairment of renal function is only moderate and a normal NPN and serum electrolyte and fluid balance can be achieved by proper preoperative medical measures, primary exploration may be possible, performing pelvic exenteration and permanent ureteroileal anastomosis in one stage. If the condition of the patient warrants, only exploration to determine resectability of the lesion and the performance of a preliminary uretero-ileal loop urinary diversion need be carried out initially, accomplishing the actual exenteration later as a second stage of the procedure, when the patient's general condition and renal status have been allowed to undergo maximal improvement.

2. If the impairment of renal function is severe, and major surgery, including even exploration and preliminary ureteroileostomy, is out of the question until renal function has been adequately restored, preliminary unilateral or, occasionally, bilateral nephrostomy will be a necessary step in the preparation of the patient for attempted radical surgical resection.

Stage IV

The same considerations with regard to the management of urinary tract impairment prior to definitive treatment apply as noted for Stage III. Because the chances of cure by radiation are less than 5 percent under the best of circumstances, the current trend is toward a primary surgical attack (anterior, posterior, or, more often, total pelvic exenteration). A second, less compelling reason for a primary surgical attack is that if rectal and/or bladder involvement is present, the development of rectovaginal or vesicovaginal fistulas following radiation therapy is likely. In spite of extensive local disease, 50 percent or more of the patients with Stage IV lesions prove to have no lymph node involvement, which is another potent argument in favor of an attempt at primary surgical excision in this stage. Continuing experience with this type of surgery has lowered the mortality and morbidity to very acceptable levels (less than 5 percent), and a most satisfactory permanent urinary diversion technique has evolved in the form of the ureteroileostomy utilizing an isolated ileal loop (Bricker pouch procedure) (see Fig. 52B). Long-term (10 or more years) end results, based in many instances on exenterations done in the early years as last-resort procedures on patients who had undergone prior irradiation or previous surgery, suggest that at least 20 to 25 percent of patients in whom at laparotomy it is found possible to carry out an exenteration with hope of cure will indeed be cured of their disease. With exenteration now being considered more often as a primary means of therapy in Stage IV, both resectability and curability rates have continued to improve.

Two points are worthy of emphasis: (1) It is rarely, if ever, possible to be absolutely certain by pelvic examination alone (even under anesthesia) whether or not a given lesion is resectable by exenteration. Hence, assuming that the general condition of the patient is satisfactory and there are no demonstrable distant metastases (as determined by negative chest and metastatic series x-ray films, normal liver chemistries, negative liver scan, and so on), all patients in whom pelvic exenteration is considered the only or the best chance for cure deserve laparotomy and exploration. Some have also advocated routine left scalene fat-pad lymph node biopsy before an exploratory operation on any patient with a view to carrying out pelvic exenteration for locally extensive cervical cancer. In a significant number of such patients, positive scalene node biopsy findings will permit recognition of remote spread and thus avoid an unnecessary laparotomy. Dissection to determine operability can be done in such a way as to permit abandoning the attempt without having done mutilating surgery, should the lesion prove unresectable. (2) Pelvic exenteration should not be carried out if it is known at the time of laparotomy to be only a palliative procedure (e.g., in the presence of liver metastases, or involved aortic nodes, or if exploratory dissection reveals that it would be necessary to cut across the tumor at the pelvic walls). In these situations the performance of pelvic exenteration has produced only unfavorable results.

An attempt at the primary radiation treatment of Stage IV lesions is still favored in some clinics, and certainly radiation therapy must be elected as the primary treatment in a number of situations: (1) in patients who are poor operative risks, though still potentially curable by radiation; (2) when exploration reveals the lesion to be unresectable by exenteration but still theoretically potentially curable by radiation; and (3) in the presence of known remote metastases, discovered either by pretreatment evaluation or at laparotomy for proposed exenteration. In this instance, radiation therapy may provide local palliation.

RESULTS OF TREATMENT

Table 5 presents the approximate average figures for the cure rates obtained in the various clinical stages of carcinoma of the cervix published in the fifteenth edition of the *Annual Report on the Results of Treatment in Carcinoma of the Uterus,* a publication sponsored by the International Federation of Gynecology and Obstetrics that includes statements of end results from 124 different institutions in 26 countries. The reported statistics concern 299,972 patients undergoing primary treatment by either radiation or radical surgery, or a combination of the two forms of therapy, during the 10-year period 1954–1963, although the vast majority were treated by radiation alone.

Table 5
Approximate Cure Rates To Be Expected for Carcinoma of the Cervix

Stage	Cure Rate (%)
0	95–100
I	77
II	56
III	31
IV	9
All stages	51

Table 6

End Results in 486 Patients Undergoing Wertheim Hysterectomy and Bilateral Pelvic Lymphadenectomy During 1939–1957 at Massachusetts General Hospital and Pondville State Cancer Hospital

Stage and Conditions of Nodes	Number	Percent	Living and Well 5 or More Years		Number of Deaths			
			Number	Percent	Died of Disease	Operative Mortality	Died of Intercurrent Disease Within 5 Years	Total
Stage I								
Negative	272	86	240	88	17	3	12	32
Positive	43	14	19	44	23	1		24
Total	315	100	259	82	40	4	12	56
Stage II								
Negative	108	63	77	71	22	2	7	31
Positive	63	37	17	27	45	1		46
Total	171	100	94	55	67	3	7	77
All patients	486		353	73	107	7	19	133

For comparison, Table 6 presents the end results following the radical Wertheim operation obtained in a series of patients with Stages I and II cervical cancer treated over a 19-year period by Meigs and associates at the Massachusetts General Hospital and the Pondville (Massachusetts Department of Public Health) State Cancer Hospital. It is apparent that the results of adequate surgery by skilled, experienced operators in the early stages of cervical cancer are at least the equal of those obtained by radiation.

Finally, in Table 7, the value of pelvic exenteration procedures in the management of many patients with advanced cervical cancer is clearly indicated by the comparable results obtained at four different institutions. It is of interest to note

Table 7

Results in the Early Years of Pelvic Exenterations for Advanced Cervical Cancer at Various Clinics

Series	Number of Cases	Positive Nodes (%)	Five-Year Survival		Operative Mortality (%)
			All Cases (%)	Primary Operation (%)	
Brunschwig [3][a]	457	50	15	21	23
Parsons [26][b]	120	35	24	32	23
M.G.H.-Pondville[c]	106	50	23		26
Ketcham et al. [21][d]	162	38	38	48	17

[a]Memorial Center for Cancer and Allied Disease, New York.
[b]Massachusetts Memorial Hospital (now University Hospital), Boston.
[c]Massachusetts General Hospital, Boston, and Pondville (Mass.) State Cancer Hospital (author's unpublished data).
[d]National Cancer Institute.

that where exenteration was done as a primary procedure rather than after previous treatment by radiation or by a lesser surgical operation, the end results were even more favorable, with 30 to 40 percent five-year survivals in some series under these circumstances.

SPECIAL PROBLEMS IN THE MANAGEMENT OF CERVICAL CANCER

Carcinoma of the Cervical Stump

Management of carcinoma of the cervical stump in accordance with the clinical stage of disease is basically the same as when the entire uterus is present. Satisfactory radium applications may be more difficult to achieve because of lack of an adequate uterine canal, and when radiation treatment is elected, the use of interstitial radium needles may often have to be substituted for the usual intracavity applicator. Complications of radiation therapy may occur more frequently as a result of the dislocation and adherence of the bladder, ureters, rectum, or small bowel produced by the previous subtotal hysterectomy. Small-bowel damage with necrosis, obstruction, or fistula formation, as well as an increased incidence of severe proctitis and rectovaginal fistulas, is encountered more frequently in attempting radiotherapy for cancer of the cervical stump. Thus treatment by radical surgery may often prove a wiser choice whenever either mode of therapy seems to offer an approximately equal chance of success.

End results should be about the same, unless it is known or can be assumed (when cancer of the residual cervix becomes manifest within one or two years) that the subtotal hysterectomy was done in the actual presence of the cervical cancer, in which case the patient's chance for ultimate cure has been seriously jeopardized. (The importance of the routine vaginal smear, speculum examination and biopsy of the suspicious cervix, and curettage prior to hysterectomy for whatever indication, particularly if abnormal bleeding is present, is again emphasized, and their use will serve to avoid this tragic occurrence.) If invasive cancer has actually been cut across, then further surgery, to be adequate, would theoretically involve exenteration, because local dissemination of tumor through some of the cleavage planes that would be utilized in performing a radical hysterectomy would have to be assumed, and the disease often would have been spread even more widely by the ill-advised supravaginal procedure. In this instance, therefore, in spite of the possible difficulties, an attempt at control by radiation therapy is frequently preferable, holding further and superradical surgery in reserve in case the response to radiotherapy is not favorable.

Inadvertent Simple Hysterectomy in the Presence of Invasive Cervical Cancer

The tragedy of the performance of simple hysterectomy in the presence of an unsuspected early invasive cervical carcinoma is a completely preventable one, as previously discussed. Unfortunately, the problem is still regularly encountered, despite the many educational programs in cancer detection for physicians and the widespread use of routine cytologic examination for the early recognition of cervical cancer. The chances for ultimate salvage of such patients are seriously jeopardized, and when recurrence is already present, the overall cure rate is roughly 20 to 25 percent. If additional, more adequate treatment is given within four months of the hysterectomy, a 40 to 65 percent cure rate may be achieved. This is still distressingly unsatisfactory in comparison with the potential 90 to 95 percent cure rate that would be expected had these patients initially received adequate treatment either by radical hysterectomy or radiotherapy for their early cervical cancers.

In managing these patients, early reoperation, when this is possible, with radical surgical removal of the residual tumor-bearing area by means of the Wertheim, Schauta, or pelvic exenteration procedures combined with pelvic lymphadenectomy, appears to offer the greatest chance for salvage, with cure rates approaching 65 percent. Radiation therapy has proved less successful in dealing with the situation, probably because of the technical obstacles to effective local application of radium posed by absence of the uterus, and five-year survivals are achieved in only about 30 percent of cases.

If the patient is referred immediately following discovery of an unsuspected cervical cancer in her simple hysterectomy specimen and as yet demonstrates no positive evidence of persistent tumor, the outlook should be somewhat better. A radical Wertheim type of dissection of the parametrial, paracervical, and paravaginal tissues, with upper vaginectomy and pelvic lymphadenectomy, is then the approach of choice and offers the best chance for cure.

Carcinoma of the Cervix in Association with Pregnancy

CARCINOMA IN SITU

Normal pregnancy is frequently accompanied by an atypical basal cell hyperplasia of the cervical epithelium that may suggest carcinoma in situ, both on cytologic smear and cervical biopsy, and that may persist for several months after termination of the pregnancy. However, most pathologists agree that the two lesions can usually be distinguished, even in the presence of pregnancy. If doubt exists, the patient should be followed closely by smears and biopsies throughout the pregnancy and for three to six months thereafter. Atypical basal cell hyperplasia simulating carcinoma in situ will regress in the involutional period, and no further treatment will be necessary. If the lesion persists and must be assumed to be true carcinoma in situ, treatment is then carried out as previously described.

If a tentative diagnosis of carcinoma in situ is made during pregnancy because of abnormal cytologic findings, or simple cervical biopsy, or both, multiple biopsies, preferably colposcopically directed, should be done (or if colposcopy is not available, cold-knife total cone biopsy should be done, accepting a small risk of complications, including resultant miscarriage), together with endocervical curettage, to be absolutely certain that one is not dealing with invasive or microinvasive carcinoma, for the presence of the latter would contraindicate vaginal delivery and require cesarean section followed by prompt treatment of the cervical carcinoma, as described subsequently. If invasive carcinoma is ruled out in this way, the pregnancy can be allowed to proceed to term, and normal vaginal delivery can be done. After an interval of six to eight weeks to allow proper involution of the uterus, a wide conization of the cervix would represent proper treatment for an intraepithelial carcinoma in any young woman in whom preservation of childbearing is desired; prolonged follow-up observation is of course essential if this more conservative management is elected. In the older patient who is not desirous of further childbearing once the current pregnancy is completed, total hysterectomy after a suitable postpartum recovery interval is frequently the management of choice.

CLINICALLY OBVIOUS INVASIVE CARCINOMA

Early and Midpregnancy

Where there is no hope of obtaining a viable fetus within a short time (a few weeks at most), the pregnancy should be ignored or suitably terminated and treatment of the malignancy according to the stage of the disease carried out as usual. (Note: Although a deliberate preliminary therapeutic abortion is not countenanced under the tenets of some religious faiths, a direct attack on a pelvic carcinoma, even though it will ultimately result in termination of a pregnancy, is considered permissible.) The method by which pregnancy is interrupted when this proves necessary will depend on the duration of pregnancy, a general guide being as follows:

Early First Trimester (0 to 8 weeks). If radiation treatment is planned, the uterus may be evacuated at the time of the first radium application, or the patient may be allowed to complete spontaneously the abortion that will inevitably follow the first radium application. Some prefer to give deep x-ray therapy initially, which will also result in spontaneous abortion, applying radium later after the course of external irradiation is completed. If radical surgery is planned (e.g., Wertheim-Meigs radical abdominal hysterectomy and pelvic lymphadenectomy), there is no contraindication to proceeding directly, without preliminary evacuation of the uterus, at this stage.

Late First, Second, and Early Third Trimesters. Termination of the pregnancy by vaginal manipulation is now contraindicated, lest the tumor be disseminated, and therefore the uterus should be emptied by cesarean hysterectomy (high classic, well away from the cervix), with treatment of the cervical cancer by radiation or radical surgery to follow after a suitable short interval. (Radical surgery can be done as late as the fifth month without preliminary uterine evacuation, however.)

Late Pregnancy. Where there is every likelihood of obtaining a viable infant within a short interval after the diagnosis of invasive cervical cancer is made, delivery by cesarean section may be elected, and treatment of the cancer begun as soon as feasible thereafter, either by radiation or radical surgery.

There is much to be said for employing radical surgery rather than radiation therapy in the management of the pregnant patient with invasive cervical cancer. Usually, the lesion is an early one, e.g., Ia (2), Ib, or IIa, and radical surgery provides a very effective approach, especially in the early trimesters, yielding cure rates that are as good or better than radiation, with fewer complications. Furthermore, the radical surgical approach usually obviates the need for prior interruption of the pregnancy and has the obvious additional advantage of not exposing this considerably younger group of women to extensive pelvic irradiation with all its potential complications for the long-term future. For more advanced lesions (Stages IIb, III), however, radiation will usually prove to be more feasible and effective, reserving possible pelvic exenteration for some of the Stage IV lesions and for patients in whom radiation fails to eradicate the tumor.

Treatment of Recurrences

The following discussion applies to cases without remote metastases that render the patients categorically incurable.

In general, if radiation treatment was used originally and the dosage employed was adequate and effectively applied, further radiation treatment of recurrent or persistent disease is unlikely to be successful and is pointless. Exceptions to this rule may occur in occasional cases in which the previous radiation is deemed to have been inadequate, or where the primary lesion itself has been controlled, the cervix and areas immediately adjacent to it being free of disease, but there is later occurrence of more peripheral disease in areas outside the zone of calculated optimal cancericidal dose (e.g., in the lower vagina or at or near the pelvic walls). A trial of additional radiotherapy may sometimes be indicated under these circumstances prior to undertaking radical surgery. However, in the case of most recurrences following radiation treatment, the patient should be carefully evaluated for and promptly offered the possibility of radical surgery (usually some form of exenteration will be required), because the disease, though unresponsive to radiation, often remains localized to the pelvis and is still resectable and potentially curable by a radical surgical attack. Roughly 15 percent of patients undergoing radical surgery for recurrence of cervical cancer following radiation therapy will survive five years. If the recurrence remains centrally located and pelvic exenteration can be done, the cure rate may approach 25 to 35 percent.

The management of recurrences following radical surgery will depend largely on the location of the recurrence. Recurrences in the central area of the pelvis are rare after a properly performed radical hysterectomy unless the operation was ill chosen for the extent of the original primary tumor. When they do occur, a trial of radiation (radium in a vaginal applicator and/or pelvic x-ray therapy) is often indicated, since pelvic exenteration can then still be offered later if the recurrence does not respond to radiation therapy. If exenteration can be done for a central pelvic recurrence following prior surgery, the expected cure rate is similar to that for exenteration performed for radiation failures, i.e., roughly 25 to 35 percent. However, recurrences following a previous operation are much less likely to occur in areas still potentially resectable by exenteration than is the case with postradiation recurrent or persistent disease. If the recurrence is peripheral and beyond the scope of pelvic exenteration, x-ray therapy will often prove of considerable palliative benefit, and an occasional patient will achieve a long-term remission.

Palliation of Incurable Disease

General supportive measures are employed for palliation of incurable cervical carcinoma, as in the management of any patient with inoperable and incurable cancer, when the conventional methods of approach by radiation and chemotherapy have been exhausted. Surprisingly enough, efforts to achieve palliation in cervical cancer by a chemotherapeutic approach have so far been notably unsuccessful. Pelvic perfusion or long-term pelvic infusion with a variety of alkylating and antimetabolic agents has failed to provide significant benefit as far as tumor regression is concerned, although some patients have experienced complete relief of pain due to a direct effect of the drug on the nonmyelinated pain fibers exposed to the perfusion. Somewhat more promising results have been obtained with some of the newer chemotherapeutic drugs such as adriamycin, but side effects have been severe and the mortality from complications excessive. Although they are employed only when absolutely necessary, certain surgical procedures such as palliative colostomy for large-bowel obstruction and posterior rhizotomy, tractotomy (recently done percutaneously using a stereotactically controlled radiofrequency current), cordotomy, or intrathecal or subdural phenol blocks for intractable pain may at times be absolutely essential and most beneficial. As mentioned previously, only rarely would one consider urinary tract diversion in the face of complete obstruction in a hopelessly incurable case.

OTHER FORMS OF CERVICAL MALIGNANT TUMORS

Although extremely rare, various types of sarcoma of the cervix are occasionally encountered, the most frequent variety being sarcoma botryoides, which characteristically occurs in infancy and childhood and which has already been discussed in Chapter 4. All the sarcomas tend to be highly malignant and to disseminate rapidly and widely; invariably, they are unresponsive to radiation, and radical surgical resection offers the only hope of cure, although the chances are remote in most cases.

Metastatic tumors of the cervix also occur occasionally, with spread from primary lesions of the ovary or rectum the most common examples; rarely, metastasis from the breast or from gastric, pancreatic, or other more remotely located primary carcinomas have been reported.

When adenocarcinoma of the endometrium extends to involve the endocervix, the lesion is classified as a separate entity and designated as carcinoma corporis et cervicis. Consideration of this special form of endometrial carcinoma and a discussion of its management are presented in Chapter 14.

REFERENCES

1. Beecham, C. T. Carcinoma in situ. *Obstet. Gynecol.* 33:125, 1969.
2. Boutselis, J. G., Ullery, J. C., and Charme, L. Diagnosis and management of Stage IA (microinvasive) carcinoma of the cervix. *Am. J. Obstet. Gynecol.* 110:984, 1971.
3. Brunschwig, A. Indications and results of pelvic exenteration. *J.A.M.A.* 194: 160, 1965.
4. Brunschwig, A., and Barber, H. R. K. Surgical treatment of carcinoma of the cervix. *Obstet. Gynecol.* 27:21, 1966.
5. Chanen, W., and Hollyock, V. E. Colposcopy and the conservative management of cervical dysplasia and carcinoma in situ. *Obstet. Gynecol.* 43:527, 1974.
6. Coppleson, M., and Reid, B. Origin of Premalignant Lesions of Cervix Uteri. In M. L. Taymor and T. H. Green, Jr. (Eds.), *Progress in Gynecology,* Vol. VI. New York: Grune & Stratton, 1975. Pp. 517–539.
7. Cramer, D. W., and Cutler, S. J. Incidence and histopathology of malignancies of the female genital organs in the United States. *Am. J. Obstet. Gynecol.* 118:443, 1974.
8. Creasman, W. T., and Rutledge, F. Carcinoma-in-situ of the cervix: An analysis of 861 patients. *Obstet. Gynecol.* 39:373, 1972.
9. Davis, J. R., and Moon, L. B. Increased incidence of adenocarcinoma of the cervix. *Obstet. Gynecol.* 45:79, 1975.
10. Declos, L., Fletcher, G. H., Suit, H. D., and Rutledge, F. After-loading vaginal irradiation. *Radiology* 96:666, 1970.
11. Finck, F. M., and Denk, M. Cervical carcinoma: Relationship between histology and survival following radiation therapy. *Obstet. Gynecol.* 35:339, 1970.
12. Gagnon, F. Contribution to the study of the etiology and prevention of cancer of the cervix of the uterus. *Am. J. Obstet. Gynecol.* 50:516, 1950.
13. Glucksmann, A., and Cherry, C. P. Incidence, histology, and response to radiation of mixed carcinomas of the uterine cervix. *Cancer* 9:971, 1956.
14. Graham, J. B., and Graham, R. M. The sensitization response in patients with cancer of the uterine cervix. *Cancer* 13:5, 1960.
15. Green, T. H., Jr. Further trial of a cytologic method for selecting either radiation or radical operation in the primary treatment of cervical cancer. *Am. J. Obstet. Gynecol.* 112:544, 1972.
16. Green, T. H., Jr. Surgical Management of Carcinoma of the Cervix in Pregnancy. In M. L. Taymor and T. H. Green, Jr. (Eds.), *Progress in Gynecology,* Vol. VI. New York: Grune & Stratton, 1975. Pp. 607–626.
17. Green, T. H., Jr., and Morse, W. J., Jr. Management of invasive cervical cancer following inadvertent simple hysterectomy. *Obstet. Gynecol.* 33:763, 1969.
18. Hollyock, V. E., and Chanen, W. The use of the colposcope in the selection of patients for cervical cone biopsy. *Am. J. Obstet. Gynecol.* 114:185, 1972.
19. Josey, W. E., Nahmias, A. J., and Naib, Z. M. Relation of Herpes Simplex Virus Type 2 Infection to Cervical Neoplasia. In M. L. Taymor and T. H. Green, Jr. (Eds.), *Progress in Gynecology,* Vol. VI. New York: Grune & Stratton, 1975. Pp. 540–557.
20. Kelso, J. W., and Funnell, J. D. Combined surgical and radiation treatment of invasive carcinoma of the cervix. *Am. J. Obstet. Gynecol.* 116:205, 1973.
21. Ketcham, A. S. Pelvic exenteration for carcinoma of the uterine cervix. *Cancer* 26:513, 1970.
22. Kyriakos, M., Kempson, R. L., and Perez, C. A. Carcinoma of the cervix in young women. *Obstet. Gynecol.* 38:930, 1971.

23. McCall, M. L. The radical vaginal operative approach in the treatment of carcinoma of the cervix. *Am. J. Obstet. Gynecol.* 78:712, 1959.
24. Meigs, J. V. (Ed.). *Surgical Treatment of Cancer of the Cervix.* New York: Grune & Stratton, 1954.
25. Meigs, J. V. Radical hysterectomy with bilateral pelvic lymph node dissection for cancer of the uterine cervix. *Clin. Obstet. Gynecol.* 1:1029, 1958.
26. Parsons, L. Pelvic exenteration. *Clin. Obstet. Gynecol.* 2:1151, 1959.
27. Reddi, P. R., Nussbaum, H., Wollin, M., and Kagan, A. R. Treatment of carcinoma of the cervix uteri with special reference to radium systems. *Obstet. Gynecol.* 43:238, 1974.
28. Savage, E. W. Microinvasive carcinoma of the cervix. *Am. J. Obstet. Gynecol.* 113:708, 1972.
29. Sedlis, A., Cohen, A., and Sall, S. The fate of cervical dysplasia. *Am. J. Obstet. Gynecol.* 107:1065, 1970.
30. Swan, D. S., and Roddick, J. W. A clinical-pathological correlation of cell type classification for cervical cancer. *Am. J. Obstet. Gynecol.* 116:666, 1973.
31. Symmonds, R. E., Pratt, J. H., and Webb, M. J. Exenterative operations: Experience with 198 patients. *Am. J. Obstet. Gynecol.* 121:907, 1975.
32. Thompson, J. D., Caputo, T. A., and Franklin, E. W., III. The surgical management of invasive cancer of the cervix in pregnancy. *Am. J. Obstet. Gynecol.* 121:853, 1975.
33. Tredway, D. R., Townsend, D. E., Hovland, D. N., and Upton, R. T. Colposcopy and cryosurgery in cervical intraepithelial neoplasia. *Am. J. Obstet. Gynecol.* 114:1020, 1972.
34. Villasanta, V. Complications of radiotherapy for carcinoma of the uterine cervix. *Am. J. Obstet. Gynecol.* 114:717, 1972.
35. Wallace, D. L., and Slankard, J. E. Teenage cervical carcinoma in situ. *Obstet. Gynecol.* 41:697, 1973.
36. Younge, P. A., Hertig, A. T., and Armstrong, D. A study of 135 cases of carcinoma in situ of the cervix at the Free Hospital for Women. *Am. J. Obstet. Gynecol.* 58:867, 1949.

14
Carcinoma of the Endometrium and Uterine Sarcomas

CARCINOMA OF THE ENDOMETRIUM

Adenocarcinoma of the endometrium arises in the body of the uterus and hence is also referred to as carcinoma of the corpus or fundus of the uterus. It represents the second most common pelvic cancer, accounting for roughly 20 to 30 percent of all malignant tumors of the female reproductive tract. During the first half of the twentieth century it was encountered approximately one-third to one-half as often as cervical cancer. Both its absolute and relative incidence have tended to increase steadily, paralleling the increased longevity of the general population. This steadily increasing incidence (refer again to Table 4), plus the fact that mass cytologic screening for the preinvasive or early invasive phases of this neoplasm has not achieved the success that was obtained for cervical cancer, bids to make endometrial cancer a greater problem in cancer control in the future than cervical cancer has been in the past. With invasive cervical cancer declining in frequency because of the early detection and treatment of the antecedent lesions, namely, carcinoma in situ and severe, persistent, or recurrent dysplasia, invasive carcinoma of the endometrium is now as common as — and in some areas of the world even more common than — invasive cervical cancer.

Etiology

The possible role in many instances of a prolonged period of abnormal, unopposed estrogenic stimulation in the genesis of endometrial carcinoma has long been suspected but is difficult to prove conclusively. Entirely compatible with this concept is the observation that the majority of patients in whom the lesion develops have in common a rather characteristic set of associated general systemic features that are consistent with this type of abnormal ovarian hormone balance. They tend to be single or nulliparous (relatively infertile and prone to functional menstrual irregularities), in the postmenopausal age group (peak incidence in the decade from age 55 to age 65), and to have had a late and prolonged menopause (age 50 to 55), one further complicated by a marked tendency to dysfunctional bleeding with recurring episodes of often profuse menometrorrhagia. The typically associated obesity, hypertension, and increased incidence of diabetes (approximately 10 to 15 percent have clinical diabetes, and 60 to 70 percent exhibit a diabetic type of response to a glucose-tolerance test) are also suggestive of a basic underlying metabolic and steroid hormonal disturbance. Finally, women with endometrial cancer are more likely than the general population to have other primary cancers, notably, carcinoma of the breast and carcinoma of the colon. The strong association between cancer of the uterine

445

corpus and breast cancer suggests the possibility that abnormal stimulation by or response to estrogen may be an important underlying factor in the etiology of both endometrial and breast cancer.

Support for the role of prolonged, unopposed estrogen stimulation in the etiology of endometrial neoplasia is also found in histologic studies of the benign areas of endometrium present in uteri removed for endometrial carcinoma. Here, too, evidence of excessive estrogenic effects is found in the form of endometrial polyps and endometrial hyperplasia, both the completely "benign" cystic type as well as the more "dysplastic" atypical and adenomatous variety. The frequent coexistence of uterine fibroids in patients with endometrial carcinoma is also cited as another manifestation of chronic hyperestrinism. Furthermore, a number of well-documented cases have been reported in which the actual progression from benign cystic hyperplasia, through the phase of atypical adenomatous hyperplasia, to endometrial carcinoma in situ, and finally to invasive cancer of the endometrium has been observed over a period of years in the same woman, the patient having undergone repeated curettages and, ultimately, hysterectomy.

In searching for the source of the continuing abnormal estrogen secretion in postmenopausal women with endometrial carcinoma, attention has been focused on the ovarian lesion designated as cortical stromal hyperplasia (see Chap. 6), which Sommers and co-workers [15, 21] and others have reported to be present at least twice as frequently (if not invariably) in the ovaries of women with cancer of the endometrium as compared with a control series of women of comparable age undergoing hysterectomy and bilateral oophorectomy for other reasons. However, the significance of these observations remains unsettled, both because they have not always been corroborated in other equally carefully studied series and because there is as yet no convincing evidence that ovaries with cortical stromal hyperplasia actually produce estrogen. Similarly, there have been a number of reports concerning the development of endometrial cancer in women who have received continuous, prolonged estrogen therapy. Such reports suggest but do not prove that the prolonged, uninterrupted administration of estrogens, particularly in large doses, may be of etiologic significance in the production of carcinoma of the endometrium in some instances. Further evidence for this relationship is to be found in reports of the development of endometrial carcinoma in several young women with gonadal dysgenesis and in one young woman with Sheehan's syndrome and complete pituitary, ovarian, adrenal, and thyroid hypofunction; all had received prolonged estrogen therapy. In some, but not all, of these women the long-term medication used had been diethylstilbestrol, introducing the possibility of a chemical carcinogenic action as well as a prolonged, unopposed estrogen effect.

The extreme rarity of endometrial carcinoma in castrated women, and the fact that as previously discussed in Chapter 6, there is a markedly increased (100 times) incidence of endometrial carcinoma in women with estrogen-secreting ovarian tumors (granulosa cell and theca cell tumors), and that when endometrial carcinoma occurs in women under the age of 40, it almost invariably does so in association with functioning ovarian tumors or more commonly in the presence of ovarian disorders such as the Stein-Leventhal syndrome or ovarian hyperthecosis, which are also accompanied by a continuous, unopposed, and prolonged estrogen excretion pattern, furnish additional, highly suggestive support for the proposed etiologic role of excessive estrogen stimulation.

Finally, the experimental production of endometrial carcinoma (and concomitant endometrial polyps and hyperplasia) in rabbits and other laboratory animals by the prolonged administration of large doses of diethylstilbestrol supplies still another link in the chain of evidence in favor of the concept that endometrial carcinoma is the end stage of a progressively increasing degree of atypical glandular proliferation induced in an endometrium exposed to abnormal amounts of estrogen over a sufficiently long period of time.

One other possible causal factor sometimes incriminated has been previous pelvic irradiation. Several reports have suggested that endometrial cancer may develop 10 to 20 years later at twice the expected rate in women treated by radiation for epidermoid carcinoma of the cervix. Furthermore, a significant number of patients have in the past been encountered in whom the development of endometrial carcinoma occurred 10 to 20 years after even small doses of intracavitary radium or x-ray therapy had been administered to control excessive premenopausal bleeding secondary to the presence of fibroids or ovarian dysfunction. It should be noted, however, that patients with this type of prolonged menopausal bleeding difficulty who were candidates for intrauterine radium in the days when it was used freely in the management of benign uterine hemorrhage correspond precisely to the type of woman in whom carcinoma of the endometrium shows a tendency to develop anyway.

Pathologic Features and Pathogenesis

The two main histologic types of endometrial carcinoma are the papillary adenocarcinomas and the purely adenomatous adenocarcinomas. The former tend to be somewhat less malignant than the latter, and within this group is included the very early, highly differentiated grade 1 lesion often termed an **adenoma malignum**. Either type may appear as a small and well-circumscribed papillary or polypoid lesion in its early stages, or later on as a more diffuse process involving most or all of the mucosal surface and projecting from it as a bulky tumor that fills and distends the entire endometrial cavity. The characteristic microscopic picture is one of a marked increase in the number of endometrial glands, which tend to replace the normal supporting stroma completely, giving the "back-to-back" glandular configuration. The glands themselves are enlarged, dilated, and poorly oriented, with the closely packed pleomorphic cells containing abundant mitoses and obviously malignant hyperchromatic nuclei. In the more anaplastic varieties, there may be partial or complete loss of the glandular pattern, the even more highly neoplastic-appearing and closely packed cells tending to grow in solid masses or columns of cells, to involve the entire endometrial lining, and to invade the underlying myometrium early and diffusely.

A third histologic type (comprising 15 to 20 percent of endometrial carcinomas)

is the adenoacanthoma, wherein there is squamous metaplasia of a varying proportion of the malignant glandular epithelium, or in which there may actually be a
malignant-appearing squamous cell component intermingling with what is otherwise
a predominately glandular type of carcinoma. In spite of an old clinical impression
to the contrary, most of the evidence indicates that adenoacanthoma is not significantly different from pure adenocarcinoma of the endometrium in its biologic
behavior, its pathologic or clinical features, or its response to therapy and subsequent
cure rate.

A fourth histologic type of endometrial cancer is the mixed adenosquamous cancer. Once only rarely seen, it appears to be increasing in incidence and now accounts
for 5 to 10 percent of endometrial cancers (30 percent in the series reported by
Reagan [27]). In contrast to the more common adenocarcinoma types, adenosquamous carcinomas of the endometrium are associated with a very poor prognosis,
with five-year survival rates of only 20 percent, as compared with 70 percent for the
other histologic types of endometrial cancer. Pure squamous cell carcinomas with
a primary origin in the endometrium have been reported but are extremely rare;
they, too, have a poor prognosis.

A fifth and even more uncommon histologic type is the clear cell carcinoma, also
of müllerian origin, though formerly sometimes erroneously called mesonephric
adenocarcinoma. When these tumors arise in the endometrium, their histologic
appearance is identical to that seen in clear cell carcinomas of the vagina, cervix,
and ovary. They occur most often in postmenopausal women with the same systemic disorders (obesity, diabetes, hypertension) that are seen in women with the
more common adenocarcinomas. However, the response to treatment of clear cell
carcinomas is considerably less favorable, a five-year survival rate of only 20 percent
having been reported in several series.

Just as in the case of cervical cancer, there is good reason to believe that invasive
carcinoma of the endometrium is probably preceded by a phase of intraepithelial
carcinoma in many, if not most, instances, and that carcinoma in situ of the endometrium is simply antedated by an atypical, adenomatous endometrial hyperplasia,
the latter clearly a microscopic change distinctly different in nature and fundamental
significance from simple cystic or "Swiss-cheese" hyperplasia, which is a temporary,
reversible lesion, not accompanied by atypical epithelial proliferation. Although this
pathogenetic sequence of events has not been documented as extensively for endometrial carcinoma as it has for cervical carcinoma, the not infrequent finding, in
early lesions, of areas of atypical adenomatous hyperplasia and carcinoma in situ
coexisting with invasive endometrial carcinoma in the same uterus and the previously
noted observations of histologic progression from adenomatous hyperplasia to intraepithelial carcinoma to invasive adenocarcinoma in the same patient over a period of
years strongly suggest its validity. Furthermore, follow-up observations of patients
in whom atypical adenomatous hyperplasia has been found at curettage reveal a
subsequent high incidence of endometrial carcinoma, though its appearance may be
delayed for a number of years. It is estimated that 3 percent of women in whom
adenomatous hyperplasia develops prior to the menopause and 25 percent of those

in whom such hyperplasia occurs postmenopausally will ultimately have endometrial carcinoma. Prophylactic hysterectomy is probably therefore often indicated in women with abnormal bleeding occurring during or shortly after the menopause in whom repeated curettage reveals this type of atypical endometrial change. This recommendation would be especially valid for those patients who also possess the typical systemic features of obesity, diabetes, and a long-standing history of irregular, anovulatory menses with dysfunctional bleeding and infertility so commonly observed in women with endometrial cancer.

Although less common during the childbearing years, atypical endometrial hyperplasia and even more severe atypicalities worthy of being termed endometrial carcinoma in situ are occasionally encountered in young women who still wish to achieve pregnancy or retain their potential for it. Most often, the endometrial atypicalities in these young women are associated with a long-standing anovulatory menstrual pattern and prolonged unopposed estrogenic stimulation of the endometrium stemming from the Stein-Leventhal syndrome, ovarian hyperthecosis, granulosa cell estrogen-producing tumors, or similar ovarian dysfunction. In this situation it may be possible to correct the ovarian dysfunction (e.g., either medically with drugs such as clomiphene, or surgically by ovarian wedge resection or removal of a functioning ovarian tumor), as well as to assist further in the resolution of the hyperplasia by the cyclic use of any of the various progestational agents or low-estrogen combination oral contraceptive drugs. Obviously, patients managed in this way must be followed very closely, and the possibility of the initial presence or subsequent development of invasive endometrial carcinoma constantly borne in mind. Such a possible progression to malignancy should be reevaluated at regular intervals by appropriate diagnostic studies, e.g., endometrial biopsies and aspiration cytology, or repeat curettage if either endometrial biopsy or cytologic findings are suspicious or if symptoms, or lack of response to the conservative therapeutic approach, or both seem to warrant it.

Although atypical adenomatous hyperplasia arises spontaneously (endogenous estrogen stimulation and/or abnormal endometrial response) in the majority of instances, it may also develop in postmenopausal women receiving prolonged estrogen therapy. In this situation the medication should be stopped and curettage repeated in three to four months. If reversion to a normal, atrophic endometrium occurs, no further treatment will be necessary, but future estrogen therapy will be contraindicated. However, should the atypical adenomatous hyperplasia persist despite cessation of estrogen therapy, hysterectomy would probably then be the indicated definitive treatment of choice.

Routes of Spread

Direct extension to involve the underlying myometrium represents the initial and most frequent pathway of extension, and to some extent its occurrence is determined by the tumor's degree of anaplasia and by the length of time it has been present. Fortunately, the majority of endometrial carcinomas are of intermediate grades of malignancy, frequently attaining considerable size before significant myometrial invasion has occurred, so that when clinically detected, the lesion is still for the most part confined to the endometrial cavity and superficial layers of the myometrium.

Once deeper, more extensive myometrial spread has occurred, tumor cells gain access to lymph channels within the uterine wall, and further extension along lymphatic pathways to involve the cervix, vagina, ovaries, and pelvic lymph nodes may then take place. Lymph node involvement is decidedly uncommon when the tumor, regardless of its size, is still essentially confined to the fundus of the uterus and is present in no more than 10 percent of such cases. In the presence of cervical involvement, however, the frequency of lymph node metastasis increases sharply, approaching 50 percent in some reported series of cases, both cervical extension and lymphatic dissemination occurring as the result of deep myometrial invasion and appearing more frequently with the more histologically malignant tumors. In fact, the presence of cervical involvement (see Fig. 53B) so affects the natural history and prognosis of carcinoma originating in the endometrium that this anatomic type of lesion was formerly classified in a completely separate category as carcinoma corporis et cervicis and, in any case, requires a different therapeutic approach, as will be discussed subsequently.

As might be expected, the lymph nodes affected by endometrial carcinoma are the same groups to which spread occurs from primary cervical cancer (see Fig. 47), namely, the paracervical and parametrial nodes first, followed by the hypogastric, obturator, and external iliac nodes of the pelvic wall, and then inguinal, common iliac, and paraaortic nodal extension occurring in the advanced stages. More direct permeation of the lymphatics along the course of the round ligaments occasionally leads to early involvement of the inguinal nodes.

Direct implantation of malignant cells at the time of surgery or metastatic spread along the submucosal lymphatic channels of the vaginal wall leads to vaginal metastases in approximately 10 to 15 percent of cases, and this type of relatively localized vaginal metastasis is prone to appear in the vaginal vault or suburethral area, both rather characteristic sites for recurrence following hysterectomy; the former is usually due to direct implantation, the latter, to lymphatic spread.

Ovarian metastases are present in 5 to 10 percent of cases and are usually the result of spread via lymphatic channels in the mesosalpinx and mesovarium, although direct extension along the tubal wall or transtubal passage and implantation of tumor cells occasionally occurs and may be responsible for generalized peritoneal seeding.

When the wall of the uterus has been completely penetrated by the tumor, direct local extension to involve the bladder or rectum may occur, although this happens much less often than is the case with primary cervical cancer. If the serosa of the fundus is perforated by tumor, diffuse peritoneal spread usually rapidly follows.

Presumably because of the greater vascularity of the uterine wall, and probably also due to the inherent nature of the tumor itself, once the tumor has penetrated the myometrium, invasion of vascular channels and distant metastasis via the bloodstream occur far more often in patients with endometrial carcinoma than in women with primary cervical cancer. Pulmonary metastases are the ones most frequently seen, but hepatic, skeletal, and cerebral metastases are also encountered.

Clinical Staging

OLD LEAGUE OF NATIONS CLASSIFICATION FOR ENDOMETRIAL CANCER

Based on a clinical estimate of the extent of the disease, an international classification comparable to the one in use for primary cancer of the cervix was also developed for carcinoma of the endometrium. The first such classification or clinical staging, The League of Nations Classification, used throughout the world until 1971, follows.

CARCINOMA OF THE CORPUS UTERI

Stage 0: Carcinoma in situ (a microscopic phase probably frequently preceding invasive malignancy in which the carcinoma remains intraepithelial and has not penetrated the basement membrane).

Stage I: The tumor is confined to the fundus of the uterus (Fig. 53A).

   Group 1: The patient's general condition is satisfactory for operation.

   Group 2: Poor general medical condition renders the patient inoperable.

Stage II: The tumor has spread outside the uterus.

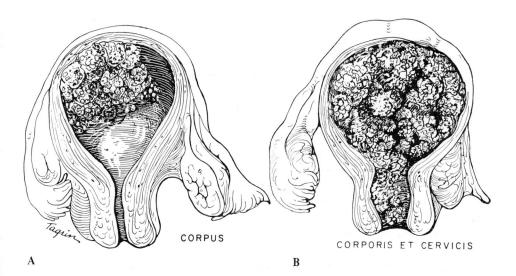

CORPUS

CORPORIS ET CERVICIS

A   B

Figure 53
Endometrial carcinoma. A. Carcinoma of the corpus. B. Carcinoma corporis et cervicis.

CARCINOMA CORPORIS ET CERVICIS

In carcinoma corporis et cervicis (Fig. 53B), the tumor has extended to involve the endocervical canal. The tumor may occupy the lower endometrial cavity and the adjacent upper cervical segment, may present as an obvious mass of cancer at the external cervical os, or may occasionally be accompanied by such extensive involvement of the entire endometrial cavity and cervix that it is difficult to establish whether the lesion is of primary cervical or endometrial origin. This type of lesion, which constitutes approximately 15 percent of all cases of endometrial carcinoma, was thus considered as a separate entity (it was also separately reported in the internationally collated *Annual Report on the Results of Treatment in Carcinoma of the Uterus*). Although in the modern clinical staging of endometrial cancer to be presented subsequently, cervical involvement is denoted simply by classifying the lesion as Stage II, it remains clear that "carcinoma corporis et cervicis" must be treated, whether by surgery, radiation, or combined radiation and surgery, essentially as if it were a primary cervical carcinoma, but with the presence of the corpus component complicating and modifying the details of therapy.

As in the case of cervical cancer, this classification of endometrial cancer by clinical stages provided a useful guide to prognosis and general plan of treatment and was essential for comparing and evaluating the results of different methods of therapy. For this purpose it was also originally deemed necessary to introduce the subgroup 2 in Stage I to take into account the fact that many patients with carcinoma of the endometrium are elderly women with serious unrelated medical disorders that often preclude the use of what would otherwise be the accepted, optimal method of treatment. Approximately 30 percent of patients with endometrial carcinoma actually fall into this category and were formerly classified Stage I—group 2.

MODERN CLASSIFICATION AND DEFINITION OF THE CLINICAL STAGES OF CARCINOMA OF THE ENDOMETRIUM

In 1970, the recommendations of the Cancer Committee of the International Federation of Gynecology and Obstetrics regarding a proposed new plan of clinical staging for endometrial cancer were approved and adopted by all the national and international societies interested in the problem. This new clinical classification, which is now more comparable to the one in use for cervical cancer and which now serves as the basis for tabulation and comparison of end-result data as published in the *Annual Report* is as follows:

Stage 0: Carcinoma in situ.
Stage I: The carcinoma is confined to the corpus.

Further subdivisions of Stage I are now employed:

Stage Ia: The length of the uterine cavity is 8 cm or less.
Stage Ib: The length of the uterine cavity is more than 8 cm.

The Stage I cases are also subgrouped with reference to the histologic type of the adenocarcinoma as follows:

G1: Highly differentiated adenomatous carcinomas.
G2: Differentiated adenomatous carcinomas with partly solid areas.
G3: Predominately solid or entirely undifferentiated carcinomas.

Stage II: The carcinoma has involved the corpus and the cervix.
Stage III: The carcinoma has extended outside the uterus but not outside the true pelvis.
Stage IV: The carcinoma has extended outside the true pelvis or has obviously involved the mucosa of the bladder or rectum.

Finally, a clinical classification proposed by Gusberg should also be mentioned; it seems particularly helpful and valid, since it specifically takes into account all three of the most important prognostic factors: the size of the tumor (or uterus), the degree of histologic anaplasia of the lesion, and whether or not extension from the uterine fundus to involve the endocervix has occurred. Gusberg's classification is as follows:

Stage 0: Carcinoma in situ.
Stage I: Uterus of normal size.
Stage II: Uterus minimally enlarged (10 cm or less in depth).
Stage III: Uterus maximally enlarged (more than 10 cm in depth).
Stage IV: Bladder or bowel involvement. Distant metastases.

Stages I, II, and III should be advanced one stage for (1) cervical involvement and/or (2) a highly anaplastic tumor on histologic examination.

The value of Gusberg's classification in planning proper therapy for each patient will also be appreciated more fully during the discussion of the treatment of endometrial cancer. As he points out, the significance of accurate staging lies in the fact that it defines the nature of the host-tumor relationship at that specific point in time: e.g., a localized, dependent tumor (Stage I); a tumor showing local geographic extension only (Stage II); a tumor beginning to show uncontrollable biologic spread with lymphatic penetration (Stage III); and a widespread, autonomous tumor (Stage IV).

Symptoms

Since the majority (75 percent) of patients with endometrial cancer are in the post-menopausal age group, postmenopausal bleeding is its most common symptom and is apt to occur very early in the course of the disease. It usually begins as occasional slight spotting and may be accompanied or even preceded by a clear, watery discharge, but ultimately the irregular bleeding becomes more frequent and profuse. Although mild uterine cramps may occasionally accompany the episodes of bleeding, pain is not a prominent feature of the clinical picture. When present, it is usually secondary to the presence of a pyometra or hematometra (the secondarily infected, necrotic tumor debris or bloody discharge accumulating behind a benign cervical stricture or an endocervical canal occluded by tumor), or it is the result of extensive spread of the disease.

When carcinoma of the fundus develops in premenopausal women, as it does in 25 percent, the abnormal bleeding takes the form of intermenstrual flow or menorrhagia. Because of the frequent occurrence of these symptoms in connection with the common functional disorders and benign lesions (e.g., polyps, fibroids) in this age group, failure to consider the possibility of endometrial cancer is unfortunately an all-too-common error in management.

Diagnosis, Determination of Extent of Disease, and General Evaluation of the Patient

In approximately 25 percent of patients with endometrial cancer the vaginal smear remains negative, apparently because recognizable malignant cells simply do not reach the vaginal pool. However, the use of endometrial smears obtained by direct aspiration of material from the uterine cavity employing any one of several available commercial kits (see Chap. 2) has markedly increased the accuracy of cytologic diagnosis, many studies reporting 95 to 100 percent of such smears positive in patients with endometrial cancer. With these improvements in technique, the cytologic method now makes it possible to establish a presumptive diagnosis in the majority of patients in whom the disease is suspected on the basis of symptoms and now provides an effective screening technique in asymptomatic patients as well.

Endometrial biopsy, a procedure that is easily done in the office or clinic, is another simple method by which a definite diagnosis can be promptly established in many patients with suggestive symptoms. An alternative method of obtaining tissue from the uterine cavity for histologic study is also available in the form of the Vabra vacuum aspirator kit (see Chap. 2). This technique requires no anesthesia and is simple, safe, and perfectly suitable for use in the office or clinic.

Curettage remains the most important and the only definitive means for either establishing a diagnosis of endometrial cancer or excluding its presence. It is important to stress that even if both the cytologic and endometrial biopsy findings are negative, a D&C is mandatory to detect or exclude the presence of carcinoma of the endometrium in the face of suggestive symptoms, most particularly in patients with postmenopausal bleeding. Among this group the differential diagnosis includes endometrial or endocervical carcinoma, endometrial or cervical polyps, atypical endometrial hyperplasia, spontaneous or estrogen-induced "benign" types of hyperplasia, and extrauterine sources of vaginal bleeding such as atrophic vaginitis or urethral caruncle.

Furthermore, curettage is nearly always essential in determining whether the tumor is confined to the uterine fundus (Stage I) or has extended to involve the endocervical canal (Stage II, formerly called carcinoma corporis et cervicis). Since treatment will be entirely different if the cervix is involved, a "fractional curettage" should be carried out with particular care to establish this point (see Chap. 2). Thus a properly performed D&C should provide the three essential items of information necessary to plan proper therapy: (1) the size of the uterus, as determined by sounding the uterine canal (also a rough index of the size of the tumor in most cases), (2) whether or not the cervix is involved, and (3) the degree of anaplasia of the tumor based on microscopic examination of the curettings. A decision whether or not to employ preoperative irradiation therapy will be based on these three factors, and knowledge that the cervix is involved may result in selection of the radical Wertheim operation rather than simple total hysterectomy as the definitive surgical procedure to be performed after preliminary irradiation therapy.

Hysteroscopy as an additional aid in the diagnosis of endometrial cancer and in the evaluation of the extent of uterine involvement has its advocates. However, it is difficult to be convinced that it offers any significant additional information useful in planning and following a program of therapy that is not already provided by a simple, properly performed fractional curettage. Furthermore, the instrument and technique are expensive, unduly complex, and cumbersome; the view is often unsatisfactory and its interpretation difficult even for trained experts; and the availability of both equipment and trained experts is decidedly limited. Most important, the hazard of uterine perforation exists, as well as the very real danger of forcing cancer cells into underlying vascular and lymphatic channels within the uterine wall, thus favoring metastatic extension, or out of the fundus through the fallopian tubes into the free peritoneal cavity. The latter complication is a potential danger whether the uterus is distended with sterile saline, dextran solution, or carbon dioxide, since pressures of 50 to 100 mm Hg are required to permit visual observation through the instrument.

Hysterosalpingography has also been suggested as another means of assessing the size of the uterine cavity and the extent and distribution of the tumor within it. Here again, the danger of dissemination is the principal objection, since injection of dye into the uterine cavity might increase the risk of lymphatic, vascular, or transtubal dissemination. A properly performed fractional curettage yields essentially the same information and is a far safer and simpler procedure.

Although careful pelvic examination in search of evidence of local extension is also important, the frequent presence of marked obesity and associated uterine fibroids in patients with endometrial cancer often limits the value and accuracy of the physical findings as an indication of the size and extent of the tumor. A chest film and metastatic skeletal survey should be routine in all patients, and in the obviously more advanced cases, additional essential studies will include cystoscopy, proctoscopy, intravenous pyelograms, and barium-enema examination.

A complete general medical evaluation is of the utmost importance in patients with endometrial cancer, with particular attention paid to an accurate assessment of their cardiovascular, renal, and pulmonary status and to screening for latent, previously unsuspected diabetes. As a group they are typically prone to premature and extensive arteriosclerotic cardiovascular disease, hypertension, and renal disorders; this consideration, together with often advanced age, marked obesity, and increased incidence of diabetes, requires that they receive extremely careful preoperative preparation and postoperative management and at times may render the operative risk prohibitive. Thus in some patients with endometrial cancer it may be the general medical condition rather than the presence and extent of the tumor that is the determining factor in the choice and details of therapy.

Treatment

Although both radiation and surgery have a role to play in the management of endometrial carcinoma, surgical removal of the uterus and adnexa is considered to be the keystone of optimal therapy in this disease, in contrast to the relatively optional choice of either radiation or radical surgery as the definitive therapy for cervical cancer, at least in the latter's earlier stages. However, radiation is used preoperatively as a routine adjunct to surgery in the standard treatment of endometrial cancer in many clinics. It is given with a view to obtaining a preliminary reduction in size of, and elimination of secondary infection in, the primary tumor. It is also employed in the hope of decreasing the likelihood of local recurrence by devitalizing any tumor cells that have already permeated or are about to enter the parametrial or vaginal lymphatics, as well as by obliterating these same channels through the effects of radiation.

Preoperative irradiation may be administered by the insertion of multiple small intrauterine radium or radioactive cobalt sources (Heyman's capsule) (Fig. 54), with or without a vaginal applicator specifically intended to destroy any microscopic tumor that might already have implanted in the submucosal vaginal lymphatics.

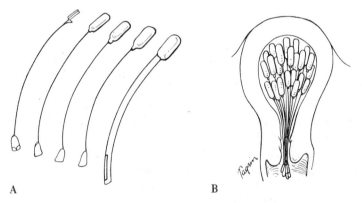

A   B

Figure 54
Heyman's capsule employed in intracavitary radiation therapy of endometrial carcinoma. A. Capsules of various sizes, the one on the right shown in position on the curved intrauterine applicator. B. Capsules in place within the uterine cavity. The use of multiple small radium sources rather than a single large radium applicator provides a more uniform distribution of radiation to all areas of the uterus.

Intrauterine radium application is effective when the uterus is of normal size or is only slightly enlarged, but when there has been significant enlargement, it is preferable to administer the preoperative irradiation by giving external x-ray therapy. The use of preoperative irradiation is probably particularly helpful and indicated in cases in which (1) the tumor is large and the chance of deep penetration great, and/or (2) the lesion is histologically highly anaplastic and can therefore be assumed to be accompanied by early and extensive myometrial (and lymphatic) invasion, and/or (3) cervical involvement is present. It is probably primarily in these three situations that the results of combined treatment will be superior to those following surgery alone. It is likely that the results of hysterectomy are not significantly improved by preoperative irradiation in the reasonably early, small, well-differentiated tumors confined to the uterine fundus and accompanied by minimal or no uterine enlargement that are encountered in the majority of patients with endometrial carcinoma, and hysterectomy alone has its advocates where this type of lesion is concerned, since it achieves an 85 to 90 percent cure rate. However, there is good evidence that even in these very favorable cases, vaginal radium application postoperatively will almost completely eliminate the late vaginal recurrences seen in 5 to 10 percent of patients who are treated by surgery alone. It is particularly important to give a postoperative vaginal radium application if there has been any myometrial invasion by the tumor, since vaginal recurrences are more common under these circumstances. If the myometrial involvement is extensive, deep, or both, a postoperative course of full-pelvic external irradiation in a dosage of 4500 R may be preferable to a postoperative vaginal radium application, since the former extends prophylactic irradiation to the much wider parauterine areas at risk when the tumor penetrates deeply into the myometrial layer.

Although radiation therapy alone can control endometrial carcinoma, particularly in its early phases, in general it has not proved to be as effective as hysterectomy, either with or without supplementary radiation, in achieving maximal curability. Its use as the sole treatment modality is therefore reserved for patients with otherwise favorable lesions who are poor operative risks, or for patients with advanced, unresectable tumors. Worthwhile palliation and even an occasional cure can be achieved in this latter group by carefully planned and administered radiotherapy. Most clinics report that radiation therapy alone achieves only a 40 to 45 percent five-year survival, whereas when surgery alone or surgery combined with adjunctive radiotherapy is used, overall cure rates of about 70 percent are obtained. (For well-differentiated tumors without uterine enlargement or significant myometrial invasion, the five-year cure rates are 90 percent or better.)

The general principles and standard programs of therapy for the various stages of endometrial cancer are briefly outlined below, and the approximate cure rates to be expected are indicated in Table 8.

STAGE I

Assuming that fractional curettage has revealed the lesion to be confined entirely to the fundus, the uterus is not enlarged, and the lesion is histologically well

Table 8
Approximate Cure Rates To Be Expected for Carcinoma of the Endometrium

Stage	Cure Rate (%)
0	90–100
I	60–90[*]
II	30–50
III	10–20
IV	5–10

[*]The five-year cure rate is 95 percent if the tumor is small, well differentiated, and confined to the endometrium, with no myometrial invasion.

differentiated, the standard operative procedure employed is a simple total hysterectomy with bilateral salpingo-oophorectomy and removal of a generous vaginal cuff. It is important to remove the adnexa because of the potential avenues of spread through the tubes and in the lymphatics of the mesosalpinx and mesovarium, as well as the known 5 to 10 percent incidence of ovarian metastases, and inclusion of an adequate margin of upper vagina with the specimen may decrease the incidence of local vaginal recurrence. Sometimes, the use of the vaginal route, if feasible, is preferable in obese, relatively high-risk patients, and more frequent use of vaginal hysterectomy as an alternative to abdominal hysterectomy might permit the benefits of the surgical approach to be offered more often in this group, reducing the number of patients relegated to the inoperable category who consequently receive only radiation therapy.

Although not all the end results in reported series have shown that radiation increases overall curability, it is commonly used as an adjunct to hysterectomy, as previously discussed, and is administered in one of two ways, either by preoperative intracavitary radiation or postoperative vaginal radiation, as follows:

1. Intracavitary radiation using a single intrauterine stem applicator, or, preferably, Heyman's capsules containing radium or radioactive cobalt (or if the uterus is significantly enlarged, 4000 R of preoperative pelvic x-ray therapy) is given first, delivering approximately 3000 to 4000 R to the uterus, and is followed in two to six weeks by total hysterectomy and bilateral salpingo-oophorectomy. Since the radiation effect on the tumor cells occurs immediately, the two- to six-week delay before undertaking hysterectomy is primarily to permit these often older, high-risk patients to recover fully from the radiotherapy program and/or the period of anesthesia and subsequent confinement to bed required if radium is used; and also to allow time enough for the shrinkage and sterilizing effects that radiation has on these enlarged uteri, with their contained necrotic and secondarily infected tumor. (The intrauterine radium is frequently supplemented by simultaneous placement of a vaginal radium applicator, the latter permitting delivery of an adequate dosage of radiation to the upper vaginal area as well.)

2. Total hysterectomy and bilateral salpingo-oophorectomy is followed in three to four weeks by application of a vaginal radium cylinder, delivering approximately 3000 R to the entire vaginal surface. (Postoperative x-ray therapy might be substituted but would involve higher dosages to the bladder and rectum.) This alternative plan is based on the fact that there is some merit in the argument that it is pointless to radiate primarily the portions of the tumor to be surgically removed, and that if the goal is prevention of vaginal lymphatic dissemination by radiation of cells potentially in transit prior to or during hysterectomy, this goal can better be realized by subsequent postoperative vaginal irradiation.

Another approach to the problem of avoiding potential vaginal recurrences due to spread via communicating submucosal lymphatics (typically on the anterior vaginal wall in the suburethral area or in the vaginal apex at or near the old suture line) is the use of radical hysterectomy and pelvic node dissection. Advocates of this approach also hope to increase curability further by the wider parametrial resection. However, in several reported series, the incidence of vaginal recurrence, though sharply reduced by preoperative or postoperative radiotherapy, has not been diminished by the radical Wertheim hysterectomy alone. Furthermore, there are cogent arguments against the routine use of the radical operation in patients with carcinoma of the endometrium:

1. Because of the frequently associated marked obesity in these patients, it is sometimes impossible to carry out a satisfactory radical dissection that assures that a sufficiently wider removal than that accomplished by simple total hysterectomy will result and make the added risk worthwhile.

2. Even assuming that a satisfactory radical hysterectomy could be accomplished every time, if the lesion is confined to the fundus, parametrial and paracervical spread and lymph node involvement are uncommon, so that a significant increase in potential curability is probably unlikely. Equally discouraging in this regard is that there have been only occasional cures in patients with lymph node metastases in spite of the addition of the pelvic lymph node dissections.

3. Patients with carcinoma of the endometrium tend to be much poorer operative risks than those with cervical carcinoma (e.g., older, obese, frequent diabetes, frequent ca. ovascular disease), and the mortality and morbidity of the more radical operation is certain to be much greater and likely to more than offset any potential increase in curability.

STAGE I, POOR MEDICAL RISK PATIENTS

Since surgery is precluded except as a last resort by the prohibitive operative risk in Stage I patients who are poor medical risks, a full course of radiotherapy is planned. If the uterus is not enlarged, therapy may begin with intracavitary radiation, usually administered in two separate applications three weeks apart of approximately 1500 milligram-hours each, followed by a course of full-pelvis x-ray therapy. If the uterus is enlarged, external irradiation is given first and then followed by one or two radium applications. Thereafter, the patient should be followed closely, preferably with routine endometrial biopsies or repeat curettages in three months, again at six months, or at any time bleeding recurs. If subsequent biopsies reveal persistent or recurrent tumor, then complete reassessment of the situation is in order, with a view to carrying out hysterectomy, despite the risks involved, in the face of failure to respond to the initial radiation treatment.

STAGE II

As already described, when extension to the cervix has occurred, the incidence of lymph node involvement approaches 50 percent. Furthermore, spread to the cervix per se invariably implies deep myometrial penetration and often is associated with the more anaplastic type of tumor, both factors tending to favor extension of the tumor along other pathways and in other directions as well. Hence it is not surprising that in the past the five-year apparent cure rate for carcinoma corporis et cervicis was at best only 25 to 30 percent, in contrast to the relatively high five-year survival rate of 60 to 70 percent when the tumor is confined to the fundus. More aggressive therapy involving preoperative irradiation and radical Wertheim hysterectomy has now increased the cure rate of Stage II endometrial cancer (carcinoma corporis et cervicis) to 50 to 60 percent in some series in recent years. As previously noted, the management of endometrial carcinoma with cervical involvement, whether by surgery or radiation, is similar in principle to the management of primary cervical cancer. A surgical approach involving radical hysterectomy and bilateral pelvic lymphadenectomy (or occasionally some type of pelvic exenteration) offers the best chance for cure and is the treatment of choice in patients in good general condition with operable lesions. Here again, the cure rate following radical hysterectomy is enhanced by preoperative full-pelvis x-ray therapy, administering 3000 to 4000 R, a dosage that should not significantly increase the risk of surgical complications. A radical Wertheim hysterectomy and bilateral pelvic lymphadenectomy is then performed one month following completion of the course of external irradiation. If after completing the external radiation, a radical hysterectomy is not feasible for medical or technical reasons (e.g., extreme obesity), a simple hysterectomy and bilateral salpingo-oophorectomy should be done instead, perhaps giving one uterovaginal radium application two to three weeks after carrying out the simple hysterectomy.

When there are medical contraindications to carrying out even a simple abdominal or vaginal hysterectomy, a radiotherapeutic approach similar to that for primary cervical cancer is employed. If the lesion is deemed potentially still curable, this will usually include two local radium applications, Heyman's capsules being substituted for the single intrauterine stem but the type of vaginal applicator remaining the same, followed by the usual course of x-ray therapy. If the tumor is large, x-ray therapy is given first, followed by the local radium applications later when the size of the lesion has been reduced.

STAGE III

If the patient with a Stage III endometrial cancer is a suitable candidate from a general medical standpoint, an attempt at surgical resection is indicated, usually after preliminary preoperative x-ray therapy to the full pelvis, since this offers a statistically greater chance for cure than does radiotherapy alone. If surgical excision does not prove feasible, palliative x-ray therapy is employed, supplemented occasionally by the use of intracavitary radium as an additional aid in the control of bleeding. As will be described, the use of hormone therapy in the form of massive doses of progesterone may also prove to be helpful for palliation in advanced disease.

STAGE IV

It is rare for endometrial cancer to invade the bladder or rectum without having become fixed to the pelvic walls or having metastasized to more distant sites. In those rare instances when local extension involves only the bladder, or rectum, or both, and there are no demonstrable distant metastases, preoperative x-ray therapy followed by some form of pelvic exenteration might be considered if the patient is reasonably young and otherwise in good health. In properly selected patients, an approximately 20 percent five-year survival rate with apparent cure may be achieved under these circumstances.

For most patients, however, palliation of the local disease is best managed by external irradiation. In addition, large doses of progesterone (see the next section) may be tried in the hope of obtaining remissions, but this type of hormone therapy has been less successful in dealing with extensive local tumor spread than with remote peripheral metastatic spread (e.g., lungs, bone) appearing a considerable time after surgery, or radiation, or both have controlled the local disease. Finally, attempts at chemotherapy with anticancer drugs have not as yet proved rewarding for endometrial cancer, though occasional trials in selected patients may be worthwhile, especially as newer, more promising agents become available.

TREATMENT OF RECURRENT AND METASTATIC ENDOMETRIAL CARCINOMA

As previously described, the most common sites of local recurrence following hysterectomy are on the anterior vaginal wall, either in the suburethral region or in the vaginal vault, or in the vaginal apical suture line itself (probable implantation recurrences). These often discrete and superficial lesions sometimes respond favorably to local radium (vaginal applicator or interstitial radium needles placed directly into the tumor) with or without supplementary x-ray treatment; occasionally, they are amenable to local excision in the form of partial vaginectomy. In any case, permanent cure of the disease results in only 20 to 30 percent of patients, and the development of vaginal recurrence is definitely an ominous prognostic sign, especially when it occurs within two years following the hysterectomy. Late vaginal recurrences after three years have a more favorable outlook and are frequently curable by radiation or even by surgical resection. The use of radiation as a supplement to hysterectomy has sharply reduced the subsequent incidence of vaginal metastases in most reported series, and this is the strongest argument in favor of its routine employment.

More extensive vaginal or central pelvic recurrences, particularly if they progress to rectal or bladder involvement or both may be an indication for some form of pelvic exenteration. Because once it extends beyond the uterus, carcinoma of the endometrium is less likely to remain localized to the central pelvis and is frequently accompanied by remote metastases, and because patients with carcinoma of the endometrium are less likely to be able to withstand pelvic exenteration, both the indications for superradical surgery and its chances of success in the management of advanced or recurrent endometrial carcinoma are considerably less than in patients with carcinoma of the cervix. If pelvic recurrence is so extensive as to be ol ʲously inoperable, palliative x-ray therapy may prove beneficial in some instances.

If remote metastases are present (pulmonary, osseous, upper abdominal), the use of large doses of progesterone should be tried. This had long been considered a possible palliative maneuver on the theoretical grounds that a hormone known to produce maturation of normal endometrium might have a favorable controlling effect on the rate of growth of endometrial carcinoma, either acting directly on the tumor or indirectly through inhibition of a pituitary-stimulating effect. With the advent of more potent, long-acting progesterone compounds, this form of palliative treatment became practical and produced favorable, occasionally dramatic responses in terms of subjective relief of symptoms in 40 to 60 percent of patients and objective evidence of decrease in size of the metastatic lesions in approximately 35 to 40 percent of patients to whom it has been given. Recent sophisticated biochemical studies of estrogen- and progesterone-binding proteins and steroid uptake by human endometrial cancer cells has shown that roughly 35 percent of endometrial cancers possess this capacity and are thus potentially "hormone-dependent."

These observations correlate well with, and perhaps account for, the 35 percent response rate observed during progesterone therapy of patients with metastatic or recurrent endometrial carcinoma. The most commonly used agents have been the following: 17-alpha-hydroxyprogesterone caproate (Delalutin) in a dosage of 0.5 to 1.0 gm intramuscularly two or three times weekly; medroxyprogesterone acetate (Depo-Provera), 3.0 to 5.0 gm intramuscularly in divided doses during the first six weeks of treatment and then 400 to 1000 mg each month; megestrol acetate (Megace), which has the advantage that it can be given orally, in a dosage of 40 to 160 mg daily in two to four divided doses; and megestrone acetate (Colprone), also an oral preparation, in a dosage of 600 mg daily in six divided doses. All these agents are given for a trial period of at least three months, and if a favorable response is obtained, treatment can be continued indefinitely thereafter, often on a reduced maintenance dosage. Evidence of regression is usually apparent within two to three months (Fig. 55), and side effects are minimal and infrequent.

The most frequent and most favorable responses have occurred in patients with well-differentiated, slowly growing tumors in whom the primary tumor has been

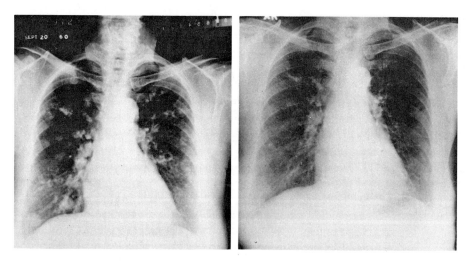

Figure 55

Progesterone therapy of pulmonary metastases in a patient with endometrial carcinoma. A persistent cough developed in a 55-year-old woman 4½ years after hysterectomy for endometrial cancer. Although there was no sign of local recurrence,
a chest x-ray film (at left) revealed multiple pulmonary metastases. Progesterone
therapy employing 17-alpha-hydroxyprogesterone caproate (Delalutin) in a dosage
of 500 mg twice weekly produced a dramatic response, with almost complete disappearance of the pulmonary lesions (the film on the right was obtained 2 months
after instituting progesterone therapy). On continuation of treatment the patient
remained in complete remission for over 10 years, dying of heart disease.

eradicated by hysterectomy, leaving them apparently cured for three or four years,
but in whom pulmonary metastases develop later. In some instances, objective
remission with complete freedom from symptoms has been observed for as long as
seven to eight years, although the average survival time of responders has been about
two years. Patients with extensive local recurrence or osseous metastases appear to
be less likely to exhibit either objective or subjective improvement, even when the
dosages of the various hormonal agents have been drastically increased. As might
be expected, patients with histologically highly undifferentiated tumors have shown
no response whatsoever.

Attempts at palliation with conventional chemotherapeutic drugs (e.g., alkylating
agents or antimetabolites) have not been particularly successful in patients with
advanced carcinoma of the endometrium.

UTERINE SARCOMAS

Sarcomatous tumors of the uterus are relatively rare lesions, constituting less than
5 percent of all uterine malignant tumors, and may arise both in the smooth muscle
of the myometrium and in the stromal cells of the endometrium. The vast majority

develop in the uterine fundus, and only occasionally is the cervix the primary site of origin. In spite of their rarity, a wide variety of histologic types has been described. This fact, together with the controversy concerning their histogenesis, the use of different nomenclatures in describing similar lesions, and the difficulties encountered in correlating microscopic appearance with clinical behavior in some varieties, has caused a certain amount of confusion in the literature on the subject. The most valid and useful classification of uterine sarcomas is the one devised by Ober and Tovell [24], which separates them into four major groups as follows:

1. Leiomyosarcoma.
2. Mesenchymal sarcoma.
3. Blood vessel sarcoma (hemangiosarcoma or hemangioendothelioma).
4. Lymphoma (recticulum cell sarcoma and lymphosarcoma).

The last two groups of tumors are extremely rare entities and will not be discussed further.

Leiomyosarcoma

Leiomyosarcomas are the sarcomas most commonly seen and constitute 50 to 75 percent of all uterine sarcomas. The majority occur in the premenopausal and perimenopausal age groups. They develop within the myometrium rather than the endometrium of the uterus, and in one third to one half or more of the cases, they appear to have arisen as a result of malignant degeneration in a previously benign fibroid. Although the chances of a malignant transformation in any given fibroid are no more than 0.5 percent, and perhaps considerably less, any apparent "fibroid" that grows rapidly, particularly any presumed "fibroid" that increases in size after the menopause, should be viewed with suspicion. Less often, the sarcomatous process apparently arises de novo within the uterine wall and, although it may remain fairly circumscribed in many cases, sometimes extends diffusely throughout the wall, producing a rapid and symmetrical uterine enlargement.

Seen grossly, these tumors are soft in consistency and present as poorly encapsulated nodules within the uterine wall or as pedunculated masses projecting into the endometrial cavity or bulging into the broad ligaments and onto the peritoneal surfaces of the uterus. On cut section they resemble meaty tissue variously described as "raw pork" or "fish flesh" in appearance, and areas of hemorrhage and necrosis are often visible. On microscopic examination the highly malignant nature of the majority of these lesions is obvious, masses of anaplastic spindle, stellate, or round cells lying within a sparse, myxomatous stroma, with frequent mitotic activity, abnormal giant cell forms, and easily demonstrated evidence of blood vessel invasion. Leiomyosarcomas that appear to have arisen in fibroids tend to be less undifferentiated in microscopic appearance and less invasive in behavior, and hence they offer a better prognosis if recognized early and treated promptly.

The usual symptoms include abnormal vaginal bleeding and malodorous discharge, awareness of an abdominal mass, and pelvic or abdominal pain as the rapidly growing tumor causes local pressure or invades adjacent organs and structures. Since these tumors are commonly necrotic and secondarily infected, an intermittent low-grade fever may also be noted. Because of the marked tendency to blood vessel invasion, rapid widespread dissemination of tumor is common, with metastases to the lung, liver, and bone appearing relatively early in the course of the disease.

Treatment in favorable cases should consist of total hysterectomy and bilateral salpingo-oophorectomy. Tumors that have extended beyond the uterus are so universally accompanied by distant metastases that more extensive radical surgery is rarely, if ever, worthwhile. In general, leiomyosarcomas are not radiosensitive, but the occasional exceptions to this rule often make a trial of radiotherapy in patients with advanced disease worthwhile in an effort to achieve some degree of temporary palliation. Chemotherapy to date has generally also been ineffective, although occasional responses have occurred to combination therapy with cyclophosphamide (Cytoxan), actinomycin D, and vincristine. The reported overall five-year survival rate following hysterectomy for leiomyosarcoma varies from 10 percent to as high as 35 percent in various series, the most favorable results being obtained when the tumor has apparently developed in a leiomyoma, and when it occurs before the menopause. In premenopausal patients whose leiomyosarcoma is still confined to the area of the myoma, whose tumor is not obviously malignant on gross examination and shows no vascular invasion on microscopic examination, cure rates of 75 percent or better are reported. Conversely, postmenopausal patients and patients whose tumors are obviously malignant on gross inspection, are not confined to a myoma, exhibit marked cellular atypicalities and a high mitotic activity, or show vascular invasion microscopically have an extremely poor prognosis.

Mesenchymal Sarcoma

Mesenchymal sarcomas arise within the endometrial stroma, and although in some varieties (the so-called carcinosarcomas) an element of epithelial malignancy is also present, it is the presence of malignant mesenchyme of stromal origin (the sarcomatous element) that characterizes these lesions and readily distinguishes them from simple endometrial adenocarcinoma. As suggested by Ober and Tovell [24], mesenchymal sarcomas can be further subdivided into the following categories:

1. Pure, homologous mesenchymal sarcoma.
   a. Endometrial stromal sarcoma.
   b. Stromatous endometriosis (also called stromal endometriosis, endolymphatic stromal myosis, stromal adenomyosis, etc.) and generally believed to be a low-grade or relatively benign variant of stromal sarcoma.
2. Pure, heterologous mesenchymal sarcoma: rhabdomyosarcoma.
3. Mixed, homologous mesenchymal sarcoma: carcinosarcoma (one variety).
4. Mixed heterologous mesenchymal sarcoma: carcinosarcoma (another variety); mixed mesenchymal sarcoma; sarcoma botryoides.

Although this classification is useful to the pathologist and serves to emphasize the common origin of all of these tumors from derivatives of the primitive mesenchymal stroma of the müllerian duct system, from a clinical standpoint it is more helpful to consider them under two broad headings, the first including only the pure homologous sarcomas, the second composed of the remaining three categories of pure heterologous, or mixed homologous or heterologous sarcomas, broadly characterized by the term **mixed mesodermal tumors.**

Stromal Endometriosis and Endometrial Stromal Sarcoma

Both types of homologous mesenchymal tumors occur in younger women, usually before or shortly after the menopause, are slow-growing, and only seldom metastasize; even in the presence of local extension or distant metastasis the clinical course is often relatively benign and protracted. Seen grossly, the uterus is usually diffusely enlarged and globular, and in the case of stromal endometriosis its cut surface is rendered coarsely irregular by protruding, yellowish, elastic, wormlike masses of tumor. Similar rubbery, polypoid masses may project into the endometrial cavity or extend beyond the wall of the uterus to involve the broad ligaments and other adjacent pelvic structures. In the case of stromal sarcoma, the tumor is usually larger and softer, its gross appearance resembling more that of a typical sarcoma of any type or location. Seen microscopically, the cells in stromal endometriosis resemble the normal stromal cells of the endometrium except for their location within the myometrium in association with endothelium-lined channels presumed to be lymphatics. In the benign form the spindle-shaped or round cells are uniform in shape, size, and staining qualities, and mitoses are absent; in the more malignant histologic types, and in the case of actual stromal sarcoma, the tumor may present a highly anaplastic microscopic appearance, the latter frequently not correlating at all with its relatively benign clinical behavior.

From the standpoint of clinical features, menometrorrhagia and pelvic pain are the usual symptoms, and uterine enlargement is often the only abnormal physical finding. Local extension, although uncommon, may result in ureteral, bladder, or rectosigmoidal involvement, with dysuria or hematuria, constipation or actual bowel obstruction, and progressive enlargement of the abdomen. Occasionally, distant metastases occur, most often to the lung, but they may remain asymptomatic and stationary or relatively slowly growing for many years.

Treatment of either stromal endometriosis or endometrial stromal sarcoma when confined to the uterus consists of total hysterectomy and bilateral salpingo-oophorectomy and offers a reasonably good chance for cure. When the tumor has extended locally, or in the face of recurrences, which often are delayed for many years, the relatively benign nature of these neoplasms makes it worthwhile to extend the primary operative procedure or carry out reexploration and removal of recurrent tumor, even though this involves resection of bowel, omentum, and other adjacent structures, since long-term survivals may be achieved in some instances. Both stromal endometriosis and stromal sarcoma are relatively radiosensitive lesions, so that radiation therapy can also be effectively utilized in the postoperative treatment of more extensive tumors or in the management of inoperable recurrent tumors or distant metastatic lesions not amenable to surgery. When the diagnosis has been established beforehand, preoperative radiation therapy followed by hysterectomy should perhaps be considered even in favorable cases when the lesion is still confined to the fundus (Stage I) in the hope of further improving the cure rates.

Occasional remissions have been observed in patients with pulmonary metastases accompanying stromal endometriosis in whom treatment with long-acting progestins has been given. It is assumed that the metastases from these well-differentiated tumors of endometrial stromal origin are responding in much the same manner as do a significant percentage of metastatic lesions in patients with well-differentiated adenocarcinoma of endometrial glandular origin.

Mixed Mesodermal Tumors

Although occasional instances of sarcoma botryoides are encountered in postmenopausal women, this is preponderantly a tumor of infants and children and has been discussed in Chapter 4. However, the pure heterologous tumors (rhabdomyosarcomas) and the mixed sarcomas (carcinosarcomas and mixed mesenchymal sarcomas) tend to occur in older, postmenopausal women. They are highly anaplastic, rapidly growing, widely metastasizing tumors in which treatment with the hope of cure is rarely possible, half the patients dying of their disease within two years of its onset, and only 15 to 30 percent in most series surviving five years. Previous pelvic irradiation (e.g., radiation therapy 5 to 25 years earlier for cervical or endometrial cancer, or, less often nowadays, the long-since abandoned radiation for "intractable, benign, functional menorrhagia" of an earlier medical era) may have been a significant etiologic factor in some cases, since roughly 20 to 30 percent of patients with mixed mesodermal tumors in various series recorded in the literature have given such a history. Carcinosarcoma is the most common form of mixed mesodermal tumor and contains an intimate mixture of carcinomatous and sarcomatous elements, both apparently derived from a primitive, multipotent type of endometrial stromal cell. Grossly, these tumors typically appear bulky and often (in 20 to 30 percent) polypoid, arising from the posterior wall of the endometrial cavity and often protruding through the secondarily dilated cervical canal as an easily bleeding, friable, necrotic mass that is secondarily infected. The initial symptoms of postmenopausal bleeding and vaginal discharge are entirely similar to those noted by patients with adenocarcinoma of the endometrium. But the rapid growth of these tumors usually leads to early and marked uterine enlargement (in 25 to 50 percent of patients) and secondary abdominal and pelvic pain, symptoms not usually present in patients with endometrial cancer. Subsequently there may be extensive local invasion of adjacent structures with omental and peritoneal spread, as well as early blood-borne or lymphatic metastases involving the pelvic and paraaortic nodes, liver, lungs, and other distant sites.

Total hysterectomy and bilateral salpingo-oophorectomy are indicated if the disease is still in the operable stage, and when the tumor is of the superficial polypoid type and is essentially confined to the endometrium within the uterine cavity, surgery may offer some hope of cure, with reported five-year survivals as high as 30 to 60 percent in this situation. As yet there is no clear-cut evidence in the literature on end results of treatment of these tumors to indicate whether or not preoperative or postoperative radiation will improve the results achieved by surgery alone. In most reported series the best five-year results have been obtained by surgery alone, but it is possible that preoperative or postoperative x-ray therapy may improve the chances of cure somewhat when the tumor is still completely confined to the uterine fundus (Stage I). Occasionally, radical hysterectomy or even pelvic exenteration may be indicated in dealing with more extensive but still resectable tumors in patients in good general condition and in whom distant metastases cannot be demonstrated to have occurred. However, once the tumor has penetrated the myometrium or has extended beyond the uterus (which is the case in 50 percent or more of patients when first seen), the prognosis for cure is essentially hopeless, although a combination of limited surgery and a course of external irradiation may be used in an effort to obtain some palliation. In general, however, the heterologous or mixed types of mesenchymal sarcoma have not proved to be radiosensitive (no five-year cures by radiation alone have ever been reported), nor have they responded to any chemotherapeutic measures so far attempted. Nevertheless, a few patients have been reported in whom long-term survivals have been achieved by radiation therapy alone, and a significant number of those apparently cured by hysterectomy had either preoperative or postoperative x-ray treatment. Therefore, in patients in whom the risk of surgery is prohibitive or the lesion is so extensive as to be technically inoperable, a trial of radiation therapy is certainly indicated as a palliative measure. Palliation with various chemotherapeutic drugs has been attempted in patients with inoperable tumors, but no evidence of significant benefit has been noted to date, although an occasional transient, partial response to cyclophosphamide and adriamycin has been reported.

The other, exceedingly rare types of mixed mesenchymal sarcomas, which may be composed of two or more of a variety of malignant mesodermal elements heterologous to the uterus, such as striated muscle, cartilage, bone, fat, or myxomatous tissue, but which lack a malignant epithelial element, are usually even more highly malignant than the carcinosarcomas. Their gross pathologic and clinical features are entirely similar, and they, too, invariably metastasize widely and pursue a rapidly fatal course. Although the majority are not amenable to any form of treatment, a few long-term survivals with apparent cure have been reported following surgical removal.

REFERENCES

1. Bettinger, H. F. Hyperplasia and carcinoma of the endometrium. *Am. J. Obstet. Gynecol.* 109:194, 1971.

2. Brown, J. M., Dockerty, M. B., Symmonds, R. E., and Banner, E. A. Vaginal recurrence of endometrial carcinoma. *Am. J. Obstet. Gynecol.* 100:544, 1968.

3. Chuang, J. T., Van Veldon, D. J. J., and Graham, J. B. Carcinosarcoma and mixed mesodermal tumors of the uterine corpus. *Obstet. Gynecol.* 35:769, 1970.

4. Cutler, B. S., Forbes, A. P., Ingersoll, F. M., and Scully, R. E. Endometrial carcinoma after stilbestrol therapy in gonadal dysgenesis. *N. Engl. J. Med.* 287:628, 1972.

5. Farrow, G. M., Coventry, M. B., and Dockerty, M. B. Endometrial sarcoma, "stromal endometriosis." *Am. J. Obstet. Gynecol.* 100:301, 1968.

6. Fehr, P. E., and Prem, K. A. Malignancy of uterine corpus following irradiation therapy for squamous cell carcinoma of the cervix. *Am. J. Obstet. Gynecol.* 119:685, 1974.

7. Frick, H. C., II, Munnell, E. W., Richart, R. M., Berger, A. P., and Lawry, M. F. Carcinoma of the endometrium. *Am. J. Obstet. Gynecol.* 115:663, 1973.

8. Garnet, J. D. Constitutional stigmas associated with endometrial carcinoma. *Am. J. Obstet. Gynecol.* 76:11, 1958.

9. Giarratano, R. C., and State, T. A. Sarcomas of the uterus. *Obstet. Gynecol.* 38:472, 1971.

10. Gilbert, H. A., Kagan, A. R., Lagasse, L., Jacobs, M. R., and Tawa, K. The value of radiation therapy in uterine sarcoma. *Obstet. Gynecol.* 45:84, 1975.

11. Gore, H., and Hertig, A. T. Carcinoma-in-situ of the endometrium. *Am. J. Obstet. Gynecol.* 94:134, 1966.

12. Graham, J. B. The value of preoperative or postoperative treatment by radium for carcinoma of the uterine body. *Surg. Gynecol. Obstet.* 132:855, 1971.

13. Gusberg, S. B. The dysfunctional and the neoplastic. Clinical investigation in the service of patient care in endometrial cancer. *Am. J. Obstet. Gynecol.* 116: 175, 1973.

14. Gusberg, S. B., and Kardon, P. Proliferative endometrial response to theca-granulosa cell tumor. *Am. J. Obstet. Gynecol.* 111:633, 1971.

15. Hertig, A. T., and Sommers, S. C. Genesis of endometrial carcinoma. *Cancer* 2:946, 1949.

16. Ingersoll, F. M. Vaginal recurrence of carcinoma of the corpus. Management and prevention. *Am. J. Surg.* 121:473, 1971.

17. Kelley, R. M., and Baker, W. H. Progestational agents in the treatment of carcinoma of the endometrium. *N. Engl. J. Med.* 264:216, 1961.

18. Kistner, R. W. The effects of progestational agents on hyperplasia and carcinoma-in-situ of the endometrium. *Int. J. Gynecol. Obstet.* 8:561, 1970.

19. Koss, L. G., Spiro, R. H., and Brunschwig, A. Endometrial stromal sarcoma. *Surg. Gynecol. Obstet.* 121:531, 1965.

20. Masterson, J. G., and Kremper, J. Mixed mesodermal tumors. *Am. J. Obstet. Gynecol.* 104:693, 1969.

21. Meissner, W. A., Sommers, S. C., and Sherman, G. Endometrial hyperplasia, endometrial carcinoma, and endometriosis produced experimentally by estrogen. *Cancer* 10:500, 1957.

22. Mortel, R., Koss, L. G., Lewis, J. L., Jr., and D'Urso, J. R. Mesodermal mixed tumors of the uterine corpus. *Obstet. Gynecol.* 43:248, 1974.

23. Norris, H. J., and Taylor, H. B. Mesenchymal tumors of the uterus. *Cancer* 19:755, 1966.

24. Ober, W. B., and Tovell, H. M. M. Mesenchymal sarcomas of the uterus. *Am. J. Obstet. Gynecol.* 77:246, 1959.

25. Peterson, E. P. Endometrial carcinoma in young women. *Obstet. Gynecol.* 31: 702, 1968.

26. Pokoly, T. A comparison of the clinical behavior of uterine adenocarcinomas and adenoacanthomas. *Am. J. Obstet. Gynecol.* 108:1080, 1970.
27. Regan, J. W. Cellular pathology and uterine cancer. *Am. J. Clin. Path.* 62:150, 1974.
28. Reid, D. E., and Shirley, R. L. Endometrial carcinoma associated with Sheehan's syndrome and stilbestrol therapy. *Am. J. Obstet. Gynecol.* 119:264, 1974.
29. Reifenstein, E. C., Jr. Hydroxyprogesterone caproate therapy in advanced endometrial cancer. *Cancer* 27:485, 1971.
30. Richardson, G. S. Endometrial cancer as an estrogen-progesterone target. *N. Engl. J. Med.* 286:645, 1972.
31. Rozier, J. C., and Underwood, P. B. Use of progestational agents in endometrial adenocarcinoma. *Obstet. Gynecol.* 44:60, 1974.
32. Rutledge, F. Mixed mesodermal sarcoma of the uterus. *Am. J. Roentgenol.* 117:632, 1973.
33. Rutledge, F., Kotz, H. L., and Chang, S. C. Mesonephric adenocarcinoma of the endometrium. *Obstet. Gynecol.* 25:362, 1965.
34. Shah, C. A., and Green, T. H., Jr. Evaluation of current management of endometrial carcinoma. *Obstet. Gynecol.* 39:500, 1972.
35. Silverberg, S. G. Leiomyosarcoma of the uterus. *Obstet. Gynecol.* 38:613, 1971.
36. Silverberg, S. G., and DeGiorgi, L. S. Clear cell carcinoma of the endometrium. *Cancer* 31:1127, 1973.
37. Stearns, H. C., and Sneeden, V. D. Leiomyosarcoma of the uterus. *Am. J. Obstet. Gynecol.* 95:374, 1966.
38. Wait, R. B. Megestrol acetate in the management of advanced endometrial carcinoma. *Obstet. Gynecol.* 41:129, 1973.
39. White, A. J., Buchsbaum, H. J., and Rodman, N. F. Accuracy of the Gravlee Jet Washer in detecting endometrial adenocarcinoma. *Am. J. Obstet. Gynecol.* 116:1169, 1973.

15
Ovarian Cysts and Benign and Malignant Ovarian Neoplasms

Ovarian enlargements of clinical significance, or **tumors** in the broad sense of the term, may be the result of disturbances in cyclic follicular activity leading to the development of functional ovarian cysts, or they may signify the presence of true benign or malignant, cystic or solid neoplasms of the ovary. One of the problems so often confronting the gynecologist is the need to differentiate the former from the latter, for the distinction is exceedingly important from the standpoint of the further management of the patient with an ovarian mass. Hence, although they have also been discussed in Chapter 5, a brief review of the nature, clinical course, and management of the ovarian cysts of functional origin is included in this chapter.

In addition to the frequent occurrence of physiologic cysts, the ovary is a common site for both benign and malignant neoplasms, and the multiplicity of cell types in the normal ovary, as well as its complex embryologic and histogenetic background, results in a sometimes confusing variety of histologic types of tumors. Figure 56 is a diagram of the fundamental origins of the various ovarian tumors, and in the following section, a simplified, although admittedly imperfect, classification is presented that may provide a helpful overall orientation before the more common cysts and tumors are considered individually in more detail.

SIMPLIFIED CLASSIFICATION OF OVARIAN CYSTS AND TUMORS (BASED ON EMBRYOLOGIC AND HISTOGENETIC DERIVATION)

1. **Anatomic origin** (embryologic development from similar mesenchymal tissue in juxtaposition with evolving kidney and adrenal).
   a. Adrenal cell—rest tumors (lipoid cell tumors).
   b. Brenner tumors (epithelial elements similar to those found in the renal pelvis or ureter and believed by some to develop from the so-called Walthard's rests of primitive kidney origin.
   c. Parovarian cysts (derived from wolffian duct remnants).
2. **Ova cells** (hindgut or germinal epithelium).
   a. Dermoid cysts (and their occasional malignant forms).
   b. Teratomas (both the many benign variants, including struma ovarii, and the various malignant forms, including teratocarcinoma, embryonal carcinoma, and the rare primary ovarian chorionepitheliomas).
3. **Epithelial cells** (müllerian duct epithelium).
   a. Simple cystomas.
   b. Serous cystadenomas and cystadenocarcinomas.
   c. Pseudomucinous cystadenomas and cystadenocarcinomas.
   d. Undifferentiated carcinoma (usually solid neoplasms).

471

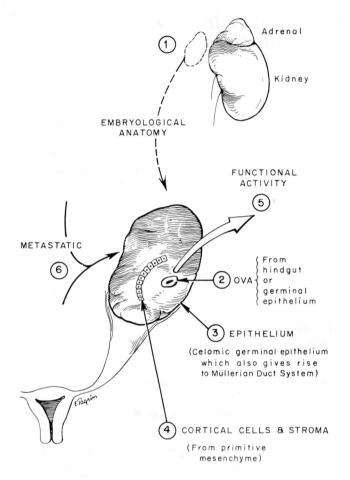

Figure 56
Origin and classification of ovarian tumors and cysts. (From T. H. Green, Jr. Gyne-
cology. In G. L. Nardi and G. D. Zuidema [Eds.], *Surgery: A Concise Guide to
Clinical Practice* [3rd ed.]. Boston: Little, Brown, 1972, Chap. 39.)

 e. Endometrioid carcinomas (and rare benign variants) of primary, de novo
  ovarian origin.

 f. Clear cell adenocarcinomas of primary, de novo ovarian origin (formerly called
  mesonephromas but now believed to be of müllerian rather than mesonephric
  origin).

 g. Endometriomas and the relatively rare primary ovarian endometrioid tumors
  (adenocarcinomas and adenoacanthomas) and clear cell adenocarcinomas that
  appear to be due to malignant change in previously benign areas of ovarian
  endometriosis.

4. **Connective tissue** (ovarian stroma).
   a. Generalized.
      (1) Fibromas (sometimes accompanied by Meigs' syndrome), fibroadenomas, papillomas, and rare angiomatous and lymphangiomatous tumors.
      (2) Sarcomas (rare, e.g., fibrosarcoma).
   b. Specialized.
      (1) Granulosa cell and theca cell tumors (and their malignant or sarcomatoid forms) **(feminizing tumors)**.
      (2) Arrhenoblastomas, Leydig cell (hilus cell) tumors, gonadoblastomas (and their malignant variants) **(masculinizing tumors)**.
      (3) Gynandroblastomas, often both **androgenic** and **estrogenic**.
      (4) Dysgerminomas.
      (5) Undifferentiated sarcomatoid or embryonal carcinomalike tumors.
5. **Functional activity**.
      Follicle cysts, corpus luteum cysts, theca-lutein cysts.
6. **Metastatic lesions**.
   a. Krukenberg tumors.
   b. Metastases from endometrial, breast, and gastrointestinal tract cancers.

PHYSIOLOGIC AND OTHER NONNEOPLASTIC OVARIAN CYSTS

FOLLICLE CYSTS

When, during the first half of the menstrual cycle, the dominant follicle does not succeed in ovulating and remains active but immature, or if any of the less-stimulated follicles fail to undergo their normal atresia, one or more follicle cysts may develop. Usually, they remain small, averaging only 1.0 to 1.5 cm in diameter, but occasionally a solitary one may attain the size of a small lemon (6 to 8 cm in diameter). Seen grossly, they are thin-walled and contain clear, serous fluid, which gives them a translucent appearance. Although increasing intracystic pressure ultimately causes atrophy of the cyst lining, microscopically it is seen to be composed of small, closely packed granulosa cells. Although the cyst fluid frequently is rich in estrogen, and although persistence of one of the larger follicle cysts is commonly associated with a period of menstrual irregularity, it is unlikely that the cysts themselves are functionally active. They invariably disappear spontaneously, either by slow resorption of fluid or by sudden rupture. Rupture of a follicle cyst or, occasionally, torsion of the ovary containing it may give rise to transient acute or chronic intermittent lower abdominal pain (see also Chap. 5). In most instances, however, conservative management suffices, and the ovary returns to normal size, with subsidence of any associated symptoms, usually within a month or two.

CORPUS LUTEUM CYSTS

Corpus luteum cysts are somewhat less common than simple follicle cysts, but are more likely to be clinically significant. They arise as a result of hemorrhage within a persistent mature corpus luteum, the accumulating hematoma producing second-ary cystic change. Grossly, they tend to attain a larger size (5 to 10 cm) than do follicle cysts and are usually purplish-red or chocolate in color due to the contained hematoma, although resorption of blood may result in a clearer, thinner type of cyst fluid. The yellowish-orange color of the cyst lining is indicative of its corpus luteal origin, and on microscopic examination the wall of the cyst is seen to consist of large, luteinized granulosa and theca cells covered by a layer of organizing blood clot.

Persistent corpus luteum cysts are prone to produce menstrual irregularities, delay in onset of the period with subsequent irregular and prolonged flow being the most typical. Furthermore, because of their larger size and a tendency to the per-sistence of intermittent bleeding within the cyst cavity, they are also more likely to be accompanied by pelvic and lower abdominal pain, usually unilateral and dull and aching in character. Finally, as the result of continued or recurrent intracystic bleed-ing, they not infrequently rupture, often with additional, sometimes massive intra-peritoneal hemorrhage. The latter event not only often simulates a ruptured ectopic pregnancy but is sometimes severe enough to constitute an acute surgical emergency in its own right. A more detailed discussion of the course and management of corpus luteum cysts is presented in Chapter 5.

THECA-LUTEIN CYSTS

Theca-lutein cysts are the least common of the physiologic cysts, and although they occasionally arise independently and may be unilateral, the vast majority occur in association with trophoblastic tumors (e.g., hydatidiform mole, chorionepithelioma), are bilateral, and often attain a considerable size (25 to 30 cm in diameter). Micro-scopically, marked luteinization of the thecal cells in the cyst wall and elsewhere in the ovarian stroma is the predominant feature; the granulosa cells may also be lutein-ized but more often undergo partial or complete atresia. These typical histologic features reflect the nature of the development of theca-lutein cysts in response to prolonged ovarian stimulation by excessive amounts of chorionic gonadotropin. The process is completely reversible, for the large, bilateral cysts undergo complete and spontaneous regression with removal of the mole or other trophoblastic lesion.

A related ovarian lesion, the so-called **pregnancy luteoma**, is a predominately solid, but sometimes partially cystic tumor of the ovary encountered occasionally in asso-ciation with normal pregnancy. It is invariably only discovered if cesarean section becomes necessary; as a result, the ovaries are actually seen and palpated at laparot-omy. Although at one time it was believed to be a true neoplasm with malignant potential, the luteoma of pregnancy is now known to be a benign hyperplastic process, whose histologic structure and steroid hormone composition resemble the normal corpus luteum or, in some instances, the theca-lutein cyst. The lesions are usually bilateral and multicentric, and they regress spontaneously following termi-nation of the pregnancy. The importance of recognizing them and avoiding unnec-essary oophorectomy for a benign, reversible, gonadotropin-induced hyperplasia is obvious.

In some instances (roughly 30 percent of cases), a luteoma of pregnancy may be the site of androgenic hormone secretion with resulting masculinization of the mother and the female fetus. Both the "tumor" and the maternal masculinization will regress when the pregnancy is completed, but approximately 65 percent of the female infants born of virilized mothers will exhibit fetal masculinization of the external genitalia.

ENDOMETRIOMAS

Ovarian endometriomas (chocolate cysts of the ovary) are another common form of nonneoplastic cyst and are discussed in detail in Chapter 10. Rarely, benign endometrioid tumors (polyps, papillary adenomas, and adenofibromas) have been encountered in endometriotic cysts, or even in the absence of ovarian endometriosis.

PAROVARIAN CYSTS

Although not actually primary ovarian lesions, parovarian cysts, usually indistinguishable clinically from true ovarian cysts, must be considered in the differential diagnosis of any cystic adnexal mass. They arise from mesonephric duct remnants and grow within the leaves of the broad ligament, displacing and distorting the tube and ovary, both of which become partially incorporated within the cyst capsule. They often reach a considerable size, occupying the entire pelvis and lower abdomen in some cases. It is usually possible to dissect and remove them from the broad ligament, guarding the ureter against harm and preserving the tube and ovary with their blood supply intact (see also Chap. 17).

BENIGN NEOPLASTIC OVARIAN CYSTS AND TUMORS

The most common benign tumors of the ovary are cystic in type and include dermoid cysts and the related benign solid teratomas, simple cystomas, and the various benign cystadenomas. Benign solid tumors occur less often, those most frequently encountered being the fibromas, the cystadenofibromas, and Brenner tumors. The ubiquitous leiomyoma, so common elsewhere in the müllerian system, is only rarely encountered in the ovary. The benign functioning ovarian tumors are discussed in Chapter 6.

Dermoid Cysts

The term **dermoid**, implying a cyst or tumor of dermal origin and content only, is actually a misnomer, for although dermal elements (e.g., cutaneous epithelium and its appendages, sebaceous fluid, hair, teeth) predominate in the majority of dermoid cysts, careful histologic study will reveal tissue derived from all three germ cell layers, confirming the true teratomatous nature of these cysts. It is now fairly well established that dermoid cysts and other types of ovarian teratomas are parthenogenic tumors that arise from a single germ cell after the first meiotic division, but before the second. They represent about 10 percent of all ovarian tumors and constitute 20 percent of all ovarian cysts; they are the most common ovarian tumor of childhood and, although they may occur at any age, usually appear during active reproductive life. They are also frequently multiple, often with several developing in the same ovary, and with bilateral ovarian involvement in 25 percent of cases.

Grossly, they usually attain only a moderate size and present as thick-walled, grayish-white, well-encapsulated, globular cysts projecting from the surface of the ovary or more often attached to it by a pedicle. The bulk of the cyst contents is usually made up of fatty, semisolid sebaceous material, which gives these cysts their characteristic doughy consistency. Collections of matted hair are also common, and well-formed teeth, often arising from a rudimentary jaw, are present in 50 percent of cases and are of course visible on x-ray films of the pelvis and abdomen (Fig. 57).

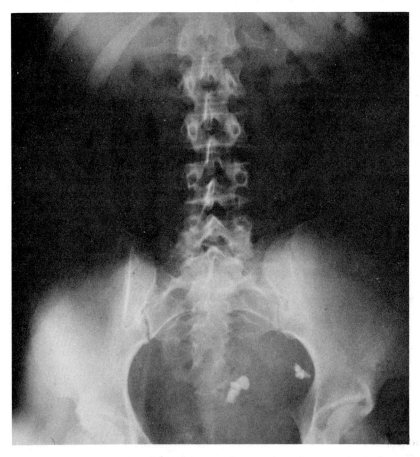

Figure 57
Plain abdominal x-ray film in patient with dermoid cyst. The typical dental structures are diagnostic of the nature of the cyst in this case.

Most of the solid components will be found arising from one localized area of thickening within the cyst wall, the inner lining of which is otherwise smooth and composed essentially of skin. Microscopically, various types and combinations of tissues representative of all three germ cell layers may be found: skin, hair, sebaceous glands, teeth, and even fingernails and rudimentary portions of the eye and the central nervous system (ectodermal); bone, cartilage, muscle, fat, and connective tissue (mesodermal); and gastrointestinal tract mucosa, respiratory epithelium, and thyroid tissue (entodermal).

Aside from their obvious presence as an ovarian mass, the most common clinical manifestations of dermoid cysts are acute pelvic and lower abdominal pain secondary to torsion, sometimes with infarction, to which their smooth, free-lying, frequently pedunculated nature predisposes them, and acute or chronic discomfort due to acute rupture or to intermittent leakage of the highly irritating cyst contents into the peritoneal cavity. Malignant change, usually squamous cell carcinoma, developing in one of the epidermal elements of the cyst, is rare, occurring in perhaps 3 percent of cases, and invariably in women well past the menopause. The development of adenocarcinomas and an occasional carcinoid tumor in dermoid cysts has also been reported, but these cases are extremely rare.

A dozen cases have been reported in which a benign cystic ovarian teratoma has been accompanied by severe hemolytic anemia of the spherocytic type, the hemolysis and anemia disappearing completely when the ovarian tumor was removed. The factors underlying this rare association are not clear.

Benign Solid Teratomas

When mesodermal and entodermal elements predominate in a dermoid type of tumor, there is little if any tendency to cystic change, and the tumor is more likely to assume the form of the so-called benign solid teratoma. These are often considerably larger, bulkier tumors, and may become adherent to surrounding structures. Although histologically similar to dermoid cysts in composition, with a mixture of tissues derived from all three germ layers in various stages of adult or embryonic development, the solid teratomas tend to proliferate more rapidly and to contain more immature cell forms. A certain proportion of tumors of this type therefore exhibit a malignant, usually sarcomatous change, which is often fortunately of low-grade potential. One specific type of benign solid teratoma composed almost entirely of adult thyroid tissue, the struma ovarii, has already been described in Chapter 6.

Simple Serous Cystomas

Simple serous cystomas are pearly-white, thin walled, translucent, smoothly rounded, and usually pedunculated. They contain a clear yellow serous fluid, and histologic examination of the cyst lining shows only a low cuboidal epithelium with no evidence of abnormal proliferative activity. There is some reason to believe that they are actually a variety of nonpapillary serous cystadenoma in which pressure atrophy of the more glandular type of epithelial lining has resulted from progressive fluid distention of the cyst. They often attain considerable size, are frequently bilateral, and because of their free-floating behavior are very prone to undergo torsion.

Pseudomucinous and Serous Cystadenomas

It is difficult to define sharply a category of benign cystadenomas and completely distinguish and separate it from the frankly malignant varieties of cystadenocarcinoma, for there are many apparently grossly benign cystadenomas that on histologic study show borderline or early malignant epithelial proliferative activity or in which the subsequent clinical course of the patient belies the relatively benign histologic appearance of the initial lesion. It is thus important at the outset to bear in mind that there is a broad spectrum of degrees of epithelial abnormality among the cystadenomatous tumors, and that between the completely benign cystadenomas and the obviously malignant cystadenocarcinomas exists a sizable group of tumors that behave like malignant tumors, although it is impossible always to predict this on the basis of their microscopic appearance.

PSEUDOMUCINOUS CYSTADENOMAS

The benign pseudomucinous cystadenoma is somewhat more common than the benign serous cystadenoma and is a less actively proliferating neoplasm. It is also less often bilateral (15 to 25 percent of cases) and less likely to be the site of malignant degeneration, which, when it occurs, is most often seen after the menopause. These cysts are characterized grossly by their sticky, gelatinous contents (this is now known to be initially secreted by the tumor cells as true mucin, chemical alterations occurring later as a result of aging) and by their being invariably multilocular on the interior due to the presence of numerous daughter cysts, which sometimes gives them a slightly lobulated appearance externally as well. They tend to become quite large; most of the enormous ovarian cysts reported as medical curiosities are of this type. In outward appearance they do not otherwise differ significantly from serous cystadenomas or other cystic tumors of the ovary.

The lining of the principal and daughter cysts is usually smooth, but in 10 percent of cases, papillary projections are found. It is in this group of papillary pseudomucinous cystadenomas that instances of a low-grade malignant potential are occasionally encountered, and undoubtedly it is in this group that malignant change occurs, approximately 5 to 10 percent of all pseudomucinous ovarian tumors being cystadenocarcinomas. Microscopically, the lining is composed of a tall, columnar, "picket-fence" type of epithelium, usually with numerous mucus-secreting goblet cells. In the uncommon papillary forms, a more proliferative, adenomatous pattern may be seen.

A rare complication, which sometimes develops if rupture of the cyst and intraabdominal spillage of its contents occur, is the diffuse seeding of peritoneal surfaces with multilocular, gelatinous, secondary implants, the condition known as **pseudo-myxoma peritonei**. Although there is no invasion of underlying structures, the process tends to be chronic, the jellylike substance continues to accumulate, is difficult to evacuate, and causes a secondary granulomatous peritonitis with adhesions, ultimately resulting in death from intestinal obstruction or inanition. (A similar condition can arise in association with a proliferative type of mucocele of the appendix.)

SEROUS CYSTADENOMAS

Although retaining a completely similar cystic outward appearance, serous cystadenomas are much more actively proliferating tumors, the majority being papillary in type. They occur almost as frequently as the pseudomucinous variety, usually during the active reproductive years, and are far more often bilateral (roughly 50 percent of the cases). Furthermore, it is among serous cystadenomas that borderline cases of histologic malignancy are so often encountered; the significance of their typical papillary nature is also emphasized by the fact that approximately 50 percent of all serous cystadenomatous lesions are frank serous cystadenocarcinomas.

Grossly, they are usually unilocular, less often compartmented, cysts containing a thin, straw-colored serous fluid, and ordinarily they attain only moderate size. The cyst lining typically is covered by numerous papillary outgrowths, and in some cases the cyst cavity is solidly filled with masses of these papillary projections. Less often, the external surface is covered by similar excrescences, but the presence of the latter usually implies malignant change. Microscopically, the connective tissue of the cyst wall and its papillary outgrowths is covered by a single layer of low cuboidal, dark-staining, nonmucus-secreting epithelial cells. In cases of borderline malignancy, the epithelium may be several cell layers thick with evidence of anaplastic cellular proliferation and even early stromal invasion. An additional and almost diagnostic microscopic feature sometimes seen in serous cystadenomas and even more common in serous cystadenocarcinomas is the presence of the so-called psammoma bodies, which represent calcium deposits within the stroma or connective-tissue core of the papillary processes, and which are more likely to be present in the more rapidly proliferating lesions. At times, psammoma body accumulations become extensive enough to be visible on x-ray films of the abdomen, and because they almost never appear in other types of abdominal or pelvic neoplasms, their histologic presence in even tiny biopsy specimens is essentially diagnostic of a serous cystadenomatous lesion, usually carcinoma.

Fibromas of the Ovary

Ovarian fibromas constitute 20 percent of all solid ovarian tumors and 5 percent of the total group of ovarian neoplasms. They are heavy, solid, pearly-white tumors composed almost entirely of pure fibrous connective tissue of ovarian stromal origin, and in 90 percent of cases they are unilateral lesions. They vary in size from small, asymptomatic nodules in the substance or on the surface of the ovary to large, melon-sized masses. The larger tumors are nearly always pedunculated and hence prone to torsion; more important, they are frequently associated with **Meigs' syndrome** (see p. 481). On cut section they are seen to have practically no capsule and to present a fairly homogeneous, fibrous, whorled appearance similar to that of a leiomyoma, except that a striking edema is often present. There may be patches of cystic, hyaline, or calcific degeneration, and in some areas a yellowish-orange streaking not unlike that seen in thecomas may be visible. In fact, there is some evidence to suggest that many fibromas were originally thecomas that subsequently degenerated and lost their hormonal function.

Cystadenofibromas

Cystadenofibromas are small fibrous tumors, usually arising within the substance of the ovary. Although grossly resembling small fibromas, they are seen histologically to contain true cystic gland spaces lined by a simple cuboidal epithelium scattered throughout a dense, fibrous stroma. They are probably related to similar warty surface growths of the ovary — the papillomas or papillary adenofibromas — and all of this group in turn are probably varieties of benign cystadenoma. They are usually asymptomatic and of significance only from the standpoint of their recognition and differentiation from other, more serious lesions. Malignant change involving the glandular epithelium of an adenofibroma and the subsequent development of adenofibrocarcinoma are extremely rare.

Brenner Tumors

Brenner tumors, which are relatively uncommon, usually appear after the menopause or occasionally in the later reproductive years, are most often unilateral, and typically are well-encapsulated, fibrous lesions resembling fibromas except for the invariable presence of many small cystic spaces within them. They are easily identified histologically by the distinctive epithelial cell nests scattered throughout their dense fibrous stroma. These cell nests resemble the Walthard's embryonic cell rests frequently found in the ovary and its vicinity and believed to be of wolffian duct origin, and the cells themselves generally resemble cells in the transitional layer of stratified squamous epithelium. The cystic spaces within the glandlike cell nests account for the cystic gross appearance of these tumors and are produced either by simple degenerative change or at times by a metaplasia of the epithelial cells and replacement by an actively secreting pseudomucinous type of epithelium with resulting distention of the gland spaces with mucus. Anaplastic change in this metaplastic epithelium may account for the occasional occurrence of malignant Brenner tumors, but the vast majority are and remain benign. Occasionally, a Brenner tumor is encountered as a separate, discrete component within the wall of a pseudomucinous cystadenoma or cystadenocarcinoma.

In clinical behavior as well as gross appearance, the Brenner tumor is entirely similar to the fibroma, and in some instances a large Brenner tumor has been accompanied by ascites and hydrothorax (Meigs' syndrome). The occasional presence of actively functioning theca cells within the stroma of a Brenner tumor sometimes results in associated abnormal vaginal bleeding.

Clinical Manifestations of Benign Ovarian Tumors and Cysts

By and large, the various types of benign ovarian lesions tend to produce similar symptoms, and although some are more prone to certain of the secondary complications than others, any of the following clinical manifestations may be encountered:

1. The presence of a totally asymptomatic lesion may simply be discovered on routine examination, the need to exclude the possibility of a malignant ovarian tumor, however, posing an immediate problem in diagnosis and management.

2. Rupture, often with secondary hemorrhage, may occur and simulate a variety of acute abdominal emergencies, often mimicking appendicitis, ectopic pregnancy, or acute pelvic inflammation. The most typical example is the ruptured, bleeding corpus luteum cyst, but other lesions that frequently rupture, or bleed, or both include endometriomas and granulosa cell tumors, and the dermoid cysts are prone to undergo intermittent leakage of their highly irritating contents.

3. Acute torsion, with or without infarction, or intermittent and recurring twists of the ovarian pedicle producing subacute distress can occur with any of the benign ovarian cysts and tumors. However, it is most commonly seen in association with the dermoid cysts, simple cystomas, cystadenomas, and fibromas, all of which are smoothly rounded, often pedunculated, and rarely adherent to neighboring structures. (This complication is uncommon with malignant ovarian tumors, presumably because, being larger and heavier, they are less mobile as well as often adherent.)

4. Secondary infection is rare but is occasionally seen in dermoid cysts and may result in a localized peritonitis.

5. Chronic intermittent pelvic discomfort, often aggravated at ovulation time, in the latter half of the cycle, or at the time of the menses, is sometimes a feature of benign ovarian lesions. This symptom is particularly common in association with physiologic cysts and endometriomas but is sometimes also encountered with dermoid cysts. The vast majority of benign cystic or solid ovarian tumors are painless, however, unless complicated by torsion or rupture.

6. Abdominal swelling and secondary pressure effects on the adjacent bladder or gastrointestinal tract due to the enlarging pelvic or abdominal mass are seen with the larger cystic tumors.

7. Meigs' syndrome.

MEIGS' SYNDROME

By definition, Meigs' syndrome is the occurrence of ascites and hydrothorax in association with fibroma of the ovary (Fig. 58), the fluid in the abdomen and chest

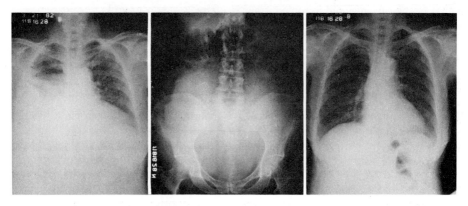

Figure 58
Chest x-rays before (on the left) and after (on the right) removal of an ovarian fibroma, in a patient with Meigs' syndrome. The plain film of the abdomen (center) demonstrates the large fibroma and the accompanying ascites.

disappearing completely and permanently following removal of the fibroma. Approximately 40 percent of fibromas larger than 6 cm in diameter are accompanied by ascites, but less than 5 percent of all fibromas give rise to Meigs' syndrome (roughly 15 percent of fibromas larger than 6 cm in diameter). The condition may also be encountered occasionally in the presence of thecomas and other fibromalike benign tumors. It should be emphasized that Meigs' syndrome does not include the development of ascites and pleural effusion secondary to metastases from ovarian or other abdominal carcinomas, although the syndrome may precisely simulate this situation, even to a malignant-appearing cachexia. Occasionally, other benign tumors and cysts of the ovary and, rarely, even large, pedunculated uterine fibroids may be accompanied by ascites and hydrothorax, a condition referred to as **pseudo-Meigs' syndrome.**

The formation of ascites may be dependent on actual fluid formation (a transudate of extracellular fluid) and leakage through the very thin capsule surrounding the myxoid tissue of the usually markedly edematous fibroma (the most widely accepted explanation) or may in part be the result of fluid formation secondary to local peritoneal irritation or even to some more generalized response similar to Selye's "alarm reaction," which alters fluid balance. The hydrothorax presumably results from the passage of excessive abdominal fluid through the lymphatics of the diaphragm.

It is important to be aware of this syndrome, for it is often highly suggestive of advanced, hopeless cancer, and many patients have been refused treatment in the past, dying of a benign, easily curable condition. The need to establish a definite histologic diagnosis in any patient with an ovarian tumor, ascites, and hydrothorax is obvious.

Diagnostic Approach

Since the general diagnostic problems and approach are essentially the same for both benign and malignant ovarian lesions, they will for the most part be discussed jointly here. There are three aspects to the problem of evaluating a pelvic mass that suggests the presence of an ovarian cyst or tumor. First is the need to establish that the mass is actually ovarian in origin. Second is the desirability of distinguishing between physiologic cysts, which will usually regress spontaneously, and true neoplastic cysts and tumors, which will require treatment. Third is the attempt to determine prior to laparotomy whether a given ovarian lesion is benign or malignant and, if malignant, the possible existence and extent of any spread beyond the ovary. A proper and accurate appraisal of the findings noted on careful, detailed abdominal, pelvic, and rectal examinations, together with a thoughtful interpretation of any associated symptoms and supplemented by any indicated additional diagnostic procedures (e.g., proctoscopy, barium enema), will usually serve to differentiate an ovarian lesion from a pelvic mass arising in some other pelvic organ or structure. The possibility that a physiologic cyst is the cause of the ovarian enlargement is usually suggested by its size and obvious cystic nature in a woman of appropriate age. In the case of definite cystic or solid tumors of the ovary, it may be impossible to establish an exact diagnosis prior to laparotomy. However, in approaching all three aspects of the problem of diagnosis, the following considerations and suggested maneuvers are often helpful.

1. **Physical findings:** The location of the lesion with respect to the uterus, mobility or adherence, consistency (cystic, doughy, firm and solid, partially cystic and partially solid), contour (smoothly rounded, irregular, or nodular), size and weight, and the presence or absence of bilateral lesions will often establish that a given mass is definitely ovarian in origin and suggest its probable nature. Thus an ovarian lesion may be distinguished from a uterine fibroid (pedunculated lateral fibroids may defy distinction on pelvic examination alone, however), pelvic inflammatory disease, or sigmoid diverticulitis, for example, and may be determined to be cystic or solid, as the case may be. The presence of an endometrioma may be suspected if the characteristic nodularity of endometriosis is palpated elsewhere in the pelvis; a dermoid cyst may be tentatively recognized by its distinctive doughy consistency; partially cystic tumors with solid components, particularly when bilateral, are more often malignant lesions, and if secondary nodules are palpable in the cul-de-sac, the presence of metastases is strongly suggested. These represent just a few examples of the way in which, with experience, the physical characteristics of the mass and the associated pelvic findings may yield valuable clues, particularly when integrated with the overall clinical picture.

2. **Laparoscopy or culdoscopy** may also prove extremely useful where there is only the suspicion of an ovarian enlargement, or where it is a matter of definitely identifying a lateral, pedunculated fibroid for which no treatment will be necessary once the possibility of an ovarian lesion has been excluded; use of this technique will avoid a certain number of unnecessary laparotomies for diagnosis only.

3. If a simple follicle or corpus luteum cyst is suspected on the basis of the physical findings, **reexamination** in four to six weeks is indicated, most physiologic cysts undergoing spontaneous regression within the next one or two menstrual cycles. If the enlargement persists, however, exploration will probably eventually be necessary.

4. **A plain x-ray** film of the abdomen may establish the diagnosis of dermoid cyst, if calcified teeth structures are present or if the typical soft-tissue laminated fat pattern produced by the sebaceous fluid is visible (see Fig. 57).

5. **Diagnostic ultrasound studies** may be very helpful in distinguishing the nature and location of pelvic masses and differentiating between solid tumors, cysts, and ascites.

6. **An intravenous pyelogram** is also often helpful in distinguishing a pelvic kidney or low-lying renal tumor and in determining whether or not there is any displacement of the ureters by the mass (see Fig. 12).

7. Since both diverticulitis and carcinoma of the sigmoid can simulate ovarian tumors, and since metastatic ovarian cancer commonly is secondary to carcinoma of the colon or stomach, **proctoscopy, barium enema, and an upper gastrointestinal series** are also often indicated in the evaluation of patients with suspected ovarian malignancy.

8. If abdominal swelling is present and is obviously fluid in nature, a large fluid-filled cyst can usually be differentiated from ascites by **abdominal percussion**, dullness over the cyst with tympany in the flanks being typical of the former, in contrast to the shifting dullness in the flanks characteristic of ascites. The umbilicus is invariably protruding and everted in the presence of ascites, remaining flat if abdominal distention is due to an ovarian cyst, another helpful differential point.

9. If definite ascites is present, **a chest roentgenogram** is indicated to reveal any associated pleural effusion or to demonstrate possible pulmonary metastases. In the presence of ascites, with or without pleural effusion, the lesion usually proves to be ovarian carcinoma with associated intraabdominal metastases, but the possibility of an ovarian fibroma with Meigs' syndrome also must be kept in mind, along with cirrhosis and other less common causes of ascites such as tuberculous peritonitis and cardiac disease. Paracentesis and cytologic examination of a sample of ascitic fluid may settle the question, or the malignant nature of the tumor may be obvious if multiple abdominal masses and/or the characteristic nodular hepatic enlargement indicative of metastatic spread are actually palpable, either before or following paracentesis.

10. **Liver scan, lung scan, bone scan,** and **lymphangiograms** may be helpful in some cases.

Treatment of Benign Ovarian Tumors and Cysts

Once it can definitely be established that they are not malignant, many benign ovarian tumors and cysts can be treated by local excision, with conservation of the involved ovary. Those in which local resection is usually indicated include all the physiologic cysts, which, because of persistent symptoms or inability to exclude the possibility of neoplasm, require operative treatment, as well as endometriomas, parovarian cysts, and simple dermoid cysts. Occasionally, however, their large size or the presence of secondary complications (e.g., rupture, hemorrhage, torsion, or secondary infection) may make unilateral salpingo-oophorectomy necessary. The cystadenomas and essentially all solid benign tumors of the ovary are best treated by unilateral salpingo-oophorectomy, because it is usually both impossible to be certain of their completely benign nature before removal as well as technically difficult to dissect them cleanly from any remaining normal ovarian substance. Occasional exceptions can be made in the case of pedunculated, obviously benign simple cystomas or fibromas.

At laparotomy the lesion should be totally removed, either by local resection or unilateral salpingo-oophorectomy. The specimen should be immediately opened and carefully examined; the opinion of the pathologist should be obtained and frozen-section studies done in the operating room if necessary before reaching the final decision whether the lesion is benign and can be treated by a conservative surgical procedure. Because many of the benign ovarian lesions also show a tendency to be bilateral, the opposite ovary must be carefully inspected and preferably bisected to avoid overlooking a similar, smaller lesion within its substance. In young women in whom a conservative operation is usually highly desirable if at all possible, and in whom a probable diagnosis of benign tumor is reached on the basis of gross appearance and microscopic findings on frozen section, it is reasonable to conclude the operation and await the results of study of the permanent histologic sections. If the final report reverses the initial impression, then reoperation and completion of an adequate cancer operation will usually be indicated. The occasional indications for and the factors involved in reaching a decision to carry out conservative surgery for a few tumors of low-grade malignant potential are further discussed in the section on treatment of malignant ovarian tumors. However, in older women approaching or beyond the menopause, even benign ovarian cysts and tumors should in general probably be treated by total hysterectomy and bilateral salpingo-oophorectomy, since little or nothing is gained by conservative management in this age group, and the risk of inadequately treating a potentially malignant lesion is thereby completely avoided.

CARCINOMA OF THE OVARY

The ovary is the third most common site of malignancy in the female reproductive tract, carcinoma of the ovary constituting 15 to 20 percent of all genital cancer. That it is a serious disease is emphasized by the fact that although ovarian cancer represents only 3 percent of all the cancers seen in the female, it causes 15 percent of the deaths from all types of cancer occurring in women, making it the fourth leading cause of cancer deaths in women. It is the number one cause of death in women with cancer of the genital tract (47 percent of all deaths from such cancers). Cancer of the ovary also appears to be slowly increasing in frequency, and the death rate from ovarian cancer is now two and one-half to three times what it was in 1930. There are now 15,000 new cases each year and roughly 10,000 deaths from ovarian cancer per year in the United States. Most ovarian cancers appear at or shortly after the menopause, the peak incidence (60 percent) being in women 40 to 60 years old, with an additional 20 percent developing in women over 60 years of age. However, 20 percent occur in women under 40 years of age and, although they may occur in any age group, the highly malignant solid teratomatous tumors, embryonal carcinomas, dysgerminomas, and the rare sarcomas are particularly prone to appear in younger women, often in adolescents or pubertal girls. Although little is known of the etiology of human ovarian cancer, recent careful epidemiologic surveys have drawn attention to several high-risk factors: namely, that nulliparous women, women who have had (or subsequently have) carcinoma of the breast, and women who are members of the rare "ovarian cancer families" (often the family history includes the majority of the females of several generations) are particularly prone to have cancer of the ovary.

Because of the poor overall prognosis for patients with ovarian cancer and because the high mortality from this disease continues despite advances in the treatment of malignant disease in general, enthusiastic support for the concept of prophylactic oophorectomy whenever hysterectomy is done has arisen from time to time over the past few decades. Although few would argue that the ovaries in menopausal or post-menopausal women undergoing hysterectomy for benign disease should, or need, be conserved, there are few if any data to justify removing them in younger women in order to protect them from ovarian cancer. There is no increased incidence of ovarian cancer developing in ovaries retained after hysterectomy; since only a small percentage of the total female population undergoes hysterectomy, routine prophylactic oophorectomy could have only an insignificant impact on the overall problem of ovarian cancer. On the other hand, routine prophylactic oophorectomy in pre-menopausal women of any age is certain to have significant, deleterious physiologic and psychological effects that will not and cannot be satisfactorily counteracted by estrogen medication in most instances.

Classification

Carcinomas of the ovary were originally simply grossly separated into the cystic and solid varieties. The former are far more common, and papillary cystadenocarcinomas account for at least 75 percent of all ovarian cancers. It is obvious, however, that carcinoma of the ovary is not a single disease entity, but that it represents a variety of epithelial tumors of ovarian origin, each of different histogenetic derivation, microscopic appearance, and clinical behavior. The three principal types of epithelial tumors of the ovary are the serous, mucinous (or pseudomucinous), and endometrioid tumors. In each category there are benign, borderline, and frankly malignant neoplasms. Based on these considerations, the histologic classification of the common primary epithelial tumors of the ovary adopted by the International Federation of Gynecology and Obstetrics and currently in use throughout the world is as follows:

I. Serous cystomas.
   a. Serous benign cystadenomas.
   b. Serous cystadenomas with proliferating activity of the epithelial cells and nuclear abnormalities but with no infiltrative destructive growth (low potential malignancy).
   c. Serous cystadenocarcinomas.
II. Mucinous cystomas.
   a. Mucinous benign cystadenomas.
   b. Mucinous cystadenomas with proliferating activity of epithelial cells and nuclear abnormalities but with no infiltrative destructive growth (low potential malignancy).
   c. Mucinous cystadenocarcinomas.
III. Endometrioid tumors (similar to adenocarcinomas in the endometrium).
   a. Endometrioid benign cysts.
   b. Endometrioid tumors with proliferating activity of the epithelial cells and nuclear abnormalities but with no infiltrative destructive growth (low potential malignancy).
   c. Endometrioid adenocarcinomas.
IV. Mesonephric tumors (clear cell adenocarcinomas, probably of müllerian origin).
   a. Benign mesonephric tumors.
   b. Mesonephric tumors with proliferating activity of the epithelial cells and nuclear abnormalities but with no infiltrative destructive growth (low potential malignancy).
   c. Mesonephric cystadenocarcinomas.
V. Concomitant carcinoma, unclassified carcinoma (tumors that cannot be allotted to one of the Groups I, II, III, or IV).

As indicated, each of the three principal types (serous, mucinous, and endometrioid) are further subdivided into their benign, borderline, and malignant varieties. The so-called unclassified carcinomas are highly malignant, often solid tumors that are so undifferentiated microscopically that it is impossible to assign them to a specific histologic category. It should be noted that both Brenner tumors (benign or malignant) as well as the clear cell adenocarcinomas of müllerian origin (formerly called mesonephromas) are also epithelial neoplasms, and finally, that some ovarian tumors will be found on microscopic examination to contain elements of two or more of the principal histologic types.

Staging

In addition to information regarding the histologic type of an ovarian cancer, knowledge of the extent of the tumor is equally important in planning treatment, estimating prognosis, and arriving at valid comparisons of the results of different programs of therapy. A useful clinical staging for this purpose, comparable to the one employed for carcinoma of the cervix but based on the findings at laparotomy is as follows:

Stage I   Lesion confined to the ovaries.
  a. Only one ovary involved; no ascites.
   (1) Capsule ruptured (invaded and breached by tumor, with surface involvement).
   (2) Capsule not ruptured.
  b. Both ovaries involved; no ascites.
   (1) Capsule ruptured.
   (2) Capsule not ruptured.
  c. One or both ovaries involved; ascites with malignant cells, or peritoneal washings positive on cytologic study, or tumor ruptured at operation.
   (1) Capsule ruptured (invaded).
   (2) Capsule not ruptured (not invaded).
Stage II   Lesion involving one or both ovaries with pelvic extension.
  a. Extension limited to uterus, tubes, opposite ovary.
  b. Extension to other pelvic tissues.
  c. In addition, ascites with malignant cells or peritoneal washings positive on cytologic study, or tumor ruptured at operation.
Stage III   Lesion involving one or both ovaries with widespread intraperitoneal metastases, including retroperitoneal nodes and omental and small-bowel involvement, even if confined within the pelvis.
Stage IV   Lesion involving one or both ovaries with distant metastases outside the peritoneal cavity but including liver metastases. Simple pleural effusion must be positive cytologically to allot a case to Stage IV.
Special category   Unexplored cases thought to be ovarian carcinoma.

Obviously, the prognosis rapidly becomes worse as the clinical stage advances. From the standpoint of tumor histology, endometrioid and mucinous carcinomas have a better prognosis than serous carcinomas, probably, in part at least, because they tend to remain localized longer and to disseminate more slowly.

Types of Ovarian Carcinomas

PAPILLARY SEROUS CYSTADENOCARCINOMA

Approximately 35 to 50 percent of ovarian cancers are papillary serous cystadenomas; the majority probably arise as the result of a progressively increasing malignant change in a serous cystadenoma and are therefore, in essence, the malignant form of the latter. Bilateral ovarian involvement is present in 50 percent of cases, a characteristic feature. In the early stages the tumor may still be completely encapsulated within the wall of the cyst, which, when opened, is found partially or completely filled with solid masses of papillary growth. At this stage it may be indistinguishable from a benign cystadenoma except by its microscopic appearance, which, though retaining the papillary pattern, is characterized by a heaping-up of obviously anaplastic cells into multiple layers around the irregular papillary processes and often by the presence of psammoma bodies. Ultimately, however, extension through the capsule leads to the appearance of typical nodular or plaquelike implants on the exterior of the cyst and eventually on the adjacent peritoneum of the pelvic walls, cul-de-sac, uterus, and rectosigmoid, the lesion becoming markedly adherent to the surrounding structures. More distant dissemination involving the omentum and the parietal and visceral surfaces throughout the peritoneal cavity rapidly leads to widespread abdominal carcinomatosis and ascites.

The distinguishing features of the serous group of ovarian carcinomas are their very rapid rates of growth and dissemination (rendering them only occasionally curable by surgical removal alone), and, from the standpoint of therapy, their moderate sensitivity to radiation and frequent responsiveness to the chemotherapeutic agents usually employed. Thus both modalities are often important in the overall management of these lesions.

PAPILLARY PSEUDOMUCINOUS CYSTADENOCARCINOMA

Papillary pseudomucinous cystadenocarcinoma accounts for approximately 10 to 15 percent of all ovarian cancers and bears a similar relationship to the benign pseudomucinous cystadenoma in terms of origin, general appearance, and histology. It is bilateral in only 25 percent of cases and tends to be somewhat more slow-growing and to extend and disseminate later and less often than the serous cystadenocarcinoma. Otherwise, it does not differ significantly in its gross appearance or clinical behavior from the latter. Microscopically, the picture varies from a moderately anaplastic, papillary type of pseudomucinous epithelial pattern to an undifferentiated form of adenocarcinoma.

From the standpoint of therapy, the important characteristics of the mucinous tumors are their slow rate of growth and dissemination (they remain totally resectable and potentially curable by surgery alone for a longer period of time) and their relative insensitivity to either radiation or chemotherapy. These same characteristics frequently make it worthwhile to reoperate on patients with mucinous carcinomas, either as a planned "second-look" procedure three to six months or more after the original surgical resection (with a view to discovery and removal of any potential residual disease that may by then have grown slowly to sufficient size to be detected) or in the deliberate management of a known recurrent tumor manifesting itself at varying intervals following the initial surgical resection.

ENDOMETRIOID CARCINOMA OF THE OVARY

Primary endometrioid cancers of the ovary are adenocarcinomas or adenoacanthomas (adenocarcinomas in which some of the neoplastic cells have differentiated into squamous elements) with a microscopic appearance entirely similar to that of adenocarcinoma or adenoacanthoma of the endometrium. Although some endometrioid tumors of the ovary (both benign and malignant forms) have convincingly been shown to have developed through malignant transformation within previously benign areas of ovarian endometriosis (as discussed in Chap. 10), the vast majority appear to have arisen de novo from the ovarian germinal epithelium, which, like the endometrium itself, is of müllerian origin. Since Long and Taylor [27], Scully and Barlow [39], and others have emphasized both the existence and relative frequency of occurrence of primary endometrioid tumors of the ovary, recognition and more accurate classification of these lesions have led to the realization that this histologic type of tumor actually accounts for 10 to 15 percent or more (in some series, 25 to 30 percent) of all primary ovarian cancers.

Seen grossly, these tumors are usually at least partially cystic, with solid papillary ingrowths or even solid extracystic components, the cysts frequently containing chocolatelike fluid; however, some are uniformly solid tumors. In about 30 percent of cases the tumors have been bilateral, less often (15 percent) with lesions of low-grade malignancy and more often (50 to 55 percent) when the tumor is highly anaplastic. Although they have been encountered over a wide range, the majority appear in women in the 50- to 60-year age group.

In a number of patients, an associated carcinoma of the endometrium has been recognized (in 10 to 15 percent of patients in most series; in some, as high as 30 percent if instances of carcinoma in situ and severe atypical adenomatous hyperplasia are included), and in some instances it has been difficult to be certain that the ovarian lesion was not a metastatic lesion. However, in many cases the endometrial cancer has been small, low grade, often microinvasive or even preinvasive. This has suggested that usually the ovarian and uterine tumors are independent primaries (neither representing a metastasis from the other) and that both the endometrium and the ovarian germinal epithelium (or occasionally an area of ovarian endometriosis) have responded to a common stimulus to neoplastic change. The excellent five-year survival rate (50 percent or better) in women with simultaneous ovarian endometrioid cancer and carcinoma of the endometrium also supports this concept.

Treatment of endometrioid carcinoma of the ovary is entirely similar to that for the more common cystadenocarcinomas of the ovary to be discussed later. It should consist of total hysterectomy and bilateral salpingo-oophorectomy, with postoperative radiation therapy if it is suspected that local disease has been left behind in the pelvis or lower abdomen, and chemotherapy if known or suspected residual disease is more widespread. Endometrioid carcinomas are usually very radiosensitive as well as moderately responsive to chemotherapy, so combined therapy should be aggressive and vigorous even in the more advanced stages and may achieve surprising results in terms of prolonged and worthwhile palliation and even apparent cures.

In general, the cure rates for endometrioid tumors of the ovary are considerably better than those for the more common serous or pseudomucinous cystadenocarcinomas, with reported overall five-year survival rates of 50 to 70 percent, suggesting that the former are usually well differentiated and considerably less malignant in their clinical behavior than the latter. The adenoacanthomas (roughly 50 percent of all the endometrioid carcinomas), in particular, are often only locally invasive and only occasionally metastasize widely, and hence they represent one of the most curable forms of ovarian cancer. However, when the ovarian endometrioid lesion is highly anaplastic, or when the tumor has spread beyond the ovary by the time of operation, the prognosis is equally ominous. Since it is well known that recurrent or metastatic endometrial cancer sometimes responds favorably to large doses of progestational agents (see Chap. 14), these agents have also been used, but without much success, in a few cases of advanced endometrioid carcinoma of the ovary.

As pointed out by Scully and Barlow [39], **clear cell adenocarcinomas** of the ovary (formerly called mesonephromas) also appear to be of müllerian (rather than mesonephric) origin and are probably variants or near relatives of the endometrioid ovarian tumors. They are entirely similar to the latter in their clinical behavior and favorable prognosis, as well as in the fact that in some instances they, too, appear to be the result of malignant change in areas of ovarian endometriosis. Despite the undoubted müllerian origin, some pathologists continue to call these tumors mesonephric or mesonephroid, because with their two main cell types, namely, the clear cell components and the tufts and tubular structures, they have some histologic resemblance to developing glomeruli and tubules.

SOLID ADENOCARCINOMAS OF THE OVARY

Solid adenocarcinomas of the ovary (roughly 10 percent of the total) constitute an unclassified group that appears to contain a variety of tumors of different histologic origin and probably includes some of the serous, pseudomucinous, and endometrioid lesions that are highly undifferentiated and have lost their cystic and secretory propensities. These tumors also vary greatly in microscopic appearance, although the descriptive terms often applied (medullary, alveolar, plexiform, scirrhous, or carcinoma simplex) have little clinical significance. Most of them show an adenocarcinomatous or papillary-adenocarcinomatous pattern.

In gross appearance, solid carcinomas of the ovary are usually of moderate size, somewhat irregularly rounded in contour, and on cut section are grayish or pinkish in color, may be stony-hard or friable and meaty in structure, depending on the amount of fibrous stroma present, and often contain areas of hemorrhage or cystic necrosis. The capsule is usually invaded early, and further and widespread peritoneal dissemination then promptly occurs. They are bilateral in over 50 percent of cases and tend to be highly malignant, pursuing a rapidly fatal course in most instances.

OTHER LESS COMMON TYPES OF OVARIAN CARCINOMA

Less common types of ovarian carcinoma are the occasional epidermoid carcinomas arising in dermoid cysts and the granulosa cell carcinomas, malignant arrhenoblastomas, adrenal cell rest carcinomas discussed in Chapter 6.

Clinical Features

Both their insidious onset and the manner in which they spread are responsible for the poor prognosis associated with the majority of ovarian carcinomas. Direct seeding by simple peritoneal diffusion once the tumor capsule has been breached is probably the most significant route of spread and rapidly leads to widespread abdominal carcinomatosis. Lymphatic and bloodstream dissemination also occurs in many cases and may lead to pelvic, paraaortic, and supraclavicular lymph node involvement as well as to distant metastases in the liver, lungs, and pleural cavity. Early diagnosis and prompt treatment when the lesion is still in the completely resectable stage currently offer the only hope of improving the curability in this disease. Every ovarian enlargement should be vigorously investigated, since approximately 40 percent of all ovarian tumors are malignant.

Diagnosis

The general diagnostic approach to any ovarian tumor or cyst is considered in the section dealing with benign ovarian lesions. In the case of ovarian carcinoma, early recognition is often hampered by the lack of any early symptoms, and a sizable tumor may lie hidden within the pelvic cavity and remain totally asymptomatic or cause only intermittent, vague distress for months or years. One should be particularly suspicious of the possible existence of an ovarian neoplasm in middle-aged women with vague pelvic or lower abdominal complaints; all too often they are inadequately examined and considered victims of psychoneurosis until, with the subsequent development of abdominal swelling, the diagnosis becomes obvious. Occasionally (in 15 to 25 percent of cases), a routine vaginal smear will be reported positive for adenocarcinoma cells or may even contain obvious psammoma bodies, but invariably by then a pelvic mass is already palpable, and the positive cytologic findings unfortunately usually indicate that the tumor has broken through its capsule and is in the stage of peritoneal seeding, tumor cells gaining access to the vaginal secretions via the patent tubes and uterine canal.

Regular, periodic examinations and early clinical detection of asymptomatic ovarian neoplasms while still in the potentially curable stage have so far been the one hope of decreasing the mortality rate from ovarian cancer. The possibility of preclinical detection of early carcinoma of the ovary by a routine screening procedure involving cytologic examination of peritoneal fluid obtained by cul-de-sac aspiration has been explored by Graham et al. [15], Keettel et al. [23], and others. Although several early ovarian cancers as well as surface lesions of borderline malignancy have already been discovered by this technique, it is still not established what percentage of early, curable, invasive cancers of the ovary will desquamate cells before they have begun actually to disseminate more widely throughout the peritoneal cavity. Perhaps the most encouraging aspect of this approach lies in the possibility that it may enable detection of preinvasive or borderline malignant ovarian lesions before they have progressed to the invasive stage. Certainly, this approach merits continued investigation. Unfortunately, however, it seems doubtful that cul-de-sac aspiration has quite the potential for development as a routine screening procedure to be used annually in millions of women, as was the case with the vaginal cytologic smear.

Various immunologic tests have been used in an attempt to find a reliable method for the very early detection of ovarian cancer, one that might also be useful in monitoring the results of therapy. Carcinoembryonic antigen (CEA) levels in the plasma of patients with ovarian carcinoma (and other gynecologic malignancies, as well) have been studied both before and after treatment, but the CEA test seems to be of no value in early diagnosis and of dubious significance in assaying therapeutic response. Alpha-fetoprotein is frequently elevated in embryonal and teratomatous tumors but only rarely in the more common epithelial tumors. On the other hand, the Regan isoenzyme of alkaline phosphatase is often detectable in increased amounts in the more common ovarian cancers. Unfortunately, it is not always present in ovarian cancer, even in patients with extensive disease, and yet it may be present in normal women as well as in association with other types of tumors. Thus neither of these immunologic techniques shows any real promise as a universally applicable screening test to achieve earlier diagnosis of ovarian cancer.

Symptoms

Symptomatic manifestations that are not necessarily specific for but are commonly associated with ovarian cancer include:

1. Vague abdominal distress and bowel and bladder irritability secondary to the enlarging pelvic mass that presses on adjacent organs.
2. Abdominal swelling or palpable tumor.
3. Irregular vaginal bleeding, which occurs in approximately 25 percent of patients and which is presumably due to an ovarian stromal hyperplasia incited by the growing tumor, with resulting secretion of steroid hormones having estrogenic activity.
4. Acute abdominal symptoms secondary to necrosis or rupture of the tumor and occasionally produced by torsion of the less common pedunculated varieties.
5. Ascites, weight loss, intestinal obstruction, or pulmonary distress due to pleural effusion, in the advanced stages of the disease. (The possibility of Meigs' syndrome must also be considered.)

It should also be noted that a number of associated paraendocrine syndromes have been reported to occur in conjunction with ovarian neoplasms, especially those of the mucinous variety, in which the tumor itself was the source of abnormal hormone production; e.g., hypercalcemia (parathyroid hormone), Cushing's syndrome (ACTH), carcinoid syndrome (catecholamines and serotonin), hypoglycemia (insulinlike substances), and Zollinger-Ellison syndrome (gastrin). Another kind of association between ovarian tumors and other clinical syndromes is exemplified by the Peutz-Jeghers syndrome, a familial syndrome in which there is a markedly increased incidence of benign and malignant ovarian neoplasms, especially granulosa cell and certain sex cord tumors, and the physician should be on the lookout for the appearance of ovarian tumors in these patients.

PHYSICAL SIGNS

Typical findings on examination, though again not always diagnostic of ovarian carcinoma, often provide a clue to the nature of the lesion. These are as follows:

1. Discovery on routine examination of an asymptomatic, nondescript ovarian enlargement (the most favorable but unfortunately the least common situation).
2. Palpation of a pelvic mass or, even more typically, bilateral adnexal tumors, with the suggestive malignant characteristics of irregular surface, partially cystic and partially solid consistency, and relative adherence or immobility, and often with palpable nodularity elsewhere in their vicinity indicative of local spread of the disease.
3. Evidence of advanced spread in the form of multiple abdominal masses, a palpable omental "cake," or nodular hepatomegaly, often with associated ascites.

Treatment

Even though the disease may seem advanced and inoperable on the basis of the clinical findings (in fact, the disease will have spread beyond the possibility of total surgical removal in 50 percent or more of the patients), almost all patients deserve exploratory laparotomy for several reasons: The tumor may not be totally resectable surgically, but the patient will usually derive considerable symptomatic benefit from removal of most of the large tumor masses. Furthermore, additional palliative therapy in the form of x-ray treatment or chemotherapeutic drugs is more likely to be effective if the bulk of the tumor is gone. There have been occasional reported instances of long-term remissions, despite extensive intraabdominal spread and even in the face of remote metastases, following x-ray therapy in patients who have undergone partial surgical removal, particularly when the ovaries with the primary tumor were included in the resection, and when any remaining tumor masses or nodules were smaller than 2 cm in diameter.

It is essential to be certain not to overlook a readily curable ovarian fibroma with accompanying Meigs' syndrome, in which ascites, pleural effusion (either may be bloody), and malignant-appearing cachexia may precisely simulate advanced ovarian malignancy. In any case, it is important to establish a definite histologic diagnosis and to determine with certainty that the tumor is primary in the ovary and not a secondary metastasis from some other abdominal organ, in which case the further management and choice of palliative agents might be entirely different.

OPERATIVE MANAGEMENT

A thorough preoperative evaluation, utilizing some or all of the possible diagnostic studies previously mentioned, may prove extremely helpful to proper operative management, particularly if advanced disease is encountered. In performing laparotomy, an adequate incision should be made, regardless of the length required, to avoid the risk of rupture and spillage during removal of a bulky, encapsulated tumor. By the same token, preliminary tapping of a cystic tumor to enable removal through a small incision is to be condemned. The following maneuvers should be carried out during laparotomy and will be extremely helpful in planning further therapy for the patient with ovarian cancer:

1. Any peritoneal fluid should be submitted for cytologic and cell block studies.
2. If no ascitic or cul-de-sac fluid is present, the cul-de-sac should be lavaged with 100 ml of normal saline and this fluid sent for cytologic studies.
3. Careful visual and palpatory exploration of the liver, diaphragm, paraaortic and pelvic nodes, any peritoneal and visceral implants, and the omentum should be done.
4. Selective biopsies of the omentum or any of the above sites should be done if involvement is suspected; suspicious areas should also be marked with dura clips.
5. Any areas of tumor adhesions should be marked on the operative specimen for special study by the pathologist, and the corresponding abdominal sites of the adhesions should be examined by biopsy and marked with dura clips. In this way, simple inflammatory adhesions can definitely be distinguished from actual penetration of the capsule by tumor, a distinction that may determine whether or not adjunctive radiation or chemotherapy is indicated.
6. Dura clips should be placed at appropriate sites to mark and outline the boundaries and extent of any known residual tumor.
7. A careful operative note is vital, describing accurately all findings, together with estimates of the location and volume of residual tumor, and a clear statement of the stage to which the case should be assigned.

If the tumor is malignant and totally excisable, the ideal operation is total hysterectomy with bilateral salpingo-oophorectomy. The entire uterus should be removed because of potential spread to it via endometrial, myometrial, and cervical lymphatics, and both ovaries should always be removed because of the frequent presence of bilateral involvement, which at times may be detectable only microscopically. If the tumor is encapsulated and there is no sign of local spread, prophylactic omental resection is probably unnecessary and unlikely to be helpful, although it is advocated by some, despite equivocal data in support of the recommendation in most series. However, the omentum should always be carefully examined and any suspicious areas examined by biopsy, since omentectomy is definitely beneficial and indicated if there is even minimal involvement by tumor.

When the tumor is not totally resectable, as much of the gross tumor as can be readily and simply removed should be excised, preferably including both ovaries, the omentum if involved by metastatic nodules, and the uterus if the tumor is adherent to it but the cul-de-sac is free of disease. On the other hand, if there is extensive pelvic seeding, it may be wisest not to perform hysterectomy, since removal of the uterus under these circumstances may only result in the rapid outgrowth of ulcerating, necrotic, bleeding tumor at the vaginal apex. Occasionally, a loop of bowel heavily involved by tumor and obviously destined to become obstructed in the near future may best be resected prophylactically at this time. Although extensive local disease might in an occasional case be potentially totally resectable by a radical Wertheim type of hysterectomy, there is usually nothing to be gained by extended, superradical operations for ovarian cancer. Because of their mode of spread, ovarian cancers are usually either potentially completely removable surgically by a standard hysterectomy and bilateral salpingo-oophorectomy, or they can no longer be completely resected surgically, and radical hysterectomy or pelvic exenteration in the more advanced stages will not improve the overall salvage.

A limited operation for a potentially malignant ovarian tumor in a young woman in whom preservation of reproductive function is desirable is occasionally possible. The factors entering into this important decision include: (1) the gross anatomy and extent of the tumor (the lesion should preferably be small, unilateral, and completely encapsulated); (2) the question of bilaterality (the opposite ovary should be bisected for thorough evaluation, before reaching a final conclusion); and (3) the histologic appearance of the tumor. The pathologist may be helpful in arriving at a diagnosis in the operating room, or the decision may have to be delayed until study of permanent histologic sections is possible. In other words, if conditions seem otherwise favorable for conservative management, but the pathologist finds it impossible to make a judgment on frozen section alone, simple unilateral salpingo-oophorectomy can be done and the operation terminated. If final pathologic study then reveals frank and extensive malignant disease, reoperation with hysterectomy and removal of the other tube and ovary will often be indicated. Table 9 lists the ovarian tumors in which conservative surgery in young women is usually or sometimes possible. Unilateral, well-encapsulated, papillary pseudomucinous carcinomas in young females and the low-grade or so-called borderline unilateral papillary serous carcinomas are the two most frequently encountered examples of ovarian epithelial tumors that can be managed conservatively by unilateral adnexectomy in young women, with excellent five-year cure rates.

POSTOPERATIVE MANAGEMENT

Radiation Therapy

If the tumor was completely encapsulated and has obviously been totally excised, there is no conclusive evidence that prophylactic postoperative irradiation treatment will increase the likelihood of cure. However, postoperative irradiation is definitely indicated in patients in whom it is known with certainty that gross disease was left behind, especially if the residual lesions are small (less than 2 cm in diameter), or in patients in whom all gross tumor was removed, but in whom the possibility of microscopic residual disease seems highly likely on the basis of penetration of the capsule by tumor, operative spillage, or the presence of even a small amount of peritoneal fluid showing positive cytologic findings. (In patients in whom there was spillage, or with malignant cells in the ascitic fluid, but with no gross disease left behind,

Table 9

Ovarian Tumors in Which Conservative Surgery in Young Women is Usually or Sometimes Possible[a]

Tumor	Can Be Safely Treated	
	Local Excision	Unilateral Oophorectomy
Dermoid cyst	Often	Always
Arrhenoblastoma	Sometimes	Nearly always
Fibroma, thecoma, Brenner tumor	Seldom (tumor usually too diffuse to permit enucleation)	Always
Granulosa cell tumor	Seldom (again, tumor usually too diffuse)	Often (incidence of malignancy low in younger age group)[b]
Dysgerminoma	Never (great tendency to local recurrence)	Fairly often[b]
"Benign" pseudomucinous cystadenoma	Never ⎫ Clinical behavior frequently at	Fairly often[b]
"Benign" serous cystadenoma	Never ⎬ variance with "benign" histologic appearance	Rarely[b]
Teratoma, sarcoma	Never	Rarely[b]

[a]This is a tentative list that individual circumstances may frequently modify. The decision is invariably influenced by the factors mentioned in the text.
[b]Nearly always involves assuming a calculated risk.

chemotherapy may be preferable.) X-ray therapy to the full pelvis and lower abdomen is administered in a total dosage of approximately 3500 to 4500 R, sometimes increasing the dose range in areas where persistent tumor is known to exist. In some clinics, the so-called moving-strip technique is employed so that radiation can be given to the entire abdomen from pelvic floor to diaphragm, delivering a moderately high dose to a different and relatively narrow strip of the abdominal cavity each day until an adequate dose has been delivered throughout. This technique permits delivery of a much larger dose to the entire abdomen over a much shorter time interval without increasing the side effects or complications significantly.

Although the radiosensitivity of the various types of ovarian cancer is highly variable and unpredictable, the further growth of known residual disease is often held completely in check for periods of one to several years, and occasional long-term remissions and even apparent cures have been attained by a combination of partial surgical removal and subsequent x-ray therapy. Endometrioid carcinomas appear to be particularly radiosensitive and mucinous carcinomas relatively radioresistant, with the radiation responsiveness of serous carcinomas falling somewhere in an intermediate range. Although intraperitoneal instillation of radioactive colloidal gold or chromic phosphate (P-32) or the use of systemic chemotherapy has had limited trials as a substitute for or to supplement x-ray therapy in the immediate postoperative management of patients with extensive disease, the results so far indicate that where residual disease is confined to the pelvis and adjacent lower abdomen (Stage II), the initial use of radiation treatment is probably preferable in most cases, withholding the chemotherapeutic agents for use later on in the course of the disease or for patients in whom there are widespread abdominal or remote metastases or both (Stages III and IV). However, in patients in whom the tumor could not be removed at operation or in whom large masses (greater than 2 cm in diameter) of residual tumor remain, systemic chemotherapy, usually with alkylating agents, will probably provide more effective palliation than radiation therapy and in some instances may result in long-term, symptom-free survival.

Palliation by Chemotherapy

Women suffering from ovarian cancer with metastases frequently survive for surprisingly long periods of time, often several years or more, in spite of extensive dissemination of their disease. The various symptoms that accompany this metastatic spread are exceedingly uncomfortable for the patient and pose a difficult problem in management for the physician, since he often must attempt to relieve them over a long period of time. The continual formation of ascitic fluid is the most frequent and distressing complication, but the painful pressure of enlarging masses and symptoms of subacute intestinal obstruction are also frequently encountered. In the palliation of the various manifestations of advancing disease following incomplete surgical removal supplemented by x-ray treatment, further radiation is usually of no benefit, and a shift to a program of chemotherapy is in order. Ovarian cancer has proved to be one of the more responsive neoplasms in trials with a variety of anticancer drugs.

Although a large number of all three of the principal types of chemotherapeutic compounds have received clinical trial, the polyfunctional alkylating agents have proved to be more effective than any of the antimetabolites (e.g., methotrexate, 5-fluorouracil) or the antibiotics (e.g., actinomycin D, sarkomycin). However, one of the more recent additions to the field, the cytotoxic antibiotic adriamycin, appears considerably more promising, either alone or especially in combination with an alkylating agent; e.g., it is often used in combination with cyclophosphamide (Cytoxan).

Polyfunctional Alkylating Agents. The following is a list of some of the alkylating agents currently available, together with the dosages and routes of administration for those which are commonly employed in the management of patients with ovarian cancer.

Nitrogen mustard (HN^2): 0.4 mg per kilogram intravenously.
Hemisulfur mustard (HSM): 600 mg intravenously, in three divided doses, or 300 mg in a single intracavitary injection.
Triethylenemelamine (TEM): 0.12 mg per kilogram intravenously; then a maintenance program of 10 to 40 mg per month in divided daily doses orally.
Triethylenethiophosphoramide (THIOTEPA): 0.8 to 1.0 mg per kilogram intravenously, or 30 to 60 mg in a single intracavitary injection.

Chlorambucil (Leukeran): 0.2 to 0.4 mg per kilogram daily orally for two to three months, or to toxicity. The course of treatment may be repeated, or the drug may be given in reduced dosage in a continuous maintenance program.

Cyclophosphamide: an initial dose of 40 to 50 mg per kilogram intravenously, given as 10 to 20 mg per kilogram per day for two to five days, as tolerated; then a maintenance dose of 1 to 5 mg per kilogram per day orally, or 10 to 15 mg per kilogram intravenously every 7 to 10 days. (Cyclophosphamide has the advantage over other alkylating agents of not affecting the platelet count.) Another standard regimen often used is 200 mg daily intravenously for five days, followed by an oral maintenance program of 50 mg twice daily.

L-**phenylalanine mustard** (melphalen): 1 mg per kilogram in divided doses for five to six days and repeated monthly as indicated and tolerated.

Other alkylating agents include: busulfan (Myleran), Nitromin, uracil mustard (U-8344), and phenylalanine mustard (PAM) (Sarcolysin).

The alkylating drugs are radiomimetic in their effects, with a selective toxicity for rapidly proliferating cells, particularly those of the bone marrow and gonadal and gastrointestinal epithelium, and for neoplastic tissue in general. Their activity is due to the introduction of alkyl groups in place of hydrogen ions in organic molecules, especially those composing nuclear genetic material, with resulting inactivation of key enzyme systems. They are thus potentially highly toxic drugs, and their administration must be carefully supervised and controlled, with the patient under close observation at all times. The chief complications are bone-marrow depression, with leukopenia, thrombocytopenia, and anemia, and the development of gastrointestinal disturbances, i.e., nausea, vomiting, diarrhea, and gastrointestinal tract bleeding. Careful hematologic control is mandatory, and if the leukocyte count falls below the 3000 to 5000 range or the platelet count below 100,000, or if the danger signs of severe stomatitis or secondary infection appear, treatment should be immediately discontinued. As in the case of radiation therapy, general supportive measures, including transfusions as indicated and attention to the nutritional status of the patient, will often minimize the side effects and increase the effectiveness of the treatment.

In view of the toxic side effects of these drugs, it is probably wise to withhold therapy until symptoms appear and to discontinue it as soon as there is early evidence of drug toxicity. Often, the dosage will have to be modified if prior radiation therapy has already produced some degree of bone-marrow depression.

Although both nitrogen mustard and hemisulfur mustard are effective drugs, the latter having proved particularly useful in the control of ascites, both must be given intravenously and both are also somewhat more toxic than the newer agents that have now largely supplanted them. Chlorambucil, which seems equally effective, has the great advantage that it can be given orally, and furthermore, that its toxic side effects are fewer and more predictable, and it is currently the drug of choice. The intracavitary use of THIOTEPA has also proved to be of some value in the relief of abdominal or pleural effusions when these fail to respond to systemic chemotherapy.

Drug Combinations. Although the alkylating agents remain the mainstay of chemotherapy for ovarian cancer, with increased knowledge of the biology of neoplastic cellular proliferation and tumor cell kinetics, chemotherapy employing multiple drugs from two or more of the main categories (alkylating agents, antimetabolites, and antibiotics) is being tried more freely, especially if there is extensive disease or if the tumor has shown a poor response to an alkylating agent alone. Among the various antitumor drugs, some affect primarily active, cycling cells (e.g., the antimetabolites), whereas others exert their effects predominantly on inactive or resting cells (e.g., the alkylating agents and antibiotics such as adriamycin) — hence the rationale for combination therapy. Furthermore, since smaller tumor masses have a greater percentage of cycling cells, the ones most susceptible to either chemotherapy or radiation, the surgical removal of large masses whenever this is feasible also makes good sense. Examples of combination chemotherapy regimens currently in use include: chlorambucil or cyclophosphamide, methotrexate, and 5-fluorouracil (5-FU); cyclophosphamide, actinomycin D, and 5-FU; chlorambucil or cyclophosphamide, adriamycin, and vincristine; and cyclophosphamide and adriamycin.

Most chemotherapy programs are now based on intermittent (or "pulsed") rather than continuous drug administration (e.g., treatment for one week at monthly intervals), since such a regimen is safer and more effective and also allows a three-week interval for the immune response mechanism to recover and even to overshoot the normal immune response.

Quinacrine. Quinacrine hydrochloride (Atabrine) is another drug that may be used in place of one of the chemotherapeutic agents for direct intracavitary instillation and is often effective in controlling recurrent ascites or pleural effusion. It has the advantage of possessing none of the hazards or complications of radiation therapy or the systemic toxic effects of the anticancer drugs. It can therefore safely be employed even when bone-marrow depression with leukopenia and thrombocytopenia are present as a result of previous radiation or chemotherapy. It apparently inhibits the effusion by producing an inflammatory reaction on the serosal surfaces (a transient chemical peritonitis or pleuritis), thus causing an obliterative fibrous thickening of the peritoneum or pleura, with decreased fluid formation. The usual dose is 50 to 100 mg for pleural injection or 100 to 200 mg for intraperitoneal instillation, repeated daily for three to five days, depending on the tolerance of the patient and the response obtained.

Attempts to increase the effectiveness of the anticancer drugs through the use of so-called regional chemotherapy, employing isolated pelvic perfusion techniques or bilateral hypogastric arterial infusions, have been unsuccessful in the case of ovarian cancer because of its tendency to diffuse dissemination.

Approximately 35 to 50 percent of patients with advanced ovarian cancer will exhibit a favorable response to chemotherapy. Beneficial effects may include diminished formation or disappearance of ascites, diminution in the size of abdominal masses, decreased pain, and increased appetite, strength, and sense of well-being, with return to more normal activity. The resulting improvement may last for from several months to several years, and, in general, if a response is obtained at all, increased longevity may be expected.

Other Measures

Another approach to the problem of recurring ascites has been the intraperitoneal instillation of a solution of radioactive colloidal gold or P-32 (radioactive chromic phosphate). In the hands of some physicians this has proved as effective as chemotherapy in decreasing the rate of fluid formation, but the frequent loculation of the effusion tends to increase the hazards of small-bowel injury and obstruction and limits the use of this technique, which furthermore affects only the superficial portions of the tumor.

A recently proposed adjunctive measure in the management of ascites is based on the assumption that much of the fluid formation is part of the pathologic physiology of the ovarian cancer itself and represents a carry-over of the function of the germinal epithelium of the ovary from which most ovarian cancers are derived. The tendency to fluid formation therefore might be expected to be potentially responsive to pituitary gonadotropins, which tend to be increasing during the premenopausal and postmenopausal decade when the majority of ovarian carcinomas appear. In the treatment of ascites due to metastatic ovarian cancer, some clinics have therefore employed large doses of testosterone, an excellent inhibitor of pituitary gonadotropin secretion, in conjunction with a course of either chemotherapy or radiation. The anabolic effects of testosterone are of additional benefit in promoting positive nitrogen balance and improving the nutritional status of the patient.

Abdominal paracentesis may also be necessary but should be done as infrequently as possible, since it is accompanied by both protein and electrolyte losses. A low-salt, high-protein diet and the judicious use of diuretics can often minimize the need for repeated paracenteses, or at least prolong the interval between them.

The management of the fortunately relatively uncommon problem of **pseudomyxoma peritonei** (or mucinous ascites) occurring in association with pseudomucinous ovarian tumors of low-grade malignancy is somewhat different. Here, radiation therapy has been shown to be totally ineffective. Best results and long-term palliation and survivals are achieved by removal of both ovaries and the appendix (mucocele of the appendix is also commonly associated with this condition), resection of the omentum, together with as many as possible of the mucinous nodules from other peritoneal sites, manual evacuation of all the thick, mucinous fluid from the peritoneal cavity, and then postoperative chemotherapy employing alkylating agents by direct intraperitoneal instillation as well as orally. In some instances the treatment of recurrences may require multiple operations and repeated courses of drug therapy over a period of years, but excellent long-term palliation can nevertheless be achieved in many of these patients.

Occasionally, further palliative surgical measures may be required, although, in general, additional operations should be avoided if possible. However, recurring episodes of small-bowel obstruction are not uncommon, and although they frequently respond to conservative management, enteroenterostomy may prove necessary for a patient not yet in the terminal phases of the disease in whom an initial trial of gastrointestinal intubation fails to relieve the obstruction. Colostomy for large-bowel obstruction due to the enlarging pelvic tumor is even less desirable and can often be avoided by maintaining the patient permanently on a low-residue diet.

SUMMARY OF GENERAL PRINCIPLES OF TREATMENT OF OVARIAN CANCER

Stage Ia

Total abdominal hysterectomy, bilateral salpingo-oophorectomy, and perhaps "prophylactic" omentectomy are performed for Stage Ia disease. Postoperative chemotherapy or intraperitoneal radioactive colloidal gold or P-32 is given if peritoneal washings are positive or if microscopic tumor is detected on the capsule surface. If the capsule is grossly invaded, or if the tumor ruptured during removal, postoperative chemotherapy or intraperitoneal radioactive colloid and/or radiation therapy should be given.

Stage Ib

Treatment is the same as for Stage Ia.

Stage Ic

Total abdominal hysterectomy and bilateral salpingo-oophorectomy are performed, and chemotherapy (or intraperitoneal radioactive colloid or abdominal irradiation by the moving-strip technique) is given.

(If the tumor is mucinous and low-grade, especially if the capsule breached or the tumor ruptured during removal, a subsequent planned second-look operation in Stage Ia, b, or c should be considered.)

Stage IIa

Total abdominal hysterectomy, bilateral salpingo-oophorectomy, and omentectomy are performed, followed by postoperative irradiation and/or chemotherapy.

Stage IIb

Usually, total abdominal hysterectomy is performed for Stage IIb lesions (unless this involves cutting across gross tumor in the cul-de-sac, in which case it may be wiser to leave the uterus), together with bilateral salpingo-oophorectomy and omentectomy, with removal of as much of any remaining gross tumor as possible, followed by postoperative irradiation and/or chemotherapy. (A second-look operation should also be considered if the tumor is histologically of the mucinous type, especially if there has been a good response to irradiation and/or chemotherapy. The operation has a twofold purpose: to remove any residual tumor and to help to determine how long chemotherapy should be continued.)

Stage IIc

Treatment for Stage IIc disease is the same as for Stage IIa and b.

Table 10
Typical Five-Year Survival Rates Following Treatment of Ovarian Cancer

Histologic Type	Five-Year Survival	
	Stage I	Overall Stages
Mucinous carcinomas	83% (57% of series)	63% (17% of series are III + IV)
Endometrioid carcinomas	81% (20% of series)	56% (17% of series are III + IV)[*]
Serous carcinomas	41% (18% of series)	15% (53% of series are III + IV)

[*]Endometrioid Stage III — 48% five-year survival.

Stage III

In Stage III, as much of the tumor is removed as possible, and the operation should include bilateral salpingo-oophorectomy plus omentectomy, if feasible, marking out the extent of residual disease with dura clips. Thereafter, postoperative chemotherapy is given, followed in some cases by irradiation. (Again, a second-look procedure should be considered if the response to chemotherapy and irradiation is good.)

Stage IV

A limited operation is performed to remove large masses and the primary tumor, where possible; it is followed by chemotherapy.

RESULTS OF TREATMENT

The overall true curability of ovarian cancer is no more than 20 percent, with five-year survivals only 25 to 30 percent at best. In the case of the most common serous cystadenocarcinomas, the five-year survival is only 10 to 15 percent, whereas for the less frequent mucinous cystadenocarcinomas and endometrioid carcinomas it is in the 55 to 65 percent range. In the unclassified group of tumors, which includes most of the solid and highly anaplastic lesions, no more than 10 to 15 percent of the patients can be expected to survive five years.

If one takes into account the extent or clinical stage of the disease, when the tumor is confined to the ovaries (Stage I), overall cure rates approach 60 to 75 percent and are even higher in the case of mucinous or endometrioid carcinomas. Cure rates then fall off rapidly with the more advanced clinical stages, and cures or even five-year survivals are uncommon (5 to 10 percent) in Stages III and IV. However, as adequate a surgical resection as possible, combined with the proper use of supplemental radiation treatment or chemotherapy, can achieve long-term remissions as well as a significant number of apparent cures in 35 to 45 percent of patients with Stage II disease. Typical five-year survival rates following treatment of the most common types of ovarian cancer are presented in Table 10.

OTHER PRIMARY MALIGNANT OVARIAN TUMORS

Although relatively uncommon, a few other types of malignant lesions not primarily of epithelial origin are encountered, all of which are solid neoplasms, and include the dysgerminoma, various types of malignant teratomas, the true sarcomas, and lymphomas. (The malignant variants of granulosa-theca cell tumors, arrhenoblastomas, gynandroblastomas, gonadoblastomas, hilus cell tumors, and the adrenal cell rest tumors are discussed in Chapter 6.)

Dysgerminoma

Dysgerminomas are relatively infrequent tumors that show a marked tendency to appear before puberty or during adolescence; roughly 75 percent occur in the second and third decades of life. They are derived from primitive germinal epithelial cells of the type found in the original asexual or neutral gonad, and analogous tumors are found in the male in the form of seminomas or embryonal carcinomas of the testis. Perhaps in keeping with their histogenesis, these tumors are somewhat more common in women with underdevelopment of the genital tract, and particularly in those exhibiting various types of pseudohermaphroditism, but many occur in patients who have normal pelvic organs and are fertile. The chief and often the only symptom is awareness of an abdominal mass, but there may be accompanying abdominal or pelvic pain, and although these tumors possess no endocrine function, there are often associated menstrual disturbances, including amenorrhea or irregular bleeding.

Seen grossly, they are solid, rubbery-firm, smooth, and initially encapsulated tumors, often bilateral, and usually of moderate size, although larger lesions that fill the pelvis or abdominal cavity have been reported. Once the growth penetrates the capsule, the originally free-lying tumor becomes adherent, and local peritoneal or retroperitoneal extension to other organs or structures may occur; distant metastases are less common. The dysgerminoma has a distinctive microscopic appearance characterized by the presence of large, clear cells with dark-staining nuclei arranged in cords or nests that are separated by thin connective-tissue septa, the latter often containing considerable lymphoid tissue. Although the majority of dysgerminomas occur in the pure form just described, in a small number, other malignant elements such as choriocarcinoma (in which case a positive human chorionic gonadotropin test may be obtained), endodermal sinus tumor, or immature teratoma may also be present. The presence of these other elements will sometimes profoundly affect the therapeutic plan and its outcome.

Although all dysgerminomas are malignant, the degree of anaplasia is highly variable, and perhaps only one third are highly malignant in their histologic appearance and clinical behavior, the bilateral lesions falling into this category. Since the majority occurring in the younger age groups are of lesser degrees of malignancy, the conservative surgical management obviously desirable in children, adolescents, and young adults is often possible. Provided that the tumor is unilateral, has not broken through its capsule, and there is no evidence of parametrial, intraperitoneal (peritoneal surfaces, omentum, liver), retroperitoneal, or paraaortic spread, simple unilateral salpingo-oophorectomy is permissible and is usually adequate treatment, although it involves a calculated risk; this risk is apparently very slight if the tumor is less than 10 cm in diameter. The opposite, apparently uninvolved ovary should be completely evaluated by wedging, with careful inspection and removal of biopsy specimens for microscopic examination of frozen sections before the final decision is made to treat the tumor by conservative unilateral operation, since in roughly 10 percent of patients the tumor is bilateral; furthermore, the possibility of retro-peritoneal lymphatic involvement should also be evaluated by a search for and excision biopsy of any suspicious paraaortic nodes. The 90 to 95 percent cure rate for these favorable lesions is not improved by more extensive surgery or by the addition of radiation therapy. Furthermore, in the small number of patients (10 to 20 percent, at most) who have a recurrence, there is still an excellent chance for ultimate cure by reoperation followed by x-ray treatment. (There is roughly a 90 percent cure rate following treatment of the few recurrent tumors that develop under these circumstances.)

If the capsule has been penetrated or ruptured at operation, if there is evidence of local or metastatic spread, or if the tumor is bilateral, total hysterectomy and bilateral salpingo-oophorectomy are definitely indicated, regardless of the age of the patient. Under these circumstances, since the tumor is usually highly radiosensitive (it is the only radiosensitive germ cell tumor of the ovary), routine postoperative x-ray therapy should always be given and may at times also be successful in controlling metastatic disease or in dealing with recurrences. In favorable, encapsulated lesions, conservative surgical removal by unilateral salpingo-oophorectomy results in cure of the disease in roughly 75 to 90 percent of patients. Nevertheless, the potentially serious nature of dysgerminomas is emphasized by reported overall cure rates varying from 25 to 75 percent.

Malignant Teratomatous Tumors

Solid teratomas are rare tumors, and the majority are highly malignant, usually containing mixtures of wildly proliferating tumor tissue derived from all three germ-cell layers but with sarcomatous elements predominating. They, too, tend to develop most often during childhood and adolescence. Histologically, these growths may also take the form of embryonal carcinoma, teratocarcinoma (an embryonal or dysgerminomalike tumor in which primitive epithelial and connective-tissue structures are formed, simulating rudimentary embryogenesis), the so-called endodermal sinus tumor (yolk sac carcinoma), the rare primary ovarian chorionepithelioma, or occasionally even mixed mesodermal types of sarcomas. Treatment should consist of radical surgical removal, but because of the tendency of these tumors to rapid dissemination and distant metastases, cure is rarely achieved by surgery alone unless the tumor is entirely encapsulated. Therefore, once surgical removal of the primary tumor and all, or as much as possible, of any local spread has been accomplished (e.g., total hysterectomy, bilateral salpingo-oophorectomy, and omentectomy), a vigorous program of postoperative treatment combining chemotherapy and radiation therapy (except in the case of endodermal sinus tumors and other radioresistant germ cell tumors) should be instituted. Chemotherapy involves the so-called *triple therapy* with methotrexate, chlorambucil, and actinomycin D, or cyclophosphamide, actinomycin D, and 5-fluorouracil. Ordinarily, three five-day courses are given, three to six weeks apart, depending on the degree of bone-marrow toxicity observed. Thereafter, a course of x-ray therapy in a dosage of 3500 to 4500 R is delivered to the full pelvis and lower abdomen, unless the lesion is one of the mixed embryonal or teratoid carcinomas known to be radioresistant. Dramatic successes with this current, more aggressive therapeutic approach to what were formerly considered hopelessly incurable neoplasms have been achieved within the past few years, and a number of long-term remissions with apparent cure have already been recorded, even when local spread or metastatic disease had been left behind at the time of initial surgery. (Results have been equally good when the same therapeutic program has been used in managing similar germinal cell tumors of the testis.)

Sarcoma

What appear to be true primary sarcomas, not arising in a malignant teratoma ("teratoid sarcoma"), are the least common of all the ovarian cancers, and although they may occur at any age, they are most likely to be encountered either at puberty or after the menopause. Histogenetically, they may be classified as having an ovarian stromal or mesenchymal origin (stromal or mesenchymal sarcomas), or as having a paramesonephric origin (paramesonephric or müllerian sarcomas — mixed mesodermal tumors, carcinosarcomas, and so on). Grossly, they tend to appear much like the larger fibromas externally and are often similarly pedunculated, but they are much more often bilateral. On cut section the occasional low-grade fibrosarcoma may resemble the benign fibroma, but the majority present the typical "raw-meat" appearance characteristic of most sarcomas, with frequent areas of hemorrhage and secondary degenerative change. Microscopically, more differentiated spindle-cell and more anaplastic round-cell variants may be recognized. In any case, they tend to grow extremely rapidly, with local extension, peritoneal implantation, lymphatic permeation, and a marked tendency to early blood vessel invasion and widespread distant metastases, usually leading to a rapidly fatal course regardless of the type of therapy given.

Lymphomas

Lymphoma of the ovary is extremely rare. It may occur as part of a more generalized pelvic or abdominal lymphoma or may be well localized and of apparent primary ovarian origin. Various histologic types are encountered and include Hodgkin's lymphoma, non-Hodgkin's lymphoma, and Burkitt's lymphoma. Treatment depends on the histologic type and on whether the ovarian involvement is primary or secondary. In selected cases of small, well-localized Hodgkin's or Burkitt's lymphoma, unilateral salpingo-oophorectomy may be sufficient for cure. For the more extensive and diffuse lesions, total hysterectomy and bilateral salpingo-oophorectomy should be done and followed by postoperative radiotherapy and/or chemotherapy, depending on the status of the paraaortic nodes, liver, and spleen, as determined by exploratory laparotomy and by liver-spleen scan and lymphangiography.

METASTATIC (SECONDARY) CARCINOMAS

Whenever an essentially solid tumor of the ovary is encountered, the possibility that it represents a metastasis from a primary carcinoma elsewhere in the body must always be considered, since the ovary is a surprisingly frequent site of metastatic involvement. The occurrence of ovarian metastases in 5 to 10 percent of patients with endometrial cancer has already been mentioned and can occur by lymphatic or direct transtubal spread. Ovarian metastases are also frequent in patients with disseminated breast cancer, being encountered in roughly 20 percent or more of women undergoing oophorectomy in the palliation of this disease. Presumably, they are the result of blood-borne metastases or of retrograde spread via the lumbar lymphatics.

Of the remaining metastatic tumors, those developing as secondary manifestations of carcinoma of the stomach and colon are the most common. The Krukenberg tumor, although originally believed by Krukenberg to be a primary ovarian neoplasm, is the classic example of metastatic malignant ovarian disease and represents a specific morphologic entity. Krukenberg's initial confusion regarding the origin of these tumors is easily explained by the fact that the primary focus, which is usually in the stomach, less often in the colon, typically is either microscopic or so small as to be asymptomatic and completely undetectable by the usual diagnostic procedures, whereas the often large and invariably bilateral ovarian metastases are the obvious presenting lesions. Seen grossly, they are firm, irregularly lobulated, sometimes huge, kidney-shaped tumors producing a symmetrical, bilateral ovarian enlargement. On cut section there may be softer areas of cystic degeneration within predominately solid granular or fibrous carcinomatous tissue that infiltrates the remaining normal ovarian stroma. The microscopic appearance of the tumor is characterized by the presence of the distinctive signet-ring cells, but an equally prominent feature of the Krukenberg tumor, as well as of many of the less specific types of metastatic ovarian carcinomas of primary gastrointestinal tract origin, is the fact that the bulk of the tumor is actually seen histologically to be composed of a marked proliferation of the ovarian stroma itself. When this is accompanied by stromal luteinization, secondary hormonal effects may become a part of the overall clinical picture, as mentioned in Chapter 6. Although dissemination through the peritoneal fluid or via the bloodstream is a potential route of transmission, it seems most likely that retrograde spread via the lumbar lymphatics is again the most reasonable explanation for the development of these usually isolated ovarian metastases. Obviously, ovarian substance must also provide a particularly favorable environment for the implantation and further growth of wandering tumor cells.

These tumors should be treated by hysterectomy and bilateral salpingo-oophorectomy, which often will completely and permanently control the pelvic manifestations of the disease, even though the ultimate prognosis is poor. If it is not already obvious at laparotomy, a careful search for the primary focus of cancer should be undertaken postoperatively. If the primary site is eventually demonstrated in the stomach or colon, a subsequent gastrectomy or colectomy may sometimes be indicated and may provide additional palliation and occasionally even long-term symptom-free survivals. No extraovarian primary site can ever be demonstrated in 10 to 20 percent of patients with histologically bona fide Krukenberg tumors, and some of these have apparently been cured by removal of the uterus and adnexa. For this reason, this small group is sometimes classified as ovarian in origin, and the tumors are presumed to arise in small, preexisting teratomas, although the possibility that an initial microscopic primary focus elsewhere remained dormant or underwent spontaneous regression can never be completely excluded.

The majority of the metastatic ovarian lesions primary in the colon or elsewhere in the gastrointestinal tract do not possess the distinctive gross and microscopic features of the Krukenberg tumor and should not be so classified. They are, however, also solid, usually bilateral, most often irregular tumor masses, roughly spherical in shape, and frequently also attain appreciable size in the absence of any symptoms referable to the primary lesion in the gastrointestinal tract; their clinical course and treatment are essentially the same.

REFERENCES

1. Asadourian, L. A., and Taylor, H. B. Dysgerminoma: An analysis of 105 cases. *Obstet. Gynecol.* 33:370, 1969.
2. Aure, C. A., Hoeg, K., and Kolstad, P. Clinical and histologic studies of ovarian carcinoma. Long term follow-up of 990 cases. *Obstet. Gynecol.* 37:1, 1971.
3. Azoury, R. S., and Woodruff, J. D. Primary ovarian sarcomas. *Obstet. Gynecol.* 37:920, 1971.
4. Barber, H. R. K., Sommers, S. C., Snyder, R., and Kwon, T. H. Histologic and nuclear grading and stromal reactions as indices for prognosis in ovarian cancer. *Am. J. Obstet. Gynecol.* 121:795, 1975.
5. Christian, C. D. Ovarian tumors: An extension of the Peutz-Jeghers syndrome. *Am. J. Obstet. Gynecol.* 111:529, 1971.
6. Cocco, A. E., and Conway, S. J. Zollinger-Ellison syndrome associated with ovarian mucinous cystadenocarcinoma. *N. Engl. J. Med.* 293:485, 1975.
7. Cruickshank, D. P., and Buchsbaum, H. J. Effects of rapid paracentesis (in patients with ovarian carcinomatosis): Cardiovascular dynamics and body fluid composition. *J.A.M.A.* 225:1361, 1973.
8. Czernobilsky, B., Silverman, B. B., and Mikuta, J. J. Endometrioid carcinoma of the ovary: A clinicopathologic study of 75 cases. *Cancer* 26:1141, 1970.
9. Decker, D. G., Webb, M. J., and Holbrook, M. A. Radiogold treatment of epithelial cancer of ovary: Late results. *Am. J. Obstet. Gynecol.* 115:751, 1973.
10. DiSaia, P. J. Immunologic aspects of gynecological malignancies. *J. Reprod. Med.* 14:17, 1975.
11. Fenn, M. E., and Abell, M. R. Carcinosarcoma of the ovary. *Am. J. Obstet. Gynecol.* 110:1066, 1971.
12. Forney, J. P., DiSaia, P. J., and Morrow, C. P. Endodermal sinus tumor. *Obstet. Gynecol.* 45:186, 1975.
13. Gall, S. A. A review of tumor antigens in gynecologic malignancies. *J. Reprod. Med.* 14:12, 1975.
14. Garcia-Bunuel, R., Berek, J. S., and Woodruff, J. D. Luteomas of pregnancy. *Obstet. Gynecol.* 45:407, 1975.
15. Graham, R. M., Schueller, E. F., and Graham, J. B. Detection of ovarian cancer at an early stage. *Obstet. Gynecol.* 26:151, 1965.

16. Green, T. H., Jr. Hemisulfur mustard in the palliation of patients with metastatic ovarian carcinoma. *Obstet. Gynecol.* 13:383, 1959.

17. Griffiths, C. T., Grogan, R. H., and Hall, T. C. Advanced ovarian cancer: Primary treatment with surgery, radiotherapy, and chemotherapy. *Cancer* 29:1, 1972.

18. Hirabayashi, K., and Graham, J. B. Genesis of ascites in ovarian cancer. *Am. J. Obstet. Gynecol.* 106:492, 1970.

19. Jens, C. A., Hoeg, K., and Kolstad, P. Mesonephroid tumors of the ovary: Clinical and histopathologic studies. *Obstet. Gynecol.* 37:860, 1971.

20. Jorgensen, E. O., Dockerty, M. B., Wilson, R. B., and Welch, J. S. Clinicopathologic study of 53 cases of Brenner's tumors of the ovary. *Am. J. Obstet. Gynecol.* 108:122, 1970.

21. Julian, C. G., and Woodruff, J. D. The biologic behavior of low grade papillary serous carcinoma of the ovary. *Obstet. Gynecol.* 40:860, 1972.

22. Kajanoja, P., and Procope, B. J. Nongenital pelvic tumors found at gynecologic operations. *Surg. Gynecol. Obstet.* 140:605, 1975.

23. Keettel, W. C., Pixley, E. E., and Buchsbaum, H. J. Experience with peritoneal cytology in the management of gynecologic malignancies. *Am. J. Obstet. Gynecol.* 120:174, 1974.

24. Kelley, R. R., and Scully, R. E. Cancer developing in dermoid cysts of the ovary. *Cancer* 14:989, 1961.

25. Linder, D., McCaw, B. K., and Hecht, F. Parthenogenic origin of benign ovarian teratomas. *N. Engl. J. Med.* 292:63, 1975.

26. Lomano, J. M., Trelford, J. D., and Ullery, J. C. Torsion of the uterine adnexa causing an acute abdomen. *Obstet. Gynecol.* 35:221, 1970.

27. Long, M. E., and Taylor, H. C., Jr. Endometrioid carcinoma of the ovary. *Am. J. Obstet. Gynecol.* 90:936, 1964.

28. Long, R. T. L., Spratt, J. S., Jr., and Dowling, E. Pseudomyxoma peritonei. New concepts in management with a report of seventeen patients. *Am. J. Surg.* 117:162, 1969.

29. Meigs, J. V. Fibroma of the ovary with ascites and hydrothorax – Meigs' syndrome. *Am. J. Obstet. Gynecol.* 67:962, 1954.

30. Munnell, E. W. The changing prognosis and treatment in cancer of the ovary. *Am. J. Obstet. Gynecol.* 100:790, 1968.

31. Munnell, E. W. Is conservative therapy ever justified in Stage I (IA) cancer of the ovary? *Am. J. Obstet. Gynecol.* 103:641, 1969.

32. O'Neill, R. T., and Mikuta, J. J. Hypoglycemia associated with serous cystadenocarcinoma of the ovary. *Obstet. Gynecol.* 35:287, 1970.

33. Pantoja, E., Rodriguez-Ibanez, I., Axtmayer, R. W., Noy, M. A., and Pelagrina, I. Complications of dermoid tumors of the ovary. *Obstet. Gynecol.* 45:89, 1975.

34. Parker, R. T., Parker, C. H., and Wilbanks, G. D. Cancer of the ovary: Survival statistics based upon operative therapy, chemotherapy, and radiotherapy. *Am. J. Obstet. Gynecol.* 108:878, 1970.

35. Piver, M. S. Radioactive colloids in the treatment of Stage IA ovarian cancer. *Obstet. Gynecol.* 40:42, 1972.

36. Piver, M. S. Guidelines for the management of patients with ovarian adenocarcinoma. *Obstet. Gynecol.* 40:411, 1972.

37. Piver, M. S., Barlow, J. J., Lee, F. T., and Vongtama, V. Sequential therapy for advanced ovarian carcinoma: Operation, chemotherapy, second-look laparotomy, and radiation therapy. *Am. J. Obstet. Gynecol.* 122:355, 1975.

38. Scully, R. E. Recent progress in ovarian cancer. *Hum. Pathol.* 1:73, 1970.

39. Scully, R. E., and Barlow, J. F. Mesonephroma of ovary: Tumor of müllerian origin related to the endometrioid carcinoma. *Cancer* 20:1405, 1967.

40. Smith, J. P., and Rutledge, F. Current Status of Therapy for Ovarian Cancer. In M. L. Taymor and T. H. Green, Jr. (Eds.), *Progress in Gynecology,* Vol VI. New York: Grune & Stratton, 1975. Pp. 627–645.
41. Smith, J. P., Rutledge, F., and Wharton, J. T. Chemotherapy of ovarian cancer: New approaches to treatment. *Cancer* 30:1565, 1972.
42. Talerman, A., Huyzinga, W. T., and Kuipers, T. Dysgerminoma: Clinicopathologic study. *Obstet. Gynecol.* 41:137, 1973.
43. Tucker, S., Buell, J., and Fisher, H. R. Luteoma of pregnancy. *Am. J. Obstet. Gynecol.* 121:282, 1975.
44. Wallach, R. C., and Blinick, G. The second look operation for carcinoma of the ovary. *Surg. Gynecol. Obstet.* 131:1085, 1970.
45. Webb, M. J., Decker, D. G., Mussey, E., and Williams, T. Factors influencing survival in Stage I carcinoma of the ovary. *Am. J. Obstet. Gynecol.* 116:222, 1973.
46. Webb, M. J., Malkasian, G. D., Jr., and Jorgensen, E. O. Factors influencing ovarian cancer survival after chemotherapy. *Obstet. Gynecol.* 44:564, 1974.
47. Wider, J. A., Marshall, J. R., Bardin, C. W., Lipsett, M. B., and Ross, G. T. Sustained remissions after chemotherapy for ovarian cancers containing choriocarcinoma. *N. Engl. J. Med.* 280:1439, 1969.
48. Woodruff, J. D., Murthy, Y. S., Bhaskar, T. N., Bordbar, F., and Tseng, S. Metastatic ovarian tumors. *Am. J. Obstet. Gynecol.* 107:202, 1970.
49. Woodruff, J. D., and Novak, E. R. The Krukenberg tumor: Study of 48 cases from the ovarian tumor registry. *Obstet. Gynecol.* 15:351, 1960.
50. Woodruff, J. D., Protos, P., and Peterson, W. F. Ovarian teratomas. *Am. J. Obstet. Gynecol.* 102:702, 1968.
51. Young, R. C., and De Vita, V. T., Jr. The design of clinical trials in the therapy of ovarian carcinoma. *Am. J. Obstet. Gynecol.* 120:1012, 1974.

16
Vulvar and Vaginal Malignancies

VULVAR NEOPLASMS

Epidermoid carcinoma of the vulva accounts for approximately 90 to 95 percent of all the vulvar malignancies and represents roughly 5 percent of all malignant neoplasms of the female genital tract. It is essentially a disease of elderly, postmenopausal women, with a peak incidence in the sixth and seventh decades. It should be one of the most curable of all malignant diseases, since it is a visible and palpable lesion on the external body surface, has prominent early symptoms and, in many cases, definite and easily detected local precursors, and is relatively slow to grow and metastasize. Furthermore, adequate therapy yields a surprisingly high cure rate even when lymph node metastases have occurred.

In actuality, it has until recently been one of the most poorly managed of all the malignancies because of patient delay in seeking medical attention (embarrassment at the nature and location of symptoms, leading to prolonged self-medication), physician delay in establishing a correct diagnosis (all too frequently it has been initially considered to be and treated as an inflammation), inadequate excision of the local lesion (all too often looked on as just another "little skin cancer"), and failure to appreciate the importance and frequency of lymphatic spread, with neglect of this important aspect of therapy.

Histologic Types and Sites of Origin

INVASIVE LESIONS

Epidermoid Carcinoma

Epidermoid carcinoma (90 to 95 percent of all cases) usually arises in the labial skin of the anterior half of the vulva. In a series of 238 cases encountered over a 25-year period at the Massachusetts General Hospital and the Pondville (Massachusetts Department of Public Health) State Cancer Hospital, the distribution of anatomic sites of origin was as follows: labia majora or minora, 183 cases; clitoris, 16 cases; vestibule, 7 cases; perineum, 7 cases; prepuce, 6 cases; too extensive to classify, 19 cases. The other pathologic features of epidermoid carcinoma of the vulva and its pattern of spread will be considered in detail in the discussion of treatment, since knowledge of them is essential to planning and executing adequate therapy. Epidermoid carcinoma may also arise in Bartholin's glands, although this is rare, and occasionally it is encountered in the distal urethra. In either case it may present as a "vulvar cancer" and will require essentially the same therapeutic approach. A rare, locally invasive, seldom metastasizing, radioresistant type of verrucous carcinoma that may grossly as well as histologically resemble and be confused with benign

511

squamous papillomas or condyloma acuminatum is occasionally seen also. Here, too, radical surgery is the treatment of choice.

ADENOCARCINOMA

Adenocarcinoma of the vulva is rare, usually arising in Bartholin's glands (however, half the cancers arising in Bartholin's gland are epidermoid in type), occasionally in the urethral and periurethral glands, or even more rarely in ectopic breast-tissue elements. The basic principles of therapy again remain the same as for squamous cell carcinoma, but these lesions are less favorable ones from the standpoint of their potential curability.

Malignant Melanoma

Malignant melanoma constitutes only roughly 2 to 3 percent of all vulvar neoplasms, but the genital skin in either female or male is one of the more common sites for melanomas in general. It has a predilection for the clitoris and adjacent mucocutaneous epithelium. As with melanomas in any location, surgical treatment is the method of choice, so that these, too, are managed according to the same operative plan as is used for epidermoid carcinoma: wide radical vulvectomy with bilateral groin (inguinofemoral) and deep pelvic (external iliac, hypogastric, common iliac, and obturator) lymph node dissections. However, their more rapid dissemination by lymphatic channels, cutaneous spread, and bloodstream invasion makes the overall prognosis for cure considerably less favorable. Overall cure rates run in the 10 to 15 percent range, with occasional reports of 30 to 50 percent five-year apparent cures in patients with small lesions and uninvolved nodes. Radiation therapy and conventional chemotherapy have yielded unsatisfactory results, but future developments in both chemotherapy and immunotherapy may lead to improvement in palliation in patients with extensive or recurrent disease.

Basal Cell Carcinoma

Basal cell carcinoma is relatively uncommon (3 to 4 percent of all cases) and like basal cell lesions of the skin elsewhere does not ordinarily metastasize. However, it is often locally extensive and invasive, and hence this lesion is prone to recurrence if not adequately excised. Wide local excision of basal cell carcinoma must therefore be practiced, and in the case of the vulva this usually implies a total vulvectomy; however, lymph node dissections need not be done.

A few related histologic types that contain a squamous cell component have been encountered, the so-called **basal-squamous carcinomas**. Since the malignant epidermoid elements can and do metastasize via the lymphatics, these lesions must be treated as if they were epidermoid cancers, and lymph node dissections should be carried out along with the wide, total vulvectomy.

Rare Forms of Vulvar Malignancy

Rare forms of malignant vulvar tumors include various types of sarcoma (e.g., myosarcoma, fibrosarcoma, liposarcoma), sweat-gland carcinomas (malignant hidradenomas), carcinomas arising in müllerian and wolffian duct remnants, malignant tumors of blood vessel origin, lymphomas and lymphosarcomas, and, occasionally, metastatic cancer from lesions primary in the cervix, endometrium, ovary, or elsewhere in the pelvis or abdomen. Sarcomas are best treated by radical surgery, though the chances of cure are low; radiation therapy has not proved helpful; chemotherapy with agents such as actinomycin D is occasionally beneficial in dealing with metastatic disease but is of no value in the palliation of local disease.

NONINVASIVE LESIONS

Two initially noninvasive malignant lesions that may eventually become invasive in character or develop superimposed malignant change are Bowen's disease of the vulva, or carcinoma in situ (an intraepithelial squamous-cell carcinoma entirely similar histologically and in its clinical behavior to carcinoma in situ of the cervix, vagina, or any other squamous epithelial surface), and Paget's disease of the vulva. The latter arises in the apocrine glandular tissue of the vulva and is similar in gross appearance, symptomatology, and histologic picture to Paget's disease of the nipple, where again it takes origin from apocrine gland elements.

Bowen's Disease

Carcinoma in situ most frequently develops in vulvar skin already afflicted with one of the so-called chronic epithelial dystrophies (including, for example, leukoplakia, lichen sclerosus et atrophicus, and basal cell hyperplasia) and probably represents an intermediate stage in the ultimate development of frankly invasive epidermoid carcinoma that nearly always follows. As is true in the cervix, carcinoma in situ of the vulva is in general encountered at an earlier age (the forties and fifties) than invasive cancer of the vulva (the sixties and seventies). Since epidermoid carcinoma of the vulva is a diffuse rather than a localized malignant change in the vulvar "skin organ," it is not uncommon to find multiple areas of both carcinoma in situ and true invasive carcinoma in the same vulva. If, however, multiple preliminary biopsies and thorough histologic examination of the resected vulva itself show only intraepithelial carcinoma with no sign of even microscopic stromal invasion, Bowen's disease is properly and adequately treated by a wide, total vulvectomy without the necessity for lymph node dissections.

Erythroplasia of Queyrat

A modification of epidermoid carcinoma in situ localized in the mucosa rather than the skin of the vulva is erythroplasia of Queyrat. Seen grossly, the mucosa of the introitus may exhibit discrete, intensely red areas, with a finely granular surface but little induration. Biologically, it differs from Bowen's disease in that it may show a much more rapid transition to invasive squamous cell carcinoma. If an invasive component has been ruled out by adequate biopsy, the treatment of erythroplasia of Queyrat is identical to that of Bowen's disease.

Paget's Disease of the Vulva

In the case of Paget's disease, the intense pruritus associated with the bright red (with scattered white patches), weeping, ulcerating, eczematoid, often extensive surface lesions, together with its known qualities as a precursor of epidermoid carcinoma, makes surgical treatment mandatory. Since it may be accompanied by invasive epidermoid carcinoma, preliminary multiple biopsies are extremely important, and if they reveal squamous cell carcinoma superimposed on the typical histologic picture of Paget's disease, then the surgical procedure must be identical with that for any epidermoid cancer of the vulva. If only Paget's disease is present on microscopic examination of the biopsy specimens as well as the final vulvectomy specimen, then the lymph node dissections can be omitted. The vulvectomy should be wide, with generous margins of normal skin about the lesions, because of the diffuse nature of the process. It should be remembered that Paget's disease of the breast is accompanied by carcinoma in a high percentage of cases (70 to 80 percent or more), and that the tumor is ordinarily an intraductal adenocarcinoma that may metastasize. In contrast, in Paget's disease of the vulva, underlying adenocarcinomatous lesions are relatively uncommon, seldom, if ever, obvious, and are even inconspicuous and difficult to demonstrate histologically. Microscopic foci of adenocarcinoma arising in the apocrine sweat glands or other vulvar skin appendages can be found in perhaps at most 10 to 20 percent of cases of Paget's disease of the vulva, and often these are glandular foci of carcinoma in situ. Thus Paget's disease of the vulva seems to originate in most instances within the epidermal cell layer and is basically an intraepithelial cancer just like epidermoid carcinoma in situ. Because its microscopic extension frequently exceeds the grossly visible abnormality, wide skin excision is required to avoid frequent local recurrence. Unless there is an extensive, clinically palpable carcinoma of the sweat gland apparatus, however, the disease remains localized to the skin, and metastases are extremely rare. However, as previously noted, the presence of the Paget's disease process in the vulva also appears to favor malignant degeneration of the squamous epithelial elements of vulvar skin in some patients.

Since the pathologic process is usually a diffuse one, local recurrences are common and may occur repeatedly over a long period of years. These can often be successfully treated by reexcision. When this is not feasible, topical 5 percent 5-fluorouracil in a cream base (Efudex) may be used, with daily applications for a three to six weeks' course, and excellent responses with complete disappearance of the lesions have been noted.

Local Precursors of Epidermoid Carcinoma of the Vulva

LEUKOPLAKIA AND RELATED "CHRONIC EPITHELIAL DYSTROPHIES"

True leukoplakia, or leukoplakic vulvitis, is the most significant of all precursors of epidermoid carcinoma of the vulva and will be found to coexist with, and to have preceded by many years the development of, vulvar cancer in 60 to 75 percent of cases. Furthermore, on the basis of a few prolonged follow-up observations in groups of patients with proved vulvar leukoplakia, it is estimated that epidermoid cancer of the vulva will ultimately develop in 10 to 25 percent of such women. It should be emphasized that true vulvar leukoplakia is considered to be a fairly definite disease entity, distinguishable from other vulvar skin changes that may superficially resemble it by its clinical appearance and by confirmatory biopsy showing the characteristic microscopic picture. The term should be applied only to the specific lesion that fulfills these definite criteria, and it is only this lesion that bears a significant precursor relationship to vulvar cancer. Thus the ancient term *kraurosis vulvae* is a misleading one and should be discarded. For some, it is still synonymous with leukoplakia, whereas in actuality it is a purely descriptive phrase connoting a shrunken, leathery vulva, the end stage of a variety of prior vulvar lesions including simple atrophy, chronic dermatologic disorders, and a "burnt-out" leukoplakic process.

Active leukoplakia is usually accompanied by grayish-white, thick, patchy lesions that are often edematous, fissured, or excoriated, and it is frequently accompanied by an intense, red, secondary inflammatory reaction. Most often, the skin changes appear after the menopause. Symptoms are usually intense and very troublesome and include pruritus, soreness, tenderness, burning on urination, and an associated disagreeable discharge of vulvovaginal origin. The histologic features include not only hyperkeratosis of the epidermis with dermal inflammatory infiltrates but, most important, varying degrees of atypical epithelial activity in the epidermal cell layers.

Although leukoplakia is the most common of all the so-called chronic vulvar epithelial dystrophies that may be precursors of squamous carcinoma of the vulva, lichen sclerosus et atrophicus, formerly believed never to be premalignant, as well as a variety of chronic vulvar dermatoses including senile hyperkeratoses and granulomatous diseases of the vulva, may occasionally be the apparent forerunners of vulvar cancer. The common denominator in these other lesions, as in leukoplakia itself, is the presence of abnormal and disorderly epithelial cell activity and growth patterns on microscopic examination. It is this variable, frequently progressive epithelial atypicality, not the commonly associated hyperkeratosis, that is of basic importance and that is responsible for the probable gradual change over a period of years from simple epithelial atypism of increasingly marked degree, through the phase of carcinoma in situ, and finally to the development of invasive epidermoid cancer. As has often been pointed out, it is more often the "red areas" rather than the "white patches" on the affected vulva that contain epithelial dysplasia, carcinoma in situ, or early invasive cancer.

From a clinical standpoint, adequate biopsy of most vulvar lesions that are not obviously acute, transient vulvar inflammations is important. Leukoplakia, lichen sclerosus et atrophicus, any of the chronic vulvar dermatoses associated with lichenification, carcinoma in situ, or even very early invasive carcinoma may often superficially resemble and erroneously be assumed to be merely a form of "vulvitis." Therefore, prompt, usually multiple biopsies of any suspicious areas or of any lesions in which the diagnosis is not clear should be done. The toluidine blue test and colposcopy (see Chap. 2) may be very helpful in selecting appropriate sites for biopsy to establish an early diagnosis of either vulvar dystrophy or intraepithelial carcinoma. Histologic examination will reveal at once the true nature of the disease if one of the atypical epithelial dystrophies or carcinoma in situ is present.

With regard to therapy, until recently there has been no really effective or curative medicinal treatment, local or systemic, for vulvar leukoplakia and the related epithelial dystrophies. If symptoms are minimal, and if the typical skin changes are mild and involve only a relatively small area, a trial of local therapy with hydrocortisone or cortisone ointments or lotions is justified and will frequently provide satisfactory symptomatic relief. Another approach involves the local application of an ointment of 2% testosterone propionate in a petrolatum base (Vulvan) two to three times daily (½ inch of the ointment as squeezed from the tube, per application) for 6 to 12 weeks or until symptoms abate, followed by a once-daily maintenance application as needed. Excellent results have been reported in terms of relief of the symptoms of pruritus, burning, and dyspareunia, a return to more normal skin texture and gross appearance, and histologic improvement in the dystrophy toward a more normal epithelium. A related approach involves the topical use of the anticancer chemotherapeutic agent, 5-fluorouracil, in a cream base (Efudex). This agent, used daily for six to eight weeks, has also proved very effective in eradicating epithelial dystrophies and even focal areas of carcinoma in situ. It has also been employed in the treatment of condyloma acuminatum.

It is important that patients treated conservatively in this manner have periodic follow-up examinations once or twice yearly, with prompt toluidine blue tests and/or colposcopic examination, if available, of the vulvar skin, followed by biopsy of any suspicious areas to detect any malignant change in its earliest stage. For most patients, however, particularly those with extensive skin changes and severe pruritus and in whom biopsy has shown atypical epithelial activity, simple vulvectomy is the treatment of choice. It not only is effective in relieving the distressing symptoms but also provides essentially complete protection against the future development of vulvar carcinoma. In performing the vulvectomy, although the plane of dissection can be kept superficial, it should be remembered that the epithelial change is a diffuse and multicentric process, and the entire vulvar skin organ must therefore be removed. Furthermore, these patients require continued, careful follow-up, because atypical changes and, less often, cancer can occasionally develop in adjacent skin areas even after an adequate simple vulvectomy.

SYPHILIS AND OTHER GRANULOMATOUS VENEREAL DISEASES

Prior luetic infection, with or without the accompanying presence of one of the granulomatous diseases such as lymphogranuloma inguinale or lymphogranuloma venereum, has been found almost invariably present in a small group of women in their thirties and forties with usually rapidly growing, highly undifferentiated vulvar carcinomas. Furthermore, syphilis is nearly always found associated with vulvar cancer in black women, in whom this particular form of malignant disease is ordinarily uncommon. It seems likely that an antecedent syphilitic infection in some way favors the development of carcinoma of the vulva, and that it may represent an even more potent precursor state than vulvar leukoplakia. This probably accounts for the much earlier age at onset of the carcinoma, the more rapidly growing, more undifferentiated type of tumor encountered, and the rarity of vulvar cancer in blacks in the absence of syphilis.

PATHOGENESIS

There is mounting evidence that carcinoma of the vulva (and dysplasia and carcinoma in situ as well) may share similar etiologic agents with carcinoma of the cervix, and that herpesvirus type 2 may act as an oncogenic virus in the vulva and vagina in much the same manner as in the cervix. If these closely related, contiguous squamous cell epithelial organs were each being exposed over a long period of time to the same oncogenic agent or accelerating factor, the frequent occurrence of independent primary epidermoid neoplasms, invasive or intraepithelial, in two or even all three of these sites would be nicely explained.

The Typical Patient

Most patients with epidermoid carcinoma share many systemic features in common, of which the following are the most significant:

1. Advanced age (70 percent over 60 years of age; 35 percent over 70 years of age). (The much rarer primary epidermoid carcinomas arising in Bartholin's glands tend to occur in women in their forties and fifties, however.)
2. High incidence of nulliparity (35 to 40 percent) and an early menopause (50 percent have ceased to menstruate by age 45).
3. Frequent obesity, premature diffuse arteriosclerotic changes, and hypertensive cardiovascular disease (60 percent).
4. Diabetes (10 percent have frank, known diabetes, and an additional significant percentage exhibit a diabetic type of glucose tolerance test).
5. Multiple cancers (13 percent of the Massachusetts General Hospital–Pondville State Cancer Hospital series of 238 patients had cancers of other sites prior or subsequent to the development of their vulvar carcinomas, the other cancers most frequently encountered being adenocarcinoma of the breast and adenocarcinoma of the endometrium; 21 percent also gave a family history of cancer).
6. Frequent association of intraepithelial carcinoma (and, to a lesser extent, invasive cancer as well) of the vulva, vagina, and cervix.

All of the typical systemic characteristics in (1) through (5) suggest an underlying metabolic or hormonal aberration of etiologic significance. From a practical standpoint, knowledge of this typical patient pattern is of value, in conjunction with an awareness of the significance of the apparent local precursors, particularly true

leukoplakia, in sharply defining a particular group of patients who should perhaps
receive special consideration from the standpoint of both prophylaxis (simple vulvectomy if they have definite, extensive, and symptomatic leukoplakia) and earlier
diagnosis of cancer of the vulva (careful, frequent follow-up observations and prompt
biopsy of any unusual vulvar skin change).

With respect to (6) there have been several reported series of epidermoid carcinoma
in situ of the vulva in which as many as 25 percent of the patients had associated,
independent intraepithelial cancers of the cervix, vagina, or both. The occurrence in
the same patient of multiple independent invasive cancers at more than one of these
three sites has also been observed, though with less frequency, probably because
either surgical or radiation therapy of the first lesion may remove the potential threat
of the development of at least one of the others and because many patients do not
survive their initial invasive tumor long enough for an independent tumor to develop
at one of the other sites. At any rate, this association perhaps is illustrative of the
phenomenon of field malignant degeneration: an entire, embryologically related
tract of squamous epithelium, probably to some extent similarly responsive to potential hormonal and metabolic influences, and in this instance including cervical,
vaginal, and vulvar epithelium, rather diffusely exhibits a multicentric tendency to
neoplastic change. Knowledge of this association in the case of the cervix, vulva,
and vagina is obviously of considerable clinical significance as well, since a patient
who presents with or has undergone prior treatment for cancer in any one of the
three should be carefully examined and followed, not only from the standpoint of
possible recurrence of the initial tumor but also because there is a very real possibility
that an independent tumor at one or both of the other two sites may be present or
will develop in the future.

TYPICAL HISTORY

The usual symptoms, often of long duration, include intense pruritus, local pain and
tenderness, an irritating, often slightly bloody discharge, "dysuria" (actually burning
discomfort in the lesion itself irritated by exposure to urine during voiding, but unfortunately sometimes treated as cystitis without examination of the patient), and awareness of a lump or ulcerated lesion on the vulva. Any of these symptoms, which may
be identical with and are often superimposed on those of leukoplakia, demand prompt
examination and biopsy of all suspicious lesions.

Diagnosis and Evaluation of Extent of Disease

The following steps should be taken to diagnose the disease and evaluate its extent:

1. Inspection and direct biopsy of any obvious tumor, taking the biopsy tissue
from the edge of the lesion to obtain a suitable histologic specimen. Where the vulva
presents a diffuse abnormality, and one is suspicious of an associated malignant
change somewhere, the toluidine blue staining technique described in Chapter 2 may
be used to pinpoint likely areas for biopsy.

2. Careful pelvic and rectal examinations to determine the local extent of the tumor.

3. Palpation of the regional node areas of both groins will sometimes demonstrate obvious, unequivocally positive nodes. However, clinical evaluation of nodal involvement is frequently inaccurate; palpable, suspicious nodes will be purely inflammatory in nature in 25 to 30 percent of cases, and even when the groin nodes are not palpably enlarged, they will be shown histologically to be involved by tumor in 35 to 40 percent of cases. Hence there is no way of clinically estimating whether or not lymphatic dissemination has occurred; rather, in view of its frequency, it must be assumed to have occurred in all cases as far as the proposed plan of treatment is concerned.

4. In 35 to 40 percent of patients with vulvar cancer the vaginal smear will be positive in the absence of independent tumors of the cervix or vagina, although as has already been noted, the latter possibility must also be considered in evaluating the significance of the positive cytologic findings. Presumably, the vulvar tumors occasionally desquamate cells into the vagina, or the desquamated cells are picked up as contaminants when the smears are taken. Where an obvious malignant lesion is visible, the additional cytologic confirmation is not of great importance; furthermore, it is equally apparent that the routine vaginal smear technique would be of limited screening value in the detection of early vulvar malignancy (carcinoma in situ), although smears prepared directly from vulvar scrapings might be more accurate and helpful for this purpose. It is obvious, however, that the vulva must be included along with the cervix, corpus, tube, vagina, and bladder, and, occasionally, even more distant intraabdominal viscera, as potential sites harboring cancers in an asymptomatic patient with no obvious disease, who is under study because a routine vaginal smear has been reported positive.

Staging

An official clinical staging utilizing the so-called TNM system has been devised for carcinoma of the vulva under the auspices of the International Federation of Gynecology and Obstetrics and is as follows:

T. Primary tumor.
- **T1** Tumor confined to the vulva: 2 cm or less in largest diameter.
- **T2** Tumor confined to the vulva: more than 2 cm in diameter.
- **T3** Tumor of any size with adjacent spread to the urethra and/or vagina and/or perineum and/or anus.
- **T4** Tumor of any size infiltrating the bladder mucosa and/or the rectal mucosa, or both, including the upper part of the urethral mucosa, and/or fixed to bone.

N. Regional lymph nodes.
- **N0** No nodes palpable.
- **N1** Nodes palpable in either groin, not enlarged, mobile (not clinically suspicious of neoplasm).

N2 Nodes palpable in either one or both groins, enlarged, firm, and mobile (clinically suspicious of neoplasm).

N3 Fixed or ulcerated nodes.

M. Distant metastases.

M0 No clinical metastases.

M1a Palpable deep pelvic lymph nodes.

M1b Other distant metastases.

Clinical Stage Groups

Stage I T1 N0 M0; T1 N1 M0.

Stage II T2 N0 M0; T2 N1 M0.

Stage III T3 N0 M0; T3 N1 M0;
T3 N2 M0; T1 N2 M0;
T2 N2 M0.

Stage IV T1 N3 M0; T2 N3 M0;
T3 N3 M0; T4 N3 M0;
T4 N0 M0; T4 N1 M0;
T4 N2 M0; all other conditions containing M1a or M1b.

If cytologic or histologic examination of the lymph nodes reveals malignant cells, the symbol + (plus) should be added to N; if such examinations do not reveal malignant cells, the symbol − (minus) should be added to N.

Treatment

The importance of prophylactic treatment in the form of simple vulvectomy in certain patients with significant amounts of leukoplakic change has already been stressed, and the management of carcinoma in situ by an adequate total vulvectomy, once invasive cancer has definitely been excluded, has also been discussed. With regard to definitive treatment for invasive epidermoid carcinoma of the vulva, it can be stated at the outset that radiation therapy is of no value in the primary treatment of this disease, and it is of little benefit even in its palliation. There is reasonable doubt as to its relative inherent effectiveness in the control of vulvar cancer as compared with its effectiveness in other skin cancers or in squamous cell cancers elsewhere in the body. Furthermore, the marked radiosensitivity of normal vulvar tissues sharply limits the dosage that can safely be applied without producing excessively damaging local effects intolerable to the patient. Finally, radiation treatment does not provide the best mode of attack against the problem of lymphatic spread, which is so frequent and of such major importance in vulvar carcinoma.

Surgery is therefore the treatment of choice, and the ideal surgical procedure offering maximal chance for cure is based on the following characteristics of the disease: (1) It is a diffuse lesion with multicentric origins (not just another localized form of skin cancer), hence inclined to recurrence and reoccurrence (new primary lesions may develop years later) if treated by local excision or partial vulvectomy and (2) it has a marked tendency to lymphatic spread (in 50 to 60 percent of cases). It should be stressed that the small lesion of low histologic grade is potentially just as dangerous in this regard as is the larger, more undifferentiated cancer, and it must therefore be treated just as vigorously. In the Massachusetts General Hospital–Pondville State Cancer Hospital series, 8 of 25 patients (32 percent) with primary tumors 1 cm or less in diameter had positive lymph nodes, and 26 of 54 patients (48 percent) with histologic grade 1 (low-grade malignancy) lesions had lymph node involvement. In the case of larger and/or more undifferentiated lesions, the frequency of lymphatic dissemination was even greater, being 65 to 70 percent in the histologic grade 2 and grade 3 lesions, and ranging from 50 percent in tumors only 2 cm in diameter to as high as 90 percent in lesions 7 cm or greater in diameter. The typical pattern of lymphatic spread as depicted in Figure 59 is as follows: (a) superficial nodes (femoral and inguinal) first; (b) Cloquet's nodes (femoral canal) next; then (c) deep pelvic nodes (external iliac, obturator, hypogastric); late spread may eventually occur to involve the common iliac, aortic, and lumbar nodes, by which time cure is no longer possible. Furthermore, because of the richness of the vulvar lymphatics, bilateral (or contralateral) spread is common (50 percent of all cases with lymphatic spread) even in the face of essentially unilateral primary tumors. Of great significance, however, is the fact that although the deep nodes are frequently involved, they are rarely if ever involved in the absence of prior superficial node involvement. Thus, though it takes place often, lymphatic spread invariably occurs in a leisurely, stepwise fashion,

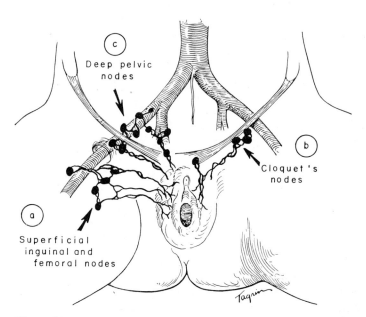

Figure 59
Routes of lymphatic spread in carcinoma of the vulva (see text, above).

and properly performed lymph node dissections can frequently encompass the area of spread.

Distant metastases are rare and usually appear late in the course of the disease, when the primary lesion and regional node spread have already reached the incurable stage. When the primary lesion and spread are untreated, death usually eventually results from massive bleeding and sepsis, often accompanied by urinary or gastro-intestinal tract obstruction, less commonly from widespread metastases.

From a consideration of these facts, it is apparent that an adequate operation for cancer of the vulva must consist of a wide radical vulvectomy in combination with bilateral groin and deep pelvic lymph node dissections. Adequate surgery is extremely effective, even in the presence of lymph node spread, but procedures less than this are nearly always followed by recurrence. There is no place in the treatment of this disease for local excision or hemivulvectomy or simple vulvectomy, nor can the lymph node dissections be omitted or limited. Although in the past the optimal procedure was customarily performed in three stages, it is now most effectively done as a single-stage procedure. A crescent type of transverse lower-abdominal, suprapubic incision allows access to the inguinal-femoral groin nodes and also permits an extraperitoneal approach to the deep pelvic nodes, both groups being bilaterally resected en bloc, with their connecting lymphatic channels and in continuity with the vulva (Fig. 60). Modern surgery (better anesthesia, antibiotics, blood replacement, improved preopera-tive and postoperative care) can maintain a very low mortality (2 to 5 percent) even in this elderly, seemingly high-risk group of patients. It should be noted parentheti-cally that in spite of their advanced age and frequently associated medical infirmities, these women tolerate this procedure of considerable magnitude exceedingly well.

With an increased awareness on the part of both patient and physician alike as to the significance of early investigation of vulvar lesions and potential premalignant disorders, vulvar cancer is now occasionally being detected in its microinvasive stage. Depending on the patient's general medical condition and the size and degree of microinvasion of her lesion, possibly a less radical operative procedure may represent adequate treatment in some of these cases, e.g., total vulvectomy, with or without bilateral superficial inguinofemoral lymph node dissections

More radical procedures (various types of pelvic exenteration) may have to be done in advanced or recurrent cases where there is involvement of the anus or peri-anal skin, urethra, bladder, vagina (extensive), or ischiorectal fossa. In properly selected cases, the results of these more extensive procedures may be highly gratify-ing. (In the 1947–1970 Massachusetts General Hospital–Pondville State Cancer Hospital series, 16 women required some form of pelvic exenteration, and 9 of these were living and well five or more years later, 6 with negative nodes after posterior exenteration, 2 with positive nodes after anterior exenteration, and 1 with positive nodes after total exenteration.) Previous inadequate treatment (all too common) may complicate the problem but does not change the basic plan of surgical therapy, and the end results of adequate treatment are often equally rewarding.

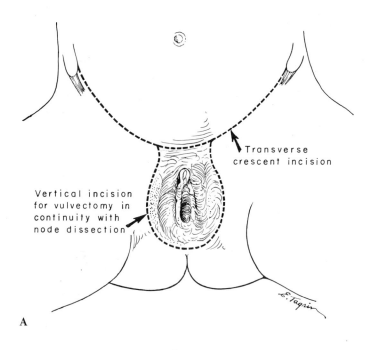

Transverse
crescent incision

Vertical incision
for vulvectomy in
continuity with
node dissection

A

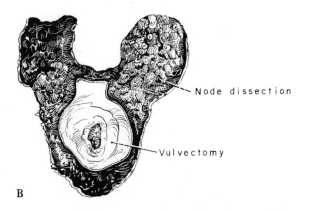

Node dissection

Vulvectomy

B

Figure 60
Radical operation for carcinoma of the vulva. A. The incision for a one-stage
approach to radical vulvectomy in continuity with bilateral groin and deep pelvic
lymph node dissections. B. The final operative specimen.

Results Following Adequate Surgery

The overall cure rate of adequately treated patients should approach 50 to 60 percent, and if the lymph nodes are histologically uninvolved, 85 to 90 percent of patients will be cured. Even more striking is that 45 to 50 percent of patients with positive lymph nodes will nevertheless be cured of their disease by what has previously been defined as an adequate operative procedure for carcinoma of the vulva. In fact, if only unilateral superficial groin node metastases have occurred, an 85 percent cure rate can still be achieved; if superficial groin node spread is present bilaterally, 60 percent of patients can be salvaged. In the presence of histologically proved, deep pelvic node spread, the cure rate falls to 10 to 15 percent. Certainly, these end result figures provide ample support for an aggressive surgical attack on this disease.

CARCINOMA OF THE URETHRA

Carcinoma of the urethra in women (usually epidermoid, occasionally adenocarcinoma, and, rarely, transitional cell carcinoma or melanoma) is often included in discussing vulvar carcinoma, because it frequently arises near the urethral meatus and hence presents as a vulvar tumor. Early lesions may masquerade as urethral caruncles, polyps, papillomas, mucosal prolapse or eversion, or erosions, and the usual symptoms are urinary frequency and vaginal bleeding that may initially be mistaken for uterine bleeding. Since the majority of women with urethral carcinoma are in the 55- to 65-year-old age group or older, "postmenopausal bleeding" is a common presenting complaint. Thus the possibility of urethral or bladder lesions should always be considered in women in whom no source for abnormal bleeding (especially postmenopausal bleeding) can be found after thorough investigation of the reproductive tract. Both the spread of urethral cancer and hence also the therapeutic approach are similar to that of vulvar cancer, with the following exceptions:

1. The primary urethral lesion, if small, may well be controlled by local interstitial radium, so that this should often be tried first; if successful, bilateral radical groin and deep pelvic node dissections should then be done.
2. If radiation treatment does not achieve control of the primary lesion, or if its size or site of origin is such that the proximal urethra or bladder has become involved or there is extensive local spread, anterior or total pelvic exenteration and deep pelvic node dissections may be necessary, the superficial groin nodes again being also bilaterally resected, usually at a second operation a few weeks later.
3. It is possible that a combination of preoperative irradiation followed by radical surgery may increase the chances for cure in the more extensive lesions.
4. The size of the initial lesion and the site and extent of urethral involvement markedly influence cure rates. Lesions involving only the anterior or distal urethra and less than 3 cm in diameter have had cure rates from 50 percent to nearly 100 percent in some series, but with extensive lesions, the cure rate is less than 10 percent, and thus early recognition of these tumors is important.

MALIGNANT TUMORS OF THE VAGINA

Carcinoma

In spite of vaginal infections, traumas, and cyclic hormonal changes, primary carcinoma of the vagina is a rare tumor, but it increases in incidence with advancing age, occurring most frequently in the 55- to 65-year-old age group. Almost invariably, it is epidermoid carcinoma (in 90 to 95 percent), although adenocarcinoma occasionally arises from mesonephric or müllerian duct remnants or ectopic cervical glands; even more rarely, it arises from areas of vaginal endometriosis. A high percentage of primary cancers of the vagina appear in patients who have also had independent primary carcinomas of the cervix or vulva, again supporting the concept that all three of these tumors originate from a multicentric process involving this entire squamous epithelial field.

Although primary carcinoma of the vagina is uncommon (1 to 2 percent of all pelvic cancers), vaginal extension or metastasis from cervical, endometrial, vulvar, and ovarian cancer is frequent, as is local spread from tumors of the rectum, bladder, or urethra. It is often impossible to be certain that one is dealing with primary carcinoma of the vagina when the lesion is situated high in the vagina and encroaches on the cervix; if doubt exists, the lesion must be classified and treated as a cervical cancer. When primary cancer of the vagina does occur, it arises most often on the posterior wall in the middle or upper vagina. The usual early symptoms are painless vaginal bleeding or foul discharge, and often there are associated urinary tract disturbances with frequency, urgency, and dysuria. The lesions are ordinarily not painful until late in the course of the disease.

As local extension and lymphatic dissemination proceed, pain, a sense of pressure or mass, constipation, and edema of the lower extremities may develop. Distant metastases are rare and late, and death is usually due to local spread complicated by hemorrhage, infection, and gastrointestinal and urinary tract obstruction. Though it occasionally remains superficial for a considerable period of time, local extension ultimately and often quite rapidly leads to involvement of the rectum, rectovaginal septum, bladder and urethra, cervix, and vulva; lymphatic involvement is also common. When located high in the vagina, vaginal cancer behaves and spreads much like a primary cervical cancer (i.e., paravaginal spread to involve pelvic wall nodes); when low in the vagina, it disseminates in a pattern similar to that of vulvar carcinoma (i.e., early inguinal and femoral node spread, with later involvement of the deep pelvic nodes).

DIAGNOSIS

From the standpoint of prompt detection, it is important to avoid overlooking the very early lesion, situated in the upper third of the posterior vaginal wall, during vaginal palpation and speculum examination. Positive vaginal cytologic findings may be the first clue, and, as previously noted, women who have been treated for either cervical or vulvar cancer, particularly of the intraepithelial type, are especially deserving of careful, frequent screening to detect the often associated, independent vaginal cancer in its earliest stages. In fact, where carcinoma in situ of the vagina is concerned, the vast majority (80 to 90 percent) of patients with this lesion will have simultaneous or antecedent cancer of the cervix or vulva. The more advanced lesions present no diagnostic problem (biopsy confirmation is readily obtained), except with respect to whether they are primary in the vagina or represent secondary extensions from cancer originating elsewhere in the pelvis.

STAGING

An official clinical staging for carcinoma of the vagina has been devised by the Cancer Committee of the International Federation of Gynecology and Obstetrics and is as follows:

Preinvasive Carcinoma
Stage   0 Carcinoma in situ or intraepithelial cancer.

Invasive Carcinoma
Stage   I The carcinoma is limited to the vaginal wall.
Stage   II The carcinoma has involved the subvaginal tissue but has not extended to the pelvic wall.
Stage III The carcinoma has extended on to the pelvic wall.
Stage IV The carcinoma has extended beyond the true pelvis or has involved the mucosa of the bladder or rectum. A bullous edema of the mucosa alone does not permit assignment of a case to Stage IV.

TREATMENT

In the past, the disease has been highly lethal, and, even today, reported cure rates in various series rarely exceed 20 to 30 percent. This is due in part to the fact that the vagina is a thin-walled organ, richly supplied with lymphatics, so that local spread and lymphatic dissemination occur early, and the disease is often in an advanced stage when the patient is first seen. Furthermore, the close proximity of both bladder and rectum creates considerable technical difficulties during treatment, whether it is by radiation therapy or radical surgery.

Radiation Therapy
Although epidermoid carcinoma of the vagina is a radiosensitive lesion, for anatomic reasons, it is often difficult to apply radium satisfactorily. Further, because of the proximity of the unprotected rectum and bladder, there are serious limitations to the dosage of either radium or x-ray that can be administered. Although reported overall results from radiation therapy reveal only a 25 to 35 percent five-year survival, if the lesion lies in the upper third of the vagina and a plan of radiation therapy similar to that used for cancer of the cervix can be employed, the results are consid-

erably better, approaching 50 to 60 percent. Anterior wall lesions and tumors of the lower two thirds of the vagina are extremely difficult to treat or cure by radiation, and the incidence of vesicovaginal or rectovaginal fistulas following radiotherapy is high.

Radical Surgery

Increasing experience with surgical extirpation of carcinoma of the vagina in recent years suggests that an operative approach in many cases may offer the greatest chance for improving the curability. Radical Wertheim hysterectomy and vaginectomy with pelvic lymphadenectomy, or radical vaginal (Schauta) hysterectomy and vaginectomy with extraperitoneal lymphadenectomy, may be done for lesions of the upper and middle thirds of the vagina without bladder or rectal involvement. If the local lesion is more extensive, posterior — or, at times, anterior or total — pelvic exenteration may have to be considered. For lesions of the lower third of the vagina, radical vulvectomy and vaginectomy combined with bilateral radical groin dissections are indicated, or some form of pelvic exenteration if the bladder or rectum is involved.

CLEAR CELL ADENOCARCINOMA OF THE VAGINA

A formerly rare histologic type of vaginal cancer, clear cell adenocarcinoma of the vagina may arise spontaneously, and its existence was known before the synthesis and clinical use of diethylstilbestrol (DES). However, the frequency of these tumors has recently been increasing, and the vast majority have appeared in adolescents and in young adult women who had been prenatally exposed to DES through administration to their mothers during the first trimester of their pregnancy as therapy for threatened or habitual abortion. Similar tumors have also been encountered in the cervix, arising in this same age group under the identical circumstances. The lesion termed **vaginal adenosis** is almost universally seen in young girls exposed to DES during fetal life. Because of this wide spectrum of resulting abnormalities, most of them benign, and all encountered primarily in childhood and adolescence, this entire subject has already been given detailed coverage in Chapter 4.

Other Malignant Vaginal Tumors

Other malignant tumors of the vagina besides carcinoma include the following: (1) sarcoma botryoides (an embryonal mixed mesodermal tumor) and endodermal sinus tumor (a variant of embryonal carcinoma of germ cell origin). These nearly always occur in infants or children (see Chap. 4); (2) other sarcomas (fibrosarcoma, leiomyosarcoma, hemangiosarcoma); and (3) malignant melanoma. Radical surgical removal offers the best hope for cure in any of these lesions, none of which are very radiosensitive, but the chances of cure are often relatively remote. For example, reported cure rates for vaginal melanoma are in the 10 to 15 percent range, at best.

REFERENCES

1. Abell, M. R., and Gosling, J. R. G. Intra-epithelial and infiltrative carcinoma of the vulva: Bowen's type. *Cancer* 14:318, 1961.
2. Blath, R. A., and Boehm, F. H. Carcinoma of the female urethra. *Surg. Gynecol. Obstet.* 136:574, 1973.
3. Breen, J. L., Neubecker, R. D., Greenwald, E., and Gregori, C. A. Basal cell carcinoma of the vulva. *Obstet. Gynecol.* 46:122, 1975.
4. Chamlian, D. L., and Taylor, H. B. Primary carcinoma of Bartholin's gland: A report of 24 patients. *Obstet. Gynecol.* 39:489, 1972.
5. Chung, A. F., Woodruff, J. M., and Lewis, J. L., Jr. Malignant melanoma of the vulva: A report of 44 cases. *Obstet. Gynecol.* 45:638, 1975.
6. DiPaola, G. R., Gomez-Rueda, N., and Arrighi, L. Relevance of microinvasion in carcinoma of the vulva. *Obstet. Gynecol.* 45:647, 1975.
7. DiSaia, P. J., Rutledge, F., and Smith, J. P. Sarcoma of the vulva: Report of 12 patients. *Obstet. Gynecol.* 38:180, 1971.
8. Fetherston, W. C., and Friedrich, E. G., Jr. The origin and significance of vulvar Paget's disease. *Obstet. Gynecol.* 39:735, 1972.
9. Franklin, E. W., III, and Rutledge, F. Prognostic factors in epidermoid carcinoma of the vulva. *Obstet. Gynecol.* 37:892, 1971.
10. Frick, H. C., II, Jacox, H. W., and Taylor, H. C., Jr. Primary carcinoma of the vagina. *Am. J. Obstet. Gynecol.* 101:695, 1968.
11. Gray, L. A., and Christopherson, W. M. In-situ and early invasive carcinoma of the vagina. *Obstet. Gynecol.* 34:226, 1969.
12. Green, T. H., Jr. Radical vulvectomy. *Clin. Obstet. Gynecol.* 8:642, 1965.
13. Green, T. H., Jr., Ulfelder, H., and Meigs, J. V. Epidermoid carcinoma of the vulva: An analysis of 238 cases. Part I. Etiology and diagnosis. Part II. Therapy and end results. *Am. J. Obstet. Gynecol.* 75:834, 1958.
14. Hansen, L. H., and Collins, C. G. Multicentric squamous cell carcinoma of the lower female genital tract. *Am. J. Obstet. Gynecol.* 98:982, 1967.
15. Herbst, A. L., Green, T. H., Jr., and Ulfelder, H. Primary carcinoma of the vagina. *Am. J. Obstet. Gynecol.* 106:210, 1970.
16. Kaufman, R. H., Gardner, H. L., Brown, D., Jr., and Beyth, Y. Vulvar dystrophies: An evaluation. *Am. J. Obstet. Gynecol.* 120:363, 1974.
17. Krupp, P. J., Lee, F. Y. L., Bohm, J. W., Batson, H. W. K., Diem, J. E., and Lemire, J. E. Prognostic parameters and clinical staging criteria in epidermoid carcinoma of the vulva. *Obstet. Gynecol.* 46:84, 1975.
18. Perez, C. A., Arneson, A. N., Dehner, L. P., and Galakatos, A. Radiation therapy in carcinoma of the vagina. *Obstet. Gynecol.* 44:862, 1974.
19. Ragni, M. V., and Tobon, H. Primary malignant melanoma of the vagina and vulva. *Obstet. Gynecol.* 43:658, 1974.
20. Thornton, W. N., Jr., and Flanagan, W. C., Jr. Pelvic exenteration in the treatment of advanced malignancy of the vulva. *Am. J. Obstet. Gynecol.* 117:774, 1973.
21. Tsukada, Y., Lopez, R. G., Pickren, J. W., Piver, M. S., and Barlow, J. P. Paget's disease of the vulva. *Obstet. Gynecol.* 45:73, 1975.
22. Way, S. Carcinoma of the vulva. *Am. J. Obstet. Gynecol.* 78:692, 1960.
23. Wharton, J. T., Gallager, S., and Rutledge, F. Microinvasive carcinoma of the vulva. *Am. J. Obstet. Gynecol.* 118:159, 1974.
24. Zelle, K. Treatment of vulvar dystrophies with topical testosterone propionate. *Am. J. Obstet. Gynecol.* 109:570, 1971.

17
Tumors of the Fallopian Tube

Benign tubal tumors are extremely rare, and primary malignant tubal neoplasms, although slightly more common, are the least frequently encountered of all the malignant tumors of the female genital tract.

BENIGN TUBAL TUMORS AND CYSTS

Although they occur infrequently, many different types of benign neoplasms originating in the fallopian tube have been encountered. Among the wide variety of histologic entities reported have been mucosal polyp, papilloma, fibroadenoma, fibroma, leiomyoma, lipoma, hemangioma, and the so-called adenomatoid tumor. These tumors may be located either within the wall of the tube or within its lumen, and not infrequently they are pedunculated and project from the fimbriated end. The majority have come to light merely as incidental findings in operative specimens removed for some other pelvic disorder and have not themselves produced symptoms. However, a few are of sufficient interest and importance to warrant brief discussion.

Adenomatoid Tumors

Adenomatoid tumors are the most common of the benign tumors of the fallopian tube. Although they are usually small and asymptomatic, they are of some importance because their histologic appearance has in the past sometimes led to an erroneous diagnosis of low-grade adenocarcinoma. At times in the past, they have also been variously identified and classified as adenomas, lymphangiomas, mesotheliomas, and even mesonephromas. It is now universally accepted that they are a distinct type of benign tumor, but there is little agreement as to their histogenesis, and it is not known whether they are of vascular, mesothelial, mesonephric, or müllerian duct origin.

They are actually less common in females than in males. In males, they usually arise in the epididymis or occasionally in the spermatic cord or testicular tunica; in females, they occur with about equal frequency in the fallopian tube and uterus. In gross appearance they are firm, discrete nodules, grayish-white or yellow in color, lying within the muscle layer of the tube and rarely exceeding 3 cm in diameter. The distinctive histologic picture is one of solid cords and glandlike spaces lined by cells that may be flattened, resembling endothelial cells, or large and vacuolated, suggesting either epithelial or mesothelial cells; hence the occasional confusion with low-grade adenocarcinoma in the past.

Benign Tubal Tumors with Clinical Significance

Occasionally, leiomyomas, fibromas, and cystic or solid teratomas may, by virtue of their size or an associated vascular or inflammatory complication, produce either acute or chronic symptoms or simply present as palpable adnexal masses of unknown nature, thus ultimately requiring surgical exploration and removal.

LEIOMYOMAS

Tubal leiomyomas are usually small, solitary, and asymptomatic, and probably many are never reported. When large, they have occasionally produced acute tubal torsion; more rarely, they have been implicated as a cause of ectopic pregnancy. They are subject to the same degenerative changes as occur in uterine fibroids, and acute or chronic symptoms may likewise result on this basis. The disparity between the low incidence of leiomyomas of the tube and their frequent occurrence in the uterus is surprising, since both are of müllerian duct origin, but it may in part be related to the relative unresponsiveness of the tubal muscle to estrogens as compared with the myometrium.

TERATOMAS

Teratomas of the fallopian tube are of the dermoid-cyst variety in the majority of instances, although solid teratomatous tumors, including struma salpingii composed entirely of adult thyroid tissue, are also encountered. Many of these tumors are small and asymptomatic and are incidental findings, usually arising by a thin intra-luminal pedicle from the mucosa of the distal portion of the tube. However, the larger teratomas frequently produce both a palpable mass and chronic symptoms as a result of either their increasing size and pressure on adjacent viscera or a secondary infection, with recurrent bouts of abdominal pain, fever, and leukorrhea simulating chronic pelvic inflammatory disease. Acute or chronic intermittent torsion may also occur; less often, there is spontaneous rupture of the cystic varieties, or, even more rarely, rupture of an associated ectopic pregnancy. Occasionally, the simultaneous occurrence of an independent ovarian dermoid cyst or teratoma has been reported, further suggesting the probability that tubal teratomas arise from primordial germ cells that have been arrested in their migration to the ovary.

Miscellaneous Tubal Cysts and Pseudotumors

Although not in any sense true neoplasms, the occasional pseudotumors produced in the wall or on the serosal surface of the fallopian tubes by adenomyosis, endo-metriosis, and so-called salpingitis isthmica nodosa are mentioned from the standpoint of differential diagnosis. The gross and microscopic pathologic findings and, in general, the clinical manifestations of endometriosis and adenomyosis are essentially the same in the tubes as in other anatomic sites in the pelvis.

SALPINGITIS ISTHMICA NODOSA

The nature and etiology of salpingitis isthmica nodosa are not entirely clear, some believing this lesion to be a benign adenomatous proliferation, others holding that it is the end stage of a prior salpingitis, usually of gonorrheal origin, with maximal chronic inflammatory changes and resulting fibrous tissue and glandular proliferation in the isthmic portions of the tubes. Still others adhere to the concept that in many instances it represents adenomyosis of the uterine cornua. Clinically, it is manifested as bilateral, symmetrical, at times multiple, nodular swellings in the isthmic and cornual portions of both tubes, the fibrous thickening of the tubal walls often completely obliterating the tubal lumen in the involved areas and leading to localized tubal obstruction. Since the remaining distal segments of each tube are often relatively normal, the resulting sterility due to bilateral tubal occlusion can sometimes be relieved by bilateral cornual resection and tubal reimplantation.

CYSTS

Finally, the commonest of all noninflammatory benign tubal lesions are the **hydatid cysts of Morgagni** (Fig. 61) and the other cystic structures of identical nature and origin that may develop within the wall of the tube, in the mesosalpinx, or within the leaves of the broad ligament (the **parovarian cyst**, which could equally well be termed a **paratubal cyst**). The latter can attain considerable size and, as a result, become clinically significant in the same fashion as any enlarging adnexal lesion by producing pain, or a palpable mass, or both, or by undergoing torsion, rupture, or secondary infection. The hydatids of Morgagni are usually small and asymptomatic, occurring as pedunculated cystic structures near the fimbriated end of the tube, and are readily excised. Rarely, intermittent torsion of and/or infarction of hydatid cysts of Morgagni may cause unexplained intermittent or acute pelvic and lower abdominal pain that is usually unilateral and colicky and may or may not be associated with nausea and vomiting, signs of peritoneal irritation, a tender adnexal mass, and low-grade fever. If symptoms are severe enough — and especially if actual torsion of the entire adnexa has been precipitated by the twisting hydatid cyst — laparotomy may be indicated; or, as is more often the case, it may be performed with a

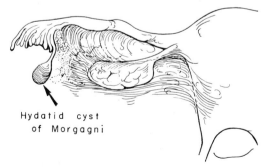

Hydatid cyst
of Morgagni

Figure 61
The common hydatid cyst of Morgagni (arrow).

mistaken preoperative diagnosis of appendicitis, twisted or ruptured ovarian cyst, or some other acute intraabdominal disorder.

All these cystic lesions are derived from leftover remnants of the wolffian or mesonephric duct system, which may give rise to retroperitoneal cysts lying postero-laterally anywhere between the lower pole of the kidney and the introitus.

PRIMARY CARCINOMA OF THE FALLOPIAN TUBE

Adenocarcinoma is by far the most common malignant fallopian tube lesion, although other primary tubal malignancies do rarely occur, including choriocarcinoma (actually a tumor arising in ectopic trophoblast), carcinosarcoma, and lymphomas and sarcomas of various types. Clinically, their symptoms and findings resemble those of primary adenocarcinomas; from the pathologic standpoint, they do not differ in gross and microscopic appearance from neoplasms of similar nature arising elsewhere in the pelvis. The incidence of primary tubal carcinomas among all female pelvic malignancies has been reported as varying from 0.1 to 1.0 percent in different institutions, and it averages about 0.5 percent.

Pathologic Features

The characteristic gross appearance of carcinoma of the fallopian tube is that of a fusiform swelling, usually involving primarily the distal portion but occasionally involving the entire length of the tube. Since the fimbriated end is often closed, and fluid or blood may accumulate in the lumen, the soft, swollen structure often externally resembles one of the more frequent benign varieties of hydrosalpinx or hematosalpinx. Often, the tumor itself is not apparent until the distended tube is opened to reveal the soft, grayish-pink, friable growth arising from the mucosal surface. The intraluminal portions of the tumor are inclined to show marked degenerative changes, and hemorrhage and characteristic yellowish areas of necrosis are often seen. In more advanced cases, however, a firmer mass may be noted when the muscular wall has been invaded, tumor may be visible on the serosal surface, or there may be obvious infiltration of the surrounding viscera or pelvic wall (Fig. 62). Less often, the tumor appears as a more localized solid or partially cystic nodule or discrete mass, again usually located in the distal portion of the tube. Although bilateral tubal carcinomas have been reported, they are relatively uncommon.

Another form of primary tubal carcinoma may show any of these aspects of the gross appearance but is continuous with similar tumor growing in the ovary, either in a confluent mass or in an ovarian cyst that communicates with the tubal lumen. In this type, it may be difficult to determine whether the tumor arose in the tube or in the ovary, but since in these cases the tube and ovary exhibit a structural unity, it is perhaps justifiable to classify these tumors as tuboovarian carcinomas, particularly when, as is often the case, the histologic appearance is more consistent with a tubal than with an ovarian origin, even though the latter possibility cannot be completely

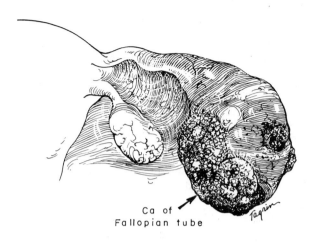

Figure 62
Typical gross appearance of primary carcinoma of the fallopian tube (arrow).

excluded. However, it is important to distinguish this category from secondary involvement of the tube by metastatic carcinoma primary in the ovary or endometrium.

The microscopic picture in tubal carcinomas is usually that of an undifferentiated neoplasm, the detailed histologic architecture varying to a great extent with the site of growth. When it is situated superficially in the tubal mucosa or has implanted on peritoneal surfaces, a papillary type of glandular carcinoma is seen; when invasion of underlying tissues has occurred or solid masses of tumor are present, the growth pattern may be either an alveolar or medullary type of adenocarcinoma. Actually, the local extent of the tumor at the time of surgery is of considerably greater prognostic significance than either the grade or histologic type of tumor. When invasion of the relatively thin tubal wall has occurred, especially if a prior pelvic inflammatory disease has produced adherence of the tube to surrounding structures, the chances of early spread are greatly increased. Even when the tumor is limited to the mucosa, there is a marked tendency for simple mechanical transplantation of fragments of viable tumor, with the development of peritoneal implants. Fortunately, the frequent occlusion of the fimbriated end of the tube secondary to antecedent pelvic inflammation often prevents this type of dissemination, which can, however, occur in the opposite direction as well, with the development of endometrial, endocervical, and even vaginal and vulvar metastases. Thus carcinoma of the fallopian tube can behave clinically, and in its growth pattern and manner of spread, almost exactly like an ovarian cancer (except that it is usually unilateral), and it is frequently impossible to distinguish it from the latter preoperatively, or, at times, even at laparotomy.

Occasional instances of carcinoma in situ of the tubal epithelium have been reported, and all were incidental findings discovered during routine pathologic study of hysterectomy specimens. The possibility that the presence of this lesion (as well as frankly invasive tubal carcinoma) might result in positive vaginal cytologic findings seems likely, however, and it should therefore be added to the list of diagnostic alternatives in cases of persistent, unexplained positive vaginal smears.

General Clinical and Etiologic Features

The vast majority of primary tubal carcinomas occur in postmenopausal women in their fifties and sixties. A past history of infertility is often obtained, and the frequent coexistence of both pelvic inflammatory disease and uterine fibroids in patients with tubal carcinoma has been noted in many reported series. The long-standing sterility of many patients, as well as the fact that in many of the early lesions the tumor is found grossly confined to tubes completely and bilaterally blocked by old pelvic inflammation, suggests that the pelvic inflammatory process antedated the malignant change and may have been an etiologic factor. That it cannot be the only factor of importance seems evident when the rarity of tubal cancer is contrasted with the frequency of salpingitis. It is also possible that a prior pelvic inflammation that has transformed the tube and ovary into a more or less continuous structure (chronic tuboovarian abscess) could account for the occurrence of many of the so-called tuboovarian cancers.

History, Findings, and Early Diagnosis

As is unfortunately also true of ovarian cancer, carcinoma of the tube is all too often in an advanced stage before symptoms sufficient to bring the patient to a physician appear. Nor is the routine yearly pelvic examination likely to improve this situation, since the early, asymptomatic tumor that is still confined to the tubal lumen and for which prompt resection still offers a reasonable chance of cure is either not palpable, or equivocal physical findings may be ascribed to old pelvic inflammatory disease or fibroids, the two lesions that so frequently coexist with tubal cancer and confuse the picture. Furthermore, when symptoms do accompany the early stage of the disease, they are often vague and intermittent, as in patients with early ovarian cancer. It is therefore important that the physician view with a high degree of suspicion vague pelvic and lower abdominal complaints in women in the fifth and sixth decades of life, particularly when accompanied by abnormal vaginal bleeding or discharge, if tubal carcinoma (or ovarian cancer) is to be recognized at a time when resection for cure may still be feasible in many instances.

Even in the face of definite symptoms and obvious, palpable adnexal disease, the correct preoperative diagnosis is rarely made. However, certain symptoms and signs do occur with sufficient frequency in association with tubal cancer to warrant seriously considering this diagnosis in their presence. An almost pathognomonic symptom of tubal carcinoma is hydrops tubae profluens, which is the intermittent occurrence of a profuse, watery, clear-yellow or bloody vaginal discharge that is characteristically abrupt in onset and accompanied by colicky pain, ceases equally rapidly, and may recur days, weeks, or months later. This phenomenon is the result of the intermittent discharge of watery, mucoid, or bloody secretions containing tumor debris from a partially obstructed, distended tube, and this symptom is almost diagnostic of tubal carcinoma, particularly if an adnexal mass is palpable on the side where the colicky pain is localized. Unfortunately, this diagnostic feature is encountered in only a minority of patients.

Far more commonly, the earliest manifestations of tubal malignancy include one or more of the triad of (1) abnormal but not dramatically episodic vaginal bleeding or discharge, (2) lower abdominal pain, and (3) abdominal swelling or a palpable mass. Postmenopausal bleeding is the most frequent symptom, and as a clue to the early diagnosis of tubal carcinoma it is especially significant when curettage fails to establish its source. In fact, the sequence of persistent bleeding after a curettage with negative findings in a postmenopausal woman has been frequently described in reported series of patients with carcinoma of the tube and should alert the physician to this possibility. In this situation, particularly if some of the other common symptoms or findings that will be described are present, exploratory laparotomy is virtually mandatory to avoid overlooking a tubal carcinoma.

A watery vaginal discharge that may be clear or mucoid and occasionally of a peculiar bright-yellow color due to the presence of cholesterol-rich tumor debris is another frequent symptom. Colicky pain due to distention of the tube and irritation of its musculature by the enlarging intraluminal mass is sometimes noted, but more commonly the discomfort is described as an intermittent, deep, aching or boring pain or a bearing-down sensation. Occasionally, bowel and bladder symptoms secondary to the pressure of the adjacent tumor on these organs accompany the pain.

Abdominal swelling or a palpable mass may be the first sign of trouble, and, not infrequently, the presence of associated uterine fibroids creates difficulty in the proper evaluation of the tubal mass. Just as is the case with ovarian cancer if its detection is to be prompt, one must beware of attributing the early symptoms and findings of tubal cancer to the incidental fibroids that so often accompany it and may obscure the diagnosis. Their presence will be misleading less often if it is remembered that fibroids rarely enlarge or cause symptoms in the postmenopausal age group, and if a high index of suspicion is maintained concerning the possibility of other lesions such as tubal or ovarian carcinomas in the presence of any or all of the preceding symptoms. In rare instances, evidences of advanced spread in the form of palpable groin nodes or ascites and pleural effusion due to metastatic implants may be the presenting complaint.

Inasmuch as the earliest and most frequent symptoms of tubal cancer, namely, abnormal discharge and bleeding, are the result of growth, ulceration, and desquamation of the tumor, earlier detection through the use of diagnostic cytology would seem possible. Indeed, some patients with tubal cancer do show positive vaginal smears, and a few early cases have recently been discovered in this way. It is to be hoped that with more widespread use of cytologic screening techniques, this will be even more true in the future. However, the vaginal cytologic findings are positive in considerably less than half of the patients with tubal carcinoma studied so far, and thus this approach does not promise to be as rewarding as it has been in the recognition of early cervical and endometrial cancer.

Treatment and Results

In view of what has been known of its patterns of dissemination, the optimal treatment for tubal carcinoma has long been considered to be total hysterectomy and bilateral salpingo-oophorectomy. Favorable results can be anticipated in patients in whom the lesion is still grossly confined to the tube, with cure rates varying from 40 to 60 percent for these localized lesions, which unfortunately represent only a small minority of the cases. Since lymphatic spread can also occur, it is possible that in these more favorable cases, performance of a radical Wertheim hysterectomy with bilateral pelvic lymphadenectomy might further increase the curability. The author has previously reported one such patient who remained free of disease until her death from other causes 7 years following this more extensive procedure for tubal carcinoma with unilateral metastasis to a pelvic wall lymph node. It is thus apparent that in the earlier lesions at least, potentially curable regional lymphatic spread can occur prior to the more usual local extension, peritoneal seeding, and distant metastases.

Unfortunately, in the vast majority of patients, the lesion is usually in an advanced stage at laparotomy, with ovarian, uterine, vaginal, rectosigmoidal, and omental extensions common, seeding or growth into the peritoneum of the cul-de-sac and pelvic walls not infrequent, and widespread peritoneal seeding occasionally present. (In the terminal stages of the disease, or at autopsy, more distant spread, with involvement of the groin nodes, liver, lungs, and pleurae is frequently seen; occasionally, skeletal and cerebral metastases are observed.) Nevertheless, if the bulk of the tumor can be removed, this should be done, and then postoperative external radiation therapy should be administered. Worthwhile results in terms of palliation, sometimes of many years' duration, will follow in a significant number of patients, although no patient with even minimal gross local spread of the primary tumor beyond the confines of the tube is likely to be cured.

In patients with residual disease outside the field of feasible postoperative irradiation, or with persistent or recurrent local disease following surgery and postoperative irradiation, or in whom more distant metastases appear, a trial of chemotherapy should be considered if the patient is still able to tolerate it. Although occasional worthwhile additional palliation may be achieved with alkylating agents or with combination drug therapy, the results of chemotherapy in the treatment of tubal cancer have generally been disappointing when compared with the more favorable response rate of ovarian cancer to the same agents.

The reported overall five-year apparent cure rates reported in the literature vary from a low of less than 5 percent to a high of 40 percent, but on the average have been between 5 and 10 percent. (In a Massachusetts General Hospital—Pondville State Cancer Hospital series of 24 patients, absolute cure was achieved in only 4 patients, or 17 percent.) Tubal carcinomas appear to be among the least curable of all female genital cancers, a reflection of the ease with which they spread and the difficulties inherent in early diagnosis.

REFERENCES

1. Boronow, R. C. Chemotherapy for disseminated tubal cancer. *Obstet. Gynecol.* 42:62, 1973.
2. Boutselis, J. G., and Thompson, J. N. Clinical aspects of primary carcinoma of the fallopian tube. *Am. J. Obstet. Gynecol.* 111:98, 1971.
3. Golden, A., and Ash, J. E. Adenomatoid tumors of the genital tract. *Am. J. Pathol.* 21:63, 1945.
4. Green, T. H., Jr., and Scully, R. E. Tumors of the fallopian tube. *Clin. Obstet. Gynecol.* 5:886, 1962.
5. Grimes, H. G., and Kornmesser, J. G. Benign cystic teratoma of the oviduct: Report of a case and review of the literature. *Obstet. Gynecol.* 16:85, 1960.
6. Hanton, E. M., Malkasian, G. D., Jr., Dahlin, D. C., and Pratt, J. H. Primary carcinoma of the fallopian tube. *Am. J. Obstet. Gynecol.* 94:832, 1966.
7. Hu, C. Y., Taymor, M. L., and Hertig, A. T. Primary carcinoma of the fallopian tube. *Am. J. Obstet. Gynecol.* 59:58, 1950.
8. Phelps, H. M., and Chapman, K. E. Role of radiation therapy in treatment of primary carcinoma of the uterine tube. *Obstet. Gynecol.* 43:669, 1973.
9. Scheffey, L. C., Lang, W. R., and Nugent, F. B. Clinical and pathologic aspects of primary sarcoma of the uterine tube. *Am. J. Obstet. Gynecol.* 52:904, 1946.
10. Schenck, S. B., and Mackles, A. Primary carcinoma of the fallopian tubes with positive smears. *Am. J. Obstet. Gynecol.* 81:782, 1961.
11. Schiller, H. M., and Silverberg, S. G. Staging and prognosis in primary carcinoma of the fallopian tube. *Cancer* 28:389, 1971.

18
Disorders of Pelvic Support

Variations in the position of the uterus, with or without accompanying shifts in the usual anatomic configuration of the vagina and the adjacent bladder, urethra, and anorectal canal, may involve simple displacement without any deficiency in the normal adequate supports. On the other hand, such variations may occur secondarily as a result of the development of a fundamental weakness and relaxation of the supporting structures of the pelvic floor and perineum. The former, which will be discussed briefly first, are most often simple anatomic variations within the so-called range of normal and are usually both asymptomatic and of no significance in terms of normal function.

SIMPLE DISPLACEMENTS

Terms such as **anteflexion** and **retroflexion**, which are sometimes employed to denote the contour of the long axis of the uterus, are purely descriptive, as are the terms **retrocession, anteversion,** and **retroversion,** which are ordinarily used to indicate the direction and location of the long axis of the uterus in relation to the pelvic basin and vaginal canal. These various positional differences are most often merely simple anatomic variations from the most frequent uterine location and axial direction in midpelvis and in moderate anteversion, approximately perpendicular to the axis of the vaginal canal. As such, they are uniformly asymptomatic and of no functional importance. Retroversion of the uterus, because it is by far the commonest of the simple displacements, and because an acquired type can be produced by cul-de-sac disease, is of some clinical significance and will be briefly considered as a specific entity.

Retroversion of the Uterus

PRIMARY, SIMPLE RETROVERSION

Simple retroversion of the uterus is encountered in 20 percent or more of otherwise normal, asymptomatic women and represents a congenital anatomic variation consisting of a short anterior vaginal wall combined with relaxed and attenuated uterosacral ligaments. Both abnormalities tend to prevent the more usual and fundamentally more normal posterior fixation of the cervix and allow, or more or less force, the fundus to fall back into the cul-de-sac. Under these circumstances it is an essentially asymptomatic entity and is usually innocent of the charge of a variety of pelvic symptoms often ascribed to it (e.g., dysmenorrhea, dyspareunia, backache, infertility, menorrhagia, pregnancy complications).

The uterus is invariably freely movable, can usually be manually placed anteriorly during pelvic examination or will fall forward spontaneously if the patient assumes the knee-chest position, and can be held there with a Smith-Hodge pessary (Fig. 63). About the only indications for attention of this type, however, are (1) to assist the uterus in rising out of the pelvis more comfortably in early pregnancy, or (2) occasionally, in an infertile couple in whom all studies are negative except for simple retroversion in the wife, to achieve a more or less constant placement of the uterus more anteriorly in the hope that a more favorable relationship between the cervical canal and the ejaculate or seminal pool may be created. (However, most women with simple retroversion conceive uneventfully, and during pregnancy the enlarging uterus ordinarily shifts spontaneously without difficulty.) The infrequent performance of uterine suspension operations nowadays and the rarity with which pessaries are now fitted for retroversion are indicative of the general awareness of the innocuousness of simple retroversion.

SECONDARY OR ACQUIRED RETROVERSION

A fixed retroversion may develop due to cul-de-sac or adnexal disease (e.g., endometriosis, chronic pelvic inflammatory disease) that produces permanent adherence of the fundus and/or adnexa posteriorly; or it may be secondary to uterine disease (e.g., large posterior fibroids) that causes the uterus to gravitate permanently in a posterior axis. Here, symptoms are due to the underlying disease, which is responsible for posterior retraction, gravitation, or adherence of the uterus. In the course of conservative surgery for these diseases with the aim of preserving and improving fertility (e.g., conservative operations for endometriosis and pelvic inflammatory disease, myomectomy), mobilization of the uterus and adnexa is an important step, and their continued maintenance in position anteriorly, away from the old or potential new area of adherence posteriorly, is essential and is probably the one most valid indication for the performance of uterine suspension.

Of the various types of uterine suspensions, the Coffey (anterior round ligament plication) or Baldy-Webster (posterior round ligament plication) is the most satisfactory and effective. (No intraabdominal traps or dangerous cul-de-sacs that might cause small-bowel obstruction are produced, and the fundus is left free to enlarge normally with pregnancy.) Obstetricians look with particular favor on the Baldy-Webster type of suspension, since the anterior surface of the fundus and cervix are left entirely free should cesarean section ever be necessary.

ANATOMY OF PELVIC SUPPORT

In terms of a better understanding of the pathologic anatomy responsible for the production of the various pelvic relaxations and the general principles of their surgical correction, it is helpful to consider first the basic structures and mechanisms involved in providing normal support for the pelvic organs. In the human female, nature is faced with the twofold problem of adequately supporting the pelvic viscera in the face of the constant gravitational stresses imposed by the upright position and other sporadic intraabdominal forces associated with coughing, defecation, and so on,

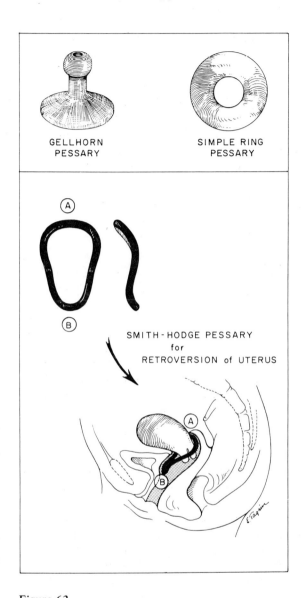

GELLHORN PESSARY

SIMPLE RING PESSARY

Ⓐ

Ⓑ

SMITH-HODGE PESSARY
for
RETROVERSION of UTERUS

Figure 63
Types of vaginal pessaries. The Gellhorn and the simple ring pessaries are employed
in the conservative management of uterine prolapse. (From T. H. Green, Jr. Gynecology. In G. L. Nardi and G. D. Zuidema [Eds.], *Surgery: A Concise Guide to
Clinical Practice* [3rd ed.]. Boston: Little, Brown, 1972, Chap. 39.)

while at the same time allowing normal egress for the urinary and gastrointestinal tracts and, most important, for normal reproductive tract function, including the ability to deliver a normal, full-term living fetus vaginally. In view of the tremendous engineering problems posed, it is indeed a miracle that a fairly satisfactory solution has been accomplished, and it is not too surprising that the supporting mechanism ultimately fails in a considerable number of women. For those interested, the probable manner in which the various supporting structures and mechanisms have undergone evolutionary adaptation from the original situation in female quadripeds to the current anatomic configuration in the bipedal human female has been well presented by Ulfelder [18].

The various structures involved in normal pelvic support are discussed in the sections that follow.

PUBIC SYMPHYSIS AND ADJACENT RAMI

As a result of the exaggerated lumbar spinal curve and accompanying downward tilt of the bony pelvis in the human, the anterior part of the bony pelvis actually rests beneath the anteriorly situated pelvic viscera or portions thereof (principally the bladder) and does in fact help to support them.

THE SACROCOCCYGEAL BONY BASIN

The widening and marked forward curve of the sacrum and coccyx that has evolved in the human female has placed them directly beneath parts of the more posteriorly located pelvic organs (principally the rectum), where they also serve as a rigid, unyielding support.

THE MUSCULAR PELVIC FLOOR

In the central pelvis, between the peripheral anterior and posterior bony segments and lateral pelvic walls, the basic problem of support for the structures directly over the pelvic outlet is ordinarily effectively solved by the bilaterally situated, fanshaped levator muscles. As depicted in Figure 64A, their separate components, the ischiococcygeus, iliococcygeus, and pubococcygeus muscles, are essentially fused on each side and also blend together in the midline, where they surround and support the three apertures or canals in the soft-tissue pelvic floor through which the terminal portions of the urinary, reproductive, and gastrointestinal tracts travel. This so-called levator sling of thick, striated muscle is admirably suited for the purpose, since it does fulfill the requirements for long-term adequate support and yet will allow for considerable temporary expansion to meet the functional demands of normal vaginal delivery and bowel evacuation. Obviously, a congenital deficiency or, more commonly, an acquired weakness of this key muscular supporting framework, with relaxation and widening of the apertures, will lead to inadequate support and ultimately to downward displacement or herniation of the pelvic viscera through the pelvic floor.

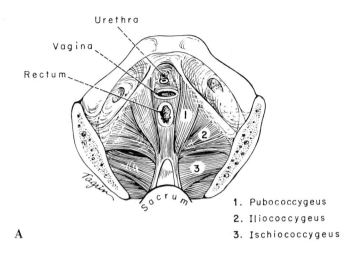

Urethra

Vagina

Rectum

1. Pubococcygeus
2. Iliococcygeus
3. Ischiococcygeus

A

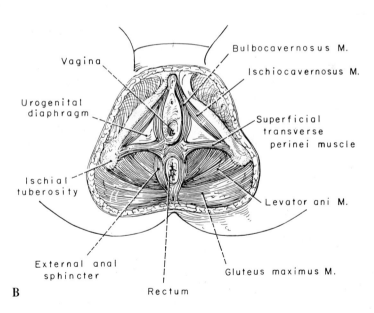

Bulbocavernosus M.

Vagina

Ischiocavernosus M.

Urogenital
diaphragm

Superficial
transverse
perinei muscle

Ischial
tuberosity

Levator ani M.

External anal
sphincter

Gluteus maximus M.

Rectum

B

Figure 64
The muscular supports of the pelvic viscera. A. Muscles of the pelvic floor. B. Perineal muscle component.

THE PERINEAL MUSCULATURE

The more superficially located muscles of the perineum, the paired ischiocavernosus, bulbocavernosus, and deep and superficial transverse perineal muscles, together with the external anal sphincter and the musculofascial tissues of the so-called urogenital diaphragm (triangular ligament), form a second hammocklike supporting mechanism basically less important than the levator sling (Fig. 64B). This second line of defense against the forces tending to produce descent of the pelvic organs is considerably less effective and rarely, if ever, will prevent the eventual continued downward displacement of the uterus, bladder, or rectum, once the levator muscle supports have been seriously weakened.

THE UTERINE LIGAMENTS AND THE "FASCIA ENDOPELVINA"

The two pairs of intrinsic uterine ligaments, the uterosacral ligaments and the round ligaments, normally play a role in the supporting mechanism, although they do not themselves actually hold the uterus up against gravitational and similar stresses tending to force it down. Rather, their function is to maintain the uterus in the proper axis relative to the vaginal canal, which passes obliquely through the muscular pelvic floor. Here, the uterosacral ligaments are the most important factor, for, if normal, they hold the cervix firmly posteriorly, with the result that the uterus remains perpendicular to the line of the vaginal canal and in a position over the thick muscular plate of the levator sling. This muscular plate can therefore effectively oppose all forces tending to drive the uterus down and out of the pelvis through the weak spot of the vaginal canal and its surrounding muscular aperture (Fig. 65). The round ligaments contribute slightly to this mechanism by tending to pull the fundus forward into the optimal position but are so elastic and easily stretched — by pregnancy, for example — that theirs is a minor role. If the uterosacral ligaments are weak and attenuated, either congenitally, as in the congenital form of uterine retroversion, or because of acquired injuries, any downward forces will cause the cervix to ride forward, and the axis of the uterus will come to rest directly over and in line with the axis of the vaginal canal. The uterus then acts as a piston or wedge when these downward forces come into play, gradually further dilating the aperture of what is usually by now an already stretched and weakened levator muscle support. Uterine prolapse and the other associated relaxations then develop.

    The broad ligaments play no supporting role and are not true ligaments in the usually accepted sense. The so-called cardinal ligaments of Mackenrodt are actually composed of the blood vessels and lymphatic channels traveling between the pelvic walls and the uterus at the level of the cervix. They gain their supportive strength, which is not inconsiderable in most cases, by virtue of the condensation around them of areolar and fibrous tissue, the so-called fascia endopelvina, which is reflected from the pelvic walls medially along all the vascular, muscular, and peritoneal tissue planes or compartments running toward the central pelvic viscera. (The term **fascia** is used rather loosely in this sense, for nowhere in the pelvis is there grossly or histologically

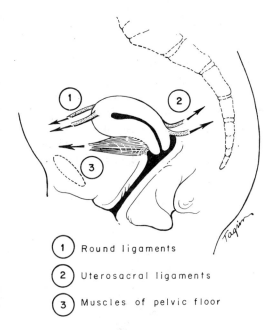

1 Round ligaments

2 Uterosacral ligaments

3 Muscles of pelvic floor

Figure 65
Role of the uterine ligaments in the mechanism of pelvic support.

any fascia in the true sense of the word, except in the case of the true muscle fascia that covers the striated muscle of the pelvic floor.) The cardinal ligaments are actually only the thickest, strongest, and most anterior sections of wider, medially running vascular "webs" that bring the blood and lymph supply from the main vessels traveling against each pelvic wall to the central pelvic organs. They may for a time maintain support for the uterine fundus, even in the face of a markedly weakened levator sling (in this situation, the poorly supported cervix below the level of the cardinal ligaments often becomes markedly elongated because of lack of support beneath it), but ultimately the cardinal ligaments will also give way, with the development of prolapse of the fundus as well, once the fundamental supporting effect of the levator sling has been impaired.

PELVIC RELAXATIONS AND ABNORMALITIES OF VISCERAL SUPPORT

The following individual types of pelvic relaxation are largely the result of obstetric injuries to the pelvic muscular floor or diaphragm (the levator sling plus the perineal musculature). Although each is a recognizable entity unto itself, it is usual for several to be present together and require simultaneous combined treatment. They are uncommon in nulliparous women, though a combination of congenitally weak musculature and the further atrophy caused by aging and specific postmenopausal changes occasionally produces simple prolapse or simple cystocele in even the virginal female.

Uterine Prolapse (Procidentia)

Prolapse of the uterus through the pelvic floor and vaginal outlet (Fig. 66) is tradi-
tionally rated as first-degree (the cervix comes down to the introitus), second-degree
(the cervix protrudes through the introitus), or third-degree (total procidentia) (the
entire uterus protrudes through the introitus). Symptoms are due to the mechanical
discomfort and inconvenience as well as to irritation of the exposed cervix and vaginal
mucous membranes. Frequently, prolapse is accompanied by marked perineal
relaxation, cystocele and rectocele, and often by enterocele. As just mentioned, in
its early stages, prolapse may sometimes consist almost entirely of a markedly

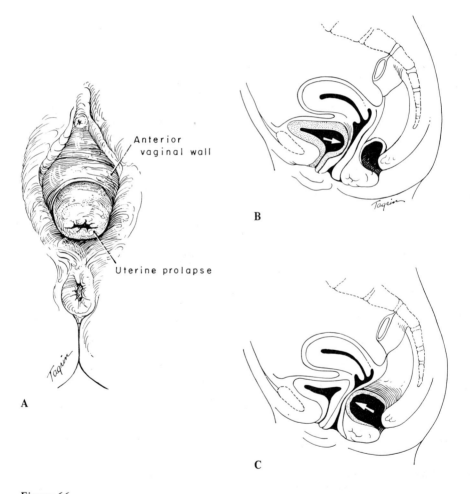

Anterior
vaginal wall

Uterine prolapse

A

B

C

Figure 66
A. Uterine prolapse. B. Cystocele. C. Rectocele. The typical gross anatomic
appearance of each of these common forms of pelvic relaxation is shown individually.
Actually, they frequently coexist.

elongated cervix, which may be 5 to 10 cm in length in contrast to the normal length of 3 cm. The protruding cervix and vaginal walls may become eroded, leading to vaginal discharge and bleeding.

Although the ideal definitive treatment is operation, conservative nonoperative management is sometimes indicated and satisfactory in certain patients. Without attempting to describe the operative procedures, the various forms of treatment will be enumerated in order of preference.

SURGICAL TREATMENT

Vaginal Hysterectomy

Vaginal hysterectomy with careful anterior and posterior colporrhaphies is the most effective and reliable method of correcting the problem of uterine prolapse, together with the frequently coexisting cystocele, rectocele, and weakness of the levator sling and perineal musculature. It usually yields excellent results in terms of restoration of normal anatomic support with preservation of and improvement in normal vaginal function as well as relief from any secondary bladder or bowel dysfunction or symptomatology. Porges [14] has published an excellent description of the basic principles of a sound method of performing vaginal hysterectomy, accompanied by an instructive discussion of how the technique can most readily be taught (and learned).

Fothergill Operation

The Fothergill operation may occasionally be preferable to vaginal hysterectomy in the older patient with a prolapse consisting almost entirely of an elongated, protruding cervix and an associated cystocele, and with a small, normal fundus, actually well supported above the level of the cardinal ligaments.

Le Fort Operation

The Le Fort operation (partial vaginal closure) is sometimes useful in elderly, high-risk patients in whom a pessary is ineffective or poorly tolerated. Good short-term results can be achieved by this simple minor and rapid plastic procedure. It should not be used unless the operative risk of vaginal hysterectomy is great, since the chief disadvantage of this operation ("burying" the uterus behind the obliterated vaginal canal) creates a very serious problem should uterine cancer develop in the future.

Abdominal Uterine Suspension Procedures

Abdominal uterine suspension procedures are mentioned only to point out their shortcomings and condemn their use in the management of uterine prolapse under any but the most exceptional circumstances. None of the uterine suspension operations provides any but the most temporary support, since they do not attack the fundamental weakness in the pelvic floor and merely substitute highly elastic structures such as the round ligaments, which rapidly become stretched and useless in holding up the uterus. Even if ventral fixation of the uterine fundus to the anterior abdominal wall is performed, the uterus simply progressively elongates due to lack of support from below, and ultimately the cervix prolapses through the introitus again, usually within a few years. Furthermore, uterine suspension is of no particular value in correcting the often associated vaginal-wall weakness (cystocele, rectocele).

About the only indication for this type of temporizing, inadequate procedure for uterine prolapse would be the rare occurrence of significant and troublesome procidentia in a young woman desirous of retaining childbearing function. Eventually, this sort of patient will undoubtedly require definitive, corrective surgery, but, in the meantime, symptomatic relief will have been temporarily achieved while she completes her family.

CONSERVATIVE THERAPY WITH A PESSARY

The use of pessaries in older, high-risk patients is probably preferable to the Le Fort operation, but a pessary is not always effective (if the pelvic floor and perineum are too badly damaged, a pessary may not be retained), nor will it always be well tolerated (discomfort, discharge, and vaginal erosion with bleeding may prevent continued use). A variety of contrivances are available (Fig. 63). Today, they are largely constructed of plastic materials that are superior to the more irritating rubber formerly used.

Techniques of Insertion

A pessary of proper diameter (usually the largest size accepted by the introitus) is selected, inserted sidewise through the levator canal, and then rotated 90 degrees to settle down flat between the posterior fornix and the pubic symphysis in much the same position as a contraceptive diaphragm, reducing and holding back the prolapse or cystocele. Because reduction of the prolapse will cause some shrinkage of the introitus and the levator muscular hiatus within a few weeks and ultimately lead to incarceration of the pessary, the patient should be seen in three to four weeks and the next smaller size inserted for permanent use. The patient is either taught to remove, clean, and replace the pessary herself (only seldom possible) or must be seen every three to four months for removal, cleaning, and replacement of the pessary; at the same time, she is checked for signs of excessive irritation.

Pessaries, particularly if too large or if left unattended and unchecked for long periods, have been known to become so incarcerated that anesthesia and morcellation of the pessary or actual episiotomy are necessary for their removal; or deep erosions, even rectovaginal fistulas, have developed. There is some evidence that the chronic irritation of the vaginal epithelium produced by prolonged use of pessaries may occasionally be an etiologic factor in the development of vaginal carcinoma.

Cystocele

When the normal striated muscular support for the vaginal canal is rendered inadequate by the permanent stretching of the oblique tunnel through the levator sling and the widening of its outlet aperture that often accompanies repeated childbirth injury, the vaginal walls and their surrounding fascia endopelvina also tend to stretch and bulge downward in response to constant gravitational forces and to the repeated intermittent stresses of coughing, lifting, straining during defecation, and so on. Ultimately, marked descent of the anterior vaginal wall and the floor of the bladder immediately deep to it may occur, with the formation of a cystocele (Fig. 66).

The chief symptoms are again the result of the mechanical inconvenience, with a sense of insecurity and an uncomfortable bearing-down sensation. Furthermore, poor bladder emptying with residual urine often produces urinary frequency and urgency as well as chronic or recurrent cystitis. However, stress incontinence is not a symptom of cystocele.

TREATMENT

The treatment for cystocele consists of anterior and posterior colporrhaphies (often combined with vaginal hysterectomy or the Fothergill operation). Occasionally, only a pessary is indicated in an elderly, poor-risk patient.

Rectocele (and Lacerated Perineum)

The posterior vaginal wall and underlying rectum commonly also tend to bulge forward and eventually protrude through the introitus when the pelvic floor and perineal muscular supports have been weakened and stretched, this anatomic abnormality being termed a *rectocele* (Fig. 66). The chief symptoms are the result of the uncomfortable protrusion and the often associated difficult emptying of the bowel, straining only exaggerating the rectocele instead of assisting defecation.

TREATMENT

Treatment of rectocele and lacerated perineum consists of posterior colporrhaphy and repair of the perineum. If the original obstetric injury was a third-degree tear, the ends of the divided external anal sphincter are also sought and resutured. Because perineal relaxation is usually marked, conservative treatment with a pessary is rarely successful.

Enterocele

Enterocele is a true hernial weakness occurring in the area between the uterosacral ligaments just posterior to the cervix (not at the very floor of the cul-de-sac, since prolapse of the floor or posterior wall of the cul-de-sac proper is simply an accompanying feature of a rectal prolapse), with the hernial sac, which often contains small bowel when the patient is standing, descending in the rectovaginal septum (Fig. 67). The hernia is often congenital (a thin-walled, narrow-necked peritoneal sac in a nullipara) or may be acquired through birth trauma; in the latter case, a larger but shorter

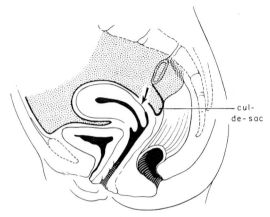

Arrow indicates area of potential hernial weakness posterior to cervix (not at floor of cul-de-sac).

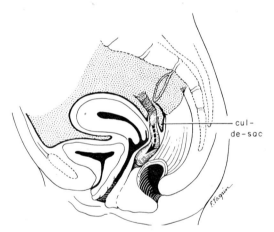

Arrow indicates hernial sac with bowel descending into rectovaginal septum.

Figure 67
Enterocele.

and blunter sac is often present. Frequently, it remains occult until the potential defect is exaggerated by the pelvic-floor injuries of childbirth; it may then go unrecognized because of failure to think of the possibility and to detect it in the face of a more obvious uterine prolapse or rectocele. Unfortunately, an enterocele occasionally first becomes apparent after a vaginal operation for rectocele, or uterine prolapse, or both, when in the immediate postoperative period both physician and patient become aware that an uncomfortable bulge and descensus are still present. This situation can be avoided by the simple diagnostic maneuvers that follow, all of which permit recognition and appropriate repair at the time of either vaginal or abdominal surgery.

PREOPERATIVE DIAGNOSIS

The examiner places his index finger in the rectum and his thumb in the vagina, the patient strains, preferably after assuming the standing position, and the bulge of the enterocele descends in the rectovaginal septum and is readily appreciated between the two fingers.

OPERATIVE DIAGNOSIS

The enterocele hernial weakness and sac can readily be searched for at the appropriate site during laparotomy and should be obvious. From the vaginal side, the enterocele sac, which lies anterior to the rectum, should be felt during any rectocele or perineal repair. During vaginal hysterectomy, when the peritoneum is first opened, digital palpation of the uterosacral ligament area and anterior wall of the cul-de-sac behind the peritoneal opening should be carried out to identify any existing enterocele defect.

TREATMENT

Enterocele repair follows the basic principles of any hernia operation: careful, complete dissection of the sac; closure at its neck and amputation of excess peritoneum; and reinforcement by closure of the available soft tissues surrounding it. This can be done from either the vaginal or the abdominal side. In the case of a huge enterocele repaired by a primary vaginal approach, additional reinforcement by the abdominal route is sometimes advisable at the same operation.

Total Prolapse of the Vagina

Total prolapse of the vagina is a relatively uncommon, very distressing sequel to progressively increasing uterine prolapse; more often, it follows vaginal hysterectomy for prolapse. It is almost invariably accompanied by enterocele and often by cystocele.

TREATMENT

It is exceedingly difficult to repair a total vaginal prolapse entirely from below with any degree of success and still preserve a functioning vaginal canal. The simplest, most effective, and most reliable therapy is total vaginal closure or obliteration (colpocleisis), and this is probably the procedure of choice in patients in whom a functioning vagina is no longer of importance. However, this situation is less common than is often believed, and in the many patients for whom it is essential to preserve a relatively normal vaginal canal, the operative approach most likely to succeed is a combined vaginal and abdominal repair. One such technique is as follows: Anterior and posterior colporrhaphies are first done in standard fashion, with repair of the frequently associated cystocele and rectocele, vaginal dissection with closure and amputation of the enterocele sac, excision of the redundant vaginal wall tissue and closure of the vaginal incision, and finally a careful perineorrhaphy. This is followed immediately by laparotomy and posterior fixation of the vaginal apex and upper vaginal canal to the lower sacrum and posterior pelvic floor. The rectosigmoid and its mesentery are first mobilized and displaced to the left, permitting placement of fascial strips or heavy silk sutures through the posterolateral vaginal walls on each side and then through the presacral and levator fascia on either side of the midline. This fixes the vaginal canal firmly in place posteriorly and to the right of the displaced rectum.

URINARY STRESS INCONTINENCE

Urinary stress incontinence is discussed in detail because the differential diagnosis, diagnostic evaluation, and choice of therapy are more complex than in other disorders of pelvic support. Although it represents a specific feature of the overall problem of obstetric trauma and resulting diminished pelvic support, the injury in this case apparently occurs sufficiently anteriorly to involve primarily the supports of the bladder neck and urethra. In contrast, the injury that subsequently leads to the development of cystocele probably weakens the supports of the more posteriorly situated portion of the bladder base. Hence, although perhaps not completely mutually exclusive, the symptom and specific anatomic defect of stress incontinence occurs most often in the absence of significant prolapse or cystocele. Simple cystocele does not result in stress incontinence.

By definition, urinary stress incontinence is the involuntary leakage of urine on coughing, sneezing, laughing, lifting, walking, and similar stresses, invariably occurring only when the patient is in the upright position but taking place regardless of the amount of urine in the bladder. It is probably an occasional symptom to a trivial degree in practically all women as a consequence of the relatively delicate supports for the female urethra and bladder neck necessary to assure an introital opening of sufficient elasticity to permit parturition. Clinically significant stress incontinence is unusual in nulliparas (although it is encountered occasionally, presumably secondary to poor pubococcygeal muscle tone, congenital weakness, or deficient innervation of the pelvic floor muscle supports) but is an extremely common problem among multiparas. Its exact incidence is difficult to estimate, since many women are loath to mention this embarrassing symptom even to a physician. This well-known reticence should be noted and remembered, and it is important to inquire specifically about the symptom of stress incontinence when eliciting the gynecologic history. It is usually a very distressing symptom, not only rendering the patient physically uncomfortable, but also often becoming a social handicap to the extent that personality disturbances sometimes develop secondarily.

Differential Diagnosis

The following possibilities should be considered in the differential diagnosis of stress incontinence:

1. True stress incontinence (deficient anatomic support of the bladder neck and urethra).
2. Detrusor dyssynergia, the disorder that most frequently masquerades as stress incontinence but is psychosomatic and functional in origin 70 to 80 percent of the time. Although frequency and urgency are the hallmarks of this condition, there may be a pseudostress incontinence in roughly 50 percent of patients. (In this situation, the stress serves to activate the hyperactive detrusor mechanism present in these patients, producing an actual "voiding" type of leakage rather than the instantaneous and brief spurt associated with the anatomically incompetent urethrovesical continence mechanism that is responsible for true stress incontinence.)
3. Pure urgency incontinence, which is most often due to a nonbacterial trigonitis and cystitis, which in turn may be secondary to an underlying trichomoniasis, candidiasis, severe endocervicitis, or, most often, atrophic vaginitis. The latter is associated with similar atrophic changes in the mucosa of the bladder and urethra, leading to marked urgency and precipitate, uncontrollable voiding.
4. Bladder neuropathies (diabetes, syphilis, multiple sclerosis, primary neurologic disorders or injuries), usually leading to an overflow type of incontinence, less often to an uninhibited detrusor type of leakage.
5. Abnormal drainage situations (ectopic ureter, urethral diverticulum, acquired vesicovaginal or urethrovaginal fistula).
6. Increased intraabdominal pressure (e.g., tumor, ascites, pregnancy) may lead to a temporary stress incontinence.
7. Primary lesions (inflammation, calculi, tumors) of the bladder, urethra, or adjacent organs (e.g., uterus, ovary, rectosigmoid), nearly always resulting in an urgency type of incontinence or to abnormal leakage due to secondary fistula formation.
8. Short urethra "total incontinence" syndrome (the abnormal shortening may be congenital or acquired, resulting in a length of less than 2 cm). Here, there is a continuous leakage, regardless of position or stress, though the symptom may be aggravated by stress.

Suggested Diagnostic Program

The following steps are suggested for confirmation of the diagnosis:

1. Taking a careful history, which will usually serve, at least tentatively, to distinguish true stress incontinence from other types of abnormal urinary leakage.
2. Pelvic and neurologic examination. There may be visible flattening of the normal, more acute urethrovesical angle; the urethral axis, normally horizontal when the

patient is in the lithotomy position, may be seen to have assumed a more vertical direction. Concomitantly, any additional pelvic disease that might influence the type of surgery selected to correct the incontinence should be noted.

3. Urinalysis and culture (to exclude urinary tract infection and secondary urgency incontinence).
4. Cystoscopy and urethroscopy (to exclude primary bladder or urethral disease as the source of abnormal urinary control).
5. Residual urine determinations.
6. Cystometrogram. This procedure and the procedure in (5) help to evaluate the possibility that either the syndrome of detrusor dyssynergia or the less common presence of a bladder neuropathy and inadequate emptying is the source of abnormal urinary leakage.
7. Intravenous pyelogram (if indicated, to rule out ectopic ureter or a secondary pathologic condition in the upper urinary tracts).
8. Vesical neck elevation test (Bonney-Read-Marchetti) (Fig. 68).
9. Urethrocystography, which is useful (1) as the best objective means of confirming the diagnosis of true stress incontinence and ruling out pseudostress or other types of incontinence and (2) as a measure of the degree of anatomic derangement and as an index of the extent and type of corrective surgical repair most suitable and most likely to achieve permanent cure.

Urethrocystography has made it apparent that patients with stress incontinence exhibit permanent changes in the urethrovesical relationships that closely resemble the temporary alterations occurring in the first stages of voiding in continent women (Figs. 69 and 70). These are:

1. Loss of the posterior urethrovesical (PUV) angle (normally approximately 90 degrees).
2. Descent and funneling of the bladder neck.
3. A variable degree of backward and downward rotation of the urethral axis.

Thus in patients with stress incontinence, the bladder and urethra are already in the anatomic position of the first stage of micturition. Any increase in downward thrust (e.g., from coughing or laughing) is sufficient to force urine to escape from the urethra. This characteristic anatomic deformity is the result of the loss of an adequate pelvic-floor muscular supporting mechanism that permits the vesical neck to plunge to the most dependent portion of the bladder base instead of remaining relatively fixed just below the symphysis. There is a consequent permanent loss of the normal posterior urethrovesical angle, and ultimately there may be a permanent rotational descent of the urethra itself. This urethral descent is of necessity a rotational one, since the distal portion of the urethra just proximal to the meatus invariably remains fixed at the level of the triangular ligament.

In the face of this characteristic abnormal urethrovesical anatomic configuration, sudden increases in intraabdominal and intravesical pressure are no longer transmitted

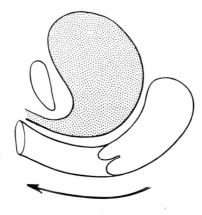

Patient in lithotomy position
straining with full bladder
demonstrates incontinence
as bladder neck descends.

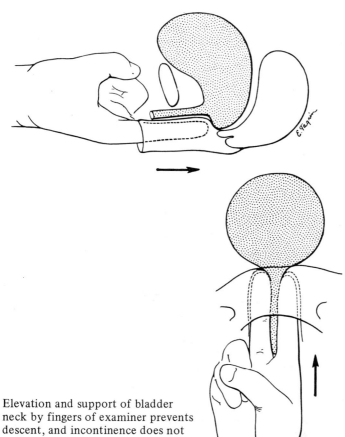

Elevation and support of bladder
neck by fingers of examiner prevents
descent, and incontinence does not
occur.

Figure 68
Vesical neck elevation test (Bonney-Read-Marchetti).

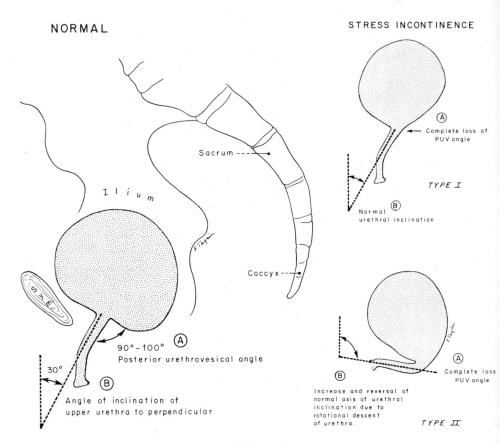

Figure 69
Diagram of urethrocystograms. Key features of urethrovesical anatomy in both the normal and the incontinent patient.

equally to the proximal urethra. Hence, during stresses such as coughing and laughing, intravesical pressure rises above intraurethral pressure, and incontinence inevitably occurs.

TECHNIQUE OF PERFORMING URETHROCYSTOGRAPHY

The equipment needed for urethrocystography includes the following:

1. Metallic, beaded chain (15 to 20 cm in length and with a strip of umbilical tape fastened to one end).
2. Longitudinally bisected No. 18 red-rubber urethral catheter.
3. Ordinary glass urethral catheter.
4. Sterile bowl.
5. Asepto syringe and bulb.
6. Michel's clips.

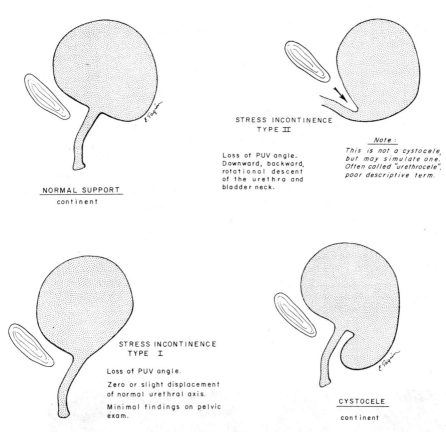

Figure 70
Urethrovesical relationships in patients with stress incontinence as contrasted with the anatomic configuration of cystocele.

After the patient voids, approximately 150 ml of 12% sodium iodide solution, warmed to body temperature, is instilled slowly into the bladder through a glass catheter, which is then removed. Almost the entire length of the metallic beaded chain is then inserted into the bladder, employing a longitudinally bisected No. 18 urethral catheter that permits the dropping-off of the chain in the bladder when the catheter is inverted and removed. The umbilical tape fastened to the end of the chain will prevent its loss in the bladder. Warm iodized oil (Lipiodol) solution, 15 ml, is then instilled slowly into the bladder to obtain optimal visualization of the vesical neck area. A small metal clip is gently affixed to the external urethral meatus to mark this site. X-ray films are then made; the lateral straining view with the patient upright is by far the most significant, but lateral resting and anteroposterior standing-straining views are also valuable.

Demonstration by these films of loss of the posterior urethrovesical angle and rotational descent of the urethra and bladder neck with a change in the axis of inclination of the urethra is diagnostic of true anatomic stress incontinence. It is convenient and extremely helpful from the standpoint of selection of the proper operative procedure to classify these patients as follows: **type 1**, where the defect involves only a loss of the posterior urethrovesical angle (Fig. 71), and **type II**, where, in addition, there is also downward-backward rotational descent of the urethra and bladder neck, with a change in the axis of inclination of the urethra (Fig. 72). Patients with this anatomic configuration usually have the most severe type of stress incontinence and are the most difficult to cure.

Note that as indicated in Figure 70, although the pelvic findings in type II stress incontinence frequently at first glance appear to simulate those of a cystocele, the two entities are basically different and should not be confused. It should be emphasized again that a cystocele does not cause stress incontinence. Actually, in many cases of huge cystocele, often with an associated complete uterine prolapse, the bladder base and urethrovesical junction may descend considerably and even come to lie outside the introitus without producing stress incontinence. In such patients, however, the normal relation between bladder and urethra is maintained, there is no funneling of the bladder neck, and a normal posterior urethrovesical angle is present, all of these being readily demonstrated by urethrocystography.

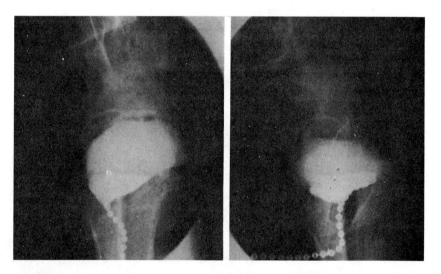

Figure 71
Urethrocystogram in type I stress incontinence. (Left) Preoperative film. (Right) Postoperative film following vaginal hysterectomy and anterior and posterior colporrhaphies. Note restoration of normal posterior urethrovesical angle postoperatively, with relief of stress incontinence.

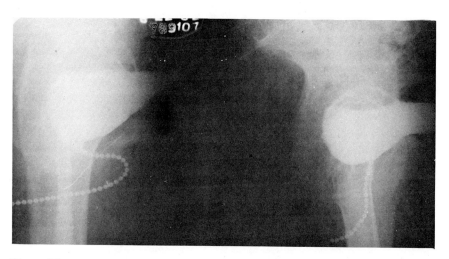

Figure 72
Urethrocystogram in type II stress incontinence. (Left) Preoperative film. (Right) Postoperative film following the Marshall-Marchetti suprapubic urethrovesical suspension operation. Note postoperative restoration of the normal posterior urethrovesical angle and the normal urethral axis of inclination, with relief of stress incontinence.

Surgical Treatment

VAGINAL REPAIR

Vaginal repair consists of anterior and posterior colporrhaphies, usually combined with a vaginal hysterectomy or Fothergill operation. Particular attention is devoted to reapproximating the supporting tissues beneath the vesical neck area in order to restore a normal posterior urethrovesical angle. The vaginal approach is suitable for type I stress incontinence and, when combined with the Marshall-Marchetti operation, for type II stress incontinence, in cases in which the overall problem makes an initial vaginal approach preferable. (Vaginal repair alone is probably not adequate for type II stress incontinence.)

URETHRAL SUSPENSION OPERATION

The Marshall-Marchetti urethral suspension operation is a highly effective procedure that can be employed to correct either type I or type II stress incontinence, particularly if other considerations dictate an abdominal approach. The approach is an abdominal, extraperitoneal one through the prevesical space of Retzius, and the urethra and vesical neck area are mobilized and snugly resuspended to the back of the pubic symphysis by a series of sutures placed through the anterior vaginal wall on either side of the urethra and then through the periosteum of the symphysis (Fig. 73A). This very effectively recreates a normal posterior urethrovesical angle

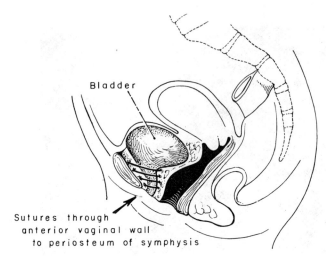

Bladder

Sutures through
anterior vaginal wall
to periosteum of symphysis

A

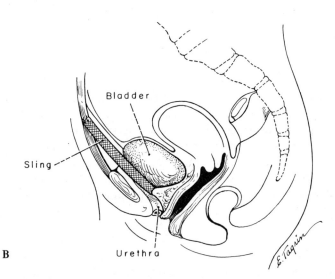

Bladder

Sling

B   Urethra

Figure 73
Operative procedures for stress incontinence. A. Marshall-Marchetti operation
(suprapubic urethrovesical suspension). B. Urethral sling operation.

and, even more important, restores the urethral axis to its normal, more vertical alignment with respect to the bladder base.

As a result of the continued widespread and successful use of the Marshall-Marchetti procedure, several variations have subsequently been introduced. Burch [4] has carried out the suprapubic urethrovesical suspension by utilizing more laterally placed sutures to approximate the anterior vaginal wall to Cooper's ligaments bilaterally rather than to the periosteum of the symphysis pubis. Bailey [1] has routinely combined a vaginal repair with a modified suspension procedure in which the operator places the vaginal-wall sutures on either side of the urethra during the final phase of the vaginal repair, an assistant having exposed the prevesical space through a separate suprapubic abdominal incision. The sutures are then passed retropubically and sutured to the periosteum of the symphysis. Pereyra and Lebherz [13] have devised a somewhat similar, though simpler procedure. It consists of a limited vaginal dissection of the paraurethral areas on each side and then passage of two sutures retropubically on either side of the urethra at the level of the vesical neck, employing a special ligature carrier introduced through a tiny suprapubic skin incision. When both sutures have been placed, they are simply tied down snugly against the anterior surface of the rectus sheath, thus serving to elevate the vesical neck and restore a normal posterior urethrovesical angle and urethral axis. The chief drawback to this operation is that it is a relatively blind procedure in which there is some hazard of inadvertent injury to adjacent structures. Furthermore, since only two sutures can be placed and the anterior vaginal wall is not actually approximated to the symphysis, it is possible that the long-term results may not be as satisfactory as those achieved by the Marshall-Marchetti procedure.

URETHRAL SLING OPERATION

The urethral sling operation is a somewhat more radical approach but is extremely useful and effective, particularly in recurrences. It involves the placement of a strip of rectus fascia beneath the urethra and bladder neck, drawing this region up against the symphysis, and fastening the ends of the fascial strip to the overlying anterior rectus sheath, making certain to achieve the desired amount of tension and support. In most cases, a combined vaginal-abdominal approach is necessary to perform this procedure properly (Fig. 73B). As clearly shown in the diagram, proper placement of the fascial sling results in excellent reestablishment of the normal posterior urethrovesical angle and normal urethral axis.

GENERAL PRINCIPLES OF THE THREE METHODS

In carrying out vaginal surgery, particular attention must be devoted to improvement in the support to the bladder neck region and to restoration of a normal posterior urethrovesical angle. A properly performed vaginal operation should be capable of curing close to 100 percent of patients with type I stress incontinence. However, clinical experience suggests that vaginal repair alone is not adequate to correct permanently with any degree of regularity the more profound anatomic derangement associated with type II stress incontinence and, in fact, will fail to do so in about 50 percent of patients. Type II stress incontinence should therefore be handled by a Marshall-Marchetti operation or one of the urethral sling procedures; or if a vaginal approach is elected, it should be supplemented by a concomitant Marshall-Marchetti vesicourethral suspension done immediately after the vaginal procedure is completed. It should be noted that even when dealing with type I stress incontinence, either the sling procedure or perhaps more often the Marshall-Marchetti urethrovesical suspension may properly be selected as the primary method of repair, if an additional abnormality dictates an abdominal approach to the pelvis. In such instances, however, a perineorrhaphy usually should be done to complete the restoration of support.

(**Note**: Urethral elongation, advancement, angulation, torsion, or narrowing procedures represent "trick" surgery and are usually done through a limited vaginal exposure. There are few indications for these procedures, and the results in general have been unsatisfactory.)

RESULTS OF OPERATIVE TREATMENT

In the past, reported results following attempts to use any one type of operative procedure for all cases fell far short of 100 percent success, few, in fact, approaching an 80 percent cure rate. However, intelligent selection and proper execution of the particular type of procedure indicated by the facts of the individual case to be the optimal one (i .e., the specific anatomic configuration [type I versus type II] ; the presence of an associated pelvic abnormality; previous attempts at surgical correction; and related factors such as age, occupation, obesity, or chronic cough) have brought an improvement in these results that now should approach the 90 to 95 percent success rate range [8]. Restoration of a normal posterior urethrovesical angle and urethral axis is the key to operative success, and postoperative urethrocystograms clearly demonstrate the complete correlation between this restoration and the relief of the symptom of stress incontinence. The importance of adequate preliminary studies before proceeding, to be certain that an anatomic defect potentially correctable by surgery is responsible for the abnormal urinary leakage, cannot be overemphasized.

Nonoperative Measures

Certain nonoperative measures may be of help in special situations, although they are useful primarily in the management of other types of functional incontinence. They are as follows:

1. Kegel exercises (pubococcygeal muscle). Although patients with a significant anatomic deformity are not greatly benefited, these exercises may help achieve control in mild cases and are useful adjuncts when surgery is refused or contraindicated, as well as in the management of patients with pseudostress incontinence.

2. Urethral dilatations and estrogen therapy are frequently very effective in relieving the urgency incontinence of atrophic vaginitis with associated abacterial cysto-urethritis.
3. Pessaries may be tried in the elderly, high-risk patient when surgical repair is con-traindicated, and they are occasionally of benefit.
4. Urecholine in appropriate doses (e.g., 10 to 40 mg four times daily) may provide some symptomatic relief for the overflow type of incontinence encountered in patients with atonic or hypotonic bladder neuropathy.
5. The administration of sedatives, tranquilizers, and anticholinergic drugs such as propantheline bromide (Pro-Banthīne) (15 mg three to four times daily) or flavox-ate hydrochloride (Urispas) (100 to 200 mg three to four times daily) often proves helpful in the management of detrusor dyssynergia or in the occasional patient with uninhibited detrusor activity accompanying an actual bladder neuropathy.
6. Weight reduction and treatment of chronic cough are also of value in many of these patients, by virtue of reducing to some extent the extrinsic forces applied to the weakened urethrovesical supports.

REFERENCES

1. Bailey, K. V. A clinical investigation into uterine prolapse with stress inconti-nence. *J. Obstet. Gynaecol. Br. Commonw.* 61:291, 1954 (Part I); 63:663, 1956 (Part II); 79:947, 1963 (Part III).
2. Bates, C. P., Loose, H., and Stanton, S. L. R. The objective study of inconti-nence after repair operations. *Surg. Gynecol. Obstet.* 136:17, 1973.
3. Beecham, C. T., and Beecham, J. B. Correction of prolapsed vagina or entero-cele with fascia lata. *Obstet. Gynecol.* 42:542, 1973.
4. Burch, J. C. Cooper's ligament urethrovesical suspension for stress incontinence. *Am. J. Obstet. Gynecol.* 100:764, 1968.
5. Green, T. H., Jr. Development of a plan for the diagnosis and treatment of uri-nary stress incontinence. *Am. J. Obstet. Gynecol.* 83:632, 1962.
6. Green, T. H., Jr. The problem of urinary stress incontinence in the female: An appraisal of its current status. *Obstet. Gynecol. Surv.* 23:603, 1968.
7. Green, T. H., Jr. Operative Management of Urinary Stress Incontinence. In P. Cooper (Ed.), *The Craft of Surgery*. Boston: Little, Brown, 1971. Chap. 118.
8. Green, T. H., Jr. Urinary stress incontinence: Differential diagnosis, patho-physiology, and management. *Am. J. Obstet. Gynecol.* 122:368, 1975.
9. Hodgkinson, C. P. Stress urinary incontinence — 1970. *Am. J. Obstet. Gynecol.* 180:1141, 1970.
10. Jeffcoate, T. N. A., and Francis, W. J. A. Urgency incontinence in the female. *Am. J. Obstet. Gynecol.* 94:604, 1966.
11. Marchetti, A. A., Marshall, V. F., and Shultis, L. D. Simple vesico-urethral sus-pension for stress incontinence of urine. *Am. J. Obstet. Gynecol.* 74:57, 1957.
12. Nichols, D. H. Types of enterocele and principles underlying choice of operation for repair. *Obstet. Gynecol.* 40:257, 1972.
13. Pereyra, A. J., and Lebherz, T. B. Combined urethrovesical suspension and vagino-urethroplasty for correction of urinary stress incontinence. *Obstet. Gynecol.* 30:537, 1967.
14. Porges, R. F. Vaginal hysterectomy at Bellevue Hospital. *Obstet. Gynecol.* 35:300, 1970.

15. Randall, C. L., and Nichols, D. H. Surgical treatment of vaginal inversion. *Obstet. Gynecol.* 38:327, 1971.
16. Ridley, J. H. Evaluation of the colpocleisis operation. *Am. J. Obstet. Gynecol.* 113:1114, 1972.
17. Te Linde, R. W. Prolapse of the uterus and allied conditions. *Am. J. Obstet. Gynecol.* 94:444, 1966.
18. Ulfelder, H. The mechanism of pelvic support in women: Deductions from a study of the comparative anatomy and physiology of the structures involved. *Am. J. Obstet. Gynecol.* 72:856, 1956.

19

The Menopause and Problems of the Premenopausal and Postmenopausal Woman

At the time of the menopause and during the years immediately preceding it, the progressive and sometimes irregular decline in ovarian function often leads to functional irregularities of the menstrual cycle not unlike those seen in the early adolescent years of ovarian function. Although the cessation of regular normal menstrual function may be abrupt and uncomplicated in some women, anovulatory cycles are commonplace and may be manifested by increasing oligomenorrhea with scanty flow, or irregular, often heavy and prolonged bleeding from a proliferative or hyperplastic endometrium, or both. The management of this type of dysfunctional bleeding during the premenopausal and menopausal phase is discussed in Chapter 5. It should be emphasized again that in the older woman it is frequently advisable to perform a diagnostic curettage (in addition to the usual cytologic studies and endometrial biopsy or suction aspiration) to exclude the possibility of malignancy before instituting a program of supplemental hormone therapy to control the episodes of abnormal bleeding. In many instances the curettage itself proves to be sufficient to prevent recurrence of abnormal bleeding. Furthermore, it should again be noted that when hormone therapy is undertaken to control dysfunctional bleeding in the premenopausal age group, estrogens may have to be employed along with progestational agents to achieve satisfactory results, since in contrast to the situation during the active reproductive years, the premenopausal woman is frequently lacking in adequate amounts of the former as well as the latter.

The hormone imbalance that characteristically results from the declining ovarian activity of the premenopausal phase is nevertheless often one of a relative excess of estrogen in the face of inadequate progesterone production. This preponderance of estrogen often leads to an exaggeration or increased frequency of some of the other cyclic functional disorders in women approaching the menopause, premenstrual tension and cystic mastitis being perhaps the most common manifestations of this tendency. The nature and management of these conditions are also discussed in Chapter 5.

AGE AT MENOPAUSE

By definition, the actual menopause is said to have occurred when there has been complete and permanent cessation of menstruation, although an interval of 6 to 12 months of amenorrhea is usually necessary to establish this fact definitely. The average age at which the menopause occurs in women currently experiencing it appears to be 49 to 50 years, although the range of normal variation spans the period of the early forties through the mid-fifties. (The phenomenon of precocious menopause occurring in the twenties and thirties is discussed in Chapter 6.) It is perhaps of some interest that during the past fifty years there has been a definite tendency to a later natural menopause; women living at the turn of the century noted its onset three or four years earlier on the average than their modern-day daughters and granddaughters. This trend has been attributed by some to the better general health and improved living conditions of women today.

PHYSIOLOGY OF THE MENOPAUSE

The primary basis for the progressive decrease in and ultimately complete termination of the cyclic function of the female reproductive organs at the time of the menopause lies in the ovary itself. When the primordial ovarian follicles have been depleted, ovulation becomes irregular and steadily more infrequent, finally ceasing altogether. As might be expected, there is an accompanying failure of progesterone production in the initial stages, and as follicle activity halts completely, a relative lack of estrogen also eventually becomes manifest in a total cessation of menstrual function due to the absence of estrogen in amounts sufficient to produce any endometrial stimulation and growth. There is evidence based on urinary excretion studies, however, that in 50 to 75 percent of women, the ovaries (for several years at least), and later on the adrenals, normally continue to secrete small amounts of estrogen for as long as 10 to 15 years after menstruation has ceased. Such small amounts of estrogen may serve a physiologic role in the body economy of postmenopausal women even though they are insufficient to produce any endometrial response. The abnormal production of larger amounts of estrogen in postmenopausal women with ovarian cortical stromal hyperplasia is an entirely different matter and is discussed in Chapter 6.

Secondarily, with removal of the reciprocal "braking effect" of estrogen, there is an increased secretion of gonadotropins by the pituitary. This permits an absolute diagnosis of the menopause to be established clinically, since the rise in the 24-hour urinary excretion of pituitary gonadotropins can be readily and accurately measured (see Chap. 2).

Because the natural menopause is initiated by the normal cessation of ovarian function in human females reaching the appropriate age, an artificial menopause such as induced by surgical or radiation castration does not differ in its fundamental physiology, nature of ensuing symptoms, or management. Inasmuch as an artificial menopause represents an abrupt change in steroid-hormone equilibrium, the resulting clinical symptoms of estrogen lack may be more pronounced and troublesome in some women, since the opportunity for gradual adjustment to declining estrogen levels ordinarily present in the natural menopause is denied them. However, the clinical differences between a natural and an artificial menopause appear to have been exaggerated and overemphasized in the past. Only a minority of women seem to experience serious difficulties in adjusting to either, and the percentage of women doing so is roughly the same in either type.

Careful biochemical studies have indicated that in the postmenopausal ovary (and adrenal as well) there is little, if any, production of estradiol (the estrogen primarily produced by the actively and cyclically functioning ovary of menstruating women during their reproductive years) and a shift instead to the production of estrone and androstenedione, the latter rapidly undergoing peripheral transformation into estrone. It has been suggested that this increased level of estrone in postmenopausal women could account for the increased incidence of both breast and endometrial cancer (and atypical endometrial hyperplasia as well) in women who have undergone a natural menopause, as compared with the much reduced incidence of these neoplastic changes in women who have undergone bilateral oophorectomy premenopausally.

Coincident with the virtual cessation of ovarian function, there appears to be an alteration in the pattern of adrenal hormone production as well. A decline in adrenal androgen secretion with normal adrenal corticosteroid excretion continuing unimpaired results in a shift in the metabolic balance that accelerates the process of protein catabolism. This same metabolic shift is probably also favored by estrogen lack.

Tissues that suffer the most from this increased protein catabolism include bone, muscle, and skin, and the addition of this catabolic effect to the normal degenerative changes produced over the years and to the simple atrophy of relative disuse encountered in the older woman results in muscular flabbiness, thinning and wrinkling of the skin, changes in the texture of the hair and nails, and varying degrees of osteoporosis. The latter is a reflection of diminished osteoblastic activity, possibly due in part to estrogen lack, as well as increased breakdown and decreased formation of protein bone matrix and impairment of its normal calcification due to the previously noted increased protein catabolism and negative nitrogen and calcium balance.

In the absence of adequate amounts of estrogen, the vaginal mucosa undergoes a characteristic thinning and atrophy. This process is not restricted to the vagina, however, but appears to be shared to some extent by mucous membranes elsewhere in the body. Clinically significant mucosal atrophy induced by estrogen lack and responding favorably to estrogen therapy is also typically seen in the urethra and trigone of the bladder and probably also occurs in the nasal, buccal, and even the gastric mucosa.

The physiologic basis for the cardinal symptoms of the menopause, namely, the flashes, hot flushes, and sweats described as a sudden sensation of heat in the face, neck, and chest with accompanying irregular flushing of the skin and profuse perspiration, probably lies in the normal role of estrogens in facilitating heat loss by favoring the process of vasodilatation at the level of the capillaries, venules, and arteriovenous anastomoses in the cutaneous circulation. In the absence of estrogen, this mechanism becomes deficient, at least for a varying period of years after the menopause, and excessive heat must therefore be dissipated by vasodilatation at the level of the arterioles instead. This alternate mechanism leads to the sudden occurrence of visible cutaneous flushes with the associated subjective hot-flash sensations, and the arteriolar dilatation is often accompanied or followed by drenching sweats, particularly at night. These phenomena may occur under a variety of circumstances whenever heat production is increased (excitement, exercise, eating, emotional tension) or heat loss is impaired (e.g., warm weather, excessive clothing, too-heavy bedclothes).

One other aspect of the systemic effects of the reduction in estrogen levels that occurs after the menopause, whether natural or artificial, concerns the role which this steroid hormone plays in the regulation of serum cholesterol, phospholipid, and lipoprotein concentrations, specific alterations of which are associated with and presumed to favor the development of atherosclerosis. Evidence in support of this potential role of estrogen in the prevention of atherosclerosis was initially found in the observation that the incidence and degree of atherosclerosis in women subjected to bilateral oophorectomy appeared to be considerably greater than in normal, non-oophorectomized controls of comparable ages, that the incidence of coronary heart disease in women appeared to rise suddenly after the menopause, and that the abnormal cholesterol and lipoprotein concentrations associated with atherosclerosis could often be reversed by administering estrogens. Recent reappraisal of this evidence has raised considerable doubt about its validity, and it now seems likely that at least some of the conclusions drawn were based on statistical artifacts. Several studies have shown that oophorectomy does not cause significant elevations of blood cholesterol or lipid levels or an increased incidence of coronary artery disease, and that the administration of various types of estrogens to oophorectomized women does not consistently or significantly lower the serum cholesterol or lipid levels or result in a decreased incidence of coronary artery disease. Equally disconcerting in this regard has been the observation of a markedly increased death rate from coronary and cerebral arteriosclerotic vascular disease among sizable groups of orchiectomized men with prostatic cancer who had received continuous estrogen therapy for many years, and a similar increased incidence of myocardial infarction in women over the age of 40 who had been receiving oral contraceptive drugs. Thus the role of estrogens in preventing atherosclerosis is still highly controversial and is certainly not sufficient reason to advocate routine estrogen replacement therapy on a permanent basis for all women undergoing the menopause, although there are some physicians who still support this kind of program. As a matter of fact, there is increasing evidence suggesting that the long-term use of estrogens may increase rather than decrease the incidence of coronary artery disease, and that estrogen therapy may also increase the incidence of thromboembolic disorders as well as foster progressive hypertension in some patients. And finally, large-scale studies have revealed that in women on estrogen therapy or receiving oral contraceptives, the risk of gallstones and other forms of gallbladder disease is two and one-half times greater than in women who have not received these medications, indicating that estrogenic substances do not appear to have the salutary effects on cholesterol and lipid metabolism that have been ascribed to them in the past.

CLINICAL MANIFESTATIONS OF THE MENOPAUSE

It is important to bear in mind at the outset that the symptoms many women experience at the time of the menopause may be divided into two categories: those that arise on an endocrinologic basis and are the result of estrogen lack and those of psychological origin. Although in the vast majority of women the symptoms are so minor that medical advice is never sought, in those 10 to 15 percent who consult a physician, the symptomatology usually represents a variable mixture of both endocrinologic and psychological components; not infrequently, the latter completely dominate the clinical picture. A number of investigators have found complete lack of correlation between either the "maturation index" of estrogenic activity in the vaginal cytologic smear or even the plasma estrogen levels and the presence or absence of postmenopausal symptoms or their degree of severity when present. This also suggests that factors other than decreased estrogen are important in the etiology of the so-called menopausal or postmenopausal syndrome.

Symptoms arising primarily on the basis of a psychological disturbance include nervousness, irritability, headaches, insomnia, inability to concentrate, spells of anxiety or depression, easy fatigability, and a general decline in physical and mental energy and sense of well-being. The origins of the psychological disturbances that may arise in some women at the time of the menopause are often multiple and complex. In some there is a history of similar emotional disturbances at other critical junctures in their lives — adolescence, marriage, pregnancy — the menopause simply representing another major alteration in the pattern of living to which they adjust with difficulty because of a fundamental underlying emotional instability. For other women, cessation of menstrual function may represent a partial loss of femininity, and hence unconsciously the menopause looms as a threat to their very existence as females and to their self-esteem. For practically every woman, the time of the menopause coincides with major changes in her family and social environment. In the case of the housewife, the children have grown up and left home, her husband is absorbed in and at the peak of his career, her once hectic and busy life and multiple home responsibilities are suddenly over, and she may feel neglected, passed by, and worst of all, no longer needed and without a worthwhile goal or purpose in life. The average healthy, emotionally well-adjusted woman rapidly finds other interests and outlets and even experiences improvement in general health and sense of well-being above and beyond the relief provided by the elimination of the physical and mental stresses involved in rearing a family. But for some the transition is extremely traumatic, and psychological disturbances of varying severity and duration appear.

Thus there appears to be no such thing as a specific postmenopausal syndrome. A variety of nonspecific symptoms often attributed to the menopausal state (e.g., palpitations, back and joint pains, headaches, irritability) have been shown in several carefully controlled clinical studies to be just as common in women (and in men, for that matter) in their thirties and early forties; furthermore, these symptoms are not relieved by estrogen therapy in most cases. There is no evidence whatsoever that estrogen therapy can maintain or restore the "cosmetic youthfulness" of skin, subcutaneous tissues, or hair, and there is no really solid support for the role of estrogen in the occurrence or management of central nervous system disorders (e.g., depression, anxiety), protection against arteriosclerosis (the reverse may be true), or even the prevention or cure of osteoporosis.

The hot flash and related vascular disturbances are probably the only symptoms of the menopause that have a true endocrinologic origin and the only ones consistently relieved by estrogen therapy. Although primarily due to estrogen deprivation, it should be remembered that the sometimes severe and distressing symptoms of vasomotor instability may both be aggravated by and serve to aggravate symptoms occurring on a psychological basis.

MANAGEMENT OF THE MENOPAUSE

From what has already been said, it should be apparent that attention to the psychological components of the symptoms of the "change of life" is usually of greater importance than hormone replacement therapy. This is best done after a careful history and thorough examination have reassured both patient and physician that no organic disease exists, emphasizing that this change in female physiology is a normal biologic event. The menopausal process and accompanying symptoms can be explained in simple terms, any misconceptions concerning harmful or undesirable effects (e.g., obesity, cancer, insanity, loss of sexual function) dispelled, and the patient given some insight into the factors other than endocrine that may be playing a role in producing those symptoms stemming from psychological maladjustment to the overall situation. At times, sympathetic explanation and reassurance must be fortified by the judicious and temporary use of sedatives or tranquilizers, but these should be discontinued as soon as fears and anxieties are allayed and the patient has been encouraged to meet and adjust realistically to her changing environment by finding new interests and activities. Occasionally, more serious emotional disorders or even psychoses may be discovered that will require psychiatric consultation and treatment.

Although vasomotor disturbances may also be helped considerably by successful management of the psychological components of the menopausal symptomatology, persistently severe hot flashes are a valid indication for estrogen therapy. The hormone replacement should be adequate but not excessive and should be given on a cyclic basis, thus avoiding prolonged, unopposed estrogen stimulation and minimizing the occurrence of endometrial hyperplasia and irregular bleeding. A regimen of Premarin, 0.625 to 1.25 mg daily, or ethinyl estradiol (Estinyl), 0.02 to 0.05 mg daily, or diethylstilbestrol, 0.5 to 1.0 mg daily, omitting the first 5 days of each calendar month, is a satisfactory one, although other variations include 30 days on medication separated by 7 days off medication, or on three weeks, off one week. Should bleeding occur during an interval off medication, it can usually be safely assumed to be estrogen withdrawal bleeding if it ceases on renewal of the drug. If doubt exists, or if the bleeding continues or occurs irregularly, curettage is usually necessary to avoid overlooking an endometrial lesion. After 6 to 12 months of such a program, the dosage can be reduced in half for another six months, subsequent reductions in dosage being made to accomplish a gradual weaning process after a year or two of therapy. In some patients, smaller initial doses and a shorter duration of therapy may suffice and will be even less likely to cause uterine bleeding. In fact, there is reason to believe that the proper dose of Premarin, for example, may be as low as 0.3 mg daily. This is based on the fact that in the normal, active menstrual cycle the average estrogen levels are equivalent to what is attained by a daily dose of 0.2 to 0.3 mg of Premarin, with a range of 0.1 mg low to a very short-lived peak high of 4.0 mg. There is no advantage to using either the once popular estrogen-androgen combinations or the newer estrogen-progesterone combinations (i.e., one of the oral contraceptives) rather than estrogen alone in managing the menopausal and post-menopausal patient with symptoms of estrogen lack. Androgens may have unpleas-ant virilizing effects (hirsutism and acne), and both the androgens and the synthetic progestogens tend to have antiestrogen effects. Furthermore, estrogen-progesterone combinations not only produce cyclic withdrawal periods, which are neither neces-sary nor desired by the menopausal or postmenopausal woman, but also appear to be associated with an increased risk of myocardial infarction, cerebrovascular acci-dents, and phlebitis, especially in this age group.

There are certain contraindications to the continued use of estrogens, including the presence of fibroids that might be stimulated to further undesirable growth, repeated episodes of estrogen-induced abnormal bleeding, significant chronic cystic mastitis that is usually aggravated by estrogen therapy, a history of thromboembolic, coronary, or cerebrovascular disease (or the presence of multiple coronary risk factors, or a family history of coronary disease, or both), and, for obvious reasons, a history of treatment for breast or endometrial cancer. Although the potential carcinogenic effects of long-term estrogen therapy remain unproved, there is enough circumstantial evidence to warrant considerable caution in prescribing it in patients with a strong family history of cancer, especially of the breast or pelvic organs, or in women with a history of a late menopause complicated by prolonged, irregular bleeding, coupled with the physical characteristics typical of patients in whom endo-metrial cancer develops, circumstances suggesting that they may be more susceptible than usual to this disease Over twice as many breast cancers occur in women in the natural postmenopausal state as in postmenopausal women who have undergone hysterectomy, or bilateral oophorectomy, or both, which raises the possibility that the continued presence of estrogen, together with the known high-risk factor of age, may be important in the genesis of breast cancer. And all the facts that strongly support the role of continuous, unopposed estrogen in the production of atypical adenomatous hyperplasia of the endometrium and ultimately in the genesis of endo-metrial carcinoma are well known and well documented and have already been set forth in detail in Chapter 14. Estrogens should probably also be avoided in patients with known cardiac and renal disease, since their tendency to promote salt and water retention may precipitate congestive heart failure. Finally, stubbornly persistent and recurring candidal vulvovaginitis develops in some women on long-term estrogen therapy, by virtue of the same increased glycogen in vaginal cells and secretions seen in pregnant and diabetic women, who also have an increased incidence of candidal infections. Although the problem may sound trivial, the symptoms may become exceedingly troublesome to the patient, and they are uncontrollable by all the usual medications until the estrogen administration is halted permanently. In any event, all patients receiving estrogens over an extended period of time should understand the need for regular periodic examinations and cytologic smears as well as the importance of reporting promptly any abnormal bleeding.

In menopausal women in whom estrogens are contraindicated but who are suffering from symptoms such as severe hot flashes, sweats, palpitation, irritability, and headache, a drug capable of stabilizing the autonomic nervous system should be tried. Excellent symptomatic relief, approximating that of estrogen replacement, has been achieved for many women with Bellergal, a combination of ergotamine tartrate, phenobarbital, and a belladonna derivative (Bellafoline), 1 tablet twice daily.

The majority of gynecologists continue to adhere to the concept that the menopause is a normal physiologic event and that estrogen therapy should not be used indiscriminately nor for more than a year or two in the management of the minority of women who require it. However, there are some physicians who maintain the point of view that the menopause is actually a disease process and that all women should receive active treatment for the resulting deficiency of ovarian steroid hormones. An article by Wilson and Wilson [10] summarizes the philosophy of this school of thought, which holds that declining ovarian function and estrogen lack lead to widespread degenerative changes with an increased susceptibility to cardiovascular and bone and joint disorders, and that intellectual and psychological as well as physical aging is unnecessarily and pathologically accelerated. Adherents of this view therefore advocate ovarian hormone replacement therapy on a permanent lifelong basis for all women after the menopause. There may be some merit in this concept, but the evidence for its universal validity remains incomplete and controversial at the present time. It certainly is abundantly clear, however, that estrogens have no effect whatsoever on the inevitable changes in skin, hair, weight distribution, breasts, joints, muscle tone, libido, and the like, induced by normal aging processes. Estrogens will not, as some women have allowed themselves to believe, maintain the perpetual bloom of youth. Nor will estrogens have any effect on the socioenvironmentally and psychologically induced symptoms that may appear at the same time that menstruation is about to cease.

It would seem that the available evidence best supports a more rational policy of an individualized estrogen replacement program for those women in whom symptoms of acute estrogen deprivation develop during the menopause (severe hot flashes and sweats) and for those who manifest signs and symptoms of estrogen deficiency (e.g., atrophic vaginitis) later on in the postmenopausal years. A dosage no larger than is necessary to relieve symptoms should be used, and the medication should be interrupted cyclically on a monthly basis to avoid estrogen-induced uterine bleeding as well as other side effects such as breast discomfort, fibrocystic changes, and excessive fluid retention frequently produced by prolonged, continuous administration. At the end of 6 to 12 months the dosage should be further reduced, and ultimately it can usually be discontinued entirely after a year or two. Avoiding too high and too prolonged a dosage regimen may facilitate the normal adrenal takeover of estrogen production that probably occurs in the majority of women and that accounts for their lack of significant symptoms or signs of estrogen deficiency until much later in life.

SPECIFIC POSTMENOPAUSAL PROBLEMS

In some women, continued estrogen lack in the postmenopausal years may lead to several different disorders of clinical significance and with sufficiently distressing symptoms to require treatment.

So-called **postmenopausal osteoporosis** (a decrease in bone mass and density due to increased resorption), possibly developing partly on the basis of the specific metabolic changes already described, may lead to disabling bone and joint symptoms, particularly back pain, and even to pathologic vertebral fractures, and in the past has often been the reason for prescribing permanent estrogen therapy. However, the role of estrogen lack in the genesis of osteoporosis is currently undergoing reappraisal, and there is now impressive evidence that long-standing negative calcium balance due to dietary inadequacy, superimposed on the normal tendency to decreased physical activity with advancing years, may be of more fundamental etiologic importance. Furthermore, a number of studies have shown that osteoporosis and decrease in bone mass is characteristic of the aging process in both men and women and does not appear to be related to any specific event in the life of women such as the menopause, at least when the latter occurs spontaneously and at the usual age. As far as the effect of oophorectomy on the incidence of osteoporosis is concerned, a recent careful study has shown that women castrated before the age of 45 may have a somewhat higher incidence of osteoporosis four years later; on the other hand, when bilateral oophorectomy is done on women over the age of 46, no effect on the mineral content and density of bone as measured radiographically can be demonstrated. Finally, there is some evidence that after an initial, possibly estrogen-facilitated, relative increase in bone formation for three to four months (estrogen probably actually decreases bone resorption by blocking the action of parathyroid hormone on bone), long-term estrogen therapy may ultimately result in decreased bone formation. This observation could well account for the initial prompt, symptomatic improvement (relief of bone pain) noted by many patients when estrogen therapy is first begun. Nevertheless, because of its inhibiting effect on bone resorption (rather than what formerly was believed to be a stimulating effect on osteoblastic activity), estrogen therapy remains a part of the total management of osteoporosis, though greater emphasis is now placed on increased dietary calcium and medications to promote calcium absorption and positive calcium balance. It is now felt that adequate calcium and vitamin D intake, together with oral fluoride medication and adequate exercise and physical activity on a regular basis to stimulate osteoblastic activity, may be far more important than estrogen therapy in the management of osteoporosis.

Atrophic vaginitis and the similar atrophic changes in the urethra and vulva that frequently accompany it are additional manifestations of estrogen lack that may cause symptoms requiring treatment in the postmenopausal woman. The clinical features and management of atrophic vaginitis and related disorders are discussed in detail in Chapter 7.

Aside from the various manifestations of the altered hormonal status, the two other most common clinical problems of a gynecologic nature encountered in the postmenopausal female are (1) the anatomic changes and symptoms resulting from **deficient pelvic support** already discussed in Chapter 18 and (2) the occurrence of **postmenopausal bleeding.** The diagnostic approach and the specific methods of treatment for the various lesions that may produce this most important symptom of potentially serious disease have been considered in detail in many of the previous chapters, but it may be helpful to enumerate again the common causes of postmenopausal bleeding and the relative frequency with which they are encountered.

Table 11 presents an analysis of 190 patients with postmenopausal bleeding encountered in the author's private practice during one 10-year period. The 30 percent incidence of malignant disease associated with bleeding after the menopause is identical with that reported by Payne et al. [5] and others, and it is in accord with the general observation that there has been an apparent decrease in the frequency with which pelvic neoplasms are found responsible for this symptom, a frequency noted to be as high as 50 to 60 percent only a few decades ago. This change may simply reflect the definitely increased incidence of bleeding secondary to estrogen therapy during the postmenopausal years, as well as the increasing tendency for women to report any and all bleeding after the menopause, the resulting prompt investigation uncovering more benign disorders. With respect to benign lesions, it is important to bear in mind that even in the presence of obvious atrophic vaginitis with hemorrhagic mucosa, cervical polyps, urethral caruncles, or a history of estrogen administration, a complete investigation including cytologic smears, cervical biopsies

Table 11
Causes of Postmenopausal Bleeding in a Consecutive Series of 190 Patients Examined, 1953–1963

Pathologic Condition Found	Number of Cases	Percentage of Cases	
Carcinoma of the cervix	35	18	⎫
Carcinoma of the endometrium	18	10	⎬ 30
Carcinoma of the vagina	4	2	⎭
Endometrial and/or cervical polyps	38	20	
Atrophic vaginitis	30	16	
Estrogen therapy	19	10	
Atrophic endometrium	9	5	
Endometrial hyperplasia	7	4	
Urethral caruncle	4	2	
Cervical stenosis with hematometrium	2	1	
Bladder tumor	1		
Unexplained	23	12	
Totals	190	100	

if indicated, and curettage is mandatory, for the benign conditions are frequently incidental findings, the actual source of the bleeding being a cervical or endometrial cancer.

The 12 percent incidence of unexplained postmenopausal bleeding in the patients presented in Table 11 also coincides with the figure reported by Payne et al. [5]. Although the vast majority of such patients are actually free of serious disease and the bleeding never recurs, a small percentage continue to have abnormal bleeding and should be investigated further by repeat curettage and ultimately by laparotomy, since small endometrial lesions missed by the previous curettage or undetected tubal or ovarian cancer may prove to be the source of persistent bleeding in some of them. The importance of keeping the "unexplained" group under surveillance is obvious. Finally, patients with postmenopausal endometrial hyperplasia, particularly of the atypical, adenomatous variety, are deserving of careful and prolonged follow-up, since an endometrial carcinoma will subsequently develop in a certain percentage (see Chap. 14).

REFERENCES

1. Aitken, J. M., Hart, D. M., Anderson, J. B., Lindsay, R., Smith, D. A., and Speirs, C. F. Osteoporosis after oophorectomy for nonmalignant disease in premenopausal women. *Br. Med. J.* 2:325, 1973.
2. Barlow, J. J., Emerson, K., Jr., and Saxena, B. N. Estradiol production after ovariectomy for carcinoma of the breast: Relevance to the treatment of menopausal women. *N. Engl. J. Med.* 280:633, 1969.
3. Davis, M. E. Estrogens and the aging process. *J.A.M.A.* 196:219, 1966.
4. Lebherz, T. B., and French, L. Nonhormonal treatment of the menopausal syndrome. *Obstet. Gynecol.* 33:795, 1969.
5. Payne, F. L., Wright, R. C., and Fetterman, H. H. Post-menopausal bleeding. *Am. J. Obstet. Gynecol.* 77:1216, 1959.
6. Randall, C. L. Ovarian function and woman after the menopause. *Am. J. Obstet. Gynecol.* 73:1000, 1957.
7. Rogers, J. Estrogens in the menopause and postmenopause. *N. Engl. J. Med.* 280:364, 1969.
8. Stone, S. C., Mickal, A., and Rye, P. H. Postmenopausal symptomatology, maturation index, and plasma estrogen levels. *Obstet. Gynecol.* 45:625, 1975.
9. Utian, W. H. Effects of oophorectomy and estrogen therapy on serum cholesterol. *Int. J. Gynecol. Obstet.* 10:95, 1972.
10. Wilson, R. A., and Wilson, T. A. The fate of the nontreated postmenopausal woman: A plea for the maintenance of adequate estrogen from puberty to the grave. *J. Am. Geriatr. Soc.* 11:347, 1963.

20

Premarital Examination, Marital Counseling, and Conception Control

PREMARITAL EXAMINATION

The original purpose of the premarital examination was simply to determine that both the prospective bride and groom were free of venereal disease. As such, it is now an established requirement for obtaining a marriage license in almost all states, although in many areas of the country, certification by the physician that a serologic test for syphilis is negative is all that is needed, and the law does not precisely stipulate that a physical examination should also be done. Nowadays, however, an increasing number of young women and their fiancés realize the importance of obtaining the full benefits of premarital counseling. These can only be secured through a complete examination, preferably of both partners, and, in particular, an adequate opportunity during the interview with the bride-to-be for a discussion of the basic facts of feminine physiology and hygiene and for explanation and advice concerning the multiple aspects of the marital relationship on which she is about to embark. Unsuspected anatomic or endocrinologic abnormalities that might seriously interfere with normal marriage or childbearing functions will occasionally be discovered in this way. Even more important, misinformation and misapprehensions concerning the sexual aspects of marriage, which are, in reality, far more likely than physical abnormalities to be the forerunners of unsatisfactory marital adjustment, may be corrected by providing proper information, general guidance, and reassurance. It is not generally appreciated that ignorance and immaturity concerning sexual matters continue to be widely prevalent among the young people of today, in spite of educational programs sponsored by school and church. The cold facts regarding the incidence in the early 1970s of illegitimacy (1 of every 20 babies born during the past decade in the United States and 20 percent of the mothers under age 17), criminal abortion (an estimated 1 million per year in the United States, and again, 20 percent or more are teenagers), the rising divorce rate (now over 500,000 per year in the United States), and the less well quantitated but undoubtedly untold numbers of profoundly unhappy marriages and homes attest to the sexual inadequacies and marital irresponsibility of a considerable segment of the population. By providing much-needed information and guidance at a time when it is normally eagerly sought and can easily be accepted as a natural step in preparation for marriage, the premarital examination, if carried out properly and on a large scale, could potentially have a tremendous impact on the various manifestations of sexual immaturity and marital unhappiness. Many of these problems could be prevented by adequate education concerning both the physiologic and psychological aspects of sexual matters as well as the adult responsibilities implicit in marriage and parenthood. Finally, the premarital examination offers the young couple an opportunity to obtain information and advice concerning conception control and family planning, information often vital to their future as well as their current happiness and success with respect to both the marriage and the husband's or wife's career.

An adequate premarital examination should, first of all, include the taking of a complete history and the performance of a complete physical examination, including a pelvic examination; a perfunctory chat during the time a blood sample is being obtained for a serologic test accomplishes little or nothing. In addition to a serologic test for syphilis, premarital serologic testing for rubella is now available and is mandatory in some states. Depending on the result, the patient then may elect immunization against rubella at some later time of convenience.

Usually, during the course of a more thorough interview or at the time the examination is done, the physician will be able to form a fairly accurate opinion as to the prospective bride's relative degree of physical and emotional maturity. At the same time, he will also gain an idea of her knowledge and sophistication regarding the anatomic, physiologic, and psychological aspects of being an adult female and participating in a sexual relationship. If she appears unduly frightened and apprehensive throughout the interview, if she timidly shrinks away and finds it impossible to relax and cooperate during the examination, or if she relates a history of severe dysmenorrhea with an obvious distaste for and severe incapacitation by menstruation, has shown inability or disinclination even to try to use tampons, or exhibits lack of any knowledge of basic feminine biology and hygiene, the warning signs are clear. Such a young woman as yet neither comprehends nor has assumed the role of a mature female, and she is almost certain, without additional help and guidance, to have sexual problems in her marriage. Help should be offered either in the form of one or more additional office visits during which she may be given the basic information and concepts she desperately needs, or by means of suggested reading on her own, with a return visit to the office if necessary for clarifying points she does not understand or to discuss questions for which she still has failed to find answers. (Appropriate books and pamphlets for this purpose are listed in the references at the end of this chapter.) Obviously, such a program cannot accomplish miracles. It cannot hope to correct completely all the misapprehensions and abnormal concepts and inhibitions engendered during a lifetime of relative ignorance and erroneous attitudes toward these matters. However, it can represent a start in the right direction, one that may be helpful enough to avoid serious marital difficulties by providing correct information, allaying groundless fears, and suggesting the proper lines of approach to the development of a more mature personality and outlook with the establishment of a normal, happy marital relationship.

Fortunately, the majority of women seen premaritally prove to be well adjusted, knowledgeable, mature, and secure and happy in being female. For these women also, an opportunity to ask questions following the initial history, physical examination, and securing of the blood sample should be provided, with suggestions for further reading if they desire. Only rarely will they require more comprehensive educational guidance and follow-up supervision.

One of the primary reasons why many young women seek premarital advice is to secure information and help regarding family planning. The wish to utilize some means of conception control is usually expressed during the preliminary interview, and this is a convenient time to discuss the various methods available, their specific advantages, disadvantages, and side effects, and the couple's own preference, if any. If use of a diaphragm is elected, it is nearly always possible to fit it properly and instruct the patient in its use during the pelvic examination that follows the interview, since vigorous participation in various athletic activities and widespread use of tampons among modern young women make it unusual not to be able to perform a satisfactory vaginal examination, including the insertion of a speculum or diaphragm, even in virgins. For those few desiring to employ a diaphragm in whom a snug hymenal orifice precludes premarital fitting, either a vaginal spermicidal jelly alone or an oral contraceptive may be temporarily prescribed, with the patient returning a month or two after the wedding for permanent fitting and instruction in the use of a diaphragm. Details of the various methods of conception control and the manner in which the patient is to be instructed and supervised in their use are completely discussed in the final section of this chapter.

Only occasionally does the pelvic examination reveal a hymenal orifice so small (or, rarely, a previously unrecognized intact hymenal membrane) that the question of whether or not premarital hymenectomy or dilatation of the hymen is indicated need be considered. In general, the performance of premarital hymenal surgery should be avoided, if possible, and if the membrane is thin and a reasonable opening present, no real problem need be anticipated. This is particularly true if the situation is explained in advance and reassurance is given to both the bride-to-be and her fiancé that, with initial gentle care and proper precoital and coital technique, no significant discomfort will be experienced.

Rarely, the presence of an abnormally thick, fibrous hymen or an extremely tiny opening will definitely indicate the advisability of preliminary dilatation (often this can be done initially in the office and continued at home by the patient using a few simple tubular dilators graduated in size) or brief hospitalization for actual hymenectomy under anesthesia. If a formal hymenectomy is deemed necessary, it should preferably be done at least six weeks prior to the wedding to allow adequate time for complete healing and freedom from any local sensitivity.

One other question frequently asked during the premarital examination concerns the matter of douching as part of the routine program of feminine hygiene for the married woman. Nowadays it is the consensus that regular, periodic douching is entirely unnecessary and that the healthy female of any age need never douche. In fact, there is some evidence that even when the most physiologic type of solution (e.g., isotonic and buffered to the proper pH) is used, douching may in some instances be detrimental because it irrigates away the normal protective mucus and bacterial flora of the vagina. Most women are pleased and relieved to learn that what once was deemed a necessity of a bygone era is no longer believed essential. The few who still feel impelled to douche occasionally should be assured that it will do them no harm, however.

MARITAL COUNSELING

Although neither space nor the scope of this book permits more than brief mention of the complex and obviously fundamentally highly important problem of marital maladjustment, it should be emphasized that the gynecologist is often the first to see its manifestations, though they may not always be initially recognized as such. When a woman complains of dyspareunia or frigidity or her husband suffers from impotence, the invariable existence of an underlying profound disturbance of the marital relationship is almost axiomatic. Less commonly appreciated is that many of the anxieties and functional complaints of women, particularly those centering around the pelvis and reproductive tract function (e.g., dysmenorrhea, premenstrual tension, functional menstrual irregularities, infertility, physiologic leukorrhea, idiopathic vulvar pruritus, the pelvic congestion syndrome, irritable bladder, low back pain, spastic colitis) are also often related, at least in part, to an unsatisfactory sexual relationship.

Although the socioeconomic aspects of marriage and family life are frequently also involved, sexual maladjustment is often the single most important factor in unhappy marriages and homes, and it is frequently the basis for many of the functional symptoms experienced by both the unfortunate partners. Sexual inadequacies in turn may stem from ignorance of proper technique or from immaturity and abnormal inhibitions, with failure to assume the normal adult role in the marital sexual relationship. Fear of an unwanted pregnancy must be included in the latter category and is a common cause of deterioration of a previously fairly satisfactory sexual relationship.

The role of the gynecologist with respect to the problem of marital disharmony is an important and twofold one. First, he must be thoroughly aware that an underlying unsatisfactory marital adjustment may be cause for a wide variety of complaints related by many patients who seek his advice. Having first carefully excluded organic disease as the sole or major cause of their symptoms, he must then be prepared and able to explore more fully the other possibility. Second, once it is apparent that an unsatisfactory marital relationship does in fact exist, he has much to contribute to the management of the problem. If sexual inadequacy is due to ignorance about sexual matters and proper coital techniques, he can supply the much-needed information to both wife and husband. If fear of pregnancy proves to be the major source of sexual maladjustment and dissatisfaction, he is able to offer advice concerning an appropriate method of conception control acceptable to the couple. If the sexual inadequacy on the part of either partner stems from a fundamental immaturity and inability or failure to assume the normal adult role in the marital relationship, he will be able to help them recognize and come to grips with the problem by seeking adequate counseling along these lines.

Obviously, more profound personality disorders or psychological disturbances frequently are the basic cause of immature emotional behavior in the marital relationship, and the more expert guidance of the psychiatrist and clinical psychologist will be required in such cases, once the existence of the problem has been defined.

Furthermore, not all unhappy marriages are due solely to sexual maladjustment; frequently, a team approach involving the additional help of a professional marriage counselor, a clergyman, and a social worker will be needed in the effort to rehabilitate the marriage.

It is nevertheless important to emphasize again that the gynecologist must be ever alert to the possible existence and significance of abnormal marital adjustment among his patients and ready to assume his share of the responsibility for helping to correct it, or in the case of the premarital patient, for endeavoring to prevent its development. Several excellent sources of more detailed information and discussion concerning sexual and other aspects of the marital relationship are included in the references at the end of the chapter.

CONCEPTION CONTROL

Efforts at birth control have been practiced since ancient times. Over the years a number of methods of varying degrees of effectiveness and social acceptance have been employed, including abstinence for long intervals, withdrawal (coitus interruptus), the rhythm method ("safe period"), the condom, special vaginal tampons, immediate postcoital douches, cervical caps, intrauterine stem pessaries, intrauterine rings, vaginal spermicidal jellies, creams, or suppositories, the vaginal diaphragm, and, within the past 20 years, ovulation-inhibiting agents. Although many of the older techniques continue to be used, particularly among underprivileged populations, they have long been known to be relatively ineffective as well as potentially harmful from both a psychological as well as a physical standpoint. Furthermore, some are simply not acceptable to most couples, since they drastically alter or interfere with normal marital sexual relationships.

During the past fifty years there has been a tremendous growth of scientific interest in the field of conception control, now of such obvious importance to the health and well-being of the individual family unit in modern society as well as to nations and the world at large. A natural outgrowth has been the assumption by the medical profession of the responsibility for providing the best possible counsel and methods for the planning and limitation of family size. Currently, the physician is able to offer advice concerning several safe and effective techniques of birth control, one or more of which will be acceptable to most couples. The ability to provide such advice represents another facet — and an important one — in the overall role that the physician of today should be able to play in improving the stability and happiness of marriage and family life among his patients. Often, fear of unwanted pregnancy or the stresses imposed by the attempt to rear and educate a larger number of children than had actually been desired or planned for are the basis for serious marital discord and unhappy, insecure homes. The unfortunate end results are all too frequently seen in terms of disabling psychosomatic or emotional disorders or are reflected in the rising incidence of abortion, divorce, and juvenile delinquency.

All the states that had them have now repealed laws prohibiting the sale of or the giving of information concerning contraceptive devices, and there is almost universal acceptance on the part of both physicians and the laity alike that this information should be available for all who desire it, whether married or single. The Roman Catholic Church condones the use of the rhythm method, but Catholic theological doctrines do not permit the use of mechanical devices, nor have they thus far sanctioned the use of ovulation-inhibiting agents for contraceptive purposes only. The physician should therefore be able to instruct his patients properly in the application of the rhythm method as well as prescribe the other contraceptive techniques and agents. As phrased in a resolution adopted in 1963 by the American College of Obstetricians and Gynecologists, there is need for "greatly expanded research" on population change and the means for its control, and "full freedom should be extended to all population groups for the selection and use of such methods for the regulation of family size as are consistent with the creed and mores of the individuals concerned."

Methods of Conception Control

Use of the condom by the male is probably the regular method employed by 10 to 20 percent of couples currently practicing birth control in this country, many of whom have never actually sought advice from a physician or clinic. Although simple for the untutored to use, its effectiveness is highly variable (70 to 90 percent protection), and in practice it often proves physically unsatisfactory or aesthetically unacceptable to many couples. For these reasons it is seldom recommended nowadays, usually only in the occasional patient who prefers that her husband take the precautions.

In the vast majority of instances, however, it is the wife who seeks contraceptive advice, and it is undoubtedly preferable that she be responsible for the program, since she is fundamentally the one most concerned and the one most likely to carry it out properly and faithfully. Before prescribing any one method, the patient should be offered a brief discussion of the several techniques available, with their advantages, disadvantages, and potential side effects. By supplying this information and answering her questions, the physician can make it easier for the patient to select the program most acceptable to her and to her husband. The following sections outline the principal methods currently in use and known to be safe and effective, together with the essential details of their application.

THE RHYTHM METHOD

By avoiding coitus during the ovulatory phase in each monthly cycle, prevention of pregnancy is possible. Difficulties in achieving complete conception control by the biologic or rhythm method stem from the fact that the exact day of ovulation is not only impossible to pinpoint but may vary considerably even in women with cycles consistently of the same length. Furthermore, 70 to 80 percent of all women vary five or more days in cycle length, and in some the variation is as much as eight or nine days. Hence to achieve any degree of reliability with respect to protection against pregnancy, the potential fertile period during which intercourse is to be avoided may of necessity be lengthy, and the corresponding "safe" period may be relatively short.

The most reliable formula for determining the fertile time and the "safe period" is the schedule proposed by Ogino, which assumes that ovulation usually occurs 12 to 16 days premenstrually, that the ovum may survive about 24 hours, and that sperm capable of ovum impregnation may survive in the female genital tract for about three days. Properly employed, the Ogino schedule provides roughly a 95 percent chance of avoiding pregnancy. Directions to the patient for effectively using the rhythm method of conception control in accordance with the Ogino formula are as follows:

1. The patient keeps a precise record of her menstrual dates (day and hour of the onset of menstruation) for at least one **year**, calculating the actual lengths of her menstrual cycles and thus determining the lengths of her shortest and longest cycles. This information is of paramount importance, inasmuch as it is impossible to predict the length of any current cycle, and all calculations of the potential fertile period must be based on the known variations in cycle length in the recent past, ovulation occurring relatively early in short cycles and late in longer cycles. Since the extent of variation in cycle length may change over the years, it is probably wise to have the patient continue to keep a careful record to be certain that all her cycles continue to fall within the initially calculated range, or to make any necessary corrections should they become longer or shorter.

2. The beginning of the potential fertile period, or the first unsafe day, is determined by subtracting 18 days from the shortest cycle length; the last unsafe day, or end of the fertile phase, is found by subtracting 10 days from the longest cycle length. There can never be less than 9 unsafe days by this formula, regardless of cycle length or variation. (Even in a woman whose cycle length is constant, these 9 days of potential fertility are accounted for by the 5-day interval during which ovulation is most likely [twelfth through sixteenth premenstrual days] plus 1 day potential ovum survival, plus 3 days potential sperm survival.)

For example: In a woman whose menstrual cycles vary between 25 and 31 days, the fertile period is calculated as extending from day 7 (25 minus 18) to day 21 (31 minus 10). The safe intervals, during which intercourse is highly unlikely ever to result in conception, include the days immediately following menstruation through day 6 (the last preovulatory safe day) of the cycle and the interval from day 22 (the first postovulatory safe day) through the onset of the next menstrual period.

Although there are a number of printed calendar devices on the market that allegedly simplify the task of calculating the safe period, nearly all are unduly complicated and expensive, and none is at all necessary. The woman's careful and continuing record of her cycles and the routine arithmetic previously described are all that are required if she has been properly instructed and understands the simple basic facts about ovulation and the menstrual cycle itself. It cannot be overemphasized, however, that her calculations must be based on prior data of cycle length and variations thereof collected over a period of at least a year (13 cycles) if she is to achieve the 95 percent protection potentially offered by the Ogino formula. The risk of conception is roughly only 0.001 per cycle under these conditions, whereas it is twice as great if computations are based on a study of nine cycles, and three to seven times as great if they are based on data obtained from only six cycles. Parenthetically, the Ogino formula for the determination of the fertile period can also be employed to increase the chances of conception in infertile couples when previously relatively infrequent or improperly timed coitus is believed to be a significant factor in their involuntary sterility.

VAGINAL DIAPHRAGMS

Use of the vaginal diaphragm continues to be the most frequent method selected by couples wishing to practice contraception. A number of pharmaceutical or medical supply houses manufacture reliable diaphragms, and, although there are minor variations in style and construction, all the devices consist basically of a thin, slightly cupshaped diaphragm of latex rubber or similar material mounted on and covering a completely flexible circular coiled spring or a flat or arching simple watch-type spring. The external diameter of the commercially available contraceptive diaphragms varies from 50 to 105 mm in gradations of 5 mm, so that an appropriate size may be chosen for each user. (The most commonly required size is 75.) A set of fitting diaphragms for office use is readily available from any of the manufacturers.

It is extremely important that the proper size be selected. The diaphragm should be as large as is comfortable for the patient, and will then extend easily over the cervix in cuplike fashion in such a way that the back rim is firmly and snugly anchored behind the cervix in the posterior fornix and the front rim similarly "locked in place" anteriorly behind the pubic symphysis (Fig. 74). (It is thus fitted in place in the identical way that a Smith-Hodge pessary is inserted in correcting uterine retroversion.) During intercourse, the properly fitted diaphragm lies snugly applied to the anterior vaginal wall, cervix, and upper portion of the posterior fornix, effectively shielding the cervical os without its presence being noted by either partner. A diaphragm that is either too small or too large may become displaced during intercourse and allow semen to gain access to the cervix. It should also be noted that the appropriate size may change after pregnancy and delivery, so that refitting six to eight weeks postpartum is desirable if the couple wishes to resume the program of family planning. Since the area of junction between the diaphragm and the vaginal walls cannot in theory ever prevent the potential passage of an organism as minute as a spermatozoon, spermicidal jelly or cream is prescribed for use as a lubricant and protective coating on the rim of the diaphragm and is applied to it just before insertion.

A complete examination should always precede a diaphragm fitting, not only to avoid overlooking unsuspected pelvic disease but also to be certain that an anatomic variation that will preclude effective use of the diaphragm method does not exist;

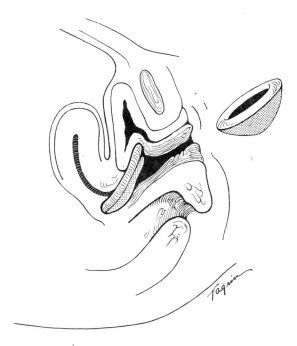

Figure 74
Proper placement of the vaginal diaphragm.

e.g., severe pelvic-floor relaxation, a large cystocele, or marked congenital retroversion with an excessively short anterior vaginal wall. The proper size is determined and the fitting diaphragm of this size inserted and checked by the physician. The patient is then helped to examine the diaphragm in place, learning the feel of the covered cervix, and particularly the feel of the front rim locked in place subpubically; the latter is her best and easiest landmark and test of proper placement. The patient should then be allowed to remove and reinsert the diaphragm herself while still on the examining table, the physician checking once more to be sure that she has mastered the procedure. Only rarely will a patient be encountered who simply cannot accomplish what is ordinarily a simple maneuver; in that event, some other means of conception control will have to be used.

The diaphragm should be coated externally with spermicidal jelly or cream, a dab of which is also placed in the center of the inner cup where it will be applied against the cervical os, and inserted before intercourse (not more than 6 to 12 hours before, however, and preferably only shortly before) and left in place for 6 to 8 hours or more after intercourse (not more than 24 to 36 hours, however, and preferably no more than 8 to 12 hours). When left in place for the recommended time interval following coitus, douching at the time of removal is unnecessary. Instructions for the cleaning and care of the diaphragm are provided by the manufacturers, who usually supply kits containing diaphragm and storage container, a tube of spermicidal jelly, and an "introducer," the latter probably not employed by the majority of users, who simply carry out insertion and removal manually. With proper care the same diaphragm will suffice for up to five to six years.

CONTRACEPTIVE JELLIES, CREAMS, AND FOAMS USED ALONE

A temporary alternative for the virginal woman about to be married for whom it is impossible to fit a diaphragm, or for the patient who for anatomic or other reasons cannot successfully insert a diaphragm, is the use of a vaginal spermicidal agent alone. These are available as suppositories, creams, jellies, and aerosol foams, the latter currently being the most popular. The various manufacturers supply syringe-type applicators designed for ready filling from the tube or container of contraceptive jelly or cream and for subsequent insertion into the vagina by the patient and delivery under moderate pressure of the recommended dose (usually 5 ml) of the agent into the upper vagina. A typical product is Preceptin Contraceptive Gel, supplied in a kit with an 82-gm tube of gel and the applicator. Insertion of the gel should be made just prior to intercourse, placing the applicator well into the vagina so that the gel is deposited near the cervix. Postcoital douching is unnecessary but, if desired, should be delayed at least 6 hours. An aerosol foam type of spermicidal agent (e.g., Emko Vaginal Foam, Dalkon Foam), is preferred by many women, and its reliability is reputedly enhanced by virtue of the foaming action and more thorough surface dispersion of the agent. Although any of these agents are reasonably effective, with an average of 80 percent protection, none appear to approach the 90 to 95 percent protection afforded by the diaphragm.

CONTRACEPTIVE DRUGS

The use of ovulation-inhibiting agents to achieve a physiologic type of conception control, as contrasted with the biologic (rhythm method) and mechanical (diaphragm and spermicidal jellies) approaches previously discussed, has received a tremendous impetus with the development during the past 20 years of the new, synthetic, highly potent oral progestogens. When administered cyclically throughout most of the menstrual cycle in proper dosage, these oral progestogens in combination or in sequence with synthetic estrogens completely suppress ovulation, presumably by inhibiting the output of pituitary gonadotropins, with the result that the normal cyclic ovarian function is totally interrupted. At the same time, the periodic short interruption of drug therapy allows an interval of withdrawal bleeding to occur that simulates the normal menstrual flow and avoids the undesirable side effects of a pseudodecidual type of endometrial hyperplasia, excessive breast stimulation, and so on, which would accompany prolonged, continuous therapy. The fascinating history of this tremendously important development in reproductive biological science is nicely summarized by Goldzieher and Rudel [12].

   If each pill contains both a progestogen and an estrogen, the drug is classified as a combination type of oral contraceptive; if the initial 14 to 16 tablets in each month's package contain only estrogen, the progestogen being added to the last 5 or 6 tablets in the treatment cycle, the product is termed a sequential oral contraceptive. The combination types were the first to be introduced and continue to be the most widely used. Sequential products were subsequently devised in the belief that they would be more physiologic, and it is claimed that their overall incidence of side effects is slightly lower. However, although both types are nearly 100 percent effective as contraceptives, the pregnancy rate for the sequential products is slightly higher (nearly all failures are in the first one or two treatment cycles).

Table 12 lists most of the oral contraceptives currently available, together with their chemical composition and dosages employed. The patient begins the oral contraceptive drug on the fifth day of the menstrual cycle, taking one tablet daily for the prescribed 20 or 21 days. Usually within 48 hours of cessation of the drug she will experience an "artificial period." On the fifth day after the onset of this withdrawal flow, she begins another 20- or 21-day treatment program. In the case of some products, the patient simply stays off the medication for 7 days after completing a 21-day pill cycle and then automatically begins the next pill cycle, regardless of when, or if, her artificial withdrawal period occurs. Most manufacturers also supply 28-tablet packages that include 7 placebo tablets at the end of the 21-day active drug tablet supply in each package, thus allowing the patient to take a tablet every day during each 28-day cycle, in the hope of avoiding mistakes in timing. In most instances, the artificial, drug-created menstrual cycle is extremely regular, more so than the patient's normal, spontaneous cycle, and the drug withdrawal menstrual flow tends to be less in amount and often of shorter duration than the flow normally experienced during her spontaneous periods, a fact which should preferably be explained in advance to the patient. Patients ordinarily suffering from menstrual cramps may also note a decrease in or even disappearance of their dysmenorrhea.

There has been a steady trend over the years in the direction of lower doses of both the progestational agent and especially the estrogenic compound used in the commercially available oral contraceptives, with a resulting decrease in side effects without compromise of the effectiveness of the product. So-called low-dose preparations have become popular but may not be satisfactory for many patients because of an increased incidence of troublesome breakthrough bleeding during each cycle. A few products containing a low dosage progestogen alone without the addition of an estrogen (the so-called mini-pill) and taken by the patient on a continuous daily basis are now on the market (Table 12). Observations so far have revealed a negligible pregnancy rate, only slightly higher (3 pregnancies per 100 woman-years) than that encountered with the standard oral contraceptives (1 pregnancy per 100 woman-years). Furthermore, the absence of estrogen seems to eliminate many side effects and should reduce the more serious potential complications of the conventional oral contraceptive agents that current statistical data suggest are due to the latter's estrogenic components. The main side effect of the mini-pill is cycle irregularity and intermittent breakthrough bleeding, and when this becomes a major inconvenience to the patient, she may find its use unsatisfactory and unacceptable, in which case a shift to a standard combination agent or to a different method entirely will be

Table 12
Currently Available Oral Contraceptives

Drug	Days	Progestogen	mg per Tablet	Estrogen	mg per Tablet
Combination drugs:					
Enovid 5 mg	20	Norethynodrel	5.0	Mestranol	0.075
Enovid-E	20	Norethynodrel	2.5	Mestranol	0.10
Ovral	21/28	Norgestrel	0.5	Ethinyl estradiol	0.05
LO/Ovral	21/28	Norgestrel	0.3	Ethinyl estradiol	0.03
Ovulen	21/28	Ethynodiol diacetate	1.0	Mestranol	0.10
Demulen	21/28	Ethynodiol diacetate	1.0	Mestranol	0.05
Norinyl 2 mg	21/28	Norethindrone	2.0	Mestranol	0.10
Norinyl 1+50	21/28	Norethindrone	1.0	Mestranol	0.05
Norinyl 1+80	21/28	Norethindrone	1.0	Mestranol	0.08
Brevicon	21	Norethindrone	0.5	Ethinyl estradiol	0.035
Norlestrin 1/50 With iron	21/28 28	Norethindrone acetate	1.0	Ethinyl estradiol	0.05
Norlestrin 2.5/50 With iron	21 28	Norethindrone acetate	2.5	Ethinyl estradiol	0.05
Loestrin 1/20	28	Norethindrone acetate	1.0	Ethinyl estradiol	0.02
Loestrin 1.5/30	28	Norethindrone acetate	1.5	Ethinyl estradiol	0.03
Ortho-Novum 1/50	21/28	Norethindrone	1.0	Mestranol	0.05
Ortho-Novum 1/80	21/28	Norethindrone	1.0	Mestranol	0.08
Ortho-Novum 2 mg	21/28	Norethindrone	2.0	Mestranol	0.10
Modi Con	21	Norethindrone	0.5	Ethinyl estradiol	0.035
Zorane 1/20	28	Norethindrone acetate	1.0	Ethinyl estradiol	0.02
Zorane 1.5/30	28	Norethindrone acetate	1.5	Ethinyl estradiol	0.03
Zorane 1/50	28	Norethindrone acetate	1.0	Ethinyl estradiol	0.05
Sequential drugs:					
Oracon	21/28	Dimethisterone	25.0	Ethinyl estradiol	0.10
Norquen	20/21	Norethindrone	2.0	Mestranol	0.08
Ortho-Novum SQ	20	Norethindrone	2.0	Mestranol	0.08
Microdose Progestogens:					
Micronor (35 tablets)	Daily	Norethindrone	0.35		
NOR-Q.D. (42 tablets)	Daily	Norethindrone	0.35		
Ovrette (28 tablets)	Daily	Norgestrel	0.075		

indicated. Furthermore, because of its slightly higher pregnancy rate, the mini-pill is not recommended if prevention of pregnancy is absolutely mandatory. In addition to probable ovulation suppression, at least some of the time, the mini-pill low-dose progestogen probably acts by producing a hostile cervical mucus that impairs sperm motility and inhibits sperm penetration and perhaps also by altering tubal function as well as by interfering with normal endometrial maturation.

If, as occasionally occurs, the usual artificially induced menstruation does not take place within two to three days of the cessation of the current treatment cycle, the patient should be instructed to begin the next course of the drug not later than seven days after she completed the last one, for in spite of the absence of menstruation, she will usually ovulate unless the cyclic treatment is resumed within a week's time.

Occasionally, so-called breakthrough bleeding indicative of inadequate endometrial hormonal support may occur during the treatment cycle, often only in the first few treatment cycles. If breakthrough bleeding remains a persistent problem, the dosage may be increased, another product tried, or the patient may elect some other contraceptive method. With currently used dosages, however, most oral contraceptive breakthrough bleeding is the result of erratic intake or faulty gastrointestinal tract absorption. If abnormal bleeding persists, organic causes should be looked for.

Other side effects, some of which are commonly noted in a small percentage of patients on an oral contraceptive program, include nausea and other gastrointestinal symptoms, abdominal pain and bloating, breast soreness and tenderness, chloasma, weight gain, edema, fatigue, headaches and exacerbation of migraines, dizziness, irritability, depression, pelvic discomfort, backache, leg cramps, changes in libido, and nervousness. These symptoms resemble a combination of those encountered in early pregnancy and in the premenstrual tension syndrome. In the majority of instances, they are mild and tolerable; furthermore, they tend to disappear after three or four months. As Table 12 indicates, some of the drugs contain greater absolute or relative amounts of the estrogenic agent. Since many of the side effects are directly related to the sodium- and water-retaining effects of the estrogen, a shift to an agent with a smaller amount of estrogen may also ameliorate some of these troublesome symptoms. However, in 5 to 10 percent of patients they are persistent and severe enough to force discontinuance of this method of contraception. Occasionally, more rapid growth of uterine fibroids has been observed in patients on oral contraceptive drugs. Therefore the known presence of fibroids may be a relative contraindication to their use. An increased incidence of candidal vulvovaginitis has also been noted, a situation not unlike that seen in pregnant women or in postmenopausal women on estrogen therapy. On occasion, the candidiasis proves so distressing and resistant to all therapy that a switch to another method of birth control becomes necessary. Finally, androgen-dominant oral contraceptives (e.g., containing norgestrel, norethindrone, or norethindrone acetate) tend to cause or aggravate acne and occasionally result in either hirsutism or mild hair loss, whereas estrogen-dominant agents (e.g., containing norethynodrel or ethynodiol diacetate) tend to improve the complexions of acne-prone women, since estrogens tend to suppress sebaceous-gland activity.

Other, potentially more serious complications, have been observed in women taking oral contraceptives, the occurrence of thromboembolic disorders being the most significant. At first, no statistically valid cause-and-effect relationship could be established between the use of the drugs and the development of phlebitis and pulmonary emboli. Furthermore, numerous investigations have revealed only minor changes in clotting time, fibrinogen, and other blood coagulation factors in women on the pill; in most instances, they were of questionable significance. However, retrospective studies in Great Britain reported in 1968 and 1969 suggested that the risk of death from thromboembolism in oral contraceptive users was 1.3 per 100,000 women as compared with 0.2 per 100,000 women in the same age group not on the pill. Comparable data released in 1969 for the United States indicate that the incidence of thromboembolic disease, including thrombophlebitis, pulmonary embolism, and cerebral thrombosis, is four times greater in pill users than in nonusers, though in actual numbers this represents only 3 to 6 per 100,000 women per year, so the risk is not an alarming one. Furthermore, in a prospective study involving 80,000 women using oral contraceptives for more than 1 million cycles, the results of which were reported in 1972 by Drill [9], no increased incidence of thromboembolic phenomena could be demonstrated. In the initial United States study, the risk appeared to be somewhat greater for women on the sequential pill, thus further suggesting that the estrogen component may play the important etiologic role in causing thromboembolic disorders. There have also been scattered reports of thrombotic vascular occlusions involving the large and small bowel.

Evidence of a small, often reversible rise in systolic blood pressure and, to a lesser extent, diastolic pressure in some women (roughly 5 percent of users over a five-year period) taking oral contraceptives has also emerged in several careful studies. A rise in plasma renin and angiotensin levels, probably estrogen-induced, as well as an increased aldosterone level with fluid retention has been observed and may be the mechanism involved. In most instances these patients had exhibited slightly elevated blood pressures before beginning an oral contraceptive program; the development of hypertension in previously normotensive women has only infrequently been observed, and in nearly all such cases, systolic and diastolic pressures returned to normal once the medication was stopped. Nevertheless, it is obvious that women who are already even mildly hypertensive should use some other form of contraception.

Another development has been the 1975 report of a study in Great Britain indicating an apparent increased risk of both nonfatal and fatal myocardial infarctions in users of oral contraceptives. In women in the 30-to-35-year age group the combined incidence of fatal and nonfatal coronary occlusions among those using oral contraceptives was 11 per 100,000 as compared with an incidence of 4 per 100,000 in age-matched controls who were nonusers; however, for women in the 40 to 44 year age group, the incidence among users was 112 per 100,000 as compared with 22 per 100,000 nonusers. Thus the average overall annual additional risk of a fatal or nonfatal myocardial infarction for women taking oral contraceptives is about 1 per 1000 in users over the age of 40. Women with other coronary risk factors such as cigarette smoking, diabetes, hypertension, a history of preeclampsia, hypercholesterolemia, and obesity are obviously at even greater risk. Inasmuch as the results of these latest British studies are at variance with previous investigations that failed to demonstrate a cause-and-effect relationship between the use of oral contraceptives and heart attacks, more extensive and long-term prospective studies will be necessary to resolve the issue completely.

Just what impact these observations should or will have on the future of oral contraception remains to be seen. Some authorities feel the problem has been overmagnified by the introduction of bias in the figures resulting from the sampling methods employed in some of these retrospective studies. Furthermore, the risk of mortality in pregnancy (22.8 deaths per 100,000 pregnant women from all causes associated with pregnancy) should not be forgotten (this risk also increases with age), nor should the psychological or sociological problems created by the constant fear of pregnancy or the need to raise an unwanted child. And also to keep in proper perspective the risk of 0.3 to 3.0 deaths from oral contraception per 100,000 woman-years, one must bear in mind the 3.2 deaths per 100,000 elective abortions and the 27 deaths from auto accidents per 100,000 person-years. In any case, the drugs should not be used in patients who have had phlebitis or thromboembolic disorders in the past, or in women over 40 with additional coronary risk factors, and the entire problem requires continued investigation and constant reevaluation.

Certain neuro-ocular complications, including retinal thrombosis and optic neuritis, have also been encountered in patients on oral contraceptives. No absolute cause-and-effect relationship has been established as yet, but immediate withdrawal of the drug is indicated if visual disturbances develop.

Changes in liver function test results as well as the occasional occurrence of cholestatic jaundice have been observed in some women taking oral contraceptives. The progestogen component of the drug appears to interfere with bile secretion in these patients, thus accounting for increased bromosulfophthalein (BSP) retention and, less often, jaundice. Since these alterations are much more likely to occur in patients with preexisting liver disease, the latter is also a contraindication to use of the pill. There also appears to be an increased tendency toward the development of gallstones in users of oral contraceptives. Other benign alterations in blood chemistry noted in women on contraceptive drugs include an elevation in protein-bound iodine (PBI) and butanol extractable iodine (BEI) (thyroid function tests) secondary to the increase of thyroxine-binding proteins (also seen in pregnancy and during estrogen administration) and a decrease in glucose tolerance, the mechanism for which remains obscure. However, there is no evidence of any fundamental effect on thyroid function (patients remain euthyroid), nor does the use of oral contraceptives in diabetic patients appear to affect the diabetic state per se or complicate its management.

As far as potential long-term deleterious effects on the organism following prolonged use of the oral contraceptive agents are concerned, it can merely be stated that in careful follow-up studies of many millions of women employing these drugs over the last 20 years, no definite ill effects of this type have so far been observed. Specifically, normal reproductive tract function and fertility are universally restored on discontinuance of the drug, and, until recently, no tendency to fetal anomalies had been demonstrated. However, there have now been reports from several centers suggesting a potential teratogenicity of progestogen-estrogen agents because of a small but definite increased incidence of multiple congenital anomalies of the type covered by the acronym **VACTERL** (vertebral-and-cardiac-tracheal-esophageal-renal-limb) in the offspring, especially male offspring, of women exposed to combined progestogen-estrogen compounds during early pregnancy. Such exposures have occurred by accident, early or late in an oral contraceptive program, or while under hormone therapy for presumed threatened or habitual abortion.

There have been scattered reports of small numbers of women who have experienced prolonged amenorrhea or oligomenorrhea following an oral contraceptive program. In most such instances, normal ovulatory menses ultimately return. Where the difficulty has persisted, it seems equally possible that the basic ovulatory disturbance may have antedated, or at least was not necessarily entirely related to, the contraceptive drug therapy. Amenorrhea or oligomenorrhea related to use of the pill is due to hypothalamic suppression and interference with the release of follicle-stimulating hormone and luteinizing hormone by the estrogenic and progestational agents in the contraceptive; therefore, treatment by cyclic therapy with estrogen and progesterone to produce artificial periods is pointless and contraindicated, since such treatment only perpetuates hypothalamic inhibition. Reassurance and watchful waiting are the best management in most such cases, although treatment with clomiphene might be considered in some cases of long standing, provided a complete endocrine evaluation has excluded all other possible causes for the amenorrhea. (Persistent lactation sometimes accompanies the amenorrhea and is presumed due to the release of inhibition of prolactin associated with hypothalamic suppression.)

No increased incidence of benign breast disorders or of pelvic or breast cancers has been noted, although the potential role of prolonged estrogen exposure in the genesis of breast and endometrial cancer in both the human female as well as certain laboratory animals has been well known for several decades. In fact, the incidence of benign breast disorders as well as the various very common functional ovarian cysts is much lower than normal in women taking oral contraceptives. However, there have been reports of an increased incidence of the previously uncommon benign hepatic cell adenomas, the majority now occurring in women taking oral contraceptives, usually first discovered when spontaneous liver rupture and secondary, often massive, intraabdominal hemorrhage occurs and requires emergency partial liver resection.

In 1969, considerable excitement was generated by a few reports concerning a possible increase in the incidence of cervical dysplasia and carcinoma in situ among women on oral contraceptives. Although data from two such follow-up series suggested that no such relationship existed, in one study involving 40,000 women using either the pill or diaphragm, a higher incidence of carcinoma in situ was detected in those on the pill. However, it is generally agreed that the significance, if any, of these observations could not be properly evaluated because of the lack of an adequate control population. In another study, cervical epithelial abnormalities suggesting dysplasia were noted but appeared to be reversible and to disappear following discontinuance of the drug. At the present time the matter is under further investigation, but, in any case, it seems unlikely that a significant risk is involved. (Mention is made in Chapter 7 of a different and unrelated benign and completely reversible, atypical endocervical hyperplasia that sometimes develops in oral contraceptive users.)

No tendency to subsequent endocrine disturbances has been noted. Although a temporary, usually transient post-pill anovulatory state occurs, prolonged amenorrhea, occasionally accompanied by galactorrhea, will be encountered in a small percentage of users and will require thorough evaluation and treatment (see Chap. 6). In the majority of these patients, a history of previous irregular cycles with episodes of amenorrhea or oligomenorrhea can be elicited. In most patients coming off the pill, however, regular cycles are resumed spontaneously within one to six months, so detailed investigation can safely be postponed until after this time. Furthermore, concern over the possibility that prolonged use of ovulation-suppressing agents might delay the onset of a normal menopause would appear to be groundless. It is fair to say, however, that the final answer to the question as to whether or not there may possibly be undesirable, long-term side effects associated with the prolonged use of oral contraceptive drugs will only come after many more years of careful follow-up studies.

Needless to say, any patient embarking on an oral contraceptive program should definitely first be given the benefits and reassurance of a careful history, complete physical examination, cytologic smear, and any other indicated laboratory studies. The opportunity presented to discover unsuspected pelvic or other diseases, as well as the need to be certain that no contraindications to the use of these agents exist, makes this preliminary survey mandatory. As brought out in the discussion of observed and potential complications, contraindications to the use of oral contraceptives include a history of phlebitis and embolic phenomena, preexisting genital or breast cancer, sizable fibroids, preexisting liver disease or a history of jaundice, or a history of coronary or cerebral vascular disease. Furthermore, patients on such a program should receive continued supervision and follow-up examinations on at least a regular yearly basis.

One of the ethical questions posed by the increasingly widespread use of oral contraceptives is whether or not the physician should prescribe them for unmarried adolescents and teenagers. In this connection, it is well to reiterate that at the present time 20 percent of all illegitimate pregnancies occur in girls under the age of 17, and that an estimated 200,000 abortions are performed annually on teenagers. Whether or not teenagers should indulge in sexual intercourse and, if they do, whether or not they should receive the pill, is a matter of "morality" only in the sense of what is best for their own emotional growth and development as adult sexual beings. There is also the practical reality that they are still not economically or educationally sufficiently independent to enter into a mature sexual relationship with an ongoing future. As a result, both the immature parents and any progeny resulting from this premature attempt at adult sexuality will in all likelihood be emotionally and socially crippled. It must be granted, therefore, that for many young people it is wise to try to help them learn and believe in the value of accepting responsibility for the physical and emotional well-being of themselves and others, so that their sexual lives will be richer and more meaningful.

Nevertheless, there are many well-adjusted, thoughtful, and responsible young women, as well as those less able to cope with the circumstances of their lives, who choose in the permissive world of today, not to postpone sexual activity. It would therefore seem desirable to prevent unwanted and undesirable pregnancy in these young women rather than to allow them to become entrapped in the difficult problem of premarital pregnancy. The latter carries with it a severely detrimental impact on their economic and educational situation, the potential for serious disruption of their emotional health and family relationships, and even today the specter of their resorting to criminal abortion with its high morbidity and mortality. Even legalized therapeutic abortion, however well justified, is an imperfect solution at best. Making an adequately supervised contraceptive program available to these young women (an estimated 41 percent of single women in the United States were taking oral contraceptives in 1974), when and if they need it, while at the same time offering them guidance in matters of overall sexuality, seems the only possible answer to the question in our society today.

INTRAUTERINE CONTRACEPTIVE DEVICES

During the past 15 years the availability of biologically inert plastic materials has revived interest in the use of mechanical intrauterine contraceptive devices (IUDs), including circular rings (modified after the original Grafenberg ring, introduced in 1929 by the German-born gynecologist Ernest Grafenberg), spiral coils, loops, and bow-shaped, M-shaped, shield-shaped and T-shaped devices. Although some of the rings are made of coiled stainless steel wire, the other types are constructed from polyethylene or similar plastic compounds, which, because of their flexible properties and ability to resume their original shape, render simple and painless the intrauterine placement of the device by means of a hollow, straight introducer passed up into the cervical canal (Fig. 75). Intrauterine devices have the great advantages of being very inexpensive and requiring no action whatsoever on the part of the user. Even more important, under favorable circumstances, they are second only to the ovulation-inhibiting oral agents among all contraceptive methods in the degree of protection they provide, with pregnancy rates as low as 2 to 4 per 100 patient-years of use. It is not clear whether the precise mechanism by which intrauterine devices prevent pregnancy is by (1) the creation of excessive myometrial contraction and deficient and altered endometrial maturation (possibly due to local release of cytotoxic products and accumulation of leukocytes produced by the endometrial surface reaction to the foreign body) that interferes with normal implantation, (2) the production of excessive tubal peristalsis that results in premature delivery of the fertilized

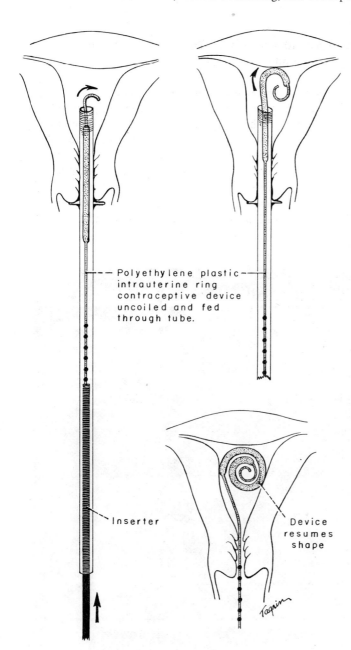

— Polyethylene plastic—
intrauterine ring
contraceptive device
uncoiled and fed
through tube.

Inserter

Device
resumes
shape

Figure 75
The intrauterine plastic ring as a contraceptive device.

ovum to the endometrial cavity with failure of implantation due to the immaturity of both the early embryo and the endometrium itself, or (3) by some combination of both mechanisms.

Within a few years after its introduction, use of the original Grafenberg ring was condemned and abandoned because of the high incidence of secondary pelvic infection, uterine perforation, pain, abnormal bleeding, and undetected expulsion of the ring leading to unwanted pregnancy. However, more recent experience in clinical trials with the modern devices indicates that the use of inert plastics and modifications in design have reduced the incidence of these undesirable side effects, although the results of the method are still not universally satisfactory. Some of the most commonly employed intrauterine contraceptive devices are illustrated in Figure 76. Among those shown in Figure 76A, the Lippes loop proved to be somewhat superior

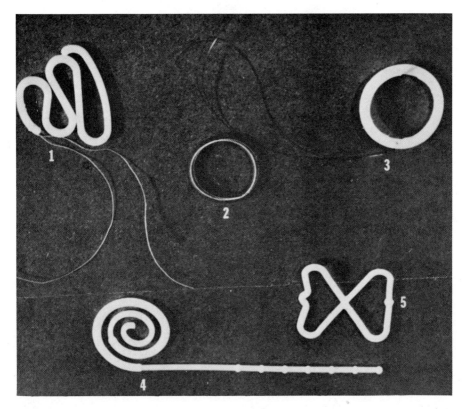

Figure 76A
Examples of early modern types of intrauterine contraceptive devices: (1) Lippes loop, (2) Hall-Stone ring, (3) H. J. Davis ring, (4) Margulies spiral, (5) Birnberg bow. (From N. J. Eastman. Intrauterine ring for conception control. *Curr. Med. Dig.,* September 1965, p. 776. © 1965 by The Williams & Wilkins Company, Baltimore, Maryland.)

to the others in having both a low pregnancy rate (1.5 to 2.5 percent), a relatively moderate expulsion rate (10 to 12 percent), and fewer complications requiring removal (10 to 15 percent). The spiral had the lowest pregnancy rate (1.8 percent) but the highest expulsion rate (22.5 percent). The rings had both high pregnancy rates (7.5 percent) and high expulsion rates (18 percent) and have been virtually abandoned. The bow had a low expulsion rate (2.4 percent) but a high pregnancy rate (5.7 percent); the bow also had a high perforation rate (1 in 300), eight times greater than any of the other devices, so that it, too, is seldom used now. Most of

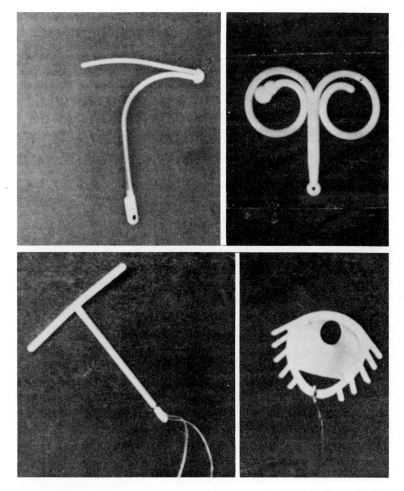

Figure 76B
Current widely employed intrauterine devices: Cu-7 (upper left), TCu-200 (lower left), Saf-T-Coil (upper right), and Dalkon Shield (lower right). The Dalkon Shield is no longer marketed, but there are still several million in use. The other IUD commonly in current use is the Lippes Loop, shown in *A*.

the devices have a polyethylene or nylon thread tail that protrudes through the cervix to permit women to check on their continued presence.

Currently, the most commonly employed IUDs are the Saf-T-Coil, the Lippes Loop, and the copper-bearing IUDs (Fig. 76B), e.g., the Copper-7 (Cu-7), the copper Tatum-T (TCu-200), and the Lippes Loop with copper. The addition of copper to the IUD itself (200 sq mm of copper wire are wound on the Cu-7 and TCu-200) stemmed from animal experiments showing copper to have a specific inhibiting effect on normal implantation. Copper may also have a spermicidal and sperm-immobilizing effect. Clinical tests were equally impressive, and copper devices are beginning to be more widely used. They appear to be 97 to 99 percent effective, and the Cu-7 and TCu-200 are smaller than the other IUDs and hence easier to insert, especially in nulligravidas, with acceptable expulsion rates of 8 and 13 percent, respectively, and with a much lower incidence of bleeding and uterine cramps. Although these newer devices appear highly promising, only further and prolonged observations in large numbers of users will permit an accurate evaluation of their true potential.

In general, IUDs are suitable only for parous women, since insertion is difficult and the expulsion and complication rates are high in nulliparas. Other contraindications to the use of an IUD include previous pelvic inflammatory disease, the presence of uterine fibroids or congenital uterine anomalies, and severe chronic cervicitis. In properly selected patients, insertion is usually readily accomplished as an office procedure but must be done carefully and atraumatically, so that the device is correctly placed in the uterus and accidental perforation is avoided. Transient slight bleeding and mild discomfort are common for a short time after insertion. Most expulsions occur within three months of insertion, usually during menstruation. Half of the women in whom the device is replaced will expel it again, so that more than two or three attempts at replacement are unwarranted. Approximately 20 to 30 percent of all expulsions are not noted by the patient, and the number of pregnancies occurring in this situation adds a highly significant 5 to 10 percent to the otherwise acceptable pregnancy rate of the method.

Complications troublesome enough eventually to require removal occur in 10 to 25 percent of women, depending on the type of device, and include persistent bleeding, uterine cramps or diffuse pelvic pain, and infection — either endometritis or acute pelvic inflammatory disease (2 to 3 percent). Some reported data suggest as high as a ninefold increased risk of acute pelvic infections among IUD wearers, and severe and repeated attacks can lead to irreparable tubal damage and sterility as well as to persistent chronic pelvic inflammatory disease, ultimately requiring hysterectomy and bilateral salpingo-oophorectomy.

More serious complications and a few deaths have been reported as a result of perforation with peritonitis or intestinal obstruction. Most perforations are probably secondary to an initial, traumatic insertion, and this complication can therefore largely be avoided by proper patient selection and careful insertion. A number of ectopic tubal and ovarian pregnancies (the rate of occurrence of the latter has been particularly increased) have also occurred in the presence of an IUD, so that this possibility must always be kept in mind.

When pregnancy occurs with an IUD in place, it is best to remove the IUD for two reasons: First, the patient is more likely to abort if the device is left in place (a 50 percent chance) than if it is removed (a 30 percent chance). There is a high incidence of fetal wastage from all causes (abortion, ectopic pregnancy, and premature labor) if the IUD is allowed to remain. Second — and even more important — there is a high incidence of premature rupture of the membranes complicated by serious intrauterine and intraamniotic sepsis as well as hemorrhage and septic abortion. A number of maternal deaths associated with shock and overwhelming sepsis in this situation have been reported (287 reported septic abortions and 39 reported deaths from 1965—1975, during which time an estimated 8 million IUDs were inserted). These reports prompted an investigation by the FDA when it appeared that one particular IUD (the Dalkon Shield) was especially prone to cause this complication, possibly because it was the only device manufactured with a polyfilament rather than a monofilament thread, the former acting like a wick and drawing fluid rich in bacteria from the vagina and cervix up into the uterine and amniotic cavities. For this reason the FDA banned the sale of Dalkon Shields for a time (although their removal from nonpregnant, asymptomatic women was not recommended). Subsequently, a new model with a monofilament thread attached was reapproved for use, but because of the previous adverse publicity and prolonged interruption in marketing, the company decided not to resume production. Since a lesser incidence of similar serious complications and fatalities have been observed in association with other IUDs (including the Lippes Loop and the Saf-T-Coil), if pregnancy does occur in the presence of an IUD, prompt removal is strongly recommended. Furthermore, early interruption of the pregnancy should perhaps be seriously considered if the problem is discovered in the first trimester.

It is apparent, then, that modern intrauterine contraceptive devices do have a place in the overall problem of population control, but it is equally clear that they have not yet fulfilled the great promise they seemed to hold when they were first reintroduced. The high rate of expulsions (12 to 15 percent or more), the significant pregnancy rate (if the pregnancies occurring as a result of unnoted expulsions are included), and the significant complication rate requiring removal appear to reduce the "use effectiveness" of the method to the point where only 50 percent of women originally fitted with an IUD will still have it in place two years later. For the roughly 50 percent of women who experience no adverse complications or side effects, the various IUDs have proved completely satisfactory and effective, and the inert plastic devices may be left in place indefinitely as long as they produce no symptoms. Copper- or progesterone-bearing devices need to be replaced at proper intervals (in two to three years for the Cu-7 and TCu-200 and one year for the progesterone-bearing T or loop) in order to maintain their effectiveness. Obviously, continued improvements in the design of the devices and further investigation of adjunctive techniques to increase effectiveness and minimize expulsion are in order in the hope of improving the effectiveness of the intrauterine contraceptive method. (Studies involving incorporation in several types of IUDs of Silastic capsules containing slow-releasing progesterone to inhibit myometrial contraction and interfere locally with normal endometrial maturation are now in progress.)

PERMANENT STERILIZATION PROCEDURES

Permanent sterility can, of course, be achieved by tubal ligation or hysterectomy in the female or by vasectomy in the male. Obviously, this is not the answer for the vast majority of young couples, because it is irreversible in most instances (although roughly 20 percent of women and 35 percent of men undergoing surgical steriliza-tion can be rendered fertile again by subsequent reparative operations). Neverthe-less, these methods should certainly receive serious consideration whenever there is need in a particular patient for permanent fertility control. Voluntary sterilization is legal in all 50 states, and in only a few are there restrictions regarding the indica-tion for its performance. In countries such as India, where national population con-trol is a particularly urgent problem, large-scale programs of voluntary sterilization have been inaugurated as a significant component of the total birth control effort.

With the increasing demand for voluntary sterilization, a number of techniques for permanent (in some cases potentially reversible) tubal occlusion have evolved, and efforts to develop simpler and safer methods continue. Laparotomy for tubal ligation is rarely necessary nowadays unless there is some additional indication for abdominal surgery or unless prior pelvic surgery or the presence of unrelated pelvic disease makes simpler approaches such as laparoscopic tubal sterilization technically impossible or dangerous. Currently, the most widely employed technique is tubal electrocoagulation and division, with or without partial resection, via laparoscopy. This approach has been highly successful and can be done on a transient operating room basis, although it requires general anesthesia in almost all cases. However, it is still not without its occasional serious complications, including hemorrhage, acci-dental electrical burns of the abdominal wall and small or large intestine (occasion-ally with resulting perforation and peritonitis), flare-up of pelvic inflammatory dis-ease, carbon dioxide embolism, and various anesthetic complications. Accordingly, attempts to substitute the laparoscopic placement of occluding tantulum metal clips or silicone rubber rings or bands for electrocautery destruction and division are currently under study.

An alternative and equally satisfactory method uses the vaginal approach. A cul-dotomy (posterior colpotomy) incision is made, and tubal ligation and fimbrial resection is done (or the Pomeroy type of ligation if the patient desires a potentially reversible method) in a few minutes and under direct vision. This procedure is also feasible in the transient operating room or outpatient setting and can even be done under local anesthesia in many patients. Culdoscopy rather than culdotomy has been used by some, but the technique of ligation under direct vision is essentially the same.

Still another potentially even simpler approach is currently being explored, namely, intrauterine occlusion of the internal cornual ostia of the tubes as visualized through the hysteroscope, employing either electrocoagulation or local application of a sclerosing agent such as quinacrine (either procedure may need to be repeated several times before complete and permanent tubal occlusion is achieved). This technique, which would probably be reversible only with great difficulty, shows great promise and would be much more easily done, but needs considerable further investigation and trial before its efficacy (currently only 90 percent successful) and safety can be established. Reversible hysteroscopic or laparoscopic tubal sterilization employing a removable silicone rubber plug introduced into the fallopian tube is also under experimental study.

Finally, for parous women who desire permanent sterilization and who, for example, also present signs and symptoms of pelvic support deficiencies (e.g., early prolapse, cystocele) or have a persistent cervical dysplasia (both exemplify a pelvic condition that in itself is not yet necessarily a sufficient indication for surgical intervention), a case can certainly be made for vaginal hysterectomy and repair, which will provide both permanent sterility and relief from current symptoms and future discomforts of inadequate pelvic support or protection against the progression from cervical dysplasia to carcinoma.

Where the male is concerned, permanent sterilization by vasectomy continues to be a simple office or transient operating room procedure, usually done under local anesthesia and with a high success rate. Ligation with division and resection of a small segment of vas, followed by burying of the divided ends, is the usual technique; electrofulgeration or injection of sclerosing agents is used by some surgeons, in which case the end result will usually not be potentially reversible by reanastamosis in the future. The couple should continue to employ their current contraceptive program for several months until complete azospermia is established and has been proved by several seminal analyses showing absence of sperm. There has been some concern about the occurrence of sperm-antibody autoimmune reactions in vasectomized men; sperm antibodies develop in 50 percent of vasectomized men and a cell-mediated immune reaction, in 20 percent, but neither appears to have any hazardous effects. There are no adverse hormonal changes whatsoever. Possible psychological complications from or contraindications to the procedure must always be borne in mind and discussed carefully during preoperative as well as postoperative counseling. Finally, efforts are being made to develop an easily reversible technique of male sterilization by intravas insertion of T-shaped devices with soft silicone and Dacron shuttle-stemmed microvalves within each vas and leaving them permanently in place, initially in the "off position," but with the possibility of readily switching them to the "on position" if desired at some future time. Thus, a husband could be literally as well as figuratively "turned on" if this experimental device should prove clinically feasible!

POSTCOITAL CONCEPTION CONTROL

Extensive studies by Morris and van Wagenen [17] and others have now established beyond question that the properly timed administration of an adequate dosage of estrogen to a woman postcoitally will prevent implantation of the fertilized ovum. Although obviously not suitable for use in a routine, long-term contraceptive program, the "morning-after pill" approach is of great value in cases of rape, ruptured condom or diaphragm, or unplanned, "accidental," unprotected intercourse under a variety of circumstances. To be effective, the estrogens must be given in the immediate postovulatory portion of the cycle or, in other words, immediately after fertilization, real or potential, has occurred but before the stage of implantation. Thus, if the past menstrual history indicates that exposure has occurred at or after midcycle, treatment should be started, preferably within 24 hours and not later than 72 hours. If unprotected intercourse has occurred during the follicular phase, it may be wiser to postpone the course of medication until just after midcycle. In either case, the patient should be warned not to have subsequent unprotected coitus in case ovulation should occur later in the cycle after the course of estrogen has been completed. Estrogen administration is not effective once implantation has occurred. Although the precise biologic mechanisms that are altered by giving large doses of estrogen are not proved (accelerated tubal transport of the ovum, abnormal endometrial maturation, and direct effects on the blastocysts are all possible factors), it is clear that failure of the implantation process is the end result.

The retroactive pill regimen consists of a five-day course of estrogen, e.g., a daily dose of 50 mg of diethylstilbestrol (DES), 30 mg of Premarin, or 5 mg of ethinylestradiol. Transient side effects due to the excessive amount of estrogen necessary are encountered and include fluid retention, breast soreness and swelling, excessive nausea, and subsequent irregular, prolonged menstrual flow. The nausea can be minimized by taking the medication with meals, together with an antiemetic drug, and the patient must be warned to take all the medication despite her nausea if the regimen is to be effective. When properly administered and timed, the postcoital estrogen therapy program is essentially 100 percent successful in preventing pregnancy. There seems to be a slightly increased incidence of ectopic pregnancy in the rare instances in which the postcoital medication program fails to prevent conception (see also Chap. 9). In all likelihood, the few failures have been associated with multiple sexual exposures, or inability to start or complete the drug program during the interval between ovulation and implantation, or inadequate estrogen dosage.

In the occasional instance of failure of the postcoital use of DES to prevent intrauterine pregnancy, therapeutic interruption would be warranted, both because it would best serve the interests of the patient with respect to an obviously undesired pregnancy and also because of the known possibility of DES-induced adverse effects on the fetus (see detailed discussions in Chapters 4 and 16). The potential creation of the latter problem in nonexistent offspring should not be construed as a valid objection to the use of the postcoital DES regimen of preventing pregnancy when it is otherwise clearly indicated, especially since it is essentially 100 percent effective in preventing pregnancy anyway.

Another approach to postcoital contraception immediately after unprotected intercourse has recently been tried, namely, the insertion of a copper-bearing IUD. Early results suggest a high degree of protection (approaching 100 percent) against subsequent pregnancy. The copper-T presumably also acts by preventing nidation and in addition may possess spermicidal activity. This technique may not be as widely applicable as the postcoital high-dose estrogen program, but it does offer a potential and highly effective alternative for some patients, many of whom might elect to retain the IUD as a permanent contraceptive.

METHODS UNDER STUDY

A number of clinical studies have been carried out using long-acting, injectable progestational agents, e.g., medroxyprogesterone acetate (Depo-Provera) given in a single intramuscular injection in dosages of 200 to 1000 mg, which appears to have prevented pregnancy for periods of 9 to 10 months in the several thousand women in whom it was tested. (The menstrual cycles are also irregular with this technique.) Variations of this approach now under study include the use of slow-release progestins such as megestrol acetate or d-norgestrel in subcutaneously implanted Silastic repositories and vaginal rings constructed of medroxyprogesterone acetate—impregnated Silastic that the patient inserts once a month in the same manner as a diaphragm, removing it on the twenty-eighth day of the cycle and replacing it with another ring after completion of withdrawal bleeding.

An entirely different approach currently being explored concerns the possibility of an immunologic method of fertility control. This work has stemmed from the observations, discussed in Chapter 11, that some cases of infertility appear to be due to the development of antisperm antibodies in the female that subsequently interfere with normal implantation of the embryo. A variety of female laboratory animals have already been successfully "immunized against pregnancy" by intradermal injection or transvaginal exposure to a homogenate of testicular tissue employed as the "vaccine." The resulting antibody titer and immunologically induced infertility has been maintained by continued coitus with its resulting reexposure to the antigens for as long as a year after the initial injections. But, most important, the immunity to pregnancy is readily reversible by allowing a definite, short period of time to elapse during which there is no further exposure to the antigens, thus permitting complete disappearance of the antisperm antibody titer. (This could be accomplished in the human by a short period of abstinence or temporary use of a condom.) Clinical trials of the immunologic method of fertility control are certain to be carried out in the near future, for if a single immunization can produce sterility and still be reversible, the method would have many obvious advantages.

Another approach currently being intensively investigated involves the development of chemical compounds that can safely be administered to males and that temporarily and reversibly render the male infertile by interfering with normal spermatogenesis. Certain of the dinitropyrroles and the recently discovered chlorohydrins have proved highly effective in this regard and without toxic side effects in laboratory animals, and their use clinically in the human male is now under trial. Indirect inhibition of spermatogenesis through male gonadotropin suppression produced by intermittent injections of long-acting progestational agents such as medroxyprogesterone acetate has also been studied. Although the sperm counts in both laboratory animals and clinical volunteers were successfully reduced to zero for periods of three to four months, androgen production and libido were also markedly depressed, rendering this method unacceptable for routine clinical use. However, a combination pill containing both a long-acting progesterone and an androgen (to avoid the loss of libido) is currently undergoing trials and appears to be effective while still maintaining normal libido. This hormonal approach requires 6 to 12 weeks to become effective, and fertility restoration, when desired, also requires several weeks or months. Finally, an immunologic approach to male contraception is also under investigation, since it has been shown in male laboratory animals that a reversible aspermatogenesis lasting for 9 to 12 months can be induced after a single injection of homologous testicular and epididymal tissue homogenates. The resulting infertility is not accompanied by any change in libido or by androgen deficiency.

REFERENCES

1. Ameriks, J. A., Thompson, N. W., Frey, C. F., Appelman, H. D., and Walter, J. F. Hepatic cell adenomas, spontaneous liver rupture, and oral contraceptives. *Arch. Surg.* 110:548, 1975.
2. Arrata, W. S. M., and Howard, A. The amenorrhea-galactorrhea syndrome following oral contraceptives. *J. Reprod. Med.* 8:139, 1972.
3. Baruch, D. W., and Miller, H. *Sex in Marriage.* New York: Hoeber Med. Div., Harper & Row, 1962.
4. Collaborative Group for the Study of Stroke in Young Women. Oral contraception and increased risk of cerebral ischemia or thrombosis. *N. Engl. J. Med.* 288:871, 1973.
5. Collaborative Group for the Study of Stroke in Young Women. Oral contraception and stroke in young women: Associated risk factors. *J.A.M.A.* 231:718, 1975.
6. Corfman, P. A., and Segal, S. J. Biologic effects of intrauterine devices. *Am. J. Obstet. Gynecol.* 100:448, 1968.
7. Dickey, R. P., and Dorr, C. H. Oral contraceptives: Selection of the proper pill. *Obstet. Gynecol.* 33:273, 1969.
8. Dreishpoon, I. H. Complications of pregnancy with an intrauterine contraceptive device in situ. *Am. J. Obstet. Gynecol.* 121:412, 1975.
9. Drill, V. A. Oral contraceptives and thromboembolic disease: Prospective and retrospective studies. *J.A.M.A.* 219:583, 1972.
10. Fisch, I. R., Freeman, S. H., and Myatt, A. V. Oral contraceptives, pregnancy, and blood pressure. *J.A.M.A.* 222:1507, 1972.
11. Goldzieher, J. W. The incidence of side effects with oral or intrauterine contraceptives. *Am. J. Obstet. Gynecol.* 102:91, 1968.
12. Goldzieher, J. W., and Rudel, H. W. How the oral contraceptives came to be developed. *J.A.M.A.* 230:421, 1974.
13. Inman, W. H. W., and Vessey, M. P. Investigation of death from pulmonary, coronary, and cerebral thrombosis and embolism in women of child-bearing age. *Br. Med. J.* 2:193, 1968.
14. Levin, M. The physician and the sexual revolution. *N. Engl. J. Med.* 273:1366, 1965.
15. Little, W. A. Current aspects of sterilization: The selection and application of various surgical methods of sterilization. *Am. J. Obstet. Gynecol.* 123:12, 1975.
16. Mann, J. I., and Inman, W. H. W. Oral contraceptives and death from myocardial infarction. *Br. Med. J.* 2:245, 1975.
17. Morris, J. M., and van Wagenen, G. Interception: The use of postovulatory estrogens to prevent implantation. *Am. J. Obstet. Gynecol.* 115:101, 1973.
18. Nelson, J. H. The use of the mini-pill in private practice. *J. Reprod. Med.* 10:139, 1973.

19. Oster, G., and Salgo, M. P. The copper intrauterine device and its mode of action. *N. Engl. J. Med.* 293:432, 1975.
20. Scott, R. B. Critical illnesses and deaths associated with intrauterine devices. *Obstet. Gynecol.* 31:322, 1968.
21. Seward, P. N., Israel, R., and Ballard, C. A. Ectopic pregnancy and intrauterine contraception: A definite relationship. *Obstet. Gynecol.* 40:214, 1972.
22. Sturgis, S. H. Opportunities and challenges of the premarital examination. *Fertil. Steril.* 13:209, 1962.
23. Tatum, H. J. Intrauterine contraception. *Am. J. Obstet. Gynecol.* 112:1000, 1972.
24. Tatum, H. J., Schmidt, F. H., Phillips, D., McCarty, M., and O'Leary, W. M. The Dalkon Shield controversy. *J.A.M.A.* 231:711, 1975.
25. Tietze, C., and Potter, R. G. Statistical evaluation of the rhythm method. *Am. J. Obstet. Gynecol.* 84:692, 1962.
26. Vessey, M. P., and Doll, R. Investigation of relation between use of oral contraceptives and thromboembolic disease: A further report. *Br. Med. J.* 2:651, 1969.
27. Weindling, H., and Henry, J. B. Laboratory test results altered by "the pill." *J.A.M.A.* 229:1762, 1974.
28. Wheeless, C. R., Jr., and Thompson, B. H. Laparoscopic sterilization: Review of 3600 cases. *Obstet. Gynecol.* 42:751, 1973.
29. Wortman, J. S., and Sciarra, J. J. Control of male fertility: Report of a workshop. *Fertil. Steril.* 26:180, 1975.
30. Yazpe, A. A., Anderson, R. J., Cohen, N. P., and West, J. L. A review of 1,035 tubal sterilizations by posterior colpotomy under local anesthesia or by laparoscopy. *J. Reprod. Med.* 13:106, 1974.

21
Role of the Gynecologist in the Management of Diseases of the Breast

It is not the purpose or intent of this chapter to present a complete or detailed description of all the known breast disorders together with a full discussion of all aspects of their medical and surgical management. Instead, emphasis will be placed primarily on the role that the gynecologist can and should play in the recognition of both benign and malignant breast diseases in his patients and on his need to be completely familiar with the various screening and diagnostic techniques and when and how to apply them. Above all, there is no question that obstetrician-gynecologists should and must play an increasingly important role in the early detection of breast cancer, and extension of the role of the adequately trained and experienced gynecologist in the management of breast problems should definitely be encouraged. Obstetrician-gynecologists currently serve not only as specialist-consultants but also as primary care physicians for the vast majority of women in the United States and, in particular, perform more periodic medical checkups for the women of today than any other category of physician. Because they see such a large number of women for regular examinations, they need to have a thorough knowledge of the natural history, symptoms, and characteristic physical findings of all the various benign and malignant breast disorders and be skilled in the proper techniques of breast examination as well as able to teach self-examination to their patients. They must also be aware of the high-risk category of women especially deserving of regular surveillance, and they should keep in mind the possibility that the long-term use of oral contraceptives and estrogens may be ill advised in this group. They must be completely familiar with all the screening and diagnostic methods available, the proper indications for their use, and their limitations.

PATIENT SCREENING AND THE EARLY DETECTION OF BREAST CANCER

History

Evaluation of the breasts is an important part of the complete gynecologic examination, whether the patient presents with what is primarily a pelvic problem, is concerned about the possibility of breast disease, or is completely asymptomatic and desires only a thorough checkup. A routine inquiry should be made concerning previous breast disorders and their medical or surgical treatment (e.g., breast abscess or mastitis, breast cyst or benign tumor) and, in the case of the parous woman, whether or not she lactated and nursed any of her infants.

If a history of recurring breast pain, tenderness, swelling, or palpable irregularity is obtained, it is important to determine whether or not these symptoms are related to the menstrual cycle. If the patient has become aware of a lump, it is helpful to find out as accurately as possible when and under what circumstances it was first discovered (e.g., did it follow an injury, was attention first drawn to it by virtue of associated pain or tenderness, or was it discovered during routine self-examination?) and, in the case of women of reproductive age, at what point in the menstrual cycle it was first noted. It is also important to inquire about the possibility of any nipple discharge, whether it is unilateral or bilateral, whether it is serous, dark in color, or bloody, and when and under what circumstances it has been noted.

In taking the history, it is also well to bear in mind that certain drugs (estrogens, certain antihypertensives, tranquilizers and other psychotropic drugs) and medication regimens (e.g., oral contraceptives and cyclic estrogen therapy) may cause breast pain, tenderness, irregular swellings, and the appearance of nipple secretion, or galactorrhea.

Finally, it is important to elicit any family history of breast cancer, specifically on the maternal side, since this may be an important factor in determining the potential risk of breast cancer in the patient and may influence the decision regarding just what screening and diagnostic studies will be undertaken and how frequently they should be repeated.

Examination and Instruction in Self-Examination

Careful examination of the breasts is the next step, including the nipples and areolar regions as well as the regional lymphatic drainage sites in the axillary and supraclavicular areas. The technique of breast examination has already been described in detail in Chapter 1. During the course of this examination, the physician should take the opportunity either to instruct the patient in the proper method for self-examination of the breasts or check her technique if she is already performing this important, potentially lifesaving, self-check on a regular basis. The proper technique for self-examination of the breasts has also been fully described in Chapter 1.

Supplementary Office Procedures

During the course of the breast examination there are several simple office diagnostic procedures that may be indicated and helpful. The most frequently called-for and useful of these is simple needle and syringe aspiration of breast cysts, the technique for which has already been described in the section on benign cyclic breast disorders in Chapter 5. If the examiner has palpated a smoothly rounded, mobile, sometimes tender, cystic or fluctuant-feeling mass in the breast, simple needle aspiration will immediately establish a definite diagnosis of simple ("blue-domed") breast cyst, a very common manifestation of the broad spectrum of so-called chronic cystic mastitis. Aspiration will at the same time provide effective and usually permanent treatment for that particular cyst, since they frequently never recur following an initial complete aspiration. If the palpable mass has completely disappeared following total aspiration of the cyst, and if the fluid is a clear or slightly turbid yellow or green in color and free of blood, the diagnosis is rarely in doubt, further studies are usually not required, and biopsy is totally unnecessary. Unless the fluid from such a cyst is bloody, there is no need to submit a specimen for cytologic examination, since essentially without exception it will prove nondiagnostic and often completely acellular; if the fluid is bloody or atypical in appearance, however, it is wisest to send it for cytologic study. Furthermore, if the fluid is bloody, or if the mass does not completely disappear following apparent total aspiration of the cyst, or if no fluid at all is obtained, then further studies are definitely indicated, and ultimately biopsy will probably be required to establish a definite diagnosis and either detect or exclude the possibility of malignancy.

A less frequently indicated and utilized office diagnostic procedure is needle aspiration biopsy, using either a Silverman needle or simply a hollow No. 18 intravenous needle and Luer-Lok syringe. This is rarely used if the patient is suspected of having a benign tumor (which will be better treated by total excisional biopsy anyway) or if malignancy is strongly suspected and the lesion is one that will probably be best handled by some type of mastectomy; in the latter case, a completely reliable open excisional or incisional surgical biopsy is greatly to be preferred. However, in cases in which malignancy is strongly suspected but is of the kind in which mastectomy or any form of local surgery is contraindicated and the treatment will be by radiation, chemotherapy, or hormonal therapy, including oophorectomy in premenopausal patients (e.g., inflammatory carcinoma of the breast or locally far-advanced and inoperable breast cancer of any type), then needle aspiration biopsy is much to be preferred. It usually permits a definite histologic diagnosis to be made, and the patient, who should promptly start radiation therapy and possibly undergo oophorectomy, is spared the potential delay required for healing and/or the subsequent wound-healing complications that may arise if open surgical biopsy is performed instead.

If the patient's chief complaint is unilateral nipple discharge, the simple maneuver of methodical, point-by-point palpation circumferentially about the nipple at or just outside the areolar margin will usually disclose just which lobular duct system contains the abnormality responsible, inasmuch as pressure over the involved group of ducts usually causes the discharge to be expressed from the nipple. This fluid should be smeared on a slide and submitted for cytologic examination, since the diagnosis of probable intraductal carcinoma can sometimes be made in this way; such a cytologic diagnosis will obviously require histologic confirmation by biopsy before proceeding with treatment.

Radiologic Screening and Diagnostic Procedures

A full discussion of **mammography** and **xeromammography** and the role and limitations of these radiographic techniques in the screening and diagnosis of breast disorders is found in Chapter 2.

From a diagnostic standpoint, mammography and xeromammography are most useful under two sets of circumstances. First, they are useful in a patient with diffuse, or multiple, or often bilateral palpable breast irregularities believed most likely to be fibrocystic disease because of (1) the characteristic findings on examination, (2) associated pain, tenderness, and swelling related to the premenstrual, menstrual, and immediate postmenstrual phase of the cycle, (3) the fact that some of the irregularities have been shown to be cystic by needle aspiration, or (4) a previous history of biopsy-proved cystic mastitis. In this situation, x-ray examination of the breasts will either show a completely benign and reassuring radiographic pattern throughout or will pinpoint any suspicious area or areas in one or both breasts that should be examined by biopsy or followed closely by repeating both the clinical and radiologic examinations in a few months. Mammography is less helpful in patients with a single, dominant, three-dimensional, breast mass, because biopsy is usually indicated in this situation, regardless of the mammographic findings.

Second, mammography and xeromammography are useful in some patients with recurring breast symptoms, with either no palpable abnormalities, or with indefinite findings, or with questionable irregularities that seem to come and go. Here, x-ray examination may resolve the issue for the patient, who is often fearful of cancer, and the physician, who is concerned about not failing to detect an early one. (In this connection it should be remembered that even in early lesions some type of pain does occur in about 25 percent of patients with breast cancer.)

From the standpoint of screening patients who have no abnormal breast symptoms or signs, periodic breast x-ray studies are indicated primarily in patients who have already had one breast cancer and those at high risk in terms of the chances that breast cancer will develop. Since breast cancer is fundamentally often a multicentric disease, roughly 10 percent of women who have had breast cancer ultimately have a second cancer in the opposite breast (this is 5 to 10 times the normal expected incidence for the general female population); it is therefore wise to screen such patients every year or two by xeromammography (oftener, if the radiographic pattern should warrant it). Screening is even more important, from the gynecologist's viewpoint, in patients over the age of 35 who fall into the so-called high-risk category because of certain features of their background and history. Among the most significant of these high risk factors are the following:

1. A family history of breast cancer, especially in the maternal line (e.g., mother, sister, maternal grandmother, maternal aunt or cousin, daughter. If one of these relatives has had the disease, the risk is increased twofold to threefold. If more than one has had the disease, the risk is increased even more, and if both the patient's mother and a sister have had the disease, the risk is nearly 50 times higher than normal.

2. Nulliparity (two to three times the usual risk) or delayed first full-term delivery until after the age of 30 (twice the usual risk). Conversely, a full-term delivery before the age of 20 is associated with a reduction in the risk by two-thirds.

3. Early menopause, or late menarche, or both. On the other hand, breast cancer rarely develops in women undergoing oophorectomy 5 to 10 years before the menopause, especially before age 35 to 40.

4. A history of lactation and nursing, once thought to protect against breast cancer, has now been shown to be statistically unrelated to the risk of its occurrence.

5. Age is an important factor. Breast cancer is rare in women under the age of 30, but the risk increases with age (the increase in risk is greatest for women 40 to 44 years old) so that breast cancer is 10 times more likely to develop in a woman of 70 than in a woman 40 years old or younger.

6. There is an increased incidence of breast cancer in women who have had any form of gynecologic cancer but especially cancer of the ovary, endometrium, cervix, and vulva.

7. Women who have at any time had breast biopsies that revealed some form of mammary dysplasia (e.g. intraductal hyperplasia, papillomatosis, or epithelial atypia) are also in a higher-risk group.

8. In patients who have had periodic mammographic surveillance, there is a group of women exhibiting a very prominent duct pattern who appear to be at a considerably greater risk than those in whom this feature is minimal or absent.

9. Miscellaneous factors include race, ethnic group, and geographical location. The current incidence of breast cancer is higher in whites than in the black, brown, or yellow races. It is higher in Jewish than in non-Jewish women, and it is six times higher in North American and European women than in African and Asian women.

10. Finally, some feel there is convincing evidence that patients with gross cystic disease of the breasts have a higher-than-normal incidence (perhaps two to four times higher) of subsequent breast cancer elsewhere in their breasts. However, this has not been accepted by all authorities on the subject or substantiated by all careful studies of the problem.

Obviously, the woman whose history reveals not one or two but a number or all of these high-risk factors is perhaps even more at risk for breast cancer and even more in need of annual or biannual breast x-rays once she reaches 35, an age before which mammography is not very reliable and the risk not very significant. One must always balance the potential risk of the development of breast cancer in the particular patient against the risk of repeated exposure to the not inconsiderable amounts of radiation required to perform either mammography or xeromammography (there is evidence that repeated exposure of the breasts to this type of irradiation may increase the incidence of carcinoma).

Nevertheless, such routine screening programs for high-risk patients are proving to be extremely valuable. An example encountered in 1975 in the author's own practice bears this out in dramatic fashion. A 50-year-old woman (gravida 1, para 1) had been followed regularly since 1955 and had been well except for known fibrocystic disease requiring a number of needle aspirations of cysts and a biopsy of the left breast in 1966. However, her cystic mastitis had been symptomatically quiescent and without palpable irregularities of any kind since her menopause in 1973. When she was seen for a routine annual checkup in early 1975, it was learned that a sister, one year older, had just undergone radical mastectomy and that two maternal cousins about the same age as the patient had died of breast cancer within the preceding two years. On the basis of this significant family history alone, and despite the complete absence of any palpable abnormalities in either breast, screening

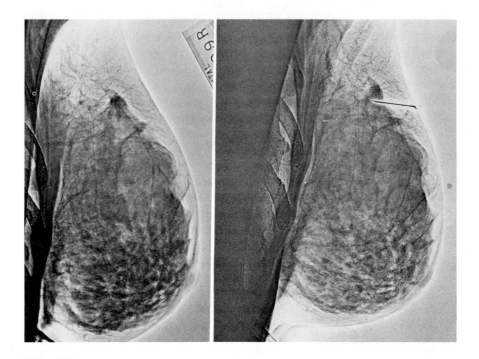

Figure 77
Xeromammography in a 50-year-old woman with unsuspected carcinoma of the right breast. The initial diagnostic xeromammogram shown on the left revealed a nonpalpable, asymptomatic irregular "mass" 1 cm in diameter in the upper outer quadrant of the right breast; the remainder of the breast parenchyma showed dysplastic changes of a mixed type. The xeromammogram on the right was made one week later immediately prior to an excisional biopsy of this suspicious area in the right breast; the No. 20 intravenous needle visible on this film was inserted under xeroradiographic control, placing the needle tip in close proximity to the lesion to localize it precisely and facilitate the complete removal of the entire mass for adequate histologic study.

xeromammograms were done and revealed a small suspicious area in the right breast (Fig. 77). Subsequent excisional biopsy of this nonpalpable lesion, aided by xeromammographic needle localization of the suspicious area (Fig. 77) revealed a tumor 8 mm in diameter that proved on frozen section to be an infiltrating intraductal carcinoma. A modified radical mastectomy was performed in March 1975, and histologic examination of the final specimen revealed negative axillary nodes and no demonstrable residual tumor in the breast itself. The patient has subsequently remained well and free of disease, and the opposite breast has remained benign, as determined by regular examinations and annual xeromammography.

Thermography

Thermography represents another and related technique for screening and diagnosis. Its chief advantage is that it avoids exposure to ionizing radiation, since it is based on a technique for the sensing and photographic recording of the skin surface infrared, or heat, radiation pattern and its variation in different areas of the breasts. Certain characteristic alterations in these patterns are produced by benign and malignant breast disorders. However, it is not nearly as accurate or reliable as mammography or xeromammography for diagnostic purposes (there is a high false-positive as well as a high false-negative rate, approaching 10 to 15 percent for both), and it is therefore primarily useful for annual screening programs. Any change or asymmetry in the baseline thermographic pattern for a given woman is an indication for prompt clinical evaluation and xeromammography, with biopsy to follow as indicated. Special and expensive equipment is required, and accurate interpretation is more difficult than is the case for mammography or xeromammography. Because of these drawbacks and the lack of diagnostic accuracy as compared with mammography and xeromammography, thermography is as yet not as widely used or available and is probably not an adequate screening maneuver unless combined with regular clinical examinations and periodic x-ray studies.

Diagnostic Ultrasound

Diagnostic ultrasound is also utilized in the diagnosis of breast disease. It, too, has the advantage of complete freedom from exposure to ionizing radiation. In addition, its low cost, noninvasive character, and ease, safety, and rapidity of performance render it well suited for screening programs. Diagnostic ultrasound appears to be highly accurate, and the technique permits correct identification of all benign cysts that are 3 mm or larger, 90 percent of all benign tumors that are 1 cm or larger, and 90 percent of all malignant tumors that are 1 cm or larger and sometimes even smaller ones near the surface of the breast.

Galactography

Finally, galactography is another, less frequently required x-ray technique that has proved useful in evaluating certain patients with abnormal nipple discharge. Using a magnifying glass to identify and gently dilate the duct opening from which the abnormal nipple discharge emanates, the duct system is painlessly injected with 0.2 to 0.5 ml of 30 percent Urografin via a lacrimal duct cannula, and soft-tissue x-rays (galactograms) are made. These will clearly demonstrate the injected portion of the milk duct system, either showing it to be normal (as in the case of galactorrhea of endocrine origin) or revealing the radiographic characteristics of some form of local intraductal disease, e.g. solitary intraductal papilloma, multiple papillomas or diffuse papillomatosis, fibrocystic disease, or noninfiltrating or infiltrating intraductal carcinomas. With the aid of this diagnostic and accurate localization technique, precise excision of the lesion is possible for histologic confirmation of the nature of the pathologic condition and a decision as to appropriate therapy.

Breast Biopsy

Since a high percentage of palpable breast abnormalities will prove to be benign, the obstetrician-gynecologist should be able to aspirate and thus prove the benign nature of simple breast cysts as well as eliminate them. He should also be able to carry out simple excision biopsy of small noncystic nodules that may be either benign or malignant; the latter procedure is now often and easily done in an outpatient or transient operating room facility, frequently under local anesthesia. Furthermore, since a significant percentage of "suspicious areas" detected by mammography or xeroradiography in either clinically normal breasts or in those in which disease is suspected will also prove to be benign, the obstetrician-gynecologist, in collaboration with the radiologist, should perhaps become proficient in the often somewhat more difficult maneuver of performing excision biopsy of these frequently subclinical lesions, particularly since frozen-section diagnosis of such small areas of abnormality is undesirable and often impossible. Rather, such biopsy specimens should be evaluated in their entirety by detailed histologic study of permanent paraffin sections. Biopsy of these asymptomatic, subclinical but suspicious lesions is usually greatly facilitated by preoperative needle placement and lesion localization under xeromammographic guidance, as illustrated in Figure 77. Obviously, should the excision biopsy performed under any of these circumstances demonstrate malignancy, the patient would then be referred to a surgeon with the requisite training and experience in the management of carcinoma of the breast. There is now abundant evidence [1, 7, 19] that a minor delay of from five to seven days to as long as two weeks between the excisional biopsy and the definitive surgery does not involve any increased risk of metastases or local recurrence, nor does it diminish the chances of cure.

On the other hand, it may prove more logical, expeditious, and helpful to the patient for the obstetrician-gynecologist to refer directly to the appropriate general surgeon any patient with a clinical lesion that has all the earmarks of a malignant tumor, or any high-risk patient with suspicious clinical or radiologic breast findings. And finally, there may be some communities or hospitals where there are particularly firmly established traditions still in existence regarding just which specialists should be responsible for decisions about both the diagnosis and management of breast disease, and it will obviously be prudent for obstetrician-gynecologists practicing in these areas to continue to monitor all their patients closely, but to refer patients with clinically or radiologically suspicious breast lesions to properly qualified general surgeons for definitive diagnostic procedures and any indicated therapy.

RECOGNITION AND MANAGEMENT OF COMMON BREAST DISORDERS

Although carcinoma of the breast is the most significant breast disease from the standpoint of the patient's overall present and future health and well-being, patients come to the physician far more frequently because of a variety of other breast disorders that are for the most part benign. Many of these benign disorders require some form of treatment for relief of symptoms, and in almost all cases the possibility of malignancy must also be excluded. Since the gynecologist is primarily concerned with the early recognition of malignancy and with the symptomatic management of benign disorders, especially those related to the endocrine physiology of the breasts, an exhaustive coverage of diseases of the breast would be out of place in this text. Instead, the following discussions will concentrate primarily on the clinical symptoms and physical findings as presented by the patient to her gynecologist. For the sake of both clarity and brevity, the fundamental information that should be of help to the clinician in arriving at a correct diagnosis and arranging for proper therapy is outlined in more or less summary form for the more common breast abnormalities and disorders.

Anomalies and Anatomic Abnormalities

SUPERNUMERARY BREASTS AND NIPPLES

Supernumerary breasts (polymastia) and supernumerary nipples (polythelia) may occur anywhere along the so-called milk lines running bilaterally from axilla to groin. Supernumerary nipples are most often unaccompanied by underlying breast tissue proper, and areas of polymastia frequently lack overlying nipples. It should be remembered that the common prolongation of breast tissue into the axilla (**tail of Spence**) is a normal finding and does not represent an accessory breast. No treatment is obligatory for either polymastia or polythelia, but for cosmetic reasons, or because supernumerary breast tissue may become persistently painful after the menarche, excision is sometimes indicated.

PRECOCIOUS PREPUBERTAL BREAST DEVELOPMENT

Precocious prepubertal breast development may be secondary to ovarian or adrenal lesions (functioning tumors or hyperplasia) or to central nervous system lesions (tumors or cysts) involving the third ventricle, especially if it occurs before the age of 8 or 9 years. Appropriate clinical and laboratory investigation to exclude these possibilities is therefore indicated. In some instances of so-called idiopathic premature breast development in children, no specific cause will be found.

PREADOLESCENT BREAST DEVELOPMENT

Preadolescent breast development before the age of 10 or 11 is usually idiopathic and can safely be simply observed, reassuring the patient and her parents. (Adolescent budding of the breasts normally has begun by age 12 in 75 percent and by age 14 in 98 percent of young women.) Occasionally, the initial development will begin in an asymmetrical fashion. Again, it is important to reassure both the young girl and her parents, and, above all, not to examine the enlarging breast by biopsy. Invariably, the other breast will begin developing normally within a few months.

BREAST HYPERTROPHY

True hypertrophy of the breasts is a rare condition, usually of unknown etiology. It can be extremely painful and disabling, with one or both mammary glands attaining huge size. Simple or partial mastectomy or reduction mammoplasty may be necessary in some cases.

Infections of the Breast

ACUTE MASTITIS

Acute mastitis is hardly ever seen except in the puerperal state or during lactation. The diagnosis is rarely in doubt, and the infection usually responds to systemic antibiotics, local application of heat, adequate breast support, and cessation of lactation. Occasionally, the septic process progresses to abscess formation and requires incision and drainage.

BREAST ABSCESS

Breast abscess may be a primary focal infection within the breast tissue or ductal system or may result from secondary infection in a breast cyst (rarely, a carcinoma may also become secondarily infected). While an abscess in a nonlactating breast may occasionally respond to local heat application and systemic antibiotics, the majority will eventually require adequate incision and drainage. If chronic infection in an old abscess cavity persists, excision of that portion of the breast may be required. Rarely, the terminal portions of the duct system may become the site of persistent infection following a breast abscess and lead to a continuing purulent discharge from the nipple. If this does not respond to vigorous antibiotic therapy, excision of the involved portion of the terminal duct system may be necessary.

It should be constantly kept in mind that inflammatory carcinoma of the breast may suggest the possibility of cellulitis and breast abscess and vice versa, that is, a breast abscess with surrounding cellulitis may simulate inflammatory carcinoma, even to the cutaneous thickening and the characteristic peau d'orange (skin dimpling resembling orange peel) of the breast skin infiltrated by an underlying carcinoma. Rarely, an ordinary noninflammatory type of breast carcinoma may become infected, with or without prior ulceration of the tumor, and present a confusing picture until biopsy clarifies the situation. (This uncommon type of secondary infection in an ordinary breast cancer is usually of a more chronic, indolent nature as compared with the acute "cellulitislike" picture seen in true inflammatory carcinoma.)

PLASMA CELL MASTITIS

Plasma cell mastitis is a rare aseptic inflammatory disorder seen primarily in young married women. It, too, may resemble carcinoma until biopsy clarification is obtained. Treatment is symptomatic, with eventual spontaneous regression.

MISCELLANEOUS CHRONIC INFECTIONS

Miscellaneous chronic infections of the breast are rare nowadays and include tuberculosis, syphilis, actinomycosis, and similar fungal and granulomatous diseases. Cultures and biopsies will be necessary to establish the diagnosis and point the way to appropriate systemic and local treatment.

Chronic Cystic Mastitis (Fibrocystic Disease)

The fundamental features and diagnosis and management of chronic cystic mastitis, which comprises a broad spectrum of mixed breast disorders, have already been covered in detail in the section on cyclic breast disorders in Chapter 5. The spectrum includes the various clinical and pathologic entities of mastodynia, periductal mastitis, adenofibrosis, microscopic and macroscopic ("blue-domed") cysts, intraductal epithelial hyperplasia, intraductal papillomas and papillomatosis, blunt duct adenosis, and sclerosing adenosis.

Despite its popular name, chronic mastitis is not fundamentally an inflammatory disease at all but is clearly the result of abnormal or exaggerated response of areas of the breasts to their usual cyclic endocrine stimulation, which in turn may be abnormal (e.g., fibrocystic disease is more common in women prone to anovulatory or progesterone-deficient cycles). Fibrocystic disease is the most common cause of the appearance of a mass in the breast, and with a few exceptions, is almost invariably the explanation for recurring breast pain.

Although not accepted by all authorities, there is some evidence that cancer of the breast may occur as much as three to five times more frequently than usual in patients with fibrocystic disease. Hence these patients are also deserving of careful, periodic surveillance.

Benign Breast Tumors

FIBROADENOMAS

Fibroadenomas are by far the most common benign breast tumors and, although they may occur at any age, are most frequently seen in young women in their late teens or early twenties. They are rarely painful or symptomatic in any way; the patient or physician simply discovers a lump. Usually, the mass is a firm, nontender, rubbery-feeling, smoothly rounded, very mobile, slippery nodule, most often found in the periareolar region; its characteristic "feel" on physical examination is almost diagnostic. They are most often solitary, although occasionally multiple lesions may be present in one or both breasts. Since they persist and sometimes continue to enlarge, local excision of these well-encapsulated tumors is the treatment of choice.

CYSTOSARCOMA PHYLLOIDES

Cystosarcoma phylloides has now been firmly established as a giant, rapidly growing fibroadenoma, and the term *cystosarcoma* is actually usually a misnomer, since these lesions are rarely, if ever, truly malignant. Rapid attainment of a large, hard, lobulated mass in the breast without evidence of adjacent soft-tissue or axillary involvement usually suggests the correct diagnosis. Wide local resection and sometimes mastectomy will be required because of the large size these tumors often attain. In rare instances a microscopically verified, truly malignant cystosarcoma phylloides may be encountered, and since axillary lymph node metastases may occur in this situation, radical mastectomy is the indicated treatment.

INTRADUCTAL PAPILLOMA

Intraductal papilloma is the second most common benign breast tumor and is the most frequent cause of a bloody discharge from the nipple, its usual presenting symptom. A papilloma most often arises in the so-called lactiferous sinus of the milk duct system, which is situated approximately at the areolar margin. The symptomatic intraductal papilloma may or may not be large enough to be palpable, but the lobular duct system containing it can usually be localized by the systematic periareolar point-by-point pressure maneuver previously described; a galactogram can also be helpful when localization is difficult. Proper treatment thereafter is removal of the breast segment from which the discharge has been demonstrated to arise or which contains the palpable mass. Removal is important both to exclude the possibility that a much less common intraductal papillary adenocarcinoma is responsible for the bloody discharge, as well as to put an end to the symptom, which is a nuisance to the patient.

MISCELLANEOUS TUMORS

Miscellaneous less common benign breast tumors include **lipomas, fibromas, sweat-gland adenomas, hamartomas,** and **hemangiomas,** all of which require local excision for definitive diagnosis and treatment. **Granular cell myoblastoma** of the breast is a very rare benign tumor and is significant primarily because it sometimes presents all the clinical signs of early breast cancer; even on cut section of a biopsy specimen it may grossly resemble a scirrhus carcinoma. As is true for all solid breast masses, biopsy and microscopic examination are essential to establish a correct diagnosis and is usually the only way a granular cell myoblastoma can be recognized as a benign lesion.

Nonneoplastic Breast Masses

HEMATOMA

The history of prior trauma usually obtained, together with the characteristic findings, often suggests the correct diagnosis of hematoma. Treatment can be expectant, with spontaneous and uncomplicated resorption usually occurring; only rarely will evacuation by aspiration or by incision and drainage be necessary. In the case of an old hematoma, the diagnosis may be in doubt and excisional biopsy necessary.

FAT NECROSIS

Fat necrosis invariably follows trauma to the breast, although the incident may not be noted or remembered by the patient. Contusion of breast tissue results in hemorrhage into and degeneration and necrosis of the fatty tissue and a hard, indurated inflammatory reaction that may closely simulate cancer, even to the presence of overlying skin dimpling or retraction. Excisional biopsy is invariably necessary to establish a correct diagnosis.

MONDOR'S DISEASE

Mondor's disease is the occurrence of acute phlebitis and periphlebitis of the veins of the chest wall directly over the breast in a manner that suggests the presence of a mass in the breast. The redness, heat, and associated dilatation of neighboring venous channels in the overlying skin are often clues to the correct diagnosis, although the picture may also resemble that of inflammatory carcinoma. When Mondor's disease is suspected, hot packs and anticoagulants may be tried and resolution awaited. If the diagnosis remains in doubt, biopsy will be indicated.

Disorders of the Nipple and Areolar Region

NIPPLE RETRACTION

Nipple inversion is most frequently a normal anatomic variation of long standing, and though most often bilateral, is also sometimes unilateral. On examination, the involved nipple can usually be manually everted and temporarily placed in the more usual erect position.

True nipple retraction is usually of recent origin, invariably unilateral, implies an underlying disease process, and is potentially an ominous sign. However, not all nipple retraction is due to breast cancer nearby; subareolar fat necrosis, chronic intraductal infection, and plasma cell mastitis can also cause irreducible nipple retraction. Biopsy is therefore usually necessary to establish a definite diagnosis.

NIPPLE ULCERATION, EROSION, OR ECZEMATOID RASH

Simple erosions occur most commonly in nursing mothers and will usually respond to conservative local measures and temporary suspension of nursing. Erosions or ulcerations can be traumatic in origin in nonlactating women, but this occurs infrequently. When the nipple and surrounding areolar area is eroded, or covered by an eczematoid, weeping lesion, or both, the possibility of Paget's disease of the nipple with an underlying intraductal adenocarcinoma (not always palpable) should be strongly suspected. Mammography and then biopsies of the skin lesion and any palpable breast mass or abnormal breast area seen on the mammogram should be done to arrive at a definite diagnosis. Radical or modified radical mastectomy is the treatment of choice.

NIPPLE DISCHARGE

Milky discharge

Milky discharge from the nipple (the sort encountered in the galactorrhea or galactorrhea-amenorrhea syndromes seen in women in their active reproductive years) is usually, though not always, bilateral. It is invariably due to an endocrine disturbance, either primary in the cyclic regulating mechanism or secondary to a medication-induced hypothalamic-pituitary dysfunction. The approach to the diagnosis and management of this problem has already been discussed in Chapter 6. However, if this type of nipple discharge should appear in a postmenopausal woman, especially if it is unilateral, careful investigation regarding possible local breast disease should be undertaken, including mammography, cytologic study of the discharge, possibly galactography, and biopsy if the discharge can be demonstrated to be originating in a focal area of the lobular system or if a mass is palpable.

Serous Discharge

Serous discharge is seen most often with benign intraductal lesions such as papillomatosis, small papillomas, or epithelial hyperplasia. Again, if no mass is palpable, mammography or galactography may be helpful. If a mass is present, or if the discharge can be shown to originate in a certain segment of the ductal system, excisional biopsy is indicated.

Bloody Discharge

Bloody discharge is most often due to an intraductal papilloma, less often to an intraductal cancer. In any case, the portion of the breast containing a mass or suspicious area that is palpable, or mammographically demonstrated, or both, or that portion of the breast from which palpation or galactography shows the discharge to be arising, should be excised to remove the lesion and establish a definite diagnosis.

Serosanguineous Discharge

Serosanguineous discharge, on the other hand, is more characteristic of an intraductal carcinoma. A palpable mass is often present, and mammography may be of additional help in localizing the lesion. Again, excisional biopsy of the segment of breast containing the palpable or radiographically demonstrated abnormality and/or that portion of the breast from which the discharge can be shown to come is clearly indicated, with definitive treatment then based on the microscopic pathologic appearance.

Mammary Duct Ectasia

A dark green or multicolored discharge that is thick and sticky and almost always bilateral is characteristic of so-called **mammary duct ectasia,** or **comedomastitis.** It is the result of dilatation of the terminal ducts, with formation of an irritating, lipid-containing fluid that produces an inflammatory reaction and hypersecretion in the nipple. Conservative treatment with cleansing detergent soaps and gentle alcohol wipes, plus avoidance of any further nipple chafing or irritation, is the proper management.

BENIGN NIPPLE AND AREOLAR SWELLINGS

Benign nipple and areolar swellings sometimes appear when inspissated secretions cause plugging and obstruction with resulting cystic dilatation of one of the nipple ducts (**galactocele**), or when a similar type of ductal obstruction occurs and results in cystic dilatation of one of the **areolar glands of Montgomery**. Often, these will drain spontaneously and subside; occasionally, they will need to be opened and drained or completely excised.

MALIGNANT TUMORS OF THE BREAST

Carcinoma of the breast is by far the most common malignant tumor, occurring eventually in approximately 1 out of every 15 women in the United States, where about 85,000 new cases are seen annually and about 30,000 deaths occur each year. The earliest manifestation is usually a small, painless breast lump, most often first discovered by the patient but not infrequently first discovered by a physician during a routine checkup. Nowadays, many early lesions are being discovered with increasing frequency by mammography or xeromammography, done either as part of a screening program or because of symptomatic or palpable breast abnormalities.

Physical Examination

Although the technique of routine breast examination has already been described in Chapter 1, there are additional features of particular significance when palpation suggests the likelihood of breast cancer. If the tumor is near the surface, there may already be slight dimpling indicative of early skin involvement and hence diagnostic of carcinoma, or the dimpling can be rendered more obvious by gentle, circumferential compression of the skin about the mass beneath it.

Retraction of the overlying skin is very common (it is seen in perhaps 80 percent of palpable breast tumors and represents involvement of the suspensory ligaments of the breast). It is not necessarily an ominous sign so long as there is not widespread skin and lymphatic involvement or fixation to the chest wall. Although skin retraction is a fairly reliable diagnostic sign of carcinoma, it is occasionally seen in association with benign breast conditions such as abscess and fat necrosis, or in the vicinity of old scars.

Shortening of **Cooper's ligaments** (the numerous fibrous septa running through the breast tissue from the underlying pectoralis muscle fascia to the overlying skin) by malignant infiltration, with resulting elevation and retraction of the breast can often be demonstrated by having the patient raise her arms. On the other hand, if the tumor is more deeply situated and there has been extension to involve the soft tissues of the chest wall proper, observing the asymmetrical motion of the involved breast (which does not fall away from the chest) in contrast to the free movement of the contralateral, uninvolved breast (which does fall away) when the patient leans forward will clearly disclose any tendency to fixation of the breast to the chest wall.

More ominous physical findings indicative of advanced and extensive local spread of the tumor and a poor prognosis include (1) the so-called peau d'orange (a pebbly dimpling and thickening of the skin with associated widening and depression of hair-follicle and sweat-gland openings indicative of the stasis and edema of the skin that results from extensive intracutaneous spread of the cancer); (2) the local anatomic appearance termed **cancer en cuirasse** (a large shieldlike palpable plaque of tumor due to widespread intracutaneous extension of cancer throughout the lymphatics of the breast, upper abdomen, and shoulder); (3) the presence of enlarged, hard, fixed axillary nodes in association with a swollen arm; and (4) the presence of skin ulceration due to extensive involvement by an underlying carcinoma.

The clinical picture of **inflammatory carcinoma** is seen in 1 to 2 percent of breast cancers and is characterized by obvious redness and local heat over a sizable area of breast skin, which is usually markedly thickened as well. The underlying breast may feel diffusely indurated or may seem to contain a large, hard mass. Nipple retraction is often present (in 50 percent of cases). It is important to recognize inflammatory carcinoma and distinguish it promptly from mastitis or breast abscess. Immediate mammography is often very helpful in establishing the diagnosis quickly, which can then be confirmed by needle aspiration biopsy, avoiding open surgical biopsy whenever possible.

Diagnosis

The additional diagnostic maneuvers commonly employed in definitely establishing a diagnosis of cancer of the breast have already been described, together with the indications for their use and their limitations. None of these studies is a substitute for surgical biopsy, especially in the presence of a single, discrete, dominant breast mass (not an easily aspirated simple cyst, of course), so that a suspicious breast mass must be examined by biopsy even when the x-ray findings are nondiagnostic for malignancy.

Management

An in-depth discussion of the treatment of breast cancer is ordinarily considered to be beyond the useful scope of a textbook of gynecology. However, since the gynecologist in his discussions with his patients needs to be knowledgeable concerning the various types of breast cancer and the general principles of their individual therapy, this chapter concludes with a brief summary thereof. Further reading relative to the surgical, medical (hormonal and chemotherapy), and radiotherapeutic management of breast cancer is strongly recommended for the gynecologist particularly interested in this field, and some useful articles selected from the current literature are included in the reference list.

CLASSIFICATION OF BREAST CANCER

There are two principal varieties of breast carcinoma, those originating within the ductal system (ductal or intraductal carcinomas), which make up about 70 percent of all breast cancers, and those arising in the glandular tissue of the mammary lobules (adenocarcinomas), which account for 25 to 30 percent of all breast cancers. In addition, Paget's disease of the nipple represents a relatively infrequent third type of carcinoma, and there is also a small group of highly undifferentiated carcinomas that do not fall into any of these three previous categories. Sarcomas of the breast are exceedingly rare. The following helpful histologic classification was proposed by Stewart [22]:

I. Paget's disease of the nipple.
II. Carcinoma of the mammary ducts.
   a. Noninfiltrating.
      1. Papillary carcinoma.
      2. Comedocarcinoma.
   b. Infiltrating.
      1. Papillary carcinoma.
      2. Comedocarcinoma.
      3. Carcinoma with fibrosis (scirrhus carcinoma).
      4. Medullary carcinoma with lymphoid infiltration.
      5. Colloid carcinoma.
III. Carcinoma of lobules (adenocarcinoma of glandular origin).
   a. Noninfiltrating (lobular carcinoma in situ).
   b. Infiltrating.
IV. Rare carcinomas: undifferentiated carcinomas; gelatinous adenocarcinomas, etc.
V. Sarcomas.

PAGET'S DISEASE OF THE NIPPLE

Paget's disease of the nipple is an eczematoid lesion entirely similar to Paget's disease of the vulva, as described in Chapter 16, but with an invariably associated underlying intraductal carcinoma. Although the intraductal carcinoma may not always be palpable, it can often be localized by mammography. In any case, biopsy of the nipple lesion will demonstrate the typical, foamy "Paget's cells," with vesicular nuclei and vacuolated cytoplasm in the epidermis. Mastectomy of the radical or modified radical type is the treatment usually indicated. Although lymph node metastases are not as frequent as with the more common types of breast cancer, they are seen often enough in patients with Paget's disease to make axillary dissection worthwhile.

CARCINOMA OF THE MAMMARY DUCTS

Noninfiltrating Carcinoma

Papillary carcinoma and comedocarcinoma, the two less malignant varieties of intraductal carcinoma, are confined within the duct, the first a fairly focal lesion, the second a more diffuse one. Unfortunately, they make up only a small percentage of clinically recognizable breast cancers, but perhaps with increasing use of screening mammography, the proportion will continue to increase. Lymphatic spread is rare until ductal carcinomas have actually infiltrated beyond the duct wall into surrounding tissues. This type of lesion is often suitable for modified radical mastectomy or occasionally even for simple mastectomy (total mastectomy without lymph node dissection). However, because of the multicentric nature of breast carcinoma in general, local excision (e.g., "lobulectomy," "quadrantectomy," or tylectomy ["lumpectomy"]) is unwise, even for these early, favorable lesions. The cure rate for these relatively noninvasive cancers following total or modified radical mastectomy should be 90 percent or better.

Infiltrating Carcinoma

Once the intraductal carcinoma infiltrates the wall and invades the surrounding tissues, the possibility of lymphatic, pectoral-muscle, and cutaneous involvement increases. However, the papillary, comedocarcinoma, and medullary varieties all tend to spread slowly and attain a large size before metastasizing. Thus they have a better-than-average cure rate if treated promptly and adequately. Scirrhus duct carcinomas are the most common of all breast cancers, making up 80 percent of the total, and typically occur in the small, atrophic breasts of elderly women. They usually present as small, rock-hard, irregular lesions beneath a slightly dimpled, flattened, or puckered overlying skin. Despite the large amount of fibrous tissue stroma comprising these tumors, they tend to spread and metastasize rather widely before they are discovered; axillary metastases are also common, and the prognosis is relatively less favorable. At the present time, radical mastectomy with complete axillary lymph node dissection is the treatment recommended by most authorities for operable lesions of the infiltrating intraductal carcinoma type.

CARCINOMA OF LOBULES (ADENOCARCINOMA OF GLANDULAR ORIGIN)

Adenocarcinomas of glandular origin tend to be slowly growing, well localized and circumscribed bulky tumors, slow to metastasize to regional nodes. They most often arise in the periphery of the breast and in a superficial location just beneath the skin (intraductal carcinomas, on the other hand, tend to arise in the central portion of the breast beneath the nipple and periareolar region); they are therefore often discovered sooner by the patient. Perhaps for these reasons, infiltrating adenocarcinomas offer a somewhat more favorable prognosis than the majority of infiltrating ductal carcinomas. Lobular carcinoma in situ can usually be safely treated by a modified or conservative type of total mastectomy. Radical or modified radical mastectomy (depending on the size and location of the lesion) is the currently accepted method of treatment for infiltrating adenocarcinomas of the breast.

GENERAL PRINCIPLES OF TREATMENT

Optimal management of the more common type of breast cancer, when detected early, has already been briefly noted. When the tumor is small and the disease still appears to be confined to the breast, routine diagnostic evaluation need not include a skeletal x-ray survey, bone scan, liver scan, or elaborate blood chemistry determinations (e.g., serum calcium, phosphorus, alkaline phosphatase, LDH, SGOT), for in this situation these studies are seldom, if ever, abnormal. Rather, these studies should be reserved for patients in whom the lesion is more extensive or in whom the history and findings suggest or disclose the presence of axillary lymph node metastases or the existence of distant spread, especially pulmonary or bony metastases. (When skeletal metastases do occur, they most frequently involve the lumbar vertebrae, pelvis, and proximal femurs.)

Radical or Modified Radical Mastectomy

In general, the treatment recommended by most authorities for so-called operable infiltrating ductal or glandular breast carcinomas is radical mastectomy or, in the case of small, early lesions (especially asymptomatic, subclinical tumors first discovered by mammography), modified radical mastectomy. Preliminary excisional biopsy is of course necessary to establish a definite diagnosis. The five-year survival rate for operable stages of breast cancer following radical mastectomy approaches 85 to 90 percent if the axillary nodes are not involved, whereas it falls to 25 to 35 percent if there is significant axillary nodal involvement. Radical mastectomy is also followed by consistently good 10-year survival rates, and there is a low incidence of local (in 5 to 10 percent) and axillary (1 to 2 percent) recurrence. However, the cosmetic result, with the axillary hollow and the occurrence of swelling of the arm in some patients (in 20 to 30 percent in some series), is not always satisfactory. Thus for the very early lesions in which the chance of lymphatic dissemination or pectoral muscle involvement is small, modified radical mastectomy with preservation of the pectoralis major muscle (sometimes sparing the pectoralis minor also) and a somewhat limited axillary dissection has much to recommend it. Subsequent plastic reconstruction of the breast can also be done successfully in many cases, if desired, following a modified radical mastectomy, whereas breast reconstruction is seldom possible or satisfactory after radical mastectomy. Modified radical mastectomy is therefore probably the procedure of choice in patients with "minimal breast cancer," i.e., noninfiltrating duct carcinoma, lobular carcinoma in situ, Paget's disease of the nipple with an underlying noninfiltrating intraductal cancer, and small, low-grade infiltrating cancers, especially those first detected by mammography or xeromammography alone. Simple mastectomy or partial mastectomy (tylectomy or "lumpectomy") is not adequate treatment for minimal breast cancer because of the known patterns of local extension and local and regional lymphatic dissemination in the first instance, and the known tendency to multicentricity of breast carcinoma in the second instance. (It should also be noted that the cosmetic end result following partial mastectomy is very unsatisfactory in a great many instances). However, simple mastectomy may sometimes be elected as appropriate treatment for early carcinoma in elderly, high-risk patients with limited life expectancy.

Alternatives to Radical or Modified Radical Mastectomy

Several alternatives to radical or modified radical mastectomy for operable lesions have recently been proposed, and the efficacy of these alternatives is under thorough trial at the present time. These include simple mastectomy followed by irradiation of the regional lymph node areas (axillary, mediastinal, and supraclavicular), and programs involving radiotherapy alone, e.g., x-ray therapy with or without supplemental interstitial irradiation to the breast and chest wall, plus external irradiation to the regional lymph node areas. To date there is no truly convincing evidence that therapy based primarily on radiation treatment yields as high cure rates as a conventional radical or modified radical mastectomy. Furthermore, there is a significant incidence of troublesome side effects following full irradiation therapy, e.g., radiation fibrosis of the lung with impaired pulmonary function and recurring pneumonitis, radiation esophagitis, adverse skin reactions (radiation dermatitis), and lymphedema of the arm. And finally, although the possibility of achieving cure of breast cancer while at the same time preserving the breast and pectoral muscles is an attractive and appealing one to both patient and physician, the cosmetic end result in terms of the final appearance of the breast following full irradiation therapy often leaves much to be desired.

Contraindications to Radical or Modified Radical Mastectomy

There are certain definite contraindications to radical mastectomy in the management of carcinoma of the breast, as follows:

1. In inflammatory breast cancer, mastectomy not only fails to cure but also often fails to be palliative and serves only to cause further dissemination of the disease. Treatment of the inflammatory carcinoma should be by radiotherapy, supplemented by oophorectomy (in premenopausal, menopausal, and early postmenopausal women), chemotherapy, and/or hormonal therapy, as indicated.
2. When distant metastases are present, oophorectomy should be done in all patients for whom this would be appropriate, with chemotherapy and/or hormonal therapy given for the generalized metastatic disease; occasionally, irradiation might be given for apparent isolated, symptomatic, distant metastasis. In addition, local irradiation or, at times, even simple mastectomy might be necessary to deal with the local disease in the breast.
3. Massive and/or fixed axillary or supraclavicular nodal metastases. For therapy, see (5).
4. Extensive axillary infiltration with swelling of the arm. For therapy, see (5).
5. Extensive fixation resulting from invasion of the chest wall. In (3), (4), and (5), an appropriate combination of irradiation, hormone therapy (estrogens, or androgens, or cortisone) or endocrine ablation therapy (oophorectomy, or adrenalectomy, or hypophysectomy), and chemotherapy should be given. Rarely, in a patient with a reasonably limited area of chest-wall invasion whose lesion was otherwise suitable for radical mastectomy, the chances for cure might be better if radical mastectomy was performed with an en bloc resection in continuity of

the involved chest wall and overlying breast and pectoral muscles, together with axillary and internal mammary node dissections ("superradical mastectomy").
6. The patient may refuse an operation, in which case she can be offered the alternative of radiation therapy.

When radical or modified radical mastectomy with axillary node dissection has been carried out, the question has arisen whether or not the cure rate might be increased by any form of supplemental therapy, specifically, oophorectomy, postoperative irradiation, and chemotherapy.

Careful prospective, randomized, and controlled studies have shown that, whether or not the axillary nodes are involved, prophylactic oophorectomy in premenopausal or menopausal women has no significant effect on the appearance of distant metastases, nor does it prolong survival in patients in whom local recurrence or distant metastasis does occur. In fact, waiting to perform oophorectomy until there is a recurrence or metastasis appears to yield equally good palliation and possibly even a longer overall worthwhile survival time.

The use of postoperative irradiation in patients in whom two or more axillary lymph nodes are found to be positive on histologic study is advocated by many. Treatment is usually directed to the axillary, mediastinal (internal mammary), and supraclavicular nodal areas, and there is some evidence that such a program may improve the five-year survival rate and the absolute curability in this group of patients.

The use of postoperative irradiation (internal mammary, mediastinal, and supraclavicular areas) in patients whose lesions have arisen in the central portion or medial quadrants of the breast (and thus can be expected to spread to the internal mammary chain of nodes with a frequency equal to or greater than their tendency to metastasize to the axillary nodes) also seems indicated in the majority of such instances. However, some authorities prefer to do internal mammary lymph node dissections as well as axillary lymph node dissections (extended radical mastectomy) rather than give routine postoperative irradiation to patients with subareolar or inner-quadrant lesions.

Prospective, randomized, controlled studies are currently still under way indicating that postoperative adjuvant chemotherapy (e.g., in one study, a short intraoperative and postoperative course of triethylenethiophosphoramide [THIOTEPA] in conjunction with radical mastectomy and in another collaborative program, a longer postoperative course of L-phenylalanine mustard) appears to increase both the 5- and 10-year survival rates and to decrease the rates of local recurrence and distant metastasis in premenopausal women with significant axillary node involvement (four or more nodes positive) [8]. Women who received adjuvant chemotherapy had a 21 percent greater 10-year survival rate and a 21 percent lower incidence of recurrent or metastatic disease.

Management of Local Recurrence and Distant Metastases

Local recurrence in the mastectomy scar or adjacent chest wall in the absence of demonstrable distant metastases, especially if it does not occur until two or three years after the mastectomy, may sometimes be treated successfully by reexcision and then close follow-up, provided that the recurrent tumor is well circumscribed and involves only a limited area. More extensive locally recurrent disease, particularly if there are multiple lesions, or the relatively infrequent axillary recurrences, will be best managed by irradiation locally, possibly supplemented by hormone therapy, when indicated (estrogen, androgen, or cortisone), endocrine ablation, when appropriate (oophorectomy, adrenalectomy, or hypophysectomy), or chemotherapy (e.g., 5-fluorouracil and/or cyclophosphamide [Cytoxan]; less often, methotrexate, vincristine, or adriamycin) when the disease does not respond to hormonal manipulations. These three modalities of treatment, usually in judiciously selected combination, are obviously the ones to be employed in the management of patients with more generalized metastatic disease.

REFERENCES

1. Abramson, D. J. 857 breast biopsies as an outpatient procedure: Delayed mastectomy in 41 cases. *Ann. Surg.* 163:478, 1966.
2. Anglem, T. J., and Leber, R. E. Characteristics of ten year survivors after radical mastectomy for cancer of the breast. *Am. J. Surg.* 121:363, 1971.
3. Bibbo, M., and Zuspan, R. P. Fine-needle aspiration of the breast in an obstetrics and gynecology hospital. *Am. J. Obstet. Gynecol.* 122:525, 1975.
4. Crile, G., Esselstyn, C. B., Hermann, R. E., and Hoerr, S. O. A new look at biopsy of the breast. *Am. J. Surg.* 126:117, 1973.
5. Dall'Olmo, C. A., Ponka, J. L., Horn, R. C., Jr., and Riu, R. Lobular carcinoma of the breast in situ: Are we too radical in its treatment? *Arch. Surg.* 110:537, 1975.
6. Donegan, W. L. Simple mastectomy for early and advanced mammary carcinoma. *Am. J. Surg.* 128:37, 1974.
7. Earle, S. S. Delayed operation for breast carcinoma. *Surg. Gynecol. Obstet.* 131:291, 1970.
8. Fisher, B., Slack, N., Katrych, D., and Wolmark, N. Ten year follow-up results of patients with carcinoma of the breast in a co-operative clinical trial evaluating surgical adjuvant chemotherapy. *Surg. Gynecol. Obstet.* 140:528, 1975.
9. Hoge, A. F., Shaw, M. T., Bottomley, R. H., and Hartsuck, J. M. Therapeutic regimens in advanced breast cancer. *J.A.M.A.* 231:1357, 1975.
10. Kline, T. S., and Neal, H. S. Role of needle aspiration biopsy in diagnosis of carcinoma of the breast. *Obstet. Gynecol.* 46:89, 1975.
11. Leis, H. P., Jr. Clinical diagnosis of breast cancer. *J. Reprod. Med.* 14:231, 1975.
12. Lewis, J. D., Milbrath, J. R., Shaffer, K. A., and DeCosse, J. J. Implications of suspicious findings in breast cancer screening. *Arch. Surg.* 110:903, 1975.
13. Madden, J. L. Modified radical mastectomy. *Surg. Gynecol. Obstet.* 121:1221, 1965.
14. McLaughlin, C. W., Jr., and Coe, J. D. Cancer of the breast. *Am. J. Surg.* 125:734, 1973.
15. Morgenstern, L., Kaufman, P. A., and Friedman, N. B. The case against tylectomy for carcinoma of the breast: The factor of multicentricity. *Am. J. Surg.* 130:251, 1975.
16. Nelson, A. J., and Montague, E. D. Resectable localized breast cancer: The rationale for combined surgery and irradiation. *J.A.M.A.* 231:189, 1975.

17. Papatestas, A. E., and Lesnick, G. J. Treatment of carcinoma of the breast by modified radical mastectomy. *Surg. Gynecol. Obstet.* 140:22, 1975.
18. Robbins, G. F., Shah, J., Rosen, P., Chu, F., and Taylor, J. Inflammatory carcinoma of the breast. *Surg. Clin. North Am.* 54:801, 1974.
19. Saltzstein, E. C., Mann, R. W., Shua, T. Y., and DeCosse, J. J. Outpatient breast biopsy. *Arch. Surg.* 109:287, 1974.
20. Segaloff, A. Hormone treatment of breast cancer. *J.A.M.A.* 234:1175, 1975.
21. Spratt, J. S., Jr., and Donegan, W. L. *Cancer of the Breast.* Philadelphia: Saunders, 1967.
22. Stewart, F. W. Tumors of the Breast. In *Atlas of Tumor Pathology,* Fascicle 34. Washington, D.C.: Armed Forces Institute of Pathology, 1950.
23. Strax, P. Breast cancer diagnosis: Mammography, thermography, and xerography: A commentary. *J. Reprod. Med.* 14:265, 1975.
24. Wanebo, H. J., Huvos, A. G., and Urban, J. A. Treatment of minimal breast cancer. *Cancer* 33:349, 1974.
25. Wever, E., and Hellman, S. Radiation as primary treatment for local control of breast carcinoma: A progress report. *J.A.M.A.* 234:608, 1975.
26. Westbrook, K. C., and Gallager, H. S. Intraductal carcinoma of the breast: A comparative study. *Am. J. Surg.* 130:667, 1975.

22

Basic Principles of Operative Gynecology and Preoperative Care

As has been indicated throughout this book, diagnostic operative procedures or surgical treatment varying in scope with the nature and extent of the disease process are frequently called for in the management of gynecologic disorders. Although the need for a diagnostic surgical procedure arises more often, actual operative therapy will be required in perhaps only 10 to 20 percent of patients undergoing treatment for pelvic conditions.

The chief indications for elective pelvic surgery are: (1) the correction of congenital anomalies or acquired structural abnormalities of the reproductive tract that interfere with normal menstrual function or that have impaired fertility or the capacity to maintain a normal pregnancy and successfully deliver a normal infant; (2) the treatment of chronic or recurrent manifestations of pelvic inflammatory disease or endometriosis; (3) the treatment of benign and malignant pelvic neoplasms or recognized premalignant disorders; (4) the repair of childbirth injuries sustained by the uterus and vagina and their supporting structures; and (5) (least often) the definitive treatment of certain persistent or recurrent functional disorders refractory to attempts at nonsurgical or minor surgical management (e.g., D&C). Emergency surgery for pelvic conditions is only occasionally indicated, usually in connection with disorders of early pregnancy, in the management of acute complications of pelvic inflammatory diseases and endometriosis, and in the treatment of vascular accidents occurring in ovarian lesions.

The essentials of the various diagnostic operative procedures are outlined in Chapter 2. The indications for, and the results that may generally be expected from, surgical treatment of the various pelvic disorders in which it may be applicable have also been presented in the appropriate chapters. While technical details of the operative procedures themselves are not within the scope of this survey of clinical gynecology, it is believed important to include a section on the fundamentals of preoperative and postoperative care, basic surgical principles essential to the proper performance of any pelvic procedure, whether by an abdominal or a vaginal approach, and the essential features of the recognition, management, and prevention of the common postoperative complications. These final chapters can thus serve to supplement any of the several excellent descriptive atlases of gynecologic operative procedures by providing additional details of the preoperative and postoperative supervision of patients undergoing pelvic operations for gynecologic disease.

PREOPERATIVE PREPARATION FOR PELVIC OPERATIONS

Vaginal Procedures

Whenever possible, existing vaginitis should be treated prior to hospitalization for elective operation. However, the use of routine cleansing douches or the local

631

application of vaginal antibiotic suppositories is unnecessary. The latter may even be harmful, having been incriminated recently as a possible cause of postoperative urinary tract infections by drug-resistant organisms. In postmenopausal women with simple atrophic changes, the prior use of estrogens locally or systemically to soften the tissues and promote healing is advocated by some but is only rarely necessary or indicated. In the case of an irreducible, edematous procidentia, often with superficially infected erosions of the cervix and adjacent vaginal mucosa, a few days of bed rest with the foot of the bed slightly elevated will resolve the congestion and edema and permit replacement of the uterus and prolapsed vagina within the vagina canal. Until reduction of the prolapse becomes possible, during the time the uterus and vagina remain exposed, warm, frequently changed saline compresses will usually suffice to clear up the superficial sepsis and even cause erosions to heal. The vaginal operation will then be considerably easier and the danger of postoperative infection or poor healing greatly reduced.

The bowel should be completely emptied by preoperative enemas to facilitate vaginal exposure and maneuvering during the operative procedure. For the same reason, the bladder should be emptied by catheter aseptically and as gently as possible during the course of preparing the vaginal field in the operating room. An empty bladder and rectosigmoid are also essential to an accurate pelvic examination under anesthesia.

Pelvic Laparotomy

The same preoperative routine is employed for pelvic laparotomy as for any lower abdominal operation. In addition, a careful vaginal preparation with antiseptics and catheterization of the bladder immediately prior to abdominal incision is essential if hysterectomy is contemplated or conceivably might be necessary. Preoperative placement of an inlying gastrointestinal suction tube (Levin, Miller-Abbott, or Harris) is rarely indicated in preparation for a simple pelvic laparotomy, with one possible exception: removal of a large pelvic tumor (e.g., huge fibroids or a giant ovarian cyst), that fills the abdomen and has compressed the entire small bowel into the limited remaining free space in the upper abdomen, since this is often followed by a prolonged ileus with profound abdominal distention, often dangerously refractory to the usual conservative measures once it has become established. This serious, occasionally nearly fatal complication can be avoided by preoperative gastrointestinal intubation, and maintenance of continuous suction postoperatively until normal peristaltic function returns will usually promote a smooth recovery in spite of the sudden, massive "decompression" of the abdomen with its attendant reflex ileus, which has been initiated by removal of the large tumor.

Rarely, preliminary cystoscopy and placement of indwelling ureteral catheters is indicated when simple total hysterectomy is contemplated in the presence of broad-ligament or cervical fibroids, extensive endometriosis, or advanced pelvic inflammatory disease. In any of these conditions, the normal anatomy may be greatly distorted, and even initial, extensive dissections of the ureters to demonstrate their course and protect them from injury may prove difficult and hazardous.

Under certain circumstances, proper timing of the laparotomy when hysterectomy is to be done is important. Obviously, the patient should be fully recovered from any recent upper respiratory or viral infection before elective hysterectomy is undertaken. But, more specifically, for example, it is wise to allow a one-month interval between completion of preoperative x-ray therapy and subsequent hysterectomy for cancer of the uterus. This interval allows the acute inflammatory reaction and increased vascularity to subside, restoring conditions more favorable for the dissection and for postoperative healing. And in the case of patients with carcinoma in situ of the cervix in whom a preliminary diagnostic conization has been necessary to exclude definitively the possible presence of invasive cancer, it has definitely been shown that unless hysterectomy is done within 48 hours of the conization, an interval of four to six weeks should elapse before proceeding [2, 6]. If hysterectomy is done in the interim instead, the risk and incidence of serious postoperative pelvic sepsis as well as abdominal wound infections is much higher.

Radical Pelvic Surgery

In radical Wertheim hysterectomy with bilateral pelvic lymphadenectomies, radical Schauta vaginal hysterectomy with or without bilateral extraperitoneal pelvic lymphadenectomies, anterior, posterior, or total pelvic exenterations, and one-stage radical vulvectomy with bilateral radical groin and pelvic node dissections, the procedures and their postoperative convalescences are facilitated by the additional routine preoperative maneuvers (exceptions as noted) detailed in the following sections.

INTESTINAL TRACT INTUBATION

Gastrointestinal intubation with a Levin, Harris, or Miller-Abbott tube, according to individual preference, the night before operation and institution of suction drainage to deflate the bowel makes packing it off from the field of radical dissection easier and less traumatic and minimizes the morbidity of the more prolonged intestinal ileus that follows these more radical procedures. (**Exceptions:** These measures are unnecessary with radical vulvectomy or with radical Schauta vaginal hysterectomy, which are essentially extraabdominal procedures and are only rarely followed by significant disturbances in gastrointestinal tract function.)

PREOPERATIVE SYSTEMIC ANTIBIOTICS

Prophylactic antibiotic therapy seems definitely indicated because of the radical nature of the dissections, the increased operating time and exposure of the wound to potential contamination from the outside, and the frequent presence of sepsis in the tumors and their lymphatic drainage areas. A combination of penicillin and streptomycin in adequate dosage continues to be the most effective routine antibiotic program for this purpose. As emphasized by the experimental studies of Burke [1] and others, the drugs must be given within a few hours of the actual start of the operation (3 to 6 hours at most) if any preventive effect whatsoever is to be achieved. They are best given initially an hour or two immediately prior to surgery, with their administration continued regularly thereafter at the standard intervals necessary to achieve constant effective drug levels during the operation and subsequent convalescence. They can usually be discontinued after four to five days. The use of preoperative prophylactic antibiotics in these procedures has markedly reduced the former high incidence of postoperative peritonitis and operative field or wound infections.

PREOPERATIVE BOWEL PREPARATION

Preoperative bowel preparation is always indicated when pelvic exenteration is contemplated and the large bowel may have to be transected. It should include mechanical cleansing with mild cathartics and enemas for several days preoperatively, a low-residue diet to obtain an empty bowel, and the oral administration of intestinal antibiotics or sulfonamides in the usual dosages to reduce the bacterial flora to a minimum.

PREPARATION OF BLADDER AND RECTUM

There are two helpful maneuvers that can be performed immediately before positioning the patient for the abdominal incision:

1. During the perineal and vaginal preparation, placement of an inlying Foley catheter to keep the bladder constantly empty and out of the way during these prolonged procedures.
2. Placement of an inlying rectal tube (unnecessary in radical vulvectomy or Schauta procedure). A No. 24 rectal tube is placed 6 to 8 inches within the rectum and taped to the buttocks, permitting any accumulation of intestinal gas that might otherwise distend the rectum and sigmoid and interfere with operative exposure to pass out or to be manually expressed from within the abdomen.

Preliminary cystoscopy and placement of ureteral catheters as a means of delineating the course of the ureters, although formerly advocated by a few physicians, appears to be rarely, if ever, necessary, since the extensive dissection required in the performance of these radical procedures readily and easily displays the ureters throughout their entire course. Furthermore, there is reason to believe that catheters lying within the ureteral lumens during their dissection may sometimes be traumatic in themselves.

ANESTHESIA FOR GYNECOLOGIC SURGERY

Neither the choice of agent nor the safe conduct of anesthesia for pelvic surgery ordinarily presents any special problem. As always, proper and conscientious evaluation of the patient preoperatively with respect to any potential anesthetic risk is essential; even if only a curettage is contemplated, complications during anesthesia are just as possible and just as likely to prove serious, if and when they occur, as in more extensive operations. Obviously, when indicated, the cardiac, pulmonary, and renal status of the patient should be thoroughly assessed, and if any degree of impairment is found, medical measures should be taken to achieve maximal preoperative improvement in the state of these vital functions wherever possible. Of particular importance in gynecologic patients is the recognition and correction of any secondary anemia or diminished blood volume before proceeding with anesthesia and surgery for the many pelvic disorders accompanied by significant acute and chronic blood loss. If not corrected, anemia and reduced blood volume pose potentially serious anesthetic hazards.

In view of the widespread use of antihypertensive agents and tranquilizers (women with certain pelvic disorders are particularly apt to have received them for systemic conditions not directly related to their pelvic disease), many of which occasion a sudden hypotension following induction of anesthesia, it is important to have obtained the history of their administration and if possible to omit them for a week or two before undertaking procedures requiring general anesthesia. If the patient has been on corticosteroids (e.g., for asthma or arthritis), it is even more vital to elicit this information, for special preoperative and postoperative corticoid supportive therapy is obviously indicated, and the anesthetist must even be prepared to proceed with the intravenous administration of supplemental hydrocortisone during anesthesia and surgery. Finally, a history of allergies, particularly of known barbiturate or procaine hydrochloride sensitivities, will nearly always contraindicate the use of certain anesthetic agents and techniques.

Under ordinary circumstances, however, almost all anesthetic agents and techniques can be suitably used. For example, ether is an extremely versatile and valuable agent, with a wide margin of safety, and it need not have the unpleasant side effects usually ascribed to it if administered properly. Cyclopropane is favored by many anesthesiologists fo emergency situations in which a low blood volume is present and cannot be completely replaced prior to the surgical procedure necessary to arrest hemorrhage (e.g., ruptured ectopic pregnancy with massive, continuing bleeding). Thiopental (Pentothal), nitrous oxide, and halothane (Fluothane) are all useful for minor procedures when profound muscle relaxation is not required. Again, none is without its own potential complications. For example, severe laryngospasm, potentially fatal unless dealt with promptly and effectively, may occur under light thiopental anesthesia. Halothane produces considerable myometrial relaxation as well as vasodilatation of the uterine vascular bed and thus should not be employed during curettage for incomplete abortion, although it is an excellent agent for D&C and other minor procedures in the nonpregnant state.

The use of muscle relaxants, e.g., curare or succinylcholine chloride (Anectine), in conjunction with agents such as thiopental or halothane, provides excellent anesthesia and muscle relaxation for major pelvic surgery. Here again, both the surgeon and the anesthesiologist must be clearly aware of the additional hazards introduced when these muscle relaxants are employed; in particular, they must be aware of the need to assure adequate pulmonary ventilation in the face of the profound generalized muscular paralysis often induced. The same considerations apply when spinal anesthesia, which provides ideal operating conditions for the pelvic surgeon, is used.

Finally, the surgeon should keep in mind the significance of the various patient positions commonly required for the performance of pelvic surgery, namely, the lithotomy position for vaginal procedures and the Trendelenburg position so often necessary and helpful in facilitating pelvic laparotomy. Either may have important physiologic effects on cardiovascular and pulmonary function, for obvious reasons, and may markedly influence pulmonary ventilation and the dynamics of cardiac output, as well as venous return to the heart. All of these factors must be taken into account in dealing with any cardiopulmonary difficulties that may arise during the course of anesthesia and surgery.

Just as important is the proper, safe placement of the patient in these positions to avoid nerve, muscle, or joint injury. When the lithotomy position is to be used, the feet and ankles should be well padded, and the stirrups should be arranged to avoid pressure against the thighs and knees, lest drop foot, secondary to peroneal nerve pressure, or muscular or joint pain develop postoperatively. When laparotomy in the steep Trendelenburg position is contemplated, a soft cloth foot tie, fastened carefully around padded feet and ankles, will most safely bear much of the weight of the patient and permit the use of a single shoulder brace with the arm at the side; only the opposite arm will be moderately abducted and supported on an arm board for the purpose of intravenous fluid administration during the procedure. In this way, the danger of producing a brachial palsy can be avoided, since this serious complication has most often occurred when the arm used for the intravenous has become hyperabducted in the presence of a shoulder brace on the same side, the full weight of the patient (and sometimes, unfortunately, a portion of the weight of the surgeon or assistant) exerting a tremendous stretching force on the vulnerable brachial plexus.

Postoperative sciatic and femoral neuropathies, usually unilateral, have been reported following vaginal hysterectomy [4, 5]. These injuries are presumed to be due to abnormal stretching of the sciatic or femoral nerves resulting from hyperextension, hyperflexion, or excessive abduction, internal rotation, or external rotation of the thighs, especially if the legs are extended at any time while the patient is in the lithotomy position. These abnormal positions may be caused by initial exaggeration of the position or by abnormal pressure on the thighs and legs if the assistants are braced or leaning against them during the operation. Occasionally, postoperative femoral neuropathy is also encountered following pelvic laparotomy, but the mechanism is entirely different and involves direct pressure on or stretching of the femoral nerve by self-retaining retractor blades. This is most commonly due to use of a retractor with blades that are too deep for the size of the patient at hand, especially if a transverse or Pfannenstiel incision has been used, allowing the blades to slide even more laterally than possible with a vertical midline incision. It is extremely important to do everything possible to avoid these nerve injuries, because although eventual recovery of motor and sensory function is usually the rule, the period of disability may last for many months or even several years.

Adequate provision for blood replacement during the procedure should be made well in advance. This is particularly true when radical pelvic surgery is in prospect and the chance of significant blood loss a definite one. It is far safer and more effective to keep abreast of blood loss as it occurs than to be faced with a sudden decline in the patient's blood pressure and general condition, only to find there will be considerable delay in obtaining much-needed blood. In the meantime, the generalized deleterious effects of prolonged hypotension will begin to exact their toll, and a situation that might have been completely avoided may rapidly become critical.

ESSENTIALS OF PELVIC LAPAROTOMY

Preliminary Anesthesia Examination and Curettage

Anesthesia examination and curettage should be done routinely as an additional, extremely valuable means of preventing errors in diagnosis and management. Even the most experienced gynecologic surgeon will occasionally find that on anesthesia examination he is unable to confirm the "adnexal mass" palpable in the office. Most important, the preliminary curettage will avoid the disaster of a pelvic operation done for some more obvious lesion but totally inadequate for the unexpected early cancer of the endocervix or fundus discovered only after the specimen is submitted to the pathologist.

Incision

The incision should be properly placed and of adequate size for the procedure contemplated. In general, a midline (paramedian is preferred by some) lower abdominal incision, extending from the symphysis to just below the umbilicus, is the most useful one for major pelvic surgery. It provides excellent exposure and routinely yields a firm, strong abdominal wall when healed, particularly if the rectus muscles are reapproximated at the time of closure. For radical pelvic surgery it will have to be extended around and above the umbilicus, with care not to extend it so high that packing off of the small bowel into the upper abdomen becomes impossible. Occasionally, in extremely obese patients, a wide transverse incision, with division of both rectus muscles at the level of the iliac spine, will provide equally good or better exposure for radical surgery and will afford better wound-healing conditions postoperatively by avoidance of the burying of large sections of a vertical incision beneath the overhanging folds of a huge panniculus. For less extensive procedures in the pelvis not involving hysterectomy (e.g., tuboplasties, myomectomies, ovarian wedge resections), a Pfannenstiel incision is often suitable and has the additional advantage of resulting in an essentially invisible scar. However, it will often not provide satisfactory exposure for more extensive procedures or in markedly obese patients. If presacral neurectomy is planned, the best incision is a right paramedian, with the junction of its upper and middle thirds centered at the umbilicus.

Exploration of the Abdomen and Pelvis

Although frequently neglected or done haphazardly and incompletely, preliminary exploration of the abdomen is extremely important and should be done immediately after the peritoneal cavity is entered. Not only will it reveal involvement of other abdominal viscera by the particular pelvic disease involved and thus possibly influence subsequent operative strategy, but it also permits the detection of unrelated disease in the abdomen (e.g., gallstones, Meckel's diverticulum), knowledge of which may prove valuable should related complications arise either in the immediate convalescence or in the future.

Pelvic exploration should include detailed inspection and palpation of the pelvic organs, their supporting ligaments, the cul-de-sac and adjacent rectosigmoid, the pelvic lymph nodes, and the parietal peritoneal areas.

Appendectomy

Routine removal of the appendix is to be strongly urged, not only in all simple, uncomplicated, pelvic laparotomies but also in most radical operations for cancer. In addition to eliminating forever the possible need of another laparotomy for appendicitis, it also removes from consideration the possibility that appendicitis may be responsible for any abdominal complications that may occur in the immediate or late convalescence. Obviously, appendectomy will be contraindicated if the pelvis and abdomen are found involved by widespread cancer. It is recommended that both abdominal exploration and appendectomy be done before packing off the intestines and beginning the pelvic operation, so that it will be unnecessary to reenter the upper abdomen after the pelvic procedure is completed. This will avoid both contamination by the bacterial flora of the vaginal canal, if the latter has been entered, and restimulation of the patient sufficient to require deepening of the anesthesia for abdominal closure.

Cardinal Principles of the Pelvic Procedure

The following are the cardinal principles to be observed when carrying out pelvic operations:

1. Adequate exposure (the usual vertical incision must be carried all the way to the pubic symphysis and must be of adequate length).
2. Complete mobilization of the pelvic viscera, if they are adherent, *before* beginning the actual dissection and removal.
3. Maintenance by the assistant of tension on the uterus, and thus on all the attached supporting and adjacent structures, throughout the dissection.
4. Observation of the usual basic principles of good surgical technique. A surgeon carrying out a pelvic procedure must have an exact knowledge of the position of the ureters and bladder (and, to a lesser extent, of the rectum and major pelvic blood vessels), and an awareness of their proximity and potential exposure to

accidental injury must always be uppermost in his mind. If pelvic disease has resulted in distorted or confused anatomy (e.g., extensive endometriosis, pelvic inflammatory disease, cervical and broad-ligament fibroids), it must be clarified precisely by preliminary mobilization and, at times, extended dissection with actual exposure of the ureters wherever their course lies close to the lesion to be removed.

Special Hemostatic Technique for Local Operations on the Uterus

The use of vasopressin as reported by Dillon [3] for injection locally into the uterine wall immediately prior to incision for myomectomy, unification procedures, or tubo-plasty of the type requiring hysterectomy, or into the cervix prior to local cervical procedures such as total cone biopsy, appears to be an excellent technique for the reduction of blood loss during certain types of gynecologic surgery. It has proved considerably more satisfactory in obtaining a relatively bloodless field and improved exposure than the usual mechanical hemostatic methods employing rubber-shod clamps or rubber-band tourniquets on or around the uterine and ovarian vessels.

The solution to be injected is prepared as follows: 4 pressor units (0.2 ml) of vasopressin (Pitressin, 20 units per milliliter) are diluted in 20 ml of normal saline to make a final vasopressin solution containing 0.2 units per milliliter. From 5 to 10 ml of this final solution is injected locally into the myometrium; blanching of the uterine wall around the site of injection is almost immediate, and an intense hemostatic effect persists for 15 to 20 minutes and then subsides.

THE APPROACH TO VAGINAL SURGERY

Preliminary examination under anesthesia and curettage is just as important in vaginal surgery as in pelvic laparotomy.

Indications and Limitations

Most vaginal operations are performed to deal with the various manifestations of deficient pelvic support, and, with a few exceptions, the vaginal approach represents either the only or the far superior route for this purpose. Because of the need to operate within the confines of a small space, exposure must be carefully assured by adequate assistance and proper retracting instruments. In the presence of pelvic relaxation, exposure is rarely a problem.

The vaginal route may also be employed for removal of the uterus for a variety of conditions in the absence of pelvic relaxation and is routinely so elected under normal circumstances by some surgeons, with excellent results. In this situation, however, in comparison with the abdominal approach, it has the disadvantage of a somewhat more difficult and limited exposure for removal of the uterus, and problems are often encountered in safely removing the adnexa when this is indicated. Furthermore, the vaginal route does not allow thorough abdominal exploration or, even more important, inspection of the pelvic viscera themselves prior to embarking on the hysterectomy. The abdominal and pelvic findings at laparotomy not infrequently dictate a necessary change in operative management from the one originally planned, an alteration impossible to foresee and make if the approach is from below. Finally, not only are there decided limitations as to the size of the uterus that can be removed vaginally, but the vaginal approach is ordinarily contraindicated and unsafe if the uterus cannot be assumed to be completely mobile and nonadherent (e.g., in the presence of extensive endometriosis or chronic pelvic inflammatory disease, or in the face of fixation following previous pelvic surgery), or if there is any suspicion of significant adnexal disease, particularly any ovarian enlargement suggesting the possible presence of a primary ovarian neoplasm of some type.

In view of these considerations, therefore, it would seem wisest to reserve the vaginal approach primarily for dealing with problems of pelvic support and, under ordinary circumstances, to employ the abdominal approach for lesions primarily intrapelvic in nature and location.

Exposure in Difficult Circumstances

If a vaginal approach is elected and exposure at operation proves limited, an extremely helpful maneuver to keep in mind is the use of the Schuchardt incision (an integral and essential part of the Schauta radical vaginal hysterectomy). Basically, this is simply an extended mediolateral episiotomy that includes partial division of the levator muscle. It can be performed at any time during a vaginal procedure when the need for more adequate exposure becomes obvious, and can be relied on to provide it.

Limited Exploration of the Pelvic Peritoneal Cavity

After vaginal removal of the uterus, the adnexa can be palpated and inspected, and unexpected abnormalities may be discovered. The cul-de-sac should also be carefully explored to determine if an enterocele is present that will require repair before peritoneal closure.

The Vaginal Procedure

The general principles of vaginal surgery are identical with those of pelvic laparotomy. As has been noted, the vaginal approach should be avoided if it is suspected that the normal pelvic anatomy has been distorted by the disease process. Nonabsorbable sutures should never be used, since excessive granulation tissue and sinus formation with prolonged suture extrusion is inevitable if they are employed. Vaginal procedures tend to be fundamentally less stressful and are accompanied by less postoperative morbidity (e.g., ileus) than abdominal procedures, and thus they are often safer in older or high-risk patients. However, it is not sufficiently appreciated that blood loss may be considerably, though unobtrusively, greater during vaginal as compared with abdominal surgery, owing to the greater vascularity of the tissues and planes of dissection. Provision for and watchful replacement of this loss is therefore important.

REFERENCES

1. Burke, J. F. The effective period of preventive antibiotic action in experimental incisions and dermal lesions. *Surgery* 50:161, 1961.
2. De Cenzo, J. A., Malo, T., and Cavanagh, D. Factors affecting cone-hysterectomy morbidity. *Am. J. Obstet. Gynecol.* 110:380, 1971.
3. Dillon, T. F. Control of blood loss during gynecologic surgery. *Obstet. Gynecol.* 19:428, 1962.
4. McQuarrie, H. G., Harris, J. W., Ellsworth, H. S., Stone, R. A., and Anderson, A. E., III. Sciatic neuropathy complicating vaginal hysterectomy. *Am. J. Obstet. Gynecol.* 113:223, 1972.
5. Sinclair, R. H., and Pratt, J. H. Femoral neuropathy after pelvic operation. *Am. J. Obstet. Gynecol.* 112:404, 1972.
6. Williams, T. J., Johnson, T. R., and Pratt, J. H. Time interval between cervical conization and hysterectomy. *Am. J. Obstet. Gynecol.* 107:790, 1970.

23

Postoperative and Postradiation Management and Treatment of Complications

MANAGEMENT AND TREATMENT OF COMPLICATIONS FOLLOWING ROUTINE PELVIC SURGERY

It seems worthwhile to present a reasonably comprehensive discussion of the principles of postoperative care and the management of the more common complications that may follow gynecologic surgery. The subject is rarely, if ever, covered in standard textbooks of gynecology, and it is often impossible to consider it in any detail even in the many excellent manuals of operative gynecology.

Bladder Care

Inasmuch as the bladder is either immediately adjacent to or actually a part of the field of dissection, detrusor tone and function are regularly temporarily impaired, and this, together with transient postoperative spasm of the supporting striated muscular structures, predisposes to difficulty in voiding or inadequate bladder emptying. In all cases, postoperative voiding should be watched carefully during the first 24 hours, and, if voiding occurs frequently and in small amounts, catheterization for retention or to check residual urine should be done promptly. This will avoid overdistention and decompensation of the detrusor musculature with development of a hypotonic or totally atonic bladder that may be a problem for days, weeks, or even months. In this way, mild temporary difficulties can be readily overcome in the first 12 to 24 hours, and normal voiding function will usually return rapidly. If the need for repeated catheterizations persists for longer than 24 hours, an indwelling Foley catheter should be placed for a few days until bladder muscle tone returns, bladder sensory irritability subsides, and spasm of the supporting musculature of the pelvic floor relaxes, permitting resumption of normal spontaneous voiding. After procedures known to be followed invariably by temporary impairment of normal voiding ability (e.g., vaginal hysterectomy, anterior and/or posterior colporrhaphy, operations for the correction of stress incontinence), it is wise to send the patient from the operating room with an indwelling catheter in place. Simple gravity drainage (routine periodic irrigation is unnecessary and may introduce bacterial contamination) is maintained for five to seven days and followed by catheter removal and a trial of normal voiding, checking the amounts voided and, when indicated, the residuals after the first few voidings until it is apparent that complete emptying is occurring. If voiding difficulties still persist, a further period of two to three days of indwelling catheter drainage may be necessary before normal voiding occurs. Resumption of normal voiding is sometimes aided by giving an oral cholinergic drug such as bethanechol chlorine (Urecholine) in a dosage of 20 to 30 mg four times daily. Less often, discharge from the hospital on prolonged constant drainage for four to eight weeks at home may be required before normal bladder tone and function are restored.

With proper equipment, properly used, significant urinary tract infection need not develop when catheter drainage of the bladder is necessary. It is important that the catheter be inserted atraumatically and with a meticulously aseptic technique. A completely closed and sterile bladder drainage apparatus should be used, and once the connection between catheter and drainage tubing is made, it should not be broken. (Repeated disconnecting and reconnecting the catheter and drainage tubing simply favor the introduction of bacteria.) Some closed drainage apparatuses now include a flutter valve to prevent accidental flow of urine from the drainage bag back into the catheter and bladder as an additional safeguard against ascent of bacteria through the tubing into the bladder. The catheter, particularly that portion nearest the urethral meatus, should be kept as clean and free of contamination as possible at all times and can periodically be rinsed or wiped off with a nonirritating antiseptic solution such as aqueous benzalkonium (Zephiran). Some physicians favor the use of a "three-way catheter" that permits constant drainage of urine as well as a continuous bladder rinse using 2 liters per 24 hours of a saline solution containing 40 mg of neomycin and 20 mg of polymyxin B per liter. Attention to these details will markedly reduce the incidence of significant bacteriuria for at least 3 to 5 days (as long as 7 to 10 days when the continuous antibiotic bladder rinse is employed). However, bacteriuria will develop in 80 to 100 percent of patients in whom an indwelling catheter is present for longer periods, regardless of the prophylactic measures employed. This only occasionally leads to a true urinary tract infection, however, and unless there is an abnormality of the urinary tract itself, the bacteriuria invariably clears promptly following the removal of the catheter.

Although administering routine prophylactic urinary antiseptics (usually one of the sulfonamides) during any period of bladder drainage has been a time-honored tradition, careful bacteriologic studies suggest that as long as the catheter is present, this prophylactic drug therapy is of little benefit and may only encourage the overgrowth of drug-resistant organisms. It is probably much wiser to start such drug therapy on the day the catheter is removed, obtaining a specimen of urine for culture and sensitivity studies at the same time, in case an organism not sensitive to sulfonamides is present and subsequently requires treatment. Thus, although bacterial contamination is potentially inherent even in a single, simple catheterization — and certainly bacteriuria always eventually develops following prolonged indwelling catheter drainage — maintenance of good fluid intake, constant observation to ensure free drainage of the catheter, and careful attention to be certain that proper emptying is achieved following removal of the catheter combine to make the occurrence of clinically significant and persistent postoperative urinary tract infections a rarity. The development of an atonic bladder through failure to utilize the catheter wisely in the postoperative period, for fear of introducing bacteria, is a far more serious matter.

Another approach to the problem of minimizing the occurrence of bacteriuria and subsequent urinary tract infection has been the introduction, or reintroduction, of suprapubic cystotomy drainage. Following the gynecologic operation, most often a vaginal procedure, the bladder is filled with 500 ml of sterile water, and suprapubic trochar puncture cystotomy is done to allow a small plastic catheter to be introduced into the bladder. This has the advantage of eliminating the urethral irritation and edema accompanying the use of the regular catheter, and bacterial contamination of the suprapubic tube is also easier to prevent. In addition, the patient is able to void spontaneously as soon as she wishes to attempt to do so; with the suprapubic tube still in place, overdistention can be prevented if voiding is incomplete, and residual urine can be checked without the need for repeated urethral catheterizations. However, there is some hazard to the actual suprapubic puncture itself, and there have been problems with plugging of the small-caliber plastic tubing as well as with dislodgment of the tubing from the bladder (the latter two problems have led to increased use of larger-bore tubing). Furthermore, bacteriologic studies have not consistently or convincingly demonstrated a significant reduction in the incidence of bacteriuria. As a result, the suprapubic catheter technique, though popular with some physicians, has not as yet been widely adopted.

If urinary tract infections occur following pelvic surgery, they ordinarily respond promptly to appropriate chemotherapy. Urine cultures and antibiotic sensitivity studies should be obtained as a guide to the selection of the proper antibiotic. A liberal fluid intake should be assured, and the possibility should be investigated that the infection might be due in part to inadequate bladder emptying, with constant residual urine; this situation can be corrected, if present, by the temporary institution of bladder drainage until normal voiding is resumed. While awaiting culture and sensitivity reports, a sulfonamide such as Gantrisin in a dosage of 1.0 to 2.0 gm four times daily may be tried for 24 to 48 hours and may often prove effective, since the usual organisms involved are commonly among the sulfonamide-sensitive coliform group. Whatever is ultimately shown to be the drug of choice should be given in adequate dosage and continued for 7 to 10 days after the temperature is normal and other urinary tract symptoms have cleared. Chronic or recurrent urinary tract infections following pelvic surgery are uncommon and, when present, are usually associated with some intrinsic pathologic condition in the urinary tract itself. They signal the need for a complete urologic investigation, including cystoscopy and intravenous or retrograde pyelography.

Postoperative Pelvic Sepsis

Wound infections may follow pelvic laparotomy, but their course and management do not differ from those occurring after any abdominal surgical procedure. However, certain relatively infrequent postoperative infections localized to the pelvis represent specific complications peculiar to gynecologic surgery.

Several excellent studies [8, 18, 21] have been carried out to determine whether or not **prophylactic antibiotic therapy** is effective in reducing the incidence of septic complications following gynecologic operations for diseases not primarily of infectious origin. There is general agreement that such therapy is probably helpful and indicated in patients undergoing radical operations for pelvic cancer. The usual choice to achieve broad-spectrum antibiotic coverage for this purpose might be penicillin G and one of the aminoglycosides such as streptomycin or kanamycin; if the anaerobic organism *Bacteroides fragilis* is known or suspected to be a potential problem, the addition of chloramphenicol or clindamycin may need to be considered. All the studies have been in agreement that the febrile morbidity and infectious complications accompanying vaginal hysterectomy can be drastically reduced by prophylactic antibiotic therapy, and most gynecologic surgeons therefore employ such a program following vaginal hysterectomy. Agents most often used include cephaloridine, or a combination of penicillin and streptomycin, and the proper timing for the prophylactic use of antibiotics consists of a short course, begun an hour or two preoperatively (so that there is adequate coverage during the operation itself), followed by a 24- to 48-hour period of antibiotic treatment postoperatively (some surgeons prefer to prolong the postoperative interval of therapy another 72 hours). Typical regimens would be: cephaloridine, 1.0 gm intravenously on call to the operating room, on return from the recovery room, and again late in the evening after the operation; or penicillin, 600,000 units, and streptomycin, 0.25 gm intramuscularly on call to the operating room and every 6 hours thereafter for four to five days postoperatively.

Where routine abdominal hysterectomy in so-called clean cases is concerned, the protective effect of antibiotics was less evident or even completely absent in several careful prospective studies. In fact, the majority of gynecologic surgeons do not employ routine prophylactic antibiotics following simple abdominal hysterectomy.

Obviously, careful preoperative preparation of the abdominal skin and vaginal area, careful walling-off of the operative field to minimize bacterial contamination, atraumatic surgery that avoids leaving behind necrotic tissue, and careful hemostasis to prevent hematoma formation (the source of most wound infections and vaginal vault abscesses) are equally, if not more, important in diminishing the chances of postoperative septic complications.

PELVIC PERITONITIS

Although pelvic peritonitis used to be common, particularly after operations for pelvic inflammatory disease or infected malignant tumors, it is seldom seen today. This is undoubtedly largely a result of the universal use of antibiotics in the preoperative and postoperative management of obviously infected lesions; in the case of chronic pelvic inflammation, it is a reflection of the modern tendency to resect rather than simply to drain the lesion. When, as occurs even more rarely, signs and symptoms of peritonitis develop unexpectedly after pelvic surgery in so-called clean cases, gross contamination with virulent outside organisms or ineffective hemostasis with secondary infection may have taken place, or more important, injury to and contamination of the pelvis from the urinary or gastrointestinal tracts should be suspected. Hence the possibility of the latter will often need to be investigated as part of the overall plan of management of this complication. Therapy should include use of the Ochsner regimen, appropriate antibiotics (covering both gram-negative aerobic as well as the anaerobic organisms so frequently present with a regimen such as intravenous penicillin and chloramphenicol), and careful attention to management of the associated ileus and to maintenance of normal fluid and electrolyte balance during the acute phase. The process will frequently completely resolve on this program, without the need for surgical drainage. In some cases, however, it may become localized and proceed to pelvic or vaginal vault abscess formation.

POSTOPERATIVE STARCH PERITONITIS

Postoperative starch peritonitis, a granulomatous, inflammatory foreign-body reaction to surgical glove powder, especially the frequently used cornstarch, can present signs and symptoms that are nearly identical with those of a septic peritonitis, complicating convalescence after pelvic or abdominal operations. This entity is being seen with increasing frequency now that there is greater awareness of its existence and nature. It is important to suspect and recognize its presence in any postlaparotomy patient with a clinical picture suggestive of peritonitis, intraperitoneal abscess, or postoperative intestinal obstruction or unusually prolonged paralytic ileus, particularly when it occurs 10 to 30 days after surgery, a characteristic time for starch peritonitis to first appear. Clinical manifestations include abdominal pain and tenderness (the former often more impressive than the latter), fever, malaise, weakness, anorexia, sometimes nausea and vomiting and other symptoms and signs suggestive of ileus or intestinal obstruction; also, there is often abdominal distention and the appearance of abdominal fluid (frequently detectable only by paracentesis) and/or palpable abdominal masses or induration (the latter representing granulomatous inflammatory nodules and masses in the omentum or on peritoneal surfaces). The leukocyte count is usually normal (there may be a moderate eosinophilia in some cases, which is another point supporting the belief that the disease is probably a cellular immune response), but the sedimentation rate is often elevated. If ascitic fluid is present, the diagnosis can be established by paracentesis, which will yield "sterile pus," a turbid fluid that exhibits an elevated protein and lymphocyte count and that on microscopic examination (either directly with polarized light or following mixing with Gram's iodine solution) reveals the diagnostic intracellular doubly refractile starch granules with their typical Maltese cross patterns. If no abdominal fluid is present, the finding of an elevated serum lysozyme, which is abnormally high in the presence of a number of granulomatous diseases, may be very helpful in confirming the clinical diagnosis of starch peritonitis and differentiating it from postoperative bacterial infections.

  If the diagnosis can be correctly made, it is possible to avoid needless reoperation (exploratory laparotomy to rule out or treat a possible intestinal obstruction or postoperative abscess) in patients with glove starch granulomatous disease, for they will eventually recover spontaneously and completely with conservative, nonoperative treatment after a variable (sometimes prolonged) period of time. (If exploratory laparotomy is done and the lesions of starch granulomatous peritonitis are found, only a small biopsy should be done; extensive dissection or attempted removal of the lesions is unnecessary and may even lead to serious complications.) If the symptoms and dysfunction are significant, a much more rapid recovery can be promoted by administering corticosteroids, e.g., prednisone, 10 mg twice daily for five to seven days, then tapering off for an additional five to seven days; intravenous or intramuscular hydrocortisone can be used at first if the severity of the disease and the patient's condition warrant. The initial favorable response to steroid therapy is often immediate and dramatic. If steroids are contraindicated, indomethacin can be tried, but in any case, the usual conservative regimen, including gastrointestinal tract suction if necessary, and intravenous fluids and even hyperalimentation if required, is the treatment indicated until spontaneous recovery occurs.

PELVIC ABSCESS

An antecedent pelvic peritonitis or, more commonly, secondary infection in a postoperative pelvic hematoma may localize and form a cul-de-sac abscess following pelvic operations of any type. A febrile course and the presence of a tender, obviously intraperitoneal cul-de-sac mass signals this development. Initial therapy with antibiotics may be necessary to prevent spreading infection, but only rarely does it cause complete resolution and may even delay localization. The development of palpable fluctuance should be patiently awaited; if the abscess does not point and drain spontaneously through the vagina shortly thereafter, simple surgical drainage may then be done at the point of maximal fluctuance in the posterior vaginal fornix, preliminary needle aspiration having confirmed the presence of pus.

VAGINAL VAULT ABSCESS

If either abdominal or vaginal hysterectomy has been done, localized pelvic sepsis usually appears in the form of a vaginal vault abscess, again most often preceded by hematoma formation in this area. This complication is less likely to occur if hemostasis is complete and if the vaginal apex is not routinely completely closed by suture at the conclusion of hysterectomy. The process is actually extraperitoneal, the collection developing between the vaginal apex and the overlying bladder-flap peritoneum and is manifested by the development of fever and a tender mass just above the vaginal vault, usually on the fifth to eighth postoperative day. At times, these localized collections primarily represent simple accumulations of blood or serum with minimal bacterial infection and systemic response, though they may cause pelvic discomfort and rectal or bladder irritability. Drainage will nearly always occur spontaneously, and it is far wiser and safer to await this event than to attempt premature evacuation surgically. In the presence of a frank abscess, antibiotics may be helpful in preserving the localized nature of the infection. Occasionally, when fluctuance is obvious but spontaneous drainage fails to occur or is inadequate, it may be initiated or promoted by gentle digital exploration of the vaginal apex.

PELVIC CELLULITIS

At times, postoperative pelvic sepsis takes the form of a diffuse cellulitis involving the retroperitoneal areolar tissues throughout the pelvis, with maximal reaction in the region of the pelvic floor, soft tissues of the lateral pelvic walls, and the para-vaginal and cardinal ligament structures centrally. Dissection of these tissue planes by infected hematomas is undoubtedly a frequent forerunner; previous pelvic inflammatory disease or prior pelvic irradiation is probably also a predisposing factor, for this particular complication is more prone to occur in these cases. A persistently febrile course with diffuse tenderness and induration throughout the pelvis, but without the development of a mass, is an early diagnostic feature. The process sometimes subsides on therapy with an effective antibiotic; or it may eventually localize, with the formation of an abscess that requires drainage through the cul-de-sac or vaginal vault or, more rarely, necessitates an inguinal or flank approach.

The most troublesome type of postoperative pelvic cellulitis is encountered following procedures performed in the face of previous extensive pelvic inflammation or after prior radiation therapy to the pelvis. The process tends to be chronic, is characterized by a diffuse woody or stony-hard induration through the entire pelvis (the term **ligneous pelvic cellulitis** is often applied), and frequently will not resolve or localize with antibiotic therapy, often requiring six months or longer to subside. The use of hydrocortisone, prednisone, or a similar corticosteroid preparation, along with antibiotics, has proved to be an extremely valuable adjunct to treatment in these cases. Prompt, dramatic resolution of the extensive brawny induration is usually achieved, with subsequent rapid clearing of the infection.

Other Local Pelvic Complications

BLEEDING FROM THE VAGINAL CUFF

Bleeding from the vaginal cuff is a relatively uncommon complication of hysterectomy that usually occurs around the seventh to twelfth postoperative day, although delayed bleeding may occasionally be encountered several weeks postoperatively. Presumably, areas in the cut margins of the vagina that were sutured to achieve hemostasis at the time of surgery undergo necrosis, with both tissue and suture dissolution leading to secondary hemorrhage as a result of the reopening of vaginal or perivaginal veins or, more often, small vaginal arterial branches. If only moderate, it may stop spontaneously on bed rest or be controlled by evacuation of all blood clots and firm vaginal tamponade with gauze packing for 24 to 48 hours. If brisk arterial bleeding is responsible, simple packing is rarely successful, and resuture of the area of the vaginal cuff involved is usually necessary and invariably requires brief anesthesia for proper exposure and relaxation to assure accurate, effective suture placement.

OSTEITIS PUBIS

Osteitis pubis, a rather infrequent complication of pelvic procedures, usually occurs following surgery that involves suprapubic dissection of the prevesical space of

Retzius, most commonly after Marshall-Marchetti urethrovesical suspensions or fascial sling procedures for urinary stress incontinence. Although an element of infection with some degree of osteomyelitis of the symphysis may at times be present, the pathologic condition in the vast majority of cases appears to be in the nature of an aseptic necrosis of periosteum and underlying bone. Presumably, these changes, which are usually visible and show a characteristic appearance of the symphysis and pubic rami on x-rays, are secondary to vascular disturbances produced by the extensive dissection of the area and the placement of sutures in the overlying periosteum. The process usually responds promptly and dramatically to the administration of cortisone or related corticosteroids with antiinflammatory action, and this is the treatment of choice. An initial dosage of 100 mg of cortisone three times daily for three days, or 10 mg of prednisone two to three times daily for three days, followed by a maintenance dosage of 50 mg of cortisone four times daily, or 5 mg of prednisone two to three times daily, until symptoms clear completely is usually sufficient, and usually the medication need be continued for no more than two weeks, at which point it should gradually be reduced and tapered off. Only rarely, in the case of frank septic osteomyelitis with persistent symptoms and suppuration, will surgical drainage and excision of nonviable bony fragments be necessary or indicated.

PROLAPSE OF THE FALLOPIAN TUBE

The relatively infrequent complication of fallopian tube prolapse is rare after abdominal hysterectomy; it is most often encountered following vaginal hysterectomy. Since both the symptoms (persistent postoperative discharge and spotting, dyspareunia, and vaginal discomfort) and the findings (a reddish, granular or polypoid, often very tender lesion visible and palpable in the vaginal apex) are entirely similar to those of the almost universal posthysterectomy vaginal vault granulations temporarily present during the postoperative healing phase, it is possible that many instances of fallopian tube prolapse are never recognized for what they are. There is often a history of factors predisposing to poor vaginal vault healing (e.g., postoperative vaginal cuff bleeding, or vaginal cuff abscess with subsequent drainage, either spontaneous or induced), resulting in a situation that favored separation of the vaginal cuff edges and the tendency for prolapse of any structures immediately above the open cuff. In most cases the problem presents itself within the first few months following the hysterectomy. Since simple granulations usually respond readily to treatment by excision and cauterization of their base with silver nitrate, whereas prolapsed tubal segments often will not disappear, the possibility of tubal prolapse should be suspected if presumed granulations persist despite this type of therapy. The diagnosis may also be suggested by visual recognition of the probable nature of the lesion, especially if it is the fimbriated end that protrudes, and should definitely be confirmed or disproved by histologic study of any "suspicious granulation tissue." Although cauterization and subsequent spontaneous healing-over of the vaginal epithelium may suffice for small areas of prolapse, more often, the prolapsed portion of the tube will need to be surgically excised via the vaginal route, with reclosure of the small opening in the vaginal vault.

Accidental Injuries to the Bladder, Ureter, and Rectum

Although inadvertent injuries to the bladder, ureter, and rectum are rare and should be avoidable, they unfortunately are occasionally encountered, and their possible occurrence must always be considered in the evaluation of any patient whose abnormal postoperative course suggests the presence of serious complications. Although vesicovaginal or rectovaginal fistulas are obviously serious, neither is an urgent problem, and both will occasionally heal spontaneously. Immediate institution of constant bladder drainage favors healing of vesicovaginal fistulas, as do adequate drainage of any soft-tissue sepsis surrounding a rectovaginal fistula and institution of a low-residue diet if the defect is tiny, or a temporary colostomy if the defect is more extensive. Definitive repair of either is best postponed for several months until local healing is complete and the postoperative reaction has subsided, so that tissues have been restored to normal pliancy. In the case of rectovaginal fistulas ultimately requiring surgical closure, a preliminary colostomy is always required. A ureterovaginal fistula is more likely to develop (usually secondary to impaired blood supply, not actual direct injury) following radical hysterectomy (see the next section for discussion and management).

However, complete or nearly complete obstruction of one ureter resulting from an accidental ligation or division requires immediate treatment if the kidney is to be salvaged (unless a fistula rapidly develops), and in bilateral ureteral injury of this type, emergency surgery is mandatory and frequently lifesaving. In the former situation, signs or symptoms may never develop, and the injury may go completely unrecognized. However, the usual manifestation is steadily increasing renal and ureteral pain, with or without chills and fever and other evidences of ascending infection. Intravenous pyelograms and cystoscopy with retrograde catheterization serve to differentiate the picture from that of simple pyelonephritis. As soon as the patient's condition permits, exploration with deligation or repair (end-to-end anastomosis, or preferably reimplantation into the bladder) of the damaged ureter should be accomplished. In the case of bilateral ureteral ligations, the diagnosis is rendered obvious by the resulting total anuria, but this, too, should be confirmed by the preceding diagnostic maneuvers, both to rule out completely a nonmechanical cause for anuria (lower nephron nephrosis or tubular necrosis syndrome) and to establish definitely the location of the block. The patient's general condition usually dictates a preliminary nephrostomy until optimal conditions for safe reopening of the abdomen are restored. Exploration with deligation, or repair, or both is then indicated without further delay.

Major Operative or Postoperative Hemorrhage

There are times during the course of pelvic surgery or in the immediate postoperative period when major bleeding from large intrapelvic branches of the hypogastric (internal iliac) arterial or venous systems is encountered. Hemorrhage may be sudden, massive, and life-threatening. Furthermore, control by simple clamp and ligation techniques may be troublesome to achieve because of difficult exposure within the confines of a narrow, deep pelvis; this is especially true when carrying out dissections in the presence of uterine or adnexal enlargement or in the face of anatomic distortion and fixation such as is produced by chronic inflammatory disease, endometriosis, pelvic cancer, or prior irradiation. The major vessels themselves still lie partially against the pelvic wall as they approach the central viscera, and furthermore they are arranged in thick vascular pedicles in such a way that it is often impossible to apply clamps safely to a single bleeding vessel without damage to and further hemorrhage from the rich collaterals in the same area. Finally, and most important, the ureters and bladder are intimately associated with this network of vessels, and blind, hasty clamping in a desperate effort to achieve control of sudden hemorrhage exposes them to a serious risk of injury.

Obviously, a careful, atraumatic surgical technique carried out along established anatomic principles and planes as well as meticulous hemostasis as the operation proceeds in an orderly, purposeful manner will do much to minimize the chance of operative or postoperative hemorrhage of significant proportions. However, it does and will occur under the best of circumstances and in the best of hands, not only in connection with radical pelvic surgery and node dissections for advanced cancer but also occasionally during difficult standard hysterectomies for benign disorders. The vascular pedicles are fragile, and even major tributaries, particularly venous trunks, tear easily and may retract out of sight yet continue to bleed profusely. In many instances, temporary gauze pressure at the bleeding site, removal of all blood and clot, and then, under good visual conditions, identification and safe ligation of the bleeding points are possible. At times, however, other techniques must be employed. Temporary aortic occlusion, either manually or by means of an aortic clamp or tourniquet, may be invaluable in controlling the hemorrhage until further dissection permits safe, accurate control of the bleeding vessel or vessels. Persistent venous ooze from pelvic wall veins that cannot be located and secured is often best managed by firm packing of the area while the operation itself proceeds to completion. Often, the ooze will have completely ceased by the time the packs are removed. Persistent, fruitless initial attempts to secure such veins, besides being ineffective, frequently lead only to extensive further blood loss, often of dangerous extent, and markedly prolong and increase the risk of the anesthesia and operation. Rarely, but particularly in the case of radical operations, the packs may be left in situ to be removed vaginally several days later if significant venous ooze persists at the end of the procedure and is still uncontrollable by individual ligation techniques.

Perhaps the most common situation encountered during simple hysterectomy is the occurrence of troublesome bleeding while attempts are being made to secure the blood supply at the level of the uterine vessels or the cervical and vaginal branches in the cardinal ligament region. The ureter is particularly close and vulnerable to injury at these points, and the blind application of clamps in a hurried effort to staunch the flow of blood is to be avoided at all costs. Instead, with the assistant maintaining temporary hemostasis by simple pressure, the surgeon will be far wiser first to expose the lower ureter adequately throughout its course from the point where it crosses the iliac vessels to well below the level of the uterine artery. This maneuver, which is illustrated in Figure 78, is one of the fundamental early steps in the radical Wertheim procedure, but it is also particularly helpful in just this situation. It not only permits a bloodless, atraumatic demonstration of the entire course of the lower ureter but also exposes the uterine artery and vein and the subjacent vessels of the cardinal ligament at their origins near the pelvic wall. Thus the surgeon, by employing this maneuver, can secure permanent hemostasis with complete safety, ligating the proximal trunks of the bleeding vessels at their origins, with the ureter under direct vision and protected from harm at all times.

Finally, when all other methods fail, bilateral hypogastric (internal iliac) artery ligations can be carried out and have proved lifesaving on many occasions in the presence of massive bleeding uncontrollable in any other way. The pressure within the distal arterial tributaries is immediately reduced, and hemorrhage either ceases completely or can readily be controlled by simple gauze packing or local application of thromboplastic foams or gels. The collateral circulation to the central pelvic organs is more than adequate to prevent any ischemic complications, even in the face of bilateral internal iliac ligations. The hypogastric arteries may be exposed in the course of surgery within the abdomen by the maneuver shown in Figure 78. They may also be approached extraperitoneally through bilateral groin incisions in postoperative patients with exsanguinating hemorrhage not responding to ordinary measures; in this situation, the dissections may even be done under local anesthesia when a retroperitoneal approach is used.

For many years, bilateral hypogastric artery ligation has proved lifesaving in a variety of circumstances. The reported indications include massive bleeding occurring (1) during or after simple hysterectomy; (2) during or after either the Wertheim procedure or radical pelvic exenteration; (3) in association with extensive carcinoma of the cervix, vagina, or endometrium, either before, during, or following radiation; and (4) in connection with certain obstetric situations complicated by massive, uncontrollable bleeding, such as uterine atony or rupture, placenta accreta or central placenta previa after cesarean section, or during precipitate labor accompanied by laceration of the broad ligament, cervix, or vagina. It is a simple, safe, and effective procedure, and it frequently will prevent a fatal outcome if employed without undue delay in the face of massive, uncontrollable pelvic hemorrhage.

Obviously, an important feature of the successful management of major operative or postoperative hemorrhage will be prompt and adequate blood replacement. This will not only frequently prove lifesaving but will also avoid serious cardiovascular and renal complications. Whenever blood transfusions must be given frequently and rapidly, the surgical team must be especially certain that every possible precaution is taken to minimize the chances for any of the several types of transfusion reactions, and they should know how to deal with an immediate reaction should one occur. A detailed discussion of this problem is beyond the scope and purpose of this book, but the reader is referred to an excellent and concise review of this subject by Baker and Nyhus [4].

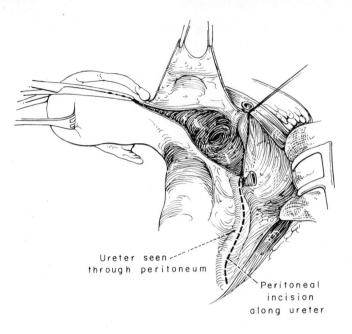

Ureter seen
through peritoneum

Peritoneal
incision
along ureter

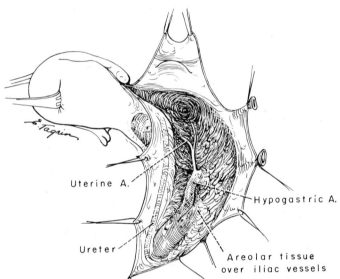

Uterine A.

Hypogastric A.

Ureter

Areolar tissue
over iliac vessels

Figure 78
Maneuver to expose the ureter and the origin of the uterine artery. With the uterus
held under tension and pulled toward the opposite side, and with traction sutures on
the round and infundibulopelvic ligaments, the iliac vessels and ureter can be seen or
palpated through the peritoneum. The peritoneum is then incised so as to leave the
ureter on the medial peritoneal flap, and the ureter is mobilized from the loose areolar
tissue and underlying iliac artery and vein. Further dissection in the lower portion of
the field will complete the freeing of the ureter and permit isolation of the uterine
artery and vein, as well as of the subjacent vessels of the cardinal ligament at their
origins. They may then safely be ligated, with the ureter in full view and protected
from harm.

654

Thromboembolic Complications

Thrombophlebitis, phlebothrombosis, and the associated embolic phenomena of minor embolization with pulmonary infarct or massive cardiopulmonary embolism have long been considered to occur somewhat more frequently following pelvic surgery than after other types of abdominal procedures. Theoretically, pelvic surgery, particularly radical pelvic procedures, would seem more likely to be accompanied by trauma to or disturbance in return blood flow in the pelvic portions of the veins of the lower extremities, thus favoring the development of phlebitis in the legs or pelvis. However, modern experience does not actually seem to indicate any significantly increased tendency to thromboembolic complications following pelvic operations as compared with other abdominal operations or procedures elsewhere in the body, particularly if prolonged bed rest is not involved during the convalescence. Furthermore, there is good evidence that the dangerous proximal thrombi that most often give rise to pulmonary emboli probably develop most often in association with and subsequent to thrombosis in the veins of the calf. Nevertheless, these potential postoperative venous complications do and will continue to occur, and the pelvic surgeon must be prepared to recognize them early and treat them appropriately. He should also thoughtfully employ preventive measures such as early ambulation, leg exercises, and the use of elastic stockings during the early days of his patient's convalescence, since the majority of venous thromboses are probably initiated within 48 hours of the operation.

The details of prophylaxis and therapy for thromboembolic complications, which cannot be considered here, are available in a number of excellent sources [1, 3, 7, 9, 13, 19, 25, 27, 33, 40]. However, a brief review of some of the highlights seems worthwhile. In addition to the mechanical methods for promoting good venous blood flow in the lower extremities previously mentioned, there is certainly a role for prophylactic anticoagulation in high-risk patients. Currently, one of the most promising of such approaches is the subcutaneous low-dose heparin regimen, consisting of the administration of 10,000 to 15,000 units daily in divided doses (5000 units two to three times daily). Such a regimen is safe, can even be started preoperatively, appears effective in preventing pulmonary emboli, and is widely applicable, even following radical pelvic procedures when the risks of postoperative bleeding might be significant if conventional programs of anticoagulation involving intravenous heparin or oral warfarin or dicumarol were used. Various antiplatelet agents have also been investigated and employed in clinical trials, e.g., the blood volume expander, low-molecular-weight dextran 40, used intravenously, as well as oral agents such as dipyridamole and aspirin. All of these agents tend to inhibit platelet release, adhesiveness, and aggregation capacity and thus reduce the incidence of spontaneous leg vein thromboses and subsequent embolization.

The pelvic surgeon should always be alert to the early clinical symptoms and signs of thrombophlebitis of the lower extremities: e.g., unilateral or bilateral swelling in the feet, ankles, or legs; calf pain and tenderness; dilated superficial veins; increased skin temperature in one or both legs; calf pain on dorsiflexion of the foot (Homans' sign), and unexplained fever during the early and middle postoperative period. Several highly accurate diagnostic methods are also available for the early detection of thrombi in the veins of the lower limbs. Phlebography (direct intravenous injection of radiopaque contrast dye into the leg veins, with fluoroscopic monitoring) is probably the most accurate and permits study of the entire venous system of the lower extremities, including the iliac veins and inferior vena cava. Another, even simpler and essentially noninvasive approach involves the use of ^{125}I-labeled fibrinogen to detect thromboses in the lower limb veins. The ^{125}I-fibrinogen technique is especially useful in detecting thrombi in the calf, popliteal area, and lower thigh but is unreliable in the upper thigh and cannot detect clots in the iliac veins. The radioactively tagged fibrinogen is injected and subsequently is incorporated into any developing thrombi, which can then be identified and localized by a standard radioactive scanning device (scintillation counter). For large thrombi in major venous trunks, the use of either the ultrasound Doppler flowmeter technique or electrical impedance plethysmography may suffice to establish the diagnosis, but neither of these diagnostic methods can completely exclude the presence of small calf-vein thrombosis, which may be the initial event in the type of thrombotic episode that ultimately results in pulmonary embolism.

Where pulmonary embolic phenomena are concerned, the development of chest pain, especially if pleuritic, or the sudden appearance of cough, especially if there is associated hemoptysis, or a sudden unexplained, simultaneous rise in temperature, pulse, and respiration (Allen's sign), should immediately suggest this possibility; it perhaps most commonly occurs in the late postoperative period on about the seventh or eighth day. A definite diagnosis can usually be established by serial chest films; it can be established even more rapidly and accurately by a four-view lung scan and by pulmonary arteriography when indicated.

In most instances, the treatment of choice for established deep-vein thrombophlebitis or for an initial pulmonary embolic episode is intravenous heparin therapy (e.g., 5000 units initially and then intermittent injection every 4 to 6 hours, or a continuous intravenous infusion of 30,000 units daily), striving to keep the partial thromboplastin time at about one and one-half to two times normal. Ultimately, the patient can be shifted to one of the oral anticoagulants if long-term therapy is indicated. If anticoagulant therapy is contraindicated, or if there is evidence of continued pulmonary embolization despite adequate anticoagulation, then ligation, plication, or clipping of the inferior vena cava should be considered; or, if the patient is too ill to tolerate this surgical procedure, a Mobin-Uddin vena caval umbrella filter may be inserted into the vena cava via the right internal jugular vein under local anesthesia.

Finally, if thrombosis has occurred and the thrombus has become well established, or when pulmonary embolism has been documented to have taken place and the patient's condition is stable, an attempt at dissolution of thrombi or emboli with so-called thrombolytic agents that enhance fibrinolysis has been shown to be worthwhile. Such an approach is bound to supplant completely the once popular femoral or iliac vein thrombectomy (careful studies eventually showed that rethrombosis and permanent obstruction almost invariably occurred following this surgical approach), and if it can be shown to be effective, will be an equally welcome improvement on the procedure of pulmonary embolectomy with its high risk and high rate of failure. A number of clinical trials with two plasminogen activators, urokinase and streptokinase, have been carried out under clinical investigational conditions, although neither drug is as yet available for routine clinical use. In all these studies, more rapid resolution of pulmonary emboli or venous thromboses than would be expected with conventional treatment using heparin alone was clearly demonstrated [13]. The properly timed combination of both a thrombolytic agent and heparin appears to be particularly effective.

One specific type of thromboembolic complication that nearly always occurs in association with gynecologic or obstetric disorders or operative procedures should be mentioned. This is the septic thrombophlebitis of the pelvic venous trunks themselves that sometimes develops in the presence of serious infectious processes involving either the pelvic organs or the soft tissues and peritoneal coverings of the pelvic walls and floor. The most frequent types of pelvic sepsis in which septic pelvic thrombophlebitis is encountered include septic abortion, postpartum sepsis, pelvic appendicitis (especially during pregnancy), acute septic complications of chronic pelvic inflammatory disease (e.g., a ruptured tuboovarian abscess), and the rare severe peritonitis that may follow any gynecologic procedure or occur after cesarean section. The most serious aspect of septic thrombophlebitis is the frequent occurrence of multiple septic pulmonary emboli. If the septic thrombotic process extends from the pelvis into the external iliac venous system, these septic emboli may be massive and immediately fatal. Even if the process remains confined to the smaller pelvic veins, the outlook if the condition is untreated is poor, since the multiplicity and septic nature of the smaller emboli will also lead to a generalized septicemia, multiple pulmonary abscesses, and ultimately a fatal outcome. Although treatment must include surgical drainage of the pelvic septic process where possible, as well as antibiotics to control the septicemia, and although anticoagulants have in some cases controlled the thrombotic and embolic aspects of the problem, in the case of continuing embolic episodes, inferior vena caval ligation is definitely indicated, will often prove lifesaving, and should be elected before the patient is in extremis. Since the ovarian veins enter the caval system above the usual site for vena caval ligation, they must be interrupted separately, as well, to eliminate completely all possibility of further septic emboli from the pelvis.

SPECIAL FEATURES IN POSTOPERATIVE MANAGEMENT AND TREATMENT OF COMPLICATIONS FOLLOWING RADICAL PELVIC SURGERY

Because of the magnitude and stressful nature of radical pelvic operations, frequently involving multiple, simultaneous procedures on the gastrointestinal, urinary, and genital tracts, as well as extensive retroperitoneal dissections, with inevitably prolonged operating and anesthesia time and proportionately greater blood loss, these patients must receive optimal immediate postoperative care and supervision. Particular attention must be paid to restoration and maintenance of normal blood volume, adequate oxygenation and ventilation, and satisfactory hydration and urine output.

Routine antibiotic therapy is indicated in the postoperative phase of all of these radical procedures, and the more prolonged ileus accompanying the radical intra-abdominal operations requires a longer period of gastrointestinal tract suction than in less radical procedures and meticulous attention to fluid and electrolyte replacement. More detailed discussion is beyond the scope of this book, but some of the more common and important specific problems are detailed in the sections that follow.

Radical Wertheim Hysterectomy

(A radical Schauta vaginal hysterectomy presents similar problems, although the postoperative morbidity is usually less and complications are generally fewer. In particular, bladder dysfunction appears to be somewhat less after the Schauta procedure.)

BLADDER FUNCTION

The extensive paravesical dissection of an adequately performed Wertheim procedure interrupts many sensory pathways, as well as a portion of the motor nerve pathways, so that the bladder is frequently rendered markedly hypotonic while the sensation of bladder fullness is simultaneously lost. Postoperative indwelling catheter drainage is therefore imperative for a minimum of several weeks, and the ideal plan to prevent the development of a markedly atonic bladder and to facilitate return of normal voiding function seems to involve prolonged constant bladder drainage for approximately two months postoperatively. The patient may be discharged from the hospital in approximately two weeks, however, on a program of 0.5 gm of sulfisoxazole (Gantrisin) four times daily and a forced fluid regimen, with ammonium chloride, 1.0 gm four times daily, if an acidifying agent seems indicated to prevent crystal and sediment formation. She may wear a plastic or rubber thigh urinal bag into which the catheter drains, thus allowing relatively normal ambulatory activities. She returns in six to eight weeks for an overnight stay in the hospital, at which time the catheter is removed and postvoiding residuals are checked until it is certain that she is actually voiding normally with satisfactory bladder emptying. It also seems likely that this plan may have the additional value of decreasing the incidence of ureterovaginal fistulas by virtue of maintaining not only the bladder but also the denuded segments of the lower ureters at complete rest and facilitating their readherence to and protection by pelvic-wall tissues during the acquisition of a new vascular supply and supporting tissue bed [16].

URETEROVAGINAL FISTULAS

Ureterovaginal fistulas used to occur in 5 to 10 percent of all reported series of large numbers of patients undergoing radical Wertheim hysterectomy, usually appearing on the eighth to tenth postoperative day. They are presumably the result of the inevitably impaired blood supply to the lower ureters, perhaps aggravated by a temporary edema at the ureterovesical junctions, both of which are secondary to the extensive dissection of these areas. If the fistula remains open, renal drainage and function invariably are excellent, and its occurrence therefore does not represent an emergency situation, except with regard to the following diagnostic and potentially therapeutic plan, which should be instituted immediately as soon as the diagnosis is suspected.

The presence of a ureteral rather than a vesical fistula should be rapidly established. This can usually be done readily by first instilling methylene blue or indigo carmine into the bladder and making certain that it does not appear on a dry sponge inserted into the vagina; it is then ascertained that indigo carmine given intravenously does appear on the dry sponge. The side on which the fistula is present should then be determined by cystoscopic examination, again employing indigo carmine intravenously if necessary (an intravenous pyelogram may also be helpful but may sometimes be misleading, actually showing better function and drainage on the side of the fistula, in contrast to the situation on the side of the intact ureter, where edema of the ureterovesical junction may retard drainage temporarily), and an attempt should be made to pass a polyethylene ureteral catheter past the site of fistula. If the attempt is successful, the catheter is left in place on gravity drainage for 14 to 21 days, and healing of the fistula frequently results. If an attempt to pass a ureteral catheter fails, a policy of watchful waiting and delayed repair is then adopted.

Occasionally, these fistulas will heal spontaneously, with or without stricture and with or without preservation of normal renal function. If healing with stricture occurs, periodic ureteral dilatation in the future may restore normal drainage and prevent recurrent pyelonephritis, or progressive decline in renal function, or both. If healing results in total ureteral obstruction, the kidney may quietly cease to function and remain asymptomatic, or nephrectomy may ultimately be required if the kidney becomes involved by recurrent or chronic pyelonephritis. If the fistula persists, definitive therapy is best delayed for several months until optimal tissue conditions are again present for repair, which should always be by reimplantation of the lower ureter into the bladder.

Fortunately, new techniques [15] of resuspending and protecting the ureter after the radical dissection is completed have been developed in recent years. As a result, the incidence of these ureteral complications has been greatly reduced, and ureterovaginal fistulas now occur in only 1 percent of cases.

VESICOVAGINAL FISTULAS

Vesicovaginal fistulas are actually relatively rare. The diagnosis is usually readily established with dye tests and cystoscopy, as described for ureterovaginal fistulas, and definitive treatment is usually best deferred for a few months as noted previously in the discussion of accidental injuries to the bladder.

MANAGEMENT OF URETEROVAGINAL OR VESICOVAGINAL FISTULAS AWAITING REPAIR

Patients awaiting repair of a ureterovaginal or vesicovaginal fistula should receive prophylactic urinary antiseptics and acidifying agents. Although sanitary napkins or the use of tampons will occasionally suffice, they are usually not entirely satisfactory in controlling the problem of constant urinary leakage. However, an ingenious method for temporary palliation is available. It involves the use of an intravaginal menstrual device, the Tassette menstrual cup (Tassette, Inc., Stamford, Conn.). A cup of appropriate size can be inserted into the vagina as a collecting receptacle, will stay in place without the need for a retaining strap or bandage, and will usually keep the patient completely dry and comfortable. The urine will be collected in the menstrual cup and drain down an attached tubing, the other end of which can be connected to a bottle at night or to a plastic or rubber thigh urinal during the day, allowing the patient to be freely ambulatory. The device may be removed daily, cleaned, and reinserted.

BOWEL FUNCTION

There is usually a somewhat greater and more prolonged ileus following the radical Wertheim procedure than after a simple abdominal hysterectomy. This can be minimized by attention to electrolyte balance, the use of gastrointestinal tract intubation-suction for 48 to 72 hours postoperatively (this promptly removes swallowed air and prevents intestinal distention), and then a gradual increase in oral intake as indicated by resumption of adequate peristaltic activity and as tolerated by the patient. The return of normal bowel function usually parallels the return of more normal general physical activity, especially ambulation. Sometimes, a tendency to flatulence and intermittent gaseous abdominal distention will persist, especially if the patient is aerophagic and unconsciously swallows large quantities of air while breathing, talking, taking fluids, or smoking. Such patients can sometimes be given symptomatic relief by simethicone (Mylicon-80) in a dosage 80 mg four times daily. This agent reduces surface tension, breaking up gas bubbles and facilitating the transport and absorption of intestinal gas.

The normal expulsive action of the rectosigmoid is usually moderately impaired as a result of the extensive pararectal dissection, and bowel function may be sluggish for months or even several years. Usually, this problem is readily managed by mild cathartics daily or every other day, and only occasionally will enemas be required.

RECTOVAGINAL FISTULAS

Rectovaginal fistulas are uncommon. Their management has been discussed under Accidental Injuries to the Bladder, Ureter, and Rectum.

Pelvic Exenteration

POSTERIOR EXENTERATION

The postoperative management and complications encountered following posterior exenteration are similar to those accompanying the Wertheim procedure, except for the additional presence of a colostomy, which usually presents no special problems.

ANTERIOR EXENTERATION

The principal additional special problem in anterior exenteration involves management of the ileal loop (Bricker pouch) or, less commonly nowadays, the uretero-sigmoidostomies, the so-called wet colostomy (see p. 662).

TOTAL EXENTERATION

Fluid Balance Problems in the Immediate Postoperative Period

Because of the extensive dissections and resections required in total pelvic exenteration, large denuded areas and dead spaces of considerable magnitude are created within the pelvis and lower abdomen from which and into which fluid, electrolyte, and protein losses inevitably take place and may assume massive proportions. This occurs even though meticulous hemostasis during the procedure may have reduced actual postoperative bleeding to a minimum. The situation is analogous to the similar extracellular fluid and protein losses in extensive burns or in the presence of severe generalized peritonitis. Furthermore, the temporary but often profound disturbances in gastrointestinal tract function may result in further intraluminal pooling of protein-rich and electrolyte-rich fluid that is also lost to the body economy, above and beyond the visible loss of intestinal fluids removed by intestinal tube drainage. Finally, since many of these patients already have some renal impairment secondary to their advanced cancer, some degree of at least temporary disturbance in urinary tract function may also be anticipated and will be accentuated by the associated surgery of the ureters during the operation.

Since it is invariably a number of days before the return of normal intestinal motility and absorptive capacity will permit oral replacement, since the "hidden losses" previously mentioned are often difficult to quantitate, and since in the face of the frequently required urinary diversion, even an accurate appraisal of the adequacy of the volume and composition of the urine output may be impossible, a potentially serious problem in the management of fluid and electrolyte balance is frequently posed. Details of replacement therapy, which should include plasma as well as blood and electrolyte solutions, and which will often require extremely large volumes of each, will not be considered here. The important point to be stressed is that the pelvic surgeon should be aware of the great likelihood of these massive losses and should, if possible, anticipate them and prevent the depletion of the patient by continuous and simultaneous restoration of fluid, protein, and electrolytes in the appropriate amounts and concentrations. At the very least, he certainly must be alert to the earliest signs of depletion, usually manifested by a tendency to hypotension, hemoconcentration, and falling urine output, readily corroborated by blood and plasma volume studies and serum protein and electrolyte determinations, and calling for prompt and vigorous replacement.

Problems Associated with Urinary Tract Diversion

Use of an isolated loop of terminal ileum (the Bricker pouch technique) as a means of conducting urine from both ureters implanted into a short (6 to 8 inches) intestinal segment brought out as an ileostomy to the skin and thence into an external bag is the most satisfactory and widely used method for handling the need for permanent urinary diversion. Healing of the ureteral anastomoses is usually uncomplicated and renal drainage excellent (normal pyelograms are invariably obtained subsequently), and problems of anastomotic stricture, pyelonephritis, or intestinal reabsorption of urine are rare. Any of the standard ileostomy appliances are satisfactory, and subsequent care by the patient is not difficult. The physician should himself be thoroughly familiar with all the details of stomal care and with all the available appliances and techniques. Even more important, he should see to it that his patient is properly equipped and carefully instructed in all phases of this care, so that she is both capable and confident and secure in her ability to manage her ileostomy and colostomy before leaving the hospital. Occasionally, anastomotic leaks may occur early in the healing phase, with the appearance of urinary leakage through the perineal wound. Healing of these temporary fistulas usually occurs spontaneously, and this is often facilitated by sump drainage of the ileal pouch itself until complete healing has occurred.

As an alternative, the surgeon may use an isolated segment of terminal sigmoid as a urinary conduit when total pelvic exenteration has been done. The sigmoid loop appears to serve equally well as an actively peristalting conduit for urine from a physiologic standpoint, although even greater care needs to be taken to assure an adequate blood supply. Use of the sigmoid loop has the great advantage of eliminating completely the need for division and reanastomosis of the small bowel. The proximal end of the sigmoid from which the sigmoid conduit segment is resected is simply brought out as the permanent sigmoid colostomy, and no bowel anastomosis is required.

With the formerly more widely used bilateral ureterosigmoidostomy procedure (either in the form of a "wet" colostomy if total exenteration has been done, or with an intact rectum and anal sphincter, as is the case with anterior exenteration), the previously noted problems are more frequent because of the concomitant presence of intestinal bacteria and the effect of intraluminal pressure within the still functioning, intact colonic segment into which the ureters have been implanted. The problem of recurrent pyelonephritis sometimes responds to prolonged antibiotic therapy, or it can occasionally be solved by performing a proximal transverse colostomy, thus separating completely the fecal and urinary streams. If stricture at the site of ureterosigmoidal anastomosis exists, however, either revision of the anastomoses or creation of an ileal loop will be necessary. If hyperchloremic acidosis develops secondary to intestinal urinary reabsorption (diagnosis by the typical clinical picture and blood studies revealing an elevated serum chloride and pH and a decreased carbon dioxide combining power), the addition of sodium bicarbonate, 0.5 to 1.0 gm four times daily, to the oral intake may solve the problem if the electrolyte disturbance is only mild, with or without additional measures to promote more rapid drainage (e.g., intermittent use of a rectal tube, correction of colostomy stricture, or a proximal colostomy to reduce the length of the absorbing colonic segment). If the problem is severe and refractory to these simpler measures, formation of an ileal loop will be necessary.

Pelvic-Floor Problems

Because of the necessary resection of the entire pelvic floor structures with all of their covering peritoneum, there is a great tendency for either ileal loops or a redundant sigmoid loop to become adherent to the raw edges of the resulting defect. This has led to serious complications in roughly 10 percent of patients, in whom intestinal obstruction, enterocutaneous fistula, or, more rarely, prolapse of a loop of small bowel through the perineal skin closure subsequently develops. Earlier efforts to avoid this complication involved the placement of a large gauze pack covered with rubber dam into the denuded cavity. The patient was then kept in bed in the Trendelenburg position and on her abdomen as much as possible for the first five to seven postoperative days, with the hope that when the pack was removed, the intestines would have become adherent above the level of the denuded, partially resected pelvic floor. Because these maneuvers failed to lower the incidence of these often disastrous complications, attention subsequently was directed toward the possibility of actually creating a new pelvic floor at the completion of the exenteration. Initial trials with sheets of synthetic materials such as tantulum mesh or nylon produced unsatisfactory results because of the tendency for these substances to become secondarily infected, with subsequent extrusion and chronic fistula formation. More recently, a technique for pelvic-floor reconstruction employing sheets of a collagen fabric film has been successfully carried out in a number of patients and shows considerably greater promise [17]. The collagen implant produces a smooth surface with no tendency to adhesions and is incorporated into the surrounding tissues with no untoward reactions or tendency to infection. Furthermore, it ultimately undergoes complete absorption and replacement by normal fibrous tissue, thus leaving no permanent foreign body. Other similar approaches [29, 32, 39] involving the transposition of nearby flaps of peritoneum or the use of pedicled flaps of omentum to cover over the raw area and create a new pelvic floor appear to be equally useful and, when feasible, avoid the need to introduce any foreign material at all.

   If obstruction or fistula does develop, either may occasionally be spontaneously relieved with the help of intestinal intubation, continuous suction, and, in the case of fistula, local sump drainage of the perineal cavity. Such a conservative approach is greatly facilitated when it is accompanied by a program of parenteral alimentation and is more likely to be successful. Intravenous hyperalimentation has proved invaluable in treating seriously ill patients under many circumstances and is especially helpful in managing patients with gastrointestinal fistulas and obstruction. The associated technical and metabolic problems, as well as the formerly more frequent complication of bacterial or fungal bloodstream infections, are now well understood and more readily prevented or managed. Nevertheless, despite these valuable adjunctive measures, subsequent laparotomy is frequently required in managing the small-bowel obstruction and/or fistula that develops after pelvic exenteration. At operation, a simple sidetracking enteroenterostomy above the point of obstruction or fistula, with division of and closure of the blind end of the adherent loop, has much to recommend it. Aside from the ease and simplicity with which this procedure can be done, avoiding an extensive, difficult dissection, it allows the blind loop to remain in place to act as a new, peritoneum-covered "pelvic floor."

Radical Vulvectomy and Bilateral Radical Groin and Pelvic Node Dissections

At the present time this combined procedure is usually carried out in one stage.

FLUID COLLECTION BENEATH MULTIPLE, WIDELY UNDERMINED SKIN FLAPS

The collection of fluid underneath multiple, widely undermined skin flaps may be largely eliminated and the overall nursing care greatly facilitated by the use of suction drainage and open management of the wound. This has proved far superior to the pressure-dressing technique, which is not only less effective in preventing fluid accumulation but also may jeopardize the viability of the skin flaps as well as promote the development of sepsis.

Two plastic catheters with five or six additional holes for drainage at suitable intervals are placed beneath the groin and lower abdominal skin flaps on each side. They are then brought out through stab wounds and connected by a Y-tube to an ordinary gastrointestinal tract suction apparatus (or to one of the simple mechanical plastic kits for combined suction and drainage that are commercially available). The wound is dressed with a sterile towel only, and suction is maintained for five to seven days (or until drainage has practically ceased), continuously at first and intermittently later, to allow reasonably early ambulation.

WOUND SEPSIS, MARGINAL NECROSIS, AND SEPARATION

Wound sepsis, marginal necrosis, and separation are also minimized by the suction-catheter wound-drainage technique. In addition, certain minor modifications in the technique and placement of the incisions for one-stage radical vulvectomy and bilateral groin dissections as outlined by Abitbol [2] are of value in preventing wound sepsis, necrosis, and separation. Should wound sepsis and necrosis develop, debridement or opening of the incision should be minimal, conservative, and carried out slowly. Sutures should remain in place regardless of the presence of necrosis of wound margins, if feasible, for two weeks and occasionally for three, lest unnecessary wound separation result. If major separation should occur, coverage should be obtained as soon as the granulating surfaces are relatively clean and free of deep sepsis, either by secondary wound closure or skin grafting, in order to avoid damage to and secondary hemorrhage from the relatively exposed underlying femoral vessels.

COMPLICATIONS OF RADIATION THERAPY

Although not strictly speaking operative complications, many of the untoward sequelae of the radiation therapy of pelvic cancers follow the operative placement of radium, usually in combination with supplementary external irradiation. Since the effect of the local radium application is often the principal factor in the subsequent development of complications, this section is a logical and convenient place in which to discuss them briefly.

Although the biologic effects of all types of ionizing radiation are identical, there are qualitative differences in radiation from different sources that influence the ways in which they can most effectively be employed and affect the nature of the undesirable side effects. The local use of radium within the uterus and vagina in anything approaching a reasonable dosage rarely produces any systemic reaction, because the falloff in dose intensity occurs so rapidly within a few centimeters of the source that there is little total body absorption. However, the adjacent bladder and rectum are very vulnerable to any significant exposure to overdosage above their inherent tolerance, since they lie within the immediate field of high intensity and may be seriously damaged by the local necrotizing effects of excessive radiation.

When external irradiation is given by standard x-ray therapy, or so-called orthovoltage therapy, falling within the 50,000 to 200,000 volt (200 kv) range, the chief risks of overdosage involve the skin and underlying superficial soft tissues, particularly bone and cartilage, lying within the portal-of-entry fields. The skin ordinarily sustains severe radiation damage with excessive doses long before the deeper tissues are so affected. The systemic reaction is often pronounced as well, even within proper, safe dosage levels, since the total amount of radiation absorbed by the patient is relatively large in comparison with the actual tumor dose, due to the considerable absorption of radiation by all the intervening tissues.

External irradiation by supervoltage x-ray therapy, in the 1 to 10 million volt (10,000 kv) range or higher, or by cobalt-60 beam therapy, where the radiation delivered is of comparable quality (shorter wavelength and greater penetrating power approximating that of 1000-kv x-ray therapy), tends to be accompanied by minimal skin and soft-tissue (including bone and cartilage) absorption; thus, even in the presence of moderate overdosage, these tissues rarely sustain serious damage. Because of the greater penetration of supervoltage x-ray or cobalt-60 beam therapy, the depth dose is proportionately increased, and a relatively greater tumor dose can therefore be achieved with a considerably lower total body dose than is possible with conventional (orthovoltage) x-ray therapy. This in turn tends also to minimize the degree of systemic reaction with the higher voltage therapy. However, it follows that the deeper, visceral tissues will now be the ones most vulnerable to overdosage, since they bear the brunt of the ischemic and necrotizing effects of any excessive radiation, maximal amounts of which accumulate well below the body surface. Not only does serious direct visceral damage occur, but subcutaneous fibrosis, or fibrosis in any area of areolar connective tissue serving as the supporting stroma of a parenchymatous organ or other body structure, is also often marked and permanent and may produce disturbances of function on a purely mechanical basis months or even years later.

These basic facts about the qualitative differences between the various radiation sources with respect to the occurrence and nature of potential undesirable side effects having been pointed out, the specific complications that may follow pelvic irradiation will now be considered briefly.

Radiation Sickness

The systemic manifestations of significant amounts of total body radiation absorption may include general malaise, anorexia, nausea, vomiting, diarrhea, and the resulting disturbances of protein metabolism and fluid and electrolyte balance. These are in part due to actual visceral damage (the mucosa of the gastrointestinal tract is particularly sensitive to radiation), in part to the systemic effects of toxic breakdown products released from the decomposing, irradiated tissues, and in part are possibly also secondary to the general "exhaustion phase" of a type of "alarm" or stress reaction induced by fundamental biologic responses to significant amounts of ionizing radiation. If bone-marrow damage is also sustained, the effects of the resulting anemia, leukopenia, and thrombocytopenia are also added to the general picture and may result in hemorrhage, decreased resistance to infection, and additional metabolic disturbances. Fortunately, significant changes in the hematopoietic system and peripheral blood elements are rarely encountered following irradiation for pelvic cancer, since the actual volume of bone marrow exposed is relatively small.

Significant radiation sickness can usually be avoided or minimized by proper preparation of the patient who is to receive therapy. Anemia should be corrected, an optimal nutritional state restored as far as is possible (including attention to protein and vitamin deficiencies), and any associated sepsis vigorously treated. These measures are just as important prior to radiation therapy as they are before surgery, and they not only increase the patient's tolerance and comfort but probably also tend to enhance the effectiveness of the therapy.

Should radiation sickness appear during therapy, its management involves the same principles. An adequate food and fluid intake must be assured, and supplementary vitamins, particularly the vitamin B group, as well as antinausea agents such as chlorpromazine (e.g., Thorazine) or prochlorperazine (e.g., Compazine) have also proved of considerable value. Transfusions and other parenteral therapy may be necessary in severe cases. The psychological reactions of the patient must not be forgotten, and explanation and reassurance, combined with mild sedatives or tranquilizers, are also an important aspect of the treatment program.

Local Complications

Skin and bone or cartilage damage has already been mentioned, but with the current techniques of pelvic irradiation they are rarely seen nowadays. Within the pelvis, complications can be conveniently classified as early, intermediate, or late, with respect to time of occurrence.

The only early complication of significance is the rapid development of pelvic cellulitis and peritonitis, with high fever and often septicemia, seen during or immediately after radium application. This results either from flare-up of the invariable low-grade pelvic sepsis accompanying an extensive, infected tumor, or from reactivation of an old, chronic pelvic inflammatory disease. It should be managed by immediate removal of the radium, if still in situ, and by vigorous treatment of the acute pelvic inflammatory process with antibiotics and a peritonitis regimen. No attempt should be made to reinsert the radium until all signs and symptoms of the pelvic infection have subsided. If an associated old, chronic pelvic inflammatory disease is suspected, bilateral salpingo-oophorectomy may have to be considered before resumption of radiation therapy. If the lesion is potentially operable, radical surgery may prove preferable to further radiation treatment.

Intermediate reactions to pelvic irradiation include the mild cystitis and mild proctitis that patients almost uniformly experience during and for a few weeks following therapy. These are due to temporary mucosal irritation, often with a low-grade associated inflammation or infection, and are manifested by urinary frequency, urgency, dysuria, and, occasionally, actual bacterial cystitis, as well as by rectal discomfort, tenesmus, and frequent, loose bowel movements with excessive mucus and occasional slight bleeding. Reassurance and symptomatic management are usually all that is required, employing urinary antiseptics and bladder antispasmodics, and a low-roughage diet, intestinal antispasmodics, and antidiarrheal drugs (e.g., Lomotil, 5 mg three times a day and/or Kaomagma, 2 ounces three or four times a day).

Late complications, typically appearing months or even years after pelvic irradiation, are often more serious and include the specific entities discussed in the sections that follow. They are due to the development of a permanent ischemic fibrosis of the submucosal and muscular layers of the organs involved, often accompanied by local areas of deep ulceration or even complete slough of the entire wall of the viscera in the region where the maximal amount of excessive radiation was absorbed.

SEVERE RADIATION PROCTITIS

Severe radiation proctitis characteristically becomes apparent 6 to 18 months following treatment, is usually associated with severe pain, diarrhea, bleeding, and stricture formation with signs and symptoms of obstruction, and not infrequently leads to rectovaginal fistula formation. A defunctioning colostomy is invariably necessary in the presence of a fistula or significant obstruction, and it may also be required if pain and bleeding are severe. Moderately severe proctitis, even with some degree of rectal stricture, can sometimes be managed by a strict low-residue diet, intestinal lubricants, stool softeners, and rectal steroid enemas, with gradual softening and restoration of a normal lumen size occurring after several years. Salicylazosulfapyridine (Azulfidine) and oral corticosteroids will also be helpful and indicated in some cases. Repair of fistulas or completely occluded areas of stricture must be delayed for several years until the adjacent tissues have regained some of their normal pliancy and healing properties. However, not infrequently, repair is never feasible, and the patient may need to be left with the colostomy and, in fact, will often elect to retain it permanently.

SEVERE RADIATION CYSTITIS

In severe radiation cystitis, deep mucosal ulcerations and submucosal changes are frequently present and often progress to vesicovaginal fistula formation, typically within three to six months of completion of therapy. Other late bladder manifestations, often not appearing for many years (as long as 5 to 20 years in some instances), are the occurrence of repeated cystitis and/or massive bleeding, as well as delayed fistula formation, due to the presence of an atrophic, telangiectatic, at times ulcerated bladder mucosa. The rigidity of the bladder wall accompanying the mucosal changes may also produce disabling urinary urgency, frequency, and dysuria, due to the reduced vesical capacity.

URETERAL DAMAGE

Although ureteral damage following radiation therapy was formerly relatively uncommon (the estimated incidence of ureteral stricture and fistulas secondary to irradiation for pelvic cancer has been only 2 to 3 percent), and although evidence of ureteral obstruction following radiation therapy signified recurrent disease rather than radiation damage in the vast majority of cases, ureteral complications are being seen with greater frequency since the introduction of supervoltage radiotherapy. Ureteral damage may be due to intrinsic injury to the mucosa and muscular wall, or it may be secondary to a periureteral fibrosis. In either case, if renal function is to be preserved, the damaged, strictured segment must either be resected and the normal proximal ureter reimplanted into the bladder, or some form of urinary diversionary procedure will have to be performed.

SMALL-BOWEL INJURY

The immediate effect of irradiation on the small bowel is to produce varying degrees of edema and hyperemia. If the effect is marked, as it may be when supervoltage therapy is given in excessively large amounts, severe bloody diarrhea may be superimposed on the usual, milder symptoms of nausea, simple diarrhea, and cramps. Rarely, multiple ulcerations and even gangrene of segments of the bowel have developed, particularly where adhesions have produced fixation of portions of the ileum. The usual mild reactions ordinarily subside within two to three weeks of the completion of therapy.

The delayed type of irradiation reaction in the small intestine is an ulcerative process complicated by stricture formation and intestinal obstruction, acute or subacute; rarely, hemorrhage from or perforation of deep penetrating ulcers may be seen, the latter complicated by peritonitis, abscess formation, or intraabdominal fistulas between neighboring viscera. If the radiation damage is diffuse rather than localized to a small segment of ileum, a syndrome may result resembling the malabsorption syndrome or sprue. Hyperalimentation and subsequently a low-fat, milk-free, and gluten-free diet may be helpful in the management of this condition. Symptoms include tenesmus, diarrhea, bloody or mucoid stools, nausea, vomiting, crampy abdominal pain, and obstipation. Symptoms of this severe type of radiation injury usually appear 6 to 12 months after therapy, but their onset can be delayed for as long as five or more years; this is especially common in the case of stricture formation and obstruction. In one large series of patients receiving a full course of radiation treatment for cervical cancer [37], small-bowel obstruction developed in 3 percent of patients; thin, diabetic, and hypertensive women appeared to be more susceptible to this complication of radiotherapy.

It is important to differentiate these manifestations of radiation damage to the bowel from those of recurrent malignant disease, and this nearly always requires exploratory laparotomy. Once a correct diagnosis has been established, treatment is surgical, usually consisting of resection of the involved segment of small bowel with reanastomosis or, more rarely, a sidetracking procedure, although the latter tends to be less satisfactory than reanastomosis in controlling all symptoms.

PYOMETRA

Endocervical stricture following radium therapy for cervical carcinoma invariably leads to complete or nearly complete obliteration of the endocervical canal. Over the course of subsequent months or years, secretions retained in the fundus may lead to the formation of a pyometra or hematometra above the point of occlusion. In addition to producing pain and, occasionally, actual symptoms of a local septic process, the appearance of the "pelvic mass" may simulate recurrence. Often, evacuation can be accomplished by dilatation of the cervix from below, followed by T-tube drainage for a month or two, and the process will then rarely recur. Occasionally, hysterectomy may be necessary.

RADIATION VAGINITIS

Epithelial atrophy and superficial erosion with resulting stenosis and often with adherence of the vaginal walls is extremely common. At first, the tendency to adhesion formation is minimal, and the areas of adherence are easily separated. If sexual intercourse is resumed within a few months of the completion of therapy, fairly satisfactory, comfortable vaginal function can be maintained, although dryness and the invariable shrinkage in caliber sometimes are troublesome. If intercourse does not take place fairly regularly, however, complete adherence with total obliteration of the vaginal canal not infrequently occurs.

PELVIC CARCINOMA FOLLOWING IRRADIATION

When a full cancericidal dose of radiation for uterine cancer has been administered, the incidence of subsequent neoplasia in other pelvic organs (e.g., ovary, rectum and sigmoid, bladder, vagina, or urethra) has been reported to be increased significantly in some, but not all, follow-up studies. However, when smaller doses of irradiation are administered, such as are occasionally employed to produce castration or formerly were used in the management of certain benign disorders (e.g., severe premenopausal functional bleeding or fibroids accompanied by excessive bleeding in patients not deemed suitable for hysterectomy), the subsequent incidence of pelvic neoplasms of different types has been shown to be definitely increased in several carefully followed and documented series of patients. It seems clearly apparent on this basis, and for other obvious reasons as well, that benign gynecologic disorders should not be treated by irradiation unless the circumstances are exceptional.

REFERENCES

1. Abernethy, E. A., and Hartsuck, J. M. Postoperative pulmonary embolism: A prospective study utilizing low dose heparin. *Am. J. Surg.* 128:739, 1974.
2. Abitbol, M. M. Carcinoma of the vulva: Improvements in the surgical approach. *Am. J. Obstet. Gynecol.* 117:483, 1973.
3. Adar, R., and Salzman, E. W. Treatment of thrombosis of veins of the lower extremities. *N. Engl. J. Med.* 292:348, 1975.
4. Baker, R. J., and Nyhus, L. M. Diagnosis and treatment of immediate transfusion reaction. *Surg. Gynecol. Obstet.* 130:665, 1970.
5. Barclay, D. L., and Roman-Lopez, J. J. Bladder dysfunction after Schauta hysterectomy. *Am. J. Obstet. Gynecol.* 123:519, 1975.
6. Bloomer, W. D., and Hellman, S. Normal tissue responses to radiation therapy. *N. Engl. J. Med.* 293:80, 1975.
7. Bohling, C., Auer, A. I., and Hershey, F. B. The Mobin-Uddin caval filter for prevention of pulmonary emboli. *Am. J. Surg.* 128:809, 1974.
8. Breeden, J. T., and Mayo, J. E. Low dose prophylactic antibiotics in vaginal hysterectomy. *Obstet. Gynecol.* 43:379, 1974.
9. Clagett, G. P., and Salzman, E. W. Prevention of venous thromboembolism in surgical patients. *N. Engl. J. Med.* 290:93, 1974.
10. Collins, C. G., Collins, J. H., Harrison, B. R., Nicholls, R. A., Hoffman, E. S., and Krupp, P. J. Early repair of vesicovaginal fistula. *Am. J. Obstet. Gynecol.* 111:524, 1971.
11. Donaldson, G. A., Linton, R. R., and Rodkey, G. V. A twenty year survey of thromboembolism at the Massachusetts General Hospital, 1939-1959. *N. Engl. J. Med.* 265:208, 1961.
12. Ellsworth, H. S., Harris, J. W., McQuarrie, H. G., Stone, R. A., and Anderson, A. E., III. Prolapse of the fallopian tube following vaginal hysterectomy. *J.A.M.A.* 224:891, 1973.
13. Fratantoni, J. C., Ness, P., and Simon, T. L. Thrombolytic therapy: Current status. *N. Engl. J. Med.* 293:1073, 1975.
14. Garibaldi, R. A., Burke, J. P., Dickinan, M. L., and Smith, C. B. Factors predisposing to bacteriuria during indwelling urethral catheterization. *N. Engl. J. Med.* 291:215, 1974.
15. Green, T. H., Jr. Ureteral suspension for prevention of ureteral complications following radical Wertheim hysterectomy. *Obstet. Gynecol.* 28:1, 1966.
16. Green, T. H., Jr., Meigs, J. V., Ulfelder, H., and Curtin, R. R. Urologic complications of radical Wertheim hysterectomy: Incidence, etiology, management and prevention. *Obstet. Gynecol.* 20:293, 1962.

17. Green, T. H., Jr., and Patterson, W. B. Collagen film pelvic floor reconstruction following total pelvic exenteration. *Surg. Gynecol. Obstet.* 126:309, 1968.
18. Harralson, J. D., van Nagell, J. R., Roddick, J. W., and Sprague, A. D. The effect of prophylactic antibiotics on pelvic infection following vaginal hysterectomy. *Am. J. Obstet. Gynecol.* 120:1046, 1974.
19. Hirsh, J., and Gallus, A. S. ^{125}I-labeled fibrinogen scanning. *J.A.M.A.* 233:970, 1975.
20. Hodgkinson, C. P., and Hodari, A. A. Trocar suprapubic cystostomy for postoperative bladder drainage in the female. *Am. J. Obstet. Gynecol.* 96:773, 1966.
21. Hunt, T. K., Alexander, J. W., Burke, J. F., and MacLean, L. D. Antibiotics in surgery. *Arch. Surg.* 110:148, 1975.
22. Ingram, J. M. Further experience with suprapubic drainage by trocar catheter. *Am. J. Obstet. Gynecol.* 121:885, 1975.
23. Josey, W. E., and Staggers, S. R., Jr. Heparin therapy in septic pelvic thrombophlebitis. *Am. J. Obstet. Gynecol.* 120:228, 1974.
24. Kirshen, E. J., Naftolin, F., and Benirschke, K. Starch glove powders and granulomatous peritonitis. *Am. J. Obstet. Gynecol.* 118:779, 1974.
25. LeQuesne, L. P. Relation between deep vein thrombosis and pulmonary embolism in surgical patients. *N. Engl. J. Med.* 291:1292, 1974.
26. MacMahon, C. E., and Row, J. W. Rectal reaction following radiation therapy of cervical carcinoma: Particular reference to subsequent occurrence of rectal carcinoma. *Am. Surg.* 173:264, 1971.
27. Mobin-Uddin, K., Trinkle, J. K., and Bryant, L. R. Present status of the inferior vena caval umbrella. *Surgery* 70:914, 1971.
28. Morales, A., and Steyn, J. Late development of vesical fistula following radiotherapy for carcinoma of the cervix. *Arch. Surg.* 104:836, 1972.
29. Morley, G. W., and Lindenauer, S. M. Peritoneal graft in total pelvic exenteration. *Am. J. Obstet. Gynecol.* 110:696, 1971.
30. Palmer, J. P., and Spratt, D. W. Pelvic carcinoma after irradiation. *Am. J. Obstet. Gynecol.* 72:497, 1956.
31. Rowbotham, J. L. Stomal care. *N. Engl. J. Med.* 279:90, 1968.
32. Ruckley, C. V., Smith, A. N., and Balfour, T. W. Perineal closure by omental graft. *Surg. Gynecol. Obstet.* 131:300, 1970.
33. Sherry, S. Low-dose heparin prophylaxis for postoperative venous thromboembolism. *N. Engl. J. Med.* 293:300, 1975.
34. Siegel, P., and Mengert. W. F. Internal iliac artery ligation in obstetrics and gynecology. *J.A.M.A.* 178:1059, 1961.
35. Sugarbaker, P. H., McReynolds, R. A., and Brooks, J. R. Glove starch granulomatous disease: An unsolved surgical problem. *Am. J. Surg.* 128:3, 1974.
36. Ulfelder, H., and Green, T. H., Jr. Special complications of gynecologic surgery. *Surg. Clin. North Am.* 43:789, 1963.
37. van Nagell, J. R., Maruyama, Y., Parker, J. C., Jr., and Dalton, W. L. Small bowel injury following radiation therapy for cervical cancer. *Am. J. Obstet. Gynecol.* 118:163, 1974.
38. Warshaw, A. L. Management of starch peritonitis without the unnecessary second operation. *Surgery* 73:681, 1973.
39. Way, S. The use of the "sac" technique in pelvic exenteration. *Gynecol. Oncol.* 2:476, 1974.
40. Williams, J. W. Venous thrombosis and pulmonary embolism. *Surg. Gynecol. Obstet.* 141:626, 1975.

Index

Abdomen. *See also* Abdominal pregnancy; Gastrointestinal tract
acute abdomen in endometriosis, 338
in acute gonorrheal inflammatory disease, 250–251
examination, 5
bidigital bimanual, 9, 10
inspection, 5
in ovarian cysts and tumors, 483, 484
exploration in pelvic surgery, 638
pain
in case history, 3
in ovarian cysts and tumors, 126, 127
roentgenograms, 49
scintiscanning, 56
Abdominal pregnancy, 286, 289, 290–291
diagnosis and management, 290–291
etiology, 290
incidence, 290
Abnormal bleeding. *See* Bleeding, abnormal; Hemorrhage
Abortion, 296–313. *See also* Induced abortion; Spontaneous abortion
classification of, 296–297
defined, 296
Abscess(es), 56
breast, 616
differential diagnosis from carcinoma, 622
fat necrosis, 619, 621
gas, degenerated leiomyomas and, 387
pelvic
culdocentesis, 263
differential diagnosis, 56
nonspecific infections and, 273
postoperative, 647, 648
retained abdominal pregnancy and, 291
as radiation therapy complication, 668
tuboovarian, 254, 255–256
vaginal vault, 647, 648

Acromegaly, 206, 209
ACTH. *See* Adrenocorticotropic hormone (ACTH)
Actinomycin D. *See* Chemotherapy
Acute retrograde menstruation, 171–172
Addison's disease, 205, 211
Adenoacanthoma(s)
endometrial, 447–448
ovarian, 473, 489–491
endometriosis and, 352
prognosis, 490
therapy, 490
Adenocarcinoma(s)
breast
described, 624
differential diagnosis, 619
incidence, 624
intraductal, 618, 619
therapy, 619, 624
cervical
diagnosis, 416
differential diagnosis, 411
incidence, 410
pathogenesis, 406
pathology, 410–411, 412
prognosis, 406, 416
clear cell, 142, 527
fetal exposure to diethylstilbestrol and, 126, 128–130, 132, 237, 240, 411–412
metastases, 132
ovarian, endometriosis and, 352–353
differential diagnosis
adenomatoid tumors, 529
cervical and endometrial, 411
vaginal smears in, 20–21
endometrial, 445, 447, 448
differential diagnosis, 411
histologic types, 453
female urethra, 524
ovarian, 472, 487, 489–491
classification of, 487
clear cell, 472, 487, 491
endometriosis and, 352–353
solid, 491
therapy, 490
tubal, 532, 533
vulvar, 512–513, 514

Adenofibromas, ovarian, 475
Adenofibrosis, breast, 179
Adenoma(s)
adrenocortical and precocious puberty, 135
breast sweat-gland, 618
endometrial, 441, 447
See also Carcinoma corporis et cervicis
ovarian, 475
of pituitary, 206
Adenoma malignum, endometrial, 447
Adenomatoid tumors
in male, 529
tubal, 529
uterine, 529
Adenomyosis
tubal, 530, 531
uterine, 328, 393–396
clinical signs, 394–395
cystic changes in, 396
differential diagnosis, 395
diffuse vs. localized, 392–394
endometriosis vs., 327, 328, 340, 393, 395
incidence, 395
pathology, 393–395
salpingitis isthmica nodosa and, 531
therapy, 396
Adenosis, vaginal
in children, 142
clear cell adenocarcinoma and, 129, 130, 237, 240
fetal exposure to diethylstilbestrol and, 120, 130–131, 237, 240, 527
Adenosquamous carcinoma, cervical, 411–412
Adnexectomy, 189
Adolescents
breasts in, 143, 615
cancer screening in, 416
cervical carcinoma in, 19
criminal abortions and illegitimate pregnancies, 577, 593
endometriosis in, 336
gynecologic and sexual education for, 143, 577

673